ANESTHESIA AND PAIN CONTROL IN THE GERIATRIC PATIENT

ANESTHESIA AND PAIN CONTROL IN THE GERIATRIC PATIENT

Editors

R. Brian Smith, M.D.
Professor and Chairman

Mary Ann Gurkowski, M.D.
Associate Professor of Anesthesiology

Christopher A. Bracken, M.D.
Associate Professor of Anesthesiology

Department of Anesthesiology
University of Texas Health Science Center at San Antonio
San Antonio, Texas

McGraw-Hill, Inc.
Health Professions Division

New York St. Louis San Francisco Auckland
Bogotá Caracas Lisbon London Madrid
Mexico City Milan Montreal New Delhi
San Juan Singapore Sydney Tokyo Toronto

Anesthesia and Pain Control in the Geriatric Patient

1234567890 DOCDOC 98765

ISBN 0-07-058642-X

This book was set in Times Roman by Northeastern Graphic Services, Inc.
The editors were Michael J. Houston and Lester A. Sheinis;
the production supervisor was Richard C. Ruzycka;
the cover designer was Marsha Cohen/Parallelogram;
the indexer was Tony Greenberg, M.D.
R. R. Donnelley & Sons Company was printer and binder.

This book is printed on acid-free paper.

Library of Congress Cataloging-in-Publication Data

Anesthesia and pain control in the geriatric patient / editors,
R. Brian Smith, Mary Ann Gurkowski, Christopher A. Bracken.
p. cm.
Includes bibliographical references and index.
ISBN 0-07-058642-X
1. Geriatric anesthesia. 2. Pain in old age. I. Smith, R. Brian. II. Gurkowski, Mary Ann. III. Bracken, Christopher A.
[DNLM: 1. Anesthesia—in old age. 2. Pain—therapy. 3. Pain—in old age. WO 445 A5765 1995]
RD145.A535 1995
617.9'6'0846—dc20
DNLM/DLC
for Library of Congress 94-27066

We wish to dedicate this book to our respective parents. We believe that their wisdom and faith was instrumental in motivating us to understand the need for this volume.

RBS
MAG
CAB

CONTENTS

CONTRIBUTORS

William E. Ackerman, M.D.
Pain Fellow
Department of Anesthesiology
Texas Tech University Health Sciences Center
Lubbock, Texas
(Chapter 24)

Amy C. Benedikt, M.D.
Pediatric Anesthesia Fellow
Children's National Medical Center
Washington, DC
(Chapter 7)

Robert F. Bossard, M.D.
Assistant Professor
Department of Anesthesiology and Pain Management
University of Texas Southwestern Medical School
Dallas, Texas
(Chapter 11)

Christopher A. Bracken, M.D., Ph.D.
Associate Professor
Department of Anesthesiology
University of Texas Health Science Center at San Antonio
San Antonio, Texas
(Chapters 2 and 15)

Lois L. Bready, M.D.
Professor
Department of Anesthesiology
University of Texas Health Science Center at San Antonio
San Antonio, Texas
(Chapter 7)

Harald Breivik, M.D., Ph.D.
Professor and Chairman
Department of Anesthesiology
University of Oslo Rikshospitalet
Oslo, Norway
(Chapter 16)

Michael S. Brown, M.D.
Assistant Professor
Department of Anesthesiology
University of Missouri
Columbia, Missouri
(Chapter 18)

Chandrasekhar Doniparthi, M.D.
Millard Fillmore Suburban Hospital
Williamsville, New York
(Chapter 25)

Dawn P. Desiderio, M.D.
Department of Anesthesiology and Critical Care Medicine
Memorial Sloan Kettering Cancer Center and Cornell University Medical College
New York, New York
(Chapter 12)

James H. Diede, M.D.
Assistant Professor
Department of Anesthesiology
Texas Tech University Health Sciences Center
Lubbock, Texas
(Chapter 24)

Diane M. L. Gilbert, M.D.
Assistant Professor
Department of Rehabilitation Medicine
University of Texas Health Science
Center at San Antonio
San Antonio, Texas
(Chapter 23)

David W. Glasser, B.S.
Department of Pharmacology
University of Texas Health Science
Center at San Antonio
San Antonio, Texas
(Chapter 6)

Mary Ann Gurkowski, M.D.
Associate Professor
Department of Anesthesiology
University of Texas Health Science
Center at San Antonio
San Antonio, Texas
(Chapters 5 and 20)

Rosemary Hickey, M.D.
Associate Professor
Department of Anesthesiology
University of Texas Health Science
Center at San Antonio
San Antonio, Texas
(Chapter 1)

David J. Jones, Ph.D.
Professor
Department of Anesthesiology
University of Texas Health Science
Center at San Antonio
San Antonio, Texas
(Chapter 6)

Girish P. Joshi, M.B.B.S., M.D., F.F.A.R.C.S.I.
Assistant Professor
Department of Anesthesiology and
Pain Management
University of Texas Southwestern
Medical Center
Dallas, Texas
(Chapter 11)

Kelly Gordon Knape, M.D.
Associate Professor
Director, Obstetrical Anesthesia
Department of Anesthesiology
University of Texas Health Science
Center at San Antonio
San Antonio, Texas
(Chapter 21)

Ronald A. Kross, M.D.
Assistant Professor
Department of Anesthesiology and
Critical Care Medicine
Memorial Sloan Kettering Cancer Center
and Cornell University Medical College
New York, New York
(Chapter 12)

Noel W. Lawson, M.D.
Assistant Professor
Department of Anesthesiology
University of Missouri
Columbia, Missouri
(Chapter 18)

Robert D. Lyons, M.D.
Assistant Professor
Department of Anesthesiology
University of Texas Health Science
Center at San Antonio
San Antonio, Texas
(Chapter 12)

John E. Morley, M.B., B.Ch.
Dammert Professor of Gerontology
Director of Geriatric Medicine
St. Louis University Medical Center
Director of Geriatric Research
Education and Clinical Center
St. Louis VA Medical Center
St. Louis, Missouri
(Chapter 4)

Joseph J. Naples, M.D.
Professor and Deputy Chairman
for Clinical Affairs
Department of Anesthesiology
University of Texas Health Science
Center at San Antonio
San Antonio, Texas
(Chapter 13)

Allen D. Noorily, M.D.
Assistant Professor
Department of Otolaryngology
University of Texas Health Science
Center at San Antonio
San Antonio, Texas
(Chapter 19)

Susan H. Noorily, M.D.
Clinical Assistant Professor
Department of Anesthesiology
University of Texas Health Science
Center at San Antonio
San Antonio, Texas
(Chapter 19)

Lauri S. Nuutinen, M.D., Ph.D.
Professor and Chairman
Department of Anesthesia
University of Kuopio
Kuopio, Finland
(Chapter 9)

Gregory D. Powell, M.D.
Assistant Professor
Department of Rehabilitation Medicine
University of Texas Health Science
Center at San Antonio
San Antonio, Texas
(Chapter 23)

Gabor Bela Racz, M.D.
Professor and Chairman
Department of Anesthesiology
Texas Tech University Health Sciences
Center
Lubbock, Texas
(Chapter 24)

James N. Rogers, M.D.
Assistant Professor
Department of Anesthesiology
University of Texas Health Science
Center at San Antonio
San Antonio, Texas
(Chapter 25)

Joseph L. Seltzer, M.D.
Professor and Chairman
Department of Anesthesiology
Thomas Jefferson University
Philadelphia, Pennsylvania
(Chapter 8)

Rahmawati Sih, M.D.
Fellow in Geriatric Medicine
St. Louis University Medical Center
St. Louis, Missouri
(Chapter 4)

Tod B. Sloan, M.D., Ph.D.
Associate Professor
Department of Anesthesiology
University of Texas Health Science
Center at San Antonio
San Antonio, Texas
(Chapter 1)

R. Brian Smith, M.D.
Professor and Chairman
Department of Anesthesiology
University of Texas Health Science
Center at San Antonio
San Antonio, Texas
(Chapters 17 and 22)

Dale E. Solomon, M.D.
Associate Professor
Department of Anesthesiology
University of Texas Health Science
Center at San Antonio
San Antonio, Texas
(Chapters 3 and 14)

Nicolas E. Walsh, M.D.
Professor and Chairman
Department of Rehabilitation Medicine
University of Texas Health Science
Center at San Antonio
San Antonio, Texas
(Chapter 23)

Charles W. Whitten, M.D.
Assistant Professor and Acting Director
Department of Anesthesiology and
Pain Management
University of Texas Southwestern
Medical Center
Dallas, Texas
(Chapter 11)

Edward A. Wilson, M.D.
Assistant Professor
Department of Anesthesiology
Texas Tech University Health Sciences
Center
Lubbock, Texas
(Chapter 10)

Thomas A. Witkowski, M.D.
Assistant Professor
Department of Anesthesiology
Thomas Jefferson University
Philadelphia, Pennsylvania
(Chapter 8)

PREFACE

The geriatric population has continued to increase both in total number and average age largely because of advancements in medicine. Because of major advances in biotechnology, diagnostics, and therapy, physicians are now performing procedures not countenanced two decades ago. Our increased knowledge of the physiological and pathological processes involved in the geriatric patient has special meaning in the field of anesthesiology where the geriatric patient must be looked upon as one who has specific needs and tolerances in terms of optimal anesthetic drug selection and delivery.

For these reasons it is the intent of this book to provide the anesthesiologist in practice and in training with an overview of the anesthetic management of the geriatric patient. The book will examine the wide variety of systemic factors that influence preoperative, perioperative, and postoperative care. With this information the book will demonstrate the pharmacological responses and physiological reactions to the large number of anesthetic agents and adjuvants used among geriatric patients. In effect, the book will develop a rational anesthetic plan for the delivery of drugs and anesthetics to this class of patients. Finally, in order to complete our approach, we have dedicated a significant portion of this book to a discussion of the many problems concerning pain in this age group with special mention to the question of pain management in the geriatric patient with cancer.

We hope that this book will not only give the reader an orientation concerning the anesthetic management of the geriatric patient but will also be useful as a source of practical information that will help him or her to bring an anesthetic or pain problem to a successful conclusion.

ACKNOWLEDGMENTS

We wish to thank Kathy Swientek for her hard work and dedication in rendering editorial assistance for completion of this book. Appreciation for secretarial contributions are also extended to Denise Wahl, Velma Lopez, and Annette Harris.

ABBREVIATIONS USED IN THIS BOOK

5HT	5-hydroxytryptamine
aPTT	Activated partial thromboplastin time
AAG	$Alpha_1$ acid glycoprotein
ABG	Arterial blood gas
ACE	Angiotensin-converting enzyme
ACT	Activated coagulation time
ACTH	Adrenocorticotropic hormone
ADH	Antidiuretic hormone
AF	Atrial fibrillation
ANH	Acute normovolemic hemodilution
ANP	Atrial natriuretic peptide
AR	Aortic regurgitation
AS	Aortic stenosis
ASHD	Arterial sclerotic heart disease
AVP	Arginine vasopressin
AVR	Aortic valve replacement
BPH	Benign prostatic hypertrophy
BSP	Bromosulphthalein
CABG	Coronary artery bypass graft
CAD	Coronary artery disease
CAT	Choline acetyltransferase
CBF	Cerebral blood flow
CHF	Congestive heart failure
CI	Cardiac index
CNS	Central nervous system
COHb	Carboxyhemoglobin
CO	Cardiac output
COP	Colloid oncotic pressure
COPD	Chronic obstructive pulmonary disease
CPAP	Continuous positive airway pressure
CPB	Cardiopulmonary bypass
CPE	Cystpanendoscopy
CPP	Cerebral perfusion pressure
CRF	Corticotropin releasing factor

CSF	Cerebral spinal fluid
CSFD	Cerebrospinal fluid drainage
CT	Computed tomography
CVA	Cerebrovascular accident
CVP	Central venous pressure
DHEA	Dihydroepiandosterone
DHT	Dihydrotestosterone
DIC	Diffuse intravascular coagulopathy
DLT	Double lumen tubes
DM	Diabetes mellitus
DREZ	Dorsal root entry zone
DVT	Deep venous thrombosis
EACA	Epsilon-aminocaproic acid
ECG	Electrocardiogram
EEG	Electroencephalogram
EDV	End-diastolic volume
EF	Ejection fraction
EKG	Electrocardiogram
ERPF	Effective renal plasma flow
ESRF	End-stage renal failure
ESWL	Extracorporeal shock wave lithotripsy
EVLW	Extravascular lung water
FFP	Fresh frozen plasma
FiO_2	Inspired oxygen content
FOB	Fiberoptic bronchoscope
FRC	Functional residual capacity
FSH	Follicle stimulating hormone
FVC	Forced vital capacity
G-CSF	Granulocyte colony stimulating factor
GM-CSF	Granulocyte-macrophage colony stimulating factor
GETA	General endotracheal anesthesia
GHRH	Growth hormone releasing hormone
GI	Gastrointestinal
GFR	Glomerular filtration rate
GnRH	Gonadotropin releasing hormone
GTP	Guanosine triphosphate
HES	Hydroxyethyl starch
HNP	Herniated nucleus pulposa
HPV	Hypoxic pulmonary vasoconstriction
HSR	Hypersensitivity reaction
IABP	Intraaortic balloon pump
IL-2	Interleukin-2
IM	Intramuscularly
IMA	Internal mammary artery
IOP	Interocular pressure
IV	Intravenous

IVP	Intravenous pyelogram
LA	Local anesthesia
LBBB	Left bundle branch block
LVEDP	Left ventricular end-diastolic pressure
LVEF	Left ventricular ejection fraction
LVH	Left ventricular hypertrophy
MAC	Monitored anesthesia care
MAO	Monoamine oxidase
MAP	Microtubular associated protein or Mean arterial pressure
MEFV	Maximum expiratory flow-volume
MI	Myocardial infarction
MR	Mitral regurgitation
MRI	Magnetic resonance imaging
MS	Mitral stenosis
MVR	Mitral valve replacement
MVV	Maximal voluntary ventilation
N_2O	Nitrous oxide
NIDDM	Non-insulin-dependent diabetes mellitus
NIF	Negative inspiratory force
NSAID	Nonsteroidal anti-inflammatory drug
NTG	Nitroglycerin
OLV	One-lung ventilation
PA	Pulmonary artery
PAC	Pulmonary artery catheter
PAE	Panacinar emphysema
PaO_2	Arterial oxygen pressure
PAOP	Pulmonary artery occlusion pressure
PCA	Patient-controlled analgesia
PCEA	Patient-controlled epidural analgesia
PCWP	Pulmonary capillary wedge pressure
PEEP	Positive end expiratory pressure
PET	Positron emission tomography
PMV	Percutaneous mitral valvuloplasty
PNH	Preoperative normovolemic hemodilution
PTCA	Percutaneous transluminal coronary angioplasty
PNS	Peripheral nervous system
PPF	Purified protein fraction
PT	Prothrombin time
PTH	Parathyroid hormone
PVC	Premature ventricular contraction
RBF	Renal blood flow
RES	Reticuloendothelial system
RFTC	Radiofrequency thermocoagulation
ROM	Range of motion
RV	Residual volume

SCC	Succinylcholine
SF6	Sulfahexafluoride
SHBG	Sex hormone binding globulin
SIADH	Syndrome of inappropriate ADH release
SLR	Straight leg raise
SMABF	Superior mesenteric artery blood flow
SN	Substantia nigra
SNP	Sodium nitroprusside
SOB	Shortness of breath
SpEP	Spinal evoked potentials
SSEP	Somatosensory evoked potential
SVR	Systemic vascular resistance
SWM	Segmental wall motion
TEA	Thoracic epidural anesthesia
TEE	Transesophageal echocardiography
TEG	Thromboelastography
TENS	Transcutaneous electrical nerve stimulation
TETT	Thallium-exercise tolerance testing
TIA	Transient ischemic attack
TLC	Total lung capacity
TMJ	Temporomandibular joint
TP	Trigger point
TPI	Trigger point injection
TRH	Thyrotropin releasing hormone
TSH	Thyroid stimulating hormone
TURP	Transurethral resection of the prostate
VC	Vital capacity
Vd	Volume of distribution

ANESTHESIA AND PAIN CONTROL IN THE GERIATRIC PATIENT

CHAPTER 1

Physiological Changes with Aging in the Central Nervous System

Rosemary Hickey
Tod B. Sloan

INTRODUCTION

The central and peripheral nervous systems deteriorate steadily after 50 years of age. Because of the intimate relation between the functioning of the nervous system and the functioning of other body systems, aging of the central nervous system (CNS) has been postulated to be a major contributor to aging of the body as a whole.[1]

Studies of aging have been confounded by two problems. First, there are marked interspecies variations, and contradictory findings are not uncommon. Second, within species there are marked differences between individuals. Despite these confounding factors, some generalizations can be made. First, there is a consistent deterioration of the central and peripheral nervous systems with age. In some individuals these changes appear to start early (age 50–60 years), while in others the processes are delayed until later (age 70–80 years). It is unclear what causes this variability with age; however, hereditary factors, the presence of medical diseases (such as cardiovascular disease and diabetes), and perhaps the individual's behavior (physical and mental activity) all appear to alter the rate of degeneration.

When degeneration begins, it primarily affects the frontal and temporal lobes. However, different individuals show changes in different regions of the nervous system in different time sequences, causing a wide spectrum of functional and neurological changes. These changes create an imbalance in the functioning of the nervous system, with a net suppression of some responses and an exaggeration of others. Overall, function deteriorates.

This chapter reviews the changes associated with aging which occur in the neural structures at macroscopic and microscopic levels in the CNS and the peripheral nervous system (PNS), the neurochemical and biochemical changes of aging, the functional changes which occur, and the resulting alterations in the neurological examination which distinguish older from younger individuals. Several common diseases of aging which appear to be exaggerations of the normal aging process are discussed, along with their implications for anesthesiology. Finally, an overview of alterations in response to inhalational, intravenous, and local anesthetics is given.

CHANGES IN CNS MORPHOLOGY WITH AGE

Gross Anatomic Changes

Vertebrate brains follow a consistent pattern of development from conception through maturation to senescence. Since neural cells do not appear to divide once they are formed, some researchers believe that neural cells are programmed to deteriorate with age.

According to the traditional view, several anatomic changes in the brain are characteristic of aging (Table 1-1). While this view has been questioned,[2] brain weight appears to decrease starting at age 40, reaching about 93 percent of the

Table 1-1 Gross anatomic changes

Decline in brain weight
Widening and deepening of sulci
Decrease in width of gyri
Increase in ventricular size
Thickening of meninges
Deterioration of choroid plexus

weight at age 20 by age 80. The decrease in brain volume results in widening and deepening of the sulci with a decrease in the width of the gyri and an increase in ventricular size. The former changes are most dramatic in the frontal lobes.[3] There is also neuronal loss in the cortex, with a reduction in lipids and water content. A concomitant increase in glial cells and glial cell processes occurs, and this may explain increases in protein, RNA, and DNA as a fraction of overall brain weight.[3,4] In addition, the meninges thicken and the choroid plexus deteriorates.[5]

Macroscopic Changes in Neurons

A variety of macroscopic changes occur in neural cells, particularly in the frontal and temporal lobes (Table 1-2). The neuronal cell populations that appear to decrease with age include granular cells, cerebellar Purkinje's cells, ganglion cells, cells in layer VI of the cerebral cortex (notably in the temporal lobe), and the pyramidal cells in layer III of the frontal lobe. Studies have revealed a 20 percent loss of nerve cells in individuals who are mentally healthy over age 70 (compared with persons age 19–28).[5] There is increased loss in diseases of aging; senile dementia 35 to 38 percent (at age 79); Alzheimer's disease, 50 percent (at age 67). Overall, the areas affected first appear to be regions of phylogenetically younger CNS formations. Neurons in subcortical regions and in the vital areas of the brainstem do not appear to decline in number, but a selective depopulation of melanin-containing neurons in the locus ceruleus and substantia nigra has been noted. This loss may be related to

Table 1-2 Neuronal changes

Macroscopic neuronal changes
Decrease in cortical neurons
Increase in glial cells
Decrease in myelinated axons
Microscopic neuronal changes
Loss of Nissl substance
Increase in lipofuscin and intracellular deposits
Nuclear atrophy with morphological changes
Granulation or fragmentation of mitochondria

cell degeneration resulting from free radical formation, since melanin exists in a free radical form.[6]

Individual neurons become elongated, somewhat irregular, and occasionally lobulated with aging. A generalized degeneration of axons occurs, especially in myelinated axons, because of a diffuse degeneration of myelin sheaths.[5] Spinal roots, for example, show a decrease in the number of myelinated fibers. The remaining axons may have a smaller diameter of the axis cylinder and myelin sheath. Degeneration of myelin results in an alteration of its normal functions, which include (1) promotion of the rate of impulse transmission, (2) enhancement of repetitive impulse transmission capacity over a given time period, and (3) conservation of nerve function energy. Thus, with aging, there is a loss of the coordination of function by myelinated axons.[7]

Within individual axons, neural dendrites appear to degenerate, with an overall loss of dendrite numbers. In some cases, arborization (branching) is more prevalent and neurofibrillary tangles occur.[5] The number of synapses per neuron decreases.[3] Extracellular heuristic plaques (senile plaques) occur in the elderly and appear to consist of a central amyloid core surrounded by degenerating neuronal processes (mainly presynaptic terminals and degenerating cellular organelles and reactive astrocytes) and an outer layer of glial cells.[4] These normal cellular changes of aging are more extensive with dementia.[8]

Changes in Neuron Interactions

Neurons do not appear to age without affecting adjacent neurons. When a neuron dies, the metabolism and activity of adjacent neurons increase sharply. This may be part of the neural adaptation to the process of aging. Neighboring cells increase their surface area, nuclear volume, number of nucleoli, and contact with blood vessels. These adaptive changes probably help maintain the functional capacity of the CNS in the face of declining neuron numbers.[1,9]

Regression of neuronal dendrites reduces cell-to-cell communication, since it leads to a decrease in the number of synapses (95 percent of the receptor surface of cortical neurons is in the dendrites).[4] Pre- and postsynaptic neurons are also altered with age; this may be related to changes in neurotransmitters (see below). Coincident with the dendrite decrease, an age-related increase in the number of terminal branches with endplates is seen (terminal sprouting). Therefore, despite the decrease in dendrite numbers, there is no net denervation.[10]

Microscopic Changes in Neurons

On microscopic examination of aging neurons, a general loss of Nissl substance (basophilic RNA-containing chromophil substance) and ribosomes is seen. A variety of organelle changes are also observed, as well as deposits of copper, iron, melanin, and pigments. Nuclear changes occur, including atrophy, changes in definition, and alterations in staining characteristics. Mitochondria and the

Golgi apparatus become granulated or fragmented. There is an increase in lipofuscin ("wear and tear pigment," "senility pigment," "chromolipid"), a pigment that is thought to be associated with aging. Its accumulation is the only constant cytological change that correlates with age, and different neuron pools accumulate the lipofuscin pigment at different rates. It has been postulated that accumulation correlates with the activity of oxidative enzymes in individual cells.[5] Lipofuscin is thought to result from the oxidation of lipids polymerized with protein and unsaturated peptides. It appears in granules that are believed to be end-stage liposomes with indigestible cellular debris.[4,6]

BIOCHEMICAL, NEUROCHEMICAL, AND PHYSIOLOGICAL CHANGES

Cerebral Blood Flow and Metabolism

A variety of cellular biochemical and physiological changes occur with aging (Table 1–3). Cerebral blood flow (CBF) with advancing age has been extensively studied.[11–13] There is disagreement about the meaning of the decline in CBF observed. Before 1960, it was commonly believed that senility is due to inadequacies of CBF. However, it is now appreciated that CBF is reduced in proportion to brain mass and metabolism.[14] A reduction in CBF is paralleled by a reduction in the cerebral metabolism of oxygen and glucose ($CMRO_2$ and CMR_{Glc}). In general, CBF is reduced by 28 percent at age 80, with more dramatic reductions in patients who exhibit intellectual deterioration. Greater changes in CBF are also seen in diseases such as dementia. In addition, individuals with diabetes, hypertension, and atherosclerotic disease clearly demonstrate CBF reductions with advancing age.[15] With age, the normal rise in regional CBF associated with local neuronal activity is blunted.[15] A loss of autoregulation also may occur in these individuals,[3] and CBF may show a reduced responsiveness to hypercapnia.[16]

Age-related changes in metabolism appear to be heterogeneous. There are marked regional variations throughout the brain, although more impressive changes are consistently seen in the frontal and temporal lobes.[8] It has been postulated that these changes are due to atherosclerotic deterioration of blood vessel walls. As blood vessels become sclerotic and thickened, the blood supply

Table 1-3 Changes in cellular biochemistry and physiology

Decreased cerebral blood flow
Loss of vascular autoregulation and responsiveness to neuronal demand and hypercapnia
Decreased cellular oxygen and glucose metabolism
Altered sodium and potassium homeostasis
Alterations in calcium homeostasis

is impaired.[1,3] CBF and $CMRO_2$ are deeply intertwined, but it appears that cerebrovascular changes may be the causative agent in reductions of both, making cerebrovascular disease a primary force in the aging process. Indeed, elderly individuals without cerebrovascular disease appear to have normal CBF.[3]

With the decrease in metabolism associated with aging, there is a decreasing supply of energy for the maintenance of cell membrane function. This leads to a slowing of the outflow of sodium from cells and of the inflow of potassium. As a result, the electrochemical potential capability of the nerve cell and its capacity for prolonged activity are limited.[1] The loss of energy may also contribute to decreases in axoplasmic flow of RNA, protein, amino acids, and other substances in neurons, leading to decreases in peripheral nerve function and consequent alterations in the organs innervated by those nerves.[1]

Calcium Metabolism

Disordered calcium ion homeostasis has been suggested to be a contributor to the aging process, with intracellular calcium levels reported to be increased in some studies and decreased in others. Studies in the hippocampus (notably CA1 cells) clearly document changes consistent with increased intracellular levels of calcium caused by reduced cellular clearance.[10] The brain may be vulnerable to injury from altered calcium homeostasis, since many neuronal processes are calcium-regulated or calcium-facilitated. In general, aging reduces calcium movement across membranes, impairing uptake and elimination; diminishes cytosolic free calcium; and alters the binding of calcium and calcium stores. Pharmacologic treatments that promote the entry of calcium into cells seem to reverse some of these effects.[17]

Uptake of calcium appears to occur through two types of cell membrane calcium channels. The fast calcium channels close quickly (1 s) after stimulation and probably play a role in neurotransmitter release. The slow channels remain open longer (15–30 s) and probably play a role in prolonged cell depolarization such as tetanic stimulation. The affinity of calcium-binding sites in some areas declines with aging, while an increase in binding sites may be seen in other areas. The net effect may be a decline in the rapid phase of synaptosomal calcium uptake.[17] Membrane depolarization stimulates calcium uptake, which normally facilitates neurotransmitter release. With the decline in calcium uptake associated with aging, neurotransmitter release is inhibited.

Nerve cell membranes have two calcium pumps to remove calcium and maintain the level of cytosolic calcium. A sodium-calcium exchanger is driven by external sodium levels moving down their transmembrane electrochemical gradient. Calcium-magnesium ATPase is an adenosine triphosphate (ATP) energy-driven and magnesium-dependent pump. With age, the function of the sodium exchange channel declines about 15 percent as a result of decreased calcium affinity. A similar change in affinity is seen in the ATPase pump. As a consequence of these changes, aging impairs the ability of neurons to remove calcium and maintain intracellular calcium homeostasis.[17]

In general, calcium binding to the plasma membranes increases with age in neural as well as nonneural tissues.[17] Age-related changes in negatively charged binding sites, sialidase activity, membrane fluidity, or gangliosides (a major binding material) could increase the affinity of binding sites.[17] Calcium binding to the cell membrane may alter the cell's structure, fluidity, and ability to communicate with other cells. Aging also alters calcium-coupled receptors, and the cell membrane may be hampered in its ability to transduce the external signals which normally bind to these receptors.[17] Altered neuronal calcium levels may also mediate other effects (Table 1-4) through altered cellular protease activity.

Neurotransmitters

A variety of changes occur in neurotransmitter function with aging. Calcium-dependent neurotransmitter release declines with age, probably as a result of reduced calcium uptake. Calcium reduction may also reduce axoplasmic transport in cells by inhibiting microtubule movement of transport vesicles.[17] Aging decreases calmodulin activity, which in turn results in an alteration of the various enzymes and cellular processes that are activated by calcium-protein binding (e.g., calmodulin). This may cause a reduction in the usual enhancement of neurotransmitter release from synaptic vesicles.[17]

In addition, an age-related "leakage" of neurotransmitters appears to occur which may be due to altered calcium levels or to displacement of calcium from membrane gangliosides.[17] This leakage phenomenon has been seen with acetylcholine, dopamine, and glutamate and could cause a minor depolarization of the postsynaptic membrane. Total brain quantities of these neurotransmitters and norepinephrine are also decreased with age.[4] Serotonin has been documented to be decreased in the caudate nucleus. These progressive but uneven declines are probably due to a general decrease in the enzymatic functions of oxidation and phosphorylation. The net effect appears to be a decrease in the amount of neurotransmitters released upon stimulation, resulting in effective synaptic depression.[10]

The progressive imbalance between various neurotransmitter systems in the brain with aging leads to altered neural system function (Table 1-5).[18] In addition to the decline in the release of various neurotransmitters, there

Table 1-4 Effects of altered neuronal calcium

Altered cell membrane structure and function
Altered cellular protease activity
Increased accumulation of intracellular deposits
Decrease in oxidative metabolism
Reduced calcium-mediated neurotransmitter release
Reduced axoplasmic transport
Reduced synaptic neurotransmitter release

Table 1-5 Proposed functional consequences of altered neurotransmitter systems in aging

Neurotransmitter	Functional change
Cholinergic system	
General decrease	Decline in cognition and memory
Reduced sympathetic and parasympathetic ganglia function	Blunted cardiovascular reflexes
Dopaminergic system	
Reduced anterior pituitary release of prolactin and luteining hormone	Senescence of estrous cycles
Reduced activity in basal ganglia	Senile gait, posture, and tremor
Norepinephrine system	
Reduced gonadotropin secretion	Endocrine senescence
Reduced sympathetic function	Blunted cardiovascular reflexes
General decrease	Depression
Serotonin system	
General decrease	Depression

are decreases in receptor binding of neurotransmitters. This decline is thought to result from a reduction in the number of receptors rather than from reduced receptor affinity. In addition, the CNS appears to be less able to increase the number of receptors (supersensitivity) when diminished stimulation occurs. Hence, the aged CNS has diminished neurotransmitter-mediated responsiveness. Specifically, this effect has been well described for both beta-adrenergic and acetylcholine receptors.[18] This altered activity of the brain's cholinergic system probably contributes to the declining cognitive and memory functions of older age.[9] The reduction in cholinergic function may be due to several causes, including a decrease in neuronal uptake of choline (the precursor), a drop in synthesis by choline acetyltransferase (CAT), a decline in acetylcholinesterase, and a diminution of receptor binding sites.[3,18,19] It is unclear if the altered acetylcholine system accounts for the increased susceptibility of older individuals to the effects of anticholinergics such as scopolamine.

Dopamine levels may decline with age because of a decrease in tyrosine hydroxylase (the enzyme responsible for the initial synthetic step for tyrosine), and increases in monoamine oxidase (responsible for dopamine metabolism) also contribute to this decline. In addition, the receptor population for dopamine declines. These changes in dopamine may be linked to several functional changes that occur with aging. For example, dopamine is believed to regulate the anterior pituitary release of prolactin and luteinizing hormone, and a reduction in this neurotransmitter or its receptors could cause senescence of estrous cycles. An age-related loss of dopaminergic function in the basal ganglia has been postulated to be the cause of abnormalities in gait and posture, which may accelerate degenerative changes in joints. Both factors may contribute to the senile gait and increased tendency toward falling seen in the elderly. Basal ganglia changes also may be responsible for a senile tremor that occurs in all limb positions. This sets the tremor apart from the tremor of Parkinson's disease (maximal with limb in repose) or cerebellar damage (maximal with limb approaching a target). Senile tremor is rarely a functional problem; it is interesting that it can usually be treated with beta blockers.[6,9]

Norepinephrine and dopamine share some synthetic and catabolic enzymes; therefore, it is not surprising that norepinephrine levels also decrease with aging. Adrenergic receptors, as was discussed above, are also reduced. Since norepinephrine is thought to play a role in gonadotropin secretion, reduced levels may be related to endocrine senescence.[19]

Although dopamine and norepinephrine levels fall with advancing age, serotonin levels appear to be rather constant.[5] The activities of gamma-aminobutyric acid (GABA) and its synthetic enzyme glutamic acid decarboxylase are reduced by age in a number of areas of the cortex. In contrast, GABA receptor-binding sites may be increased.[9] This may contribute to an alteration in the response to agents which act through GABA-mediated channels (e.g., benzodiazepines and barbiturates).

Cellular Neurophysiology

In addition to neurotransmitter changes, cellular neuroelectrophysiology is altered with age (Table 1-6). Although membrane potentials are not altered, action potential duration increases as a result of the reduced membrane activity in ion transport noted above. Interneuron thresholds for spinal reflexes also change. In general, electrical excitability is decreased. However, some areas become more excitable, and this may explain the lowered threshold for seizure activity seen with a number of convulsant drugs.[1] Changes in excitability also lead to altered reflex activity, resulting in modification of the functional state of other organs innervated by autonomic pathways. In general, the difference between the most and least excitable structures decreases with

Table 1-6 Alterations in cellular electrophysiology

Cellular
Increased action potential duration
General decrease in excitability
Decreased peripheral nerve conduction velocity
Imbalance of inhibitory and facilitory influences
Altered reflex responses
Reduced peripheral nerve function
Electroencephalogram
Slowing: generalized and focal
Hypersynchronization and spindle activity
Evoked potentials
Increased latency

age, and CNS responses to widely different stimuli become more generalized and stereotypical.

A variety of changes occur in descending facilitory and inhibitory neural pathways. Some reflex responses are activated, while others are inhibited.[1] In general, the most important manifestation of change in the CNS is a weakening of inhibition at the various levels of its organization. Since inhibitory influences play an important role in coordinating and integrating CNS function, this leads to overall changes in reflex activity and a disorganization of highly coordinated activities.[1]

Neuroendocrine Function

The homeostasis of the entire organism is altered by changes in the neurohumoral system that maintains the internal milieu (Table 1-7). Therefore, disturbances leading to altered blood pressure, blood sugar, and acid-base balance are tolerated less well than they are in young individuals. This can lead to pathological processes that would not occur in younger individuals whose bodies are confronted with otherwise innocuous stimuli.[1]

The function of the hypothalamic-pituitary system is modified with age, altering peripheral organ function: Some organs increase their activity, while others decrease it. Many investigators believe that changes in hypothalamic function are a leading cause of aging in the entire body. In general, anterior hypothalamic activity appears to decrease with age, but this is not uniform. In addition, the anterior hypothalamus becomes less responsive to hormonal control. This dysfunction of the anterior hypothalamus leads to changes in peripheral organ systems, tending to send the whole body out of homeostatic control.[1] In addition, a decrease in the sensitivity of the hypothalamic system to the inhibitory action of various hormones (particularly estrogen and corticosteroids) may lead to hypertension, atherosclerosis, obesity, and diabetes.[1]

One of the most typical characteristics of aging is a reduction in the power of the organism to adapt to environmental changes. The response to stress of various types is less effective. For example, age changes in the hypothalamic-

Table 1-7 Autonomic and homeostatic changes

Decreased anterior hypothalamic activity
Decreased sensitivity of hypothalamus to inhibitory hormones
Increased threshold of vagal and sympathetic nerves
Altered sympathetic and parasympathetic function
Reduced control and responsiveness of cardiovascular tone
Reduced temperature regulation
Orthostatic hypotension
Chronic constipation
Decreased sympathetic function (slowed heart rate and decreased blood pressure)

pituitary-adrenal axis lead to reductions in the ability to respond to external stresses such as cold, pain, and immobilization. In addition, changes in the levels of catecholamines and stimulation of the limbic system are tolerated less well. This leads to an altered ability to regulate body temperature during heating and cooling.[1]

The unequal aging process of brain structures which regulate the cardiovascular and respiratory systems leads to circulatory pathology and altered cardiovascular and ventilatory responses. Weakening of nervous control of the cardiovascular system is a general phenomenon. For example, the thresholds for stimulation of the vagus and sympathetic nerves are raised, causing hemodynamic changes. Aging results in a reduction in the excitability of the sympathetic and parasympathetic ganglia caused by reductions in the synthesis and hydrolysis of acetylcholine. As a consequence, significant CNS changes are not as vigorously translated into peripheral changes in cardiovascular tone.[1] As a result, responses to surgical pain may be blunted so that hypotension occurs with minimal anesthesia or in the face of hypovolemia. As neural control of the periphery by the CNS weakens, there are also changes in sensitivity to humoral factors. Many reactions in old age become prolonged and protracted.[1] Therefore, mild cardiovascular disturbances such as blood loss may be poorly tolerated.

BEHAVIORAL AND FUNCTIONAL CHANGES

Normal functional changes in the geriatric nervous system are a result of aging of the neural systems, as was described above (Table 1-8). Some functions decline, others appear to be unaffected, and still others improve with age. Several clearly definable functions decline with age and are responsible for dependency.[3] In individuals over 65 years of age, 93 percent of those dependent on others for care have problems identifiable as neurological disease. Among those who are disabled, 48 percent have neurological disease. Among individuals disabled by neurological disease, the most common causes are

Table 1-8 Behavioral and functional changes

Slowed reaction time
Dysfunction in learning
Reduced information retrieval (especially short-term memory)
Slower peripheral information acquisition time
Decrease in intelligence
Decline in language skills
Depression
Decreased sensory function
Reduced visual sensitivity to short wavelengths
High-frequency hearing loss
Decreased proprioception and vibration

movement disorders (20.5 percent), dementia (16.4 percent), and strokes or transient ischemic attacks (TIAs) (16 percent).[20]

Behavior and Memory

Most types of behavior slow with age. There is a 15 to 20 percent increase in reaction time between 20 and 60 years of age.[3] This increase appears to be due primarily to a change in neural processing, with a general slowing of the speed of response. The increased reaction time appears to affect most activities, including task-oriented responses.[3]

Alterations in behavior may also be due in part to changes in memory and learning. Dysfunction in learning and memory is repeatedly shown in psychometric studies of older individuals and is a common complaint in the elderly.[3] The most striking change in memory is reduced information retrieval. Of interest, there is no decline in the ability to recognize items, even when recognition requires memorization.[3]

The speed and consistency of short-term memory appear to decline most with age.[3] Learning appears to change in the elderly; individuals learn better when learning patterns have some element of previously learned material (i.e., already in memory). As a consequence, the elderly may have trouble coping in new environments where they must adapt to situations that were not previously encountered.[21] The elderly require more trials to learn lists, and this may be related to difficulty in encoding items in memory. The elderly appear to be forgetful in everyday activities, probably as a consequence of difficulty with memory retrieval.[3] Above age 70, memory retrieval deficits (identified as errors in naming objects) become more noticeable. By age 75 years, 25 percent of the elderly show memory deficits (50 percent do so by age 80).[4] The acquisition speed for environmental information is slowed, and this also contributes to the decline in learning and memory.

Intelligence, Cognition, and Emotion

A variety of changes in cognition, personality, and emotion occur normally with age.[21] Intelligence appears to decline linearly, beginning as early as adolescence.[3] Cognitive function declines with age.[3] Information processing is clearly affected, with changes in both peripheral and central information.[3] Language skills such as naming and defining begin to decline after age 70, but this appears to be related to forgetting rather than to lack of understanding.[21] Emotional problems of many varieties increase with age; the most common is depression. A variety of studies suggest that this may be related to altered levels of neurotransmitter substances (notably norepinephrine and serotonin), neuronal sodium accumulation, and possibly altered hormonal levels.[18] Studies are not clear, however, since reductions in motivation are commonly seen in the elderly, resulting from behavioral slowness. This leads to dependence on group opinion and may be interpreted as depression.[3]

Sensory Function

Normal changes with aging generally result in the deterioration of sensory modalities (distal extremities), with muscle wasting, a decline in strength, and an absence of or decrease in tendon reflexes.[22] Visual acuity appears to decline, with increases in light threshold, a decrease in visual task performance, and a reduction of the ability to appreciate shorter wavelengths. These changes are thought to be related primarily to processes in the eye.[3] A loss of auditory acuity also occurs with age. This appears to be related to changes in the ear, although the decline in speech perception is probably due to central changes.[3] These changes are reflected in diagnostic electrophysiological studies (see below).

Peripheral Nervous System Function

By age 50 years, 20 percent of individuals have abnormal neurological findings on examination (Table 1-9). Common changes include reduced rate and amount of motor activity, impaired fine coordination and agility, slowed reaction time, slowed and narrowed perception, decreased vibratory sense in the feet and toes, and reduced Achilles tendon reflexes. Patients 55 to 75 years of age constitute the largest group of individuals with peripheral neuropathy. The most commonly cited causes are diabetes, malignancy, alcohol, drugs, demyelination, autoimmune diseases, and nutritional deficiencies. Aging itself is re-

Table 1-9 Common neurological changes in the elderly

Cognition	
Memory	Modest decline in short-term memory
Verbal intelligence	Decline after seventh decade
Processing speech	Decline with age
Sensory, motor	
Vision	Smaller pupils, slow reactivity, progressive limitation of upward gaze, presbyopia (loss of lens elasticity)
Hearing	Decreased acuity at high frequencies (presbycusis)
Vibratory sense	Decline in function of distal extremities
Spinal reflexes	Ankle jerks decreased or absent, increased primitive reflexes (glabella, palmomental, snout)
Gait/posture	Slowed, forward-flexed, and mildly unsteady
Motor	Decline in grip strength and mild state of extrapyramidal dysfunction

sponsible for loss and damage of the component nerve fibers (motor, sensory, and autonomic).[22]

A variety of changes cause a decrease in the information transmitted along nerve pathways to peripheral locations. These changes include a decline of nerve endings and receptors, a decrease in the number of neurons in the brain, and a reduction in the number of fibers in nerve trunks. Changes in metabolism and transport mechanisms within nerve cells and slowing of the velocity of impulse conduction also contribute.[1] It has been estimated that about 25 percent of lumbosacral anterior horn cells and spinal sensory ganglia are lost with aging.[4] This appears to correlate with reductions in reaction time. It is of note that individuals who exercise regularly have faster reaction times. A variety of evidence suggests that the decline in physical activity parallels the decline in mental activity.[3]

Loss of motor and sensory axons is most prominent in the legs. This results in a reduction in conduction velocity in sensory nerves to the greatest extent and in motor neurons to a lesser extent. There is a progressive fall in the number of functional motor sites in the peripheral nervous system over age 60, and the majority of the remaining fibers innervate slow (type 1) muscles.[9] Motor and sensory nerve conduction velocity slows after age 60, particularly in the distal parts of axons.[9] The decline in physical fitness and athletic ability appears to be related to aging of the CNS,[3] with a decrease in conduction velocity contributing to a slowed response time.[4] Proprioceptive and vibratory senses are reduced, probably as a result of peripheral changes.[3]

Autonomic Function

Age-related changes in the autonomic nervous system produce a functional neuropathy that may result in clinical disease by altering the maintenance and integration of visceral functions or by causing subclinical changes that diminish the safety margin for physiological insults (Table 1-7). Deterioration in the autonomic nervous system leads to difficulties with homeostasis as organ coordination is lost. Autonomic dysfunction is due to a variety of effects, including dysfunction in the dorsal nucleus of the vagus, hypothalamus, intermediolateral columns of the spinal cord, and sympathetic ganglia,[23] as well as altered sensitivity of the baroreceptors, decreases in compliance of the blood vessels, loss of fibers, and slowed nerve conduction velocity.[24]

These autonomic changes lead to several disturbances. Postural hypotension, which is uncommon in middle age (1 percent), is far more common in old age (18 percent of those over 65 years of age).[24] Diminished sympathetic function is thought to occur, and this may explain a decrease in heart rate and blood pressure in the absence of vascular disease. The reduced sympathetic function may be due to a decrease in norepinephrine in the neural system, decreased receptor responsiveness, axonal degeneration (thought to be due to loss of postganglionic sympathetic neurons), decreased vasoreceptor sensitivity, and decreased adrenergic responsiveness of the heart.

Blood pressure is normally regulated by the autonomic nervous system through alterations in vascular tone and myocardial function. This occurs via sensors in the vasoreceptors of the great vessels and the carotid sinus, with neural input to the brainstem through the glossopharyngeal nerve and carotid sinus nerves. Mediation occurs through the nuclei of the tractus solitarius and the paramedian nuclei, with efferents to higher centers and to preganglionic sympathetic cells of the spinal cord. Postganglionic fibers of sympathetic and parasympathetic nature then radiate to the vascular system.[24] Autonomic dysfunction leads to impaired activity of this complex system, impaired thermoregulation (caused by impairment of sweating and diminished vasoconstriction upon cooling), and chronic constipation (disordered bowel motility).

EEG/Evoked Potentials

A variety of electrophysiological changes occur in the brain, paralleling functional and neurophysiological changes (Table 1-6). A general slowing in the electroencephalogram (EEG) has been observed.[3] This frequency change appears to be related to general activity and health; older individuals may have predominant frequencies in the theta range [4–7 Hertz (Hz)], resembling the slow record of childhood, with more active individuals having frequencies in the alpha range (8–12 Hz), similar to younger adults. The generalized EEG slowing is also associated with the reduced CBF and $CMRO_2$ seen with aging.[3] More diffuse slowing, with ventral replacement of normal EEG activity, is most common in patients with dementia or psychiatric disease and has a strong relation with significant intellectual deterioration.[3]

In addition to the generalized EEG changes, focal slowing occurs, with localized sharp waves or spikes which are not normally associated with epileptiform discharges. These focal changes are seen most commonly in the temporal lobes.[3] EEG changes of hypersynchronization and spindle activity or disorganization probably can be explained by alterations in the number and properties of neurons, reduction of CBF, changes in cortical-subcortical relations, and a reduction in the flow of afferent impulses.[1]

Consistent with decreased proprioception, somatosensory evoked potentials are commonly increased in latency. Auditory evoked potentials usually are not altered unless there is high-frequency hearing loss. Visual evoked responses usually show a decline in amplitude of the cortical waves that may be related to a decrease in attention.[6]

COMMON DISEASES OF AGING

Neurological disorders are the most common causes of disability in the elderly, accounting for about 50 percent of functional problems. As was discussed above, declines in memory, cognition, perception, and motor function occur with age, but they are usually not a source of significant impairment. A normal neurological exam is likely to reveal changes from those of younger patients (Table 1-9).[6]

A variety of diseases are more common in the elderly. In some cases this occurs because these diseases do not appear to occur in younger individuals or because the changes associated with aging appear to unmask or exaggerate the disease symptomatology. In some cases, the symptoms of the diseases may be such that a subtle transition occurs from normal elderly changes to the disease state, making identification of the disease difficult. This is particularly true of diseases characterized by deterioration in memory, dementia, or motor function. Thus, these disease states often masquerade as exaggerated aging.

Dementia

Dementia is the most serious pathological process affecting the elderly and is a good predictor of mortality. Dementia is characterized as a decline in all levels of mental functioning. The most common cause is Alzheimer's disease, which is an age-dependent process leading to total brain dysfunction. The diagnosis is based on deterioration in orientation and memory and a decline in intellect. Ultimately, daily acts of living cannot be performed.[3] This disorder is the most frequent cause of chronic institutionalization of the elderly.[20]

Dementia has many causes. Approximately half the cases are due to a vascular pathology such as atherosclerosis. Vascular disease contributes through several mechanisms, including multiple lacunar infarcts (usually associated with arterial hypertension), Binswanger's disease (possibly a disorder of microcirculatory regulation of blood flow), and a variety of focal vascular lesions (usually bilateral in pathology).[25] The metabolic causes of dementia are hypothyroidism, pernicious anemia, lupus erythmatosus, adrenal insufficiency, renal failure, disorders of calcium metabolism, and Wilson's disease.[3]

Cerebrovascular insufficiency and dementia are clearly related. CBF decreases diffusely, with areas of stroke showing even more dramatic reductions. Memory disturbances appear to correlate with reductions of CBF in the temporal lobes. Regional changes are associated with specific neurological symptoms, and decreases in CBF correlate with diminished performance on psychological tests.[3]

Dementia may go unnoticed unless it is specifically evaluated. The abbreviated mental test score may allow an evaluation, provided that the patient is not deaf, dysphasic, depressed, or medically debilitated. This test includes recall of age, an address for recall at the end of the test, year, name of hospital, recognition of two persons, date of birth, year of first world war, current President, and ability to count backward from 20.[26] Personality changes are uncommon in dementia associated with normal aging (90 percent without changes). In contrast, dementia associated with Alzheimer's disease commonly shows changes in personality (80 percent), including impaired emotional control, diminished initiative, and withdrawal.

The anesthetic management of a patient with dementia should take into consideration the reduced anesthetic requirement seen in elderly patients (see below). The cause of the dementia should be noted, as this may affect anesthetic management. Family members and previous medical records may supplement patient history in the preoperative evaluation. Coexisting diseases and drug therapy should be noted, as they may influence the anesthetic course.

Alzheimer's Disease

Alzheimer's disease includes pathological processes which are very specific and are not simply an exaggeration of normal aging. The differential diagnosis includes tumor, infection, hydrocephalus, cerebrovascular disease, metabolic diseases, chronic intoxications, trauma, depression, and Pick's disease. Alzheimer's disease is associated with frontal and temporal lobe atrophy with plaques, intracytoplasmic neurofibrillary tangles, and occasionally granulovascular degeneration. These symptoms seem to be related to cholinergic deficiencies in presynaptic components.[18]

In addition to changes in dopaminergic neurotransmitter systems, major losses in glutamatergic receptors are seen. It has been postulated that the latter changes may be responsible for the cognitive impairment.[27] Despite all the changes that have been observed, the actual cause of Alzheimer's disease is not known. Several environmental risk factors and the discovery of several linked genetic loci and point mutations associated with the disease suggest a genetic contribution.[28] Several mechanisms of disease as consequences of genetic alterations have been proposed, including defective DNA repair[29] and abnormal proteolytic processing of proteins leading to intracellular amyloidosis.[30] It is of interest that the latter processes would lead to intracellular accumulation of materials, which is seen with normal aging and several diseases as well as in Alzheimer's disease.

The anesthetic management of a patient with Alzheimer's disease should take into consideration the possible difficulty of dealing with a patient unable to fully comprehend the environment or cooperate with those around him or her. Centrally acting anticholinergic drugs are omitted from the premedication because of the possibility of cortical cholinergic deficiency. Possible drug interactions should be considered in patients receiving anticholinesterase drugs for treatment of Alzheimer's disease. The reduced anesthetic requirement of geriatric patients necessitates careful titration of inhalational and intravenous agents.

Parkinson's Disease

Parkinson's disease, like dementia, is essentially a disorder of aging, with a negligible incidence below age 50 years and a prevalance of 25 in 100,000 in individuals age 50 to 59. The incidence is over 3000 per 100,000 above age 70.[20] Parkinsonian syndromes are characterized by extrapyramidal hypertonia, akinesia, and involuntary tremor. Parkinson's disease appears to be due to a selective degeneration of the nigrostriatal system.[18] This is related to an imbalance of dopamine and acetylcholine in the dopaminergic system, with nerve cell loss in the substantia nigra. Although it can be caused by substantia nigra lesions, the degenerative form occurs most commonly among patients over age 70 (75–88 percent).[23] Pharmacologic therapy to restore function with L-dopa suggests that the neurochemical balance can be partially restored.[19]

Management of anesthesia is based on knowledge of the disease process and potential adverse drug effects. Phenothiazines, butyrophenones (droperidol), and metoclopramide are avoided because of their ability to antagonize the effects of dopamine in the basal ganglia. Anesthetic agents that sensitize the heart to arrhythmias, such as halothane, are excluded because of the concern that halothane could precipitate cardiac dysrhythmias in patients receiving levodopa, although this has not been documented. There has been one case report of a hyperkalemic response after succinylcholine administration in a patient with Parkinson's disease, but this report was clouded by the complex nature of the case.[31] A subsequent series of seven patients with severe Parkinson's disease who received succinylcholine during surgery for adrenal medullary to caudate transplantation did not develop hyperkalemia after the succinylcholine.[32] There has also been one case report of an acute dystonic reaction after alfentanil in a patient with untreated Parkinson's disease.[33] The monoamine oxidase (MAO) inhibitor selegiline has been used to prevent degradation of dopamine in the brain of patients with Parkinson's disease. It is an MAO type B inhibitor (intestinal MAO is type A, while most of that in brain is type B). Although drug interactions may be less common with this drug than with nonselective MAO inhibitors, there has been one case report of a severe adverse reaction (agitation, stupor, muscle rigidity, hyperthermia) between selegiline and the narcotic meperidine (pethidine).[34]

Autonomic dysfunction may be seen in patients with Parkinson's disease. Gastrointestinal dysfunction may be manifested by difficulties in swallowing saliva and, in more advanced cases, solid foods. The most common cardiovascular symptom is orthostatic hypotension, which may be exacerbated by antiparkinsonian drugs (levodopa, bromocriptine). Postoperatively, patients with Parkinson's disease have been shown to be more susceptible to developing confusion and hallucinations.[35] Drug therapy is resumed as soon as possible in the postoperative period to avoid recurrent extrapyramidal symptoms.

Other Diseases

Demyelinating diseases are seen more commonly with advancing age, perhaps because of the normal changes in myelinated axons (loss of myelin as well as fiber loss). Part of the increased incidence is related to a loss of redundancy in fiber pathways that may be degenerating. It has been estimated that a patient may be asymptomatic until 80 percent of a pathway becomes pathologically altered.[7]

Strokes are relatively common in older individuals. Over age 55, the incidence is about 1 in 200 per year, increasing to 1 in 125 over age 65 and to about

1 in 50 over age 75 (average for all ages, about 1 in 500 per year). Vascular disease is a common accompaniment of stroke.[20]

Finally, the appearance of slow-growing tumors may be more apparent as the decline in the CNS occurs. The most common brain tumors in the elderly are meningiomas and gliomas. Meningiomas are usually hemispheric tumors attached to the undersurface of the dura and derived from the pia, arachnoid, and dura.[36] Gliomas are tumors arising from astrocytes, oligodendroglia, and ependymal cells. Among these tumors, astrocytes are the most common (60 percent).[36]

CHANGES IN ANESTHETIC AND ANALGESIC REQUIREMENTS

The decline in CNS function associated with aging is accompanied by a reduced anesthetic and analgesic requirement. Although the precise neuroanatomic basis for these changes is unknown, many of the anatomic and functional changes described above have been theorized to play a role. For example, the gradual decline in cortical neuron density and the decrease in synaptic transmission may play a role. The reduction in neuronal density is accompanied by a decline in hemispheric CBF and $CMRO_2$. Also theorized to play a role is the age-related decrease in the rate of synthesis of, and the corresponding reduction in the brain levels of, neurotransmitters. A reduction in the number of receptor sites and a decrease in the sensitivity to biogenic amines (e.g., catecholamines) also have been proposed as an explanation for the greater sensitivity of elderly patients to the depressant effects of drugs that act on the CNS. In the peripheral nervous system, the reduction in the axonal population and the deterioration of the myelin sheath may contribute to the progressive slowing of peripheral motor and sensory nerve conduction velocities seen with advancing age.

The reduced anesthetic requirements for geriatric patients apply to inhalational, intravenous, and local anesthetics. Although alterations in many other systems may affect these requirements, this discussion will focus primarily on the CNS effects of these drugs.

Inhalational Drugs

The MAC (minimum alveolar concentration of a drug that prevents movement on skin incision in 50 percent of patients) decreases with advancing age. This has been shown repeatedly for different inhalational agents. Gregory and associates[37] noted that the MAC of halothane is highest in the newborn and lowest in the elderly. Studying halothane in different age groups, Nicodemus and coworkers[38] found that halothane is 1.28 and 1.12 times more potent in producing anesthesia in adults than it is in the 0- to 6-month and 6- to 24-month age groups, respectively. Stevens and associates[39] studied patients 19 years of age and older and noted a reduction in isoflurane MAC with increasing age. The MAC of the newer inhalational agents desflurane and sevoflurane has also been shown to be age-related. Rampil and colleagues[40] noted that for patients between the third and fifth decades, the desflurane anesthetic requirement declined to 83 percent of third-decade MAC. Smaller MAC values of sevoflurane have also been noted in elderly patients[41] compared with the values reported for children and adults.[42–44]

To test the thesis that aging has a general effect on the anesthetic requirement for all agents, Munson and associates[45] compared the age-related changes in halothane and isoflurane MAC to those found with cyclopropane, an anesthetic with solvent and pharmacologic properties significantly different from those of halothane and isoflurane. They noted that the slope of the relation between MAC and age for cyclopropane paralleled those previously noted for halothane and isoflurane. These results were consistent with the thesis that aging has a general effect on the anesthetic requirement for all agents. To obtain a rough estimate of MAC in geriatric patients, the published MAC value of inhalational agents is decreased by 4 percent for every decade of age over 40 years.[46] For example, the MAC of halothane in an 80-year-old is obtained by multiplying by 84 percent, which was derived from the formula [100% − (4% × 4 decades)] times the published halothane MAC value of 0.76, to equal 0.64.[46]

Intravenous Drugs

The apparent sensitivity of the CNS to intravenous drugs is also increased in elderly patients. Both pharmacodynamic (plasma concentration–drug response relation) and pharmacokinetic (drug uptake, tissue distribution, hepatic metabolism, and renal elimination) factors may play a role, the balance of which depends on the particular drug involved.

For thiopental sodium and etomidate, the dose required to reach a uniform EEG endpoint decreases significantly with increasing age.[47,48] However, it has been suggested that the increased sensitivity to these drugs with aging relates more to differences in pharmacokinetics than to pharmacodynamics. For example, a reduction in the initial distribution volume for both thiopental and etomidate in an elderly patient results in higher serum concentrations after a given dose.[47,48] This contributes to the lower dose requirements in elderly patients. An increase in the volume of distribution at steady state has been shown for thiopental sodium, producing an increase in the terminal elimination half-life.[49] A decrease in the clearance of etomidate is consistent with the decline in hepatic blood flow in the elderly, since etomidate clearance depends on hepatic blood flow.[48]

The plasma concentration of diazepam required to achieve a desired pharmacologic effect is lower in elderly patients (pharmacodynamic response).[50] A prolonged terminal elimination half-life of diazepam reflects an increased volume of distribution (pharmacokinetic response). Sensitivity to midazolam is also increased in elderly patients. For example, a dose of 0.3 mg/kg was adequate for anesthetic induction in 100 percent of unpremedicated elderly patients (age 60 years or over), whereas 0.5 mg/kg did not adequately induce anesthesia in 40 percent of young unpremedicated patients.[51] Elimination half-life is longer and total clearance of midazolam is reduced in elderly versus young males.[52]

The dose requirement of narcotics decreases significantly in the elderly. The dose requirement of fentanyl or alfentanil decreases 50 percent from age 20 to age 89.[53] The alteration in dose requirement is primarily a function of altered brain sensitivity (pharmacodynamic response). Elderly patients have an increased brain sensitivity to fentanyl and alfentanil, as demonstrated by a study relating spectral edge frequency to narcotic serum concentrations.[53] Some changes in pharmacokinetic parameters have also been noted, including a decrease in plasma clearance and an increase in terminal elimination half-life.[54,55]

Local Anesthetics

Reduced requirements for local anesthetics may be seen in elderly patients. For example, there is a greater segmental spread of local anesthetic in elderly patients undergoing epidural anesthesia.[56] Serum levels of local anesthetics are increased, and thus it is suggested that the dose of local anesthetic for epidural anesthesia should be reduced in an elderly patient. Similarly, for spinal anesthesia, it has been demonstrated that the time to maximum spread is shorter and the sensory spinal blockade is slightly higher in older patients.[57] A number of reasons have been postulated for reduced local anesthetic requirements, including (1) progressive occlusion of the intervertebral foramina with increasing age so that local anesthetic solutions injected epidurally have a greater longitudinal spread, (2) reduced vertebral column height lowering dose requirements for spinal anesthesia, (3) deterioration of myelin sheaths, (4) decreased CNS neuronal population, (5) decreased number of axons in peripheral nerves, and (6) alterations in the pharmacokinetics of local anesthetics in elderly patients.

SUMMARY

The rate of normal aging differs among individuals, with variability among individuals in regard to the specific effects. A global decrease in neural function is a general process. However, the hallmark of aging neural function is the development of processes that lead to an imbalance in the various systems that control neural and visceral functioning. In general, older individuals share (1) reduced short-term memory, (2) a need for basing learning patterns on previously learned material, (3) a tendency to depression, (4) reduced visual, auditory, and peripheral nerve function, (5) altered gait and tremor with loss of fine motor coordination, and (6) reduced homeostatic control, making them more susceptible to physiological disturbances that would be easily accommodated by a younger individual. The decline in CNS function in elderly patients is accompanied by a reduction in requirements for inhalational, intravenous, and local anesthetics. This may be due to alterations in pharmacodynamic and/or pharmacokinetic responses. The greater sensitivity to anesthetic agents may lead to decreased dose requirements, slowed onset, prolonged duration of action, and exaggerated side effects.

REFERENCES

1. Frol'kis VV, Bezrukov VV: Aging of the central nervous system. *Hum Physiol* 78:478, 1978.
2. Duckett S: The normal aging human brain, in Duckett S (ed): *The Pathology of the Aging Human Nervous System.* Philadelphia: Lea & Febiger, 1991, pp 1–19.
3. Long DM: Aging in the nervous system. *Neurosurgery* 17:348, 1985.
4. Boss BJ: Normal aging in the nervous system: Implications for SCI nurses. *SCI Nurs* 8:42, 1991.
5. Berlin M, Wallace RB: Aging and the central nervous system. *Exp Aging Res* 2:125, 1976.
6. Morris JC, McManus DQ: The neurology of aging: Normal versus pathologic change. *Geriatrics* 46:47, 1991.
7. Knobler RL: Demyelinating disorders of the aged brain, in Duckett S (ed): *The Pathology of the Aging Human Nervous System.* Philadelphia: Lea & Febiger, 1991, pp 317–335.
8. Duara R, London ED, Rapoport SI: Changes in structure and energy metabolism of the aging brain, in Finch CE, Schneider EL (eds): *Handbook of the Biology of Aging*, 2d ed. New York: Van Nostrand Reinhold, 1985, pp 595–616.
9. Hubbard BM, Squier M: The physical ageing of the neuromuscular system, in Tallis R (ed): *The Clinical Neurology of Old Age.* Chichester: J Wiley, 1989, pp 3–26.
10. Smith DO: Cellular and molecular correlates of aging in the nervous system. *Exp Gerontol* 23:399, 1988.
11. Gustafson L, Brun A, Ingvar DH: Presenile dementia: Clinical symptoms, pathoanatomical findings and cerebral blood flow, in Meyer JS, Lechner H, Reivich M (eds): *Cerebral Vascular Disease.* Amsterdam: Excerpta Medica, 1976, pp 5–9.
12. Gustafson L, Hagberg B, Ingvar DH: Speech disturbances in presenile dementia related to local cerebral blood flow abnormalities in the dominant hemisphere. *Brain Lang* 5:103, 1978.
13. Gustafson T, Risberg J: Regional cerebral blood flow measurements by the ^{133}Xe inhalation technique in differential diagnosis of dementia. *Acta Neurol Scand* 72:546, 1979.
14. Strehler BL: Fundamental mechanisms of neuronal aging, in Cervos-Navarro J, Sarkander H-I (eds): *Brain Aging: Neuropathology and Neuropharmacology.* New York: Raven Press, 1983, pp 75–95.
15. Arnold KG: Cerebral blood flow in geriatrics—a review. *Age Ageing* 10:5, 1981.
16. Deshmukh VD, Meyer JS: *Noninvasive Measurement of Regional Cerebral Blood Flow in Man.* S P Medical Scientific Books. New York: Spectrum, 1978.
17. Gibson GE, Peterson C: Calcium and the aging nervous system. *Neurobiol Aging* 8:329, 1987.
18. Samorajski T: Normal and pathologic aging of the brain, in Enna SJ, Samorajski T, Beer B (eds): *Brain Neurotransmitters and Receptors in Aging and Age-Related Disorders.* New York: Raven Press, 1981, pp 1–12.
19. Rogers J, Bloom FE: Neurotransmitter metabolism and function in the aging

central nervous system, in Finch CE, Schneider EL (eds): *Handbook of the Biology of Aging*, 2d ed. New York: Van Nostrand Reinhold, 1985, pp 645–691.
20. Broe GA: The neuroepidemiology of old age, in Tallis R (ed): *The Clinical Neurology of Old Age*. Chichester, UK: Wiley, 1989, pp 51–65.
21. Binks M: Changes in mental functioning associated with normal ageing, in Tallis R (ed): *The Clinical Neurology of Old Age*. Chichester, UK: Wiley, 1989, pp 27–39.
22. Vital C, Vital A: Peripheral neuropathy, in Duckett S (ed): *The Pathology of the Aging Human Nervous System*. Philadelphia: Lea & Febiger, 1991, pp 393–432.
23. Gray F, Poirier J, Scaravilli F: Parkinson's disease and Parkinsonian syndromes, in Duckett S (ed): *The Pathology of the Aging Human Nervous System*. Philadelphia: Lea & Febiger, 1991, pp 179–199.
24. Lye M: Autonomic dysfunction and abnormal vascular reflexes, in Tallis R (ed): *The Clinical Neurology of Old Age*. Chichester, UK: Wiley, 1989, pp 191–211.
25. Brion S, Mikol J, Plas J, Bereanu A: Dementia, in Duckett S (ed): *The Pathology of the Aging Human Nervous System*. Philadelphia: Lea & Febiger, 1991, pp 77–87.
26. George J: The neurological examination of the elderly patient, in Tallis R (ed): *The Clinical Neurology of Old Age*. Chichester, UK: Wiley, 1989, pp 67–88.
27. Myhrer T: Animal models of Alzheimer's disease: Glutamatergic denervation as an alternative approach to cholinergic denervation. *Neurosci Biobehav Rev* 17:195, 1993.
28. Breitner JC, Gatz M, Bergem AL, et al: Use of twin cohorts for research in Alzheimer's disease. *Neurology* 43:261, 1993.
29. Boerrigter ME, Wei JY, Vijg J: DNA repair and Alzheimer's disease. *J Gerontol* 47:B177, 1992.
30. Kosik KS: Alzheimer's disease: A cell biological perspective. *Science* 256(5058):780, 1992.
31. Gravlee GP: Succinylcholine-induced hyperkalemia in a patient with Parkinson's disease. *Anesth Analg* 59:444, 1980.
32. Muzzi DA, Black S, Cucchiara RF: The lack of effect of succinylcholine on serum potassium in patients with Parkinson's disease. *Anesthesiology* 71:322, 1989.
33. Mets B: Acute dystonia after alfentanil in untreated Parkinson's disease. *Anesth Analg* 72:557, 1991.
34. Zornberg GL, Bodkin JA, Cohen BM: Severe adverse interaction between pethidine and selegiline. *Lancet* 337:246, 1991.
35. Golden WE, Lavender RC, Metzer S: Acute postoperative confusion and hallucinations in Parkinson's disease. *Ann Intern Med* 111:218, 1989.
36. Alvord EC Jr, Shaw C-M: Neoplasms affecting the nervous system of the elderly, in Duckett S (ed): *The Pathology of the Aging Human Nervous System*. Philadelphia: Lea & Febiger, 1991, pp 210–286.
37. Gregory GA, Eger EI, Munson ES: The relationship between age and halothane requirement in man. *Anesthesiology* 30:488, 1969.
38. Nicodemus HF, Nassiri-Rahimi CN, Bachman L, Smith TC: Median effective doses (ED_{50}) of halothane in adults and children. *Anesthesiology* 31:344, 1969.
39. Stevens WC, Dolan WM, Gibbons RT, et al: Minimum alveolar concentrations (MAC) of isoflurane with and without nitrous oxide in patients of various ages. *Anesthesiology* 42:197, 1975.
40. Rampil IJ, Lockhart SH, Zwass MS, et al: Clinical characteristics of desflurane in surgical patients: Minimum alveolar concentration. *Anesthesiology* 74:429, 1991.
41. Nakajima R, Nakajima Y, Ikeda K: Minimum alveolar concentration of sevoflurane in elderly patients. *Br J Anaesth* 70:273, 1993.

42. Katoh T, Ikeda K: Minimum alveolar concentrations of sevoflurane in children. *Br J Anaesth* 68:139, 1992.
43. Katoh T, Ikeda K: The minimum alveolar concentration (MAC) of sevoflurane in humans. *Anesthesiology* 66:301, 1987.
44. Scheller MS, Saidman LJ, Partridge BL: MAC of sevoflurane in humans and the New Zealand white rabbit. *Can J Anaesth* 35:153, 1988.
45. Munson ES, Hoffman JC, Eger EI: Use of cyclopropane to test generality of anesthetic requirement in the elderly. *Anesth Analg* 63:998, 1984.
46. Hilgenberg JC: Inhalational and intravenous drugs in the elderly patient. *Semin Anesth* V:44, 1986.
47. Homer TD, Stanski DR: The effect of increasing age on thiopental distribution and anesthetic requirement. *Anesthesiology* 62:714, 1985.
48. Arden JR, Holley FO, Stanski DR: Increased sensitivity to etomidate in the elderly: Initial distribution versus altered brain response. *Anesthesiology* 65:19, 1986.
49. Jung D, Mayersohn M, Perrier D, et al: Thiopental disposition as a function of age in female patients undergoing surgery. *Anesthesiology* 56:263, 1982.
50. Reidenberg MM, Levy M, Warner H, et al: Relationship between diazepam dose, plasma level, age, and central nervous system depression. *Clin Pharmacol Ther* 23:371, 1978.
51. Gamble JAS, Kawar P, Dundee JW, et al: Evaluation of midazolam as an intravenous induction agent. *Anaesthesia* 36:868, 1981.
52. Greenblatt DJ, Abernethy DR, Locniskar A, et al: Effect of age, gender and obesity on midazolam kinetics. *Anesthesiology* 61:27, 1984.
53. Scott JC, Stanski DR: Decreased fentanyl and alfentanil dose requirements with age: A simultaneous pharmacokinetic and pharmacodynamic evaluation. *J Pharmacol Exp Ther* 240:159, 1987.
54. Helmers H, Peer AV, Woestenborghs R, et al: Alfentanil kinetics in the elderly. *Clin Pharmacol Ther* 36:239, 1984.
55. Bentley JB, Borel JD, Nenad RE: Influence of age on the pharmacokinetics of fentanyl. *Anesth Analg* 61:171, 1982.
56. Finucane BT, Hammonds WD, Welch MB: Influence of age on vascular absorption of lidocaine from the epidural space. *Anesth Analg* 66:843, 1987.
57. Racle JP, Benkhadra A, Poy JY, Gleizal B: Spinal analgesia with hyperbaric bupivacaine: Influence of age. *Br J Anaesth* 60:508, 1988.

CHAPTER 2

Physiological Changes with Aging in the Respiratory System

Christopher A. Bracken

INTRODUCTION

In the operating room, the anesthesiologist serves as the patient's acute-care internal medicine doctor. This requires extensive knowledge of all organ system functions, particularly an awareness of respiratory system function, as the airway always comes first in the anesthesiologist's list of differential diagnoses. As a function of most deep anesthetics, the patient's autoregulatory ability is impaired. Therefore, the anesthesiologist must assume the responsibility for maintaining homeostasis during a period of surgical stress. Aging in general impairs the ability of the organism (the patient) to handle stress, since a significant portion of the functional reserve that normally deals with stressful situations is lost. It thus behooves a prudent anesthesiologist to take these alterations of physiological function into consideration when planning and carrying out anesthesia in a geriatric patient. This chapter discusses the alterations in respiratory anatomy and function that occur with aging and may affect the course of an anesthetic.

SUCCESSFUL AGING

Geriatrics is not defined by age alone. There is a continuum of decreasing physiological function, beginning at about age 30, which results in an increasing vulnerability to challenges and stresses. Individuals, and indeed organ systems within a given individual, "age" at various rates and must be evaluated on a case-by-case basis. It is thus important to differentiate patients who have undergone what has been termed "successful aging," meaning an elderly person who has retained most of the physiological functions associated with youth, from elderly patients who have undergone "accelerated aging," meaning physiological processes that have deteriorated more rapidly than would be anticipated from the statistical norms.[1]

STRUCTURAL AND MORPHOLOGICAL CHANGES

As a consequence of the aging process, the respiratory system experiences anatomic as well as functional changes that result in a decreased functional reserve. The muscles of respiration lose strength, and chest wall compliance decreases. There is a net increase in small airway closure after the loss of elastic fiber attachments. The resulting increase in functional residual capacity (FRC), which is due to an increase in residual volume (RV), reflects air trapped in peripheral airways. Although RV/TLC increases with age, total lung capacity (TLC) does not routinely change with age; thus, the increased RV comes at the expense of vital capacity (VC).[2] The fall in VC averages 20 ml/year after age 30 years, as is shown in Fig. 2-1. "The aging effect appears to be statistically

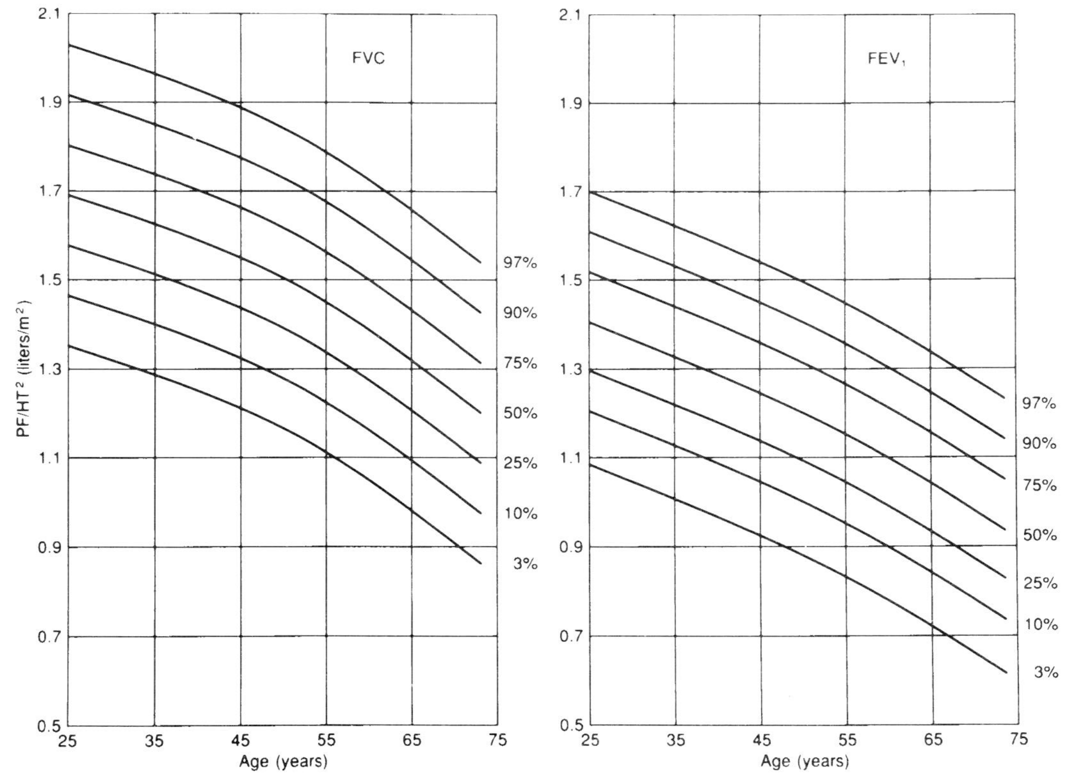

Figure 2-1 Percentile charts for height-standardized pulmonary function of men. The "percentiles" of pulmonary function (liters) divided by height (meters) squared (PF/HT^2) presented here are based on measurements of white nonsmokers who reported no respiratory symptoms and were drawn from a random sample of adults in six U.S. cities. (*Reprinted with permission from Tockman MS: Aging of the respiratory system, in Hazzard WR, Andes R, Bierman EL, Blass JP (eds): Principles of Geriatric Medicine and Gerontology, 2d ed. New York: McGraw-Hill, 1990, pp 499–508.*)

significant and inexorable but yet not very profound."[3] Figure 2-2 shows the changes in the component lung volumes that can be observed at different ages.

Mechanical Function

In general, aging adversely affects the speed and strength of muscle contraction. The respiratory muscles are affected, along with other muscle groups, perhaps by as much as 35 percent by age 70 years. Both inspiratory effort and expiratory maximal effort are significantly decreased. For example, the phenomenon of postobstructive negative-pressure pulmonary edema is almost unknown in the geriatric population but is a concern in the younger population. Intrinsic contributing factors may include a general reduction in muscle mass, a selective decrease in type 2 fibers, and a loss of high-energy phosphate storage capacity. Skeletal factors may contribute. Rib attachment cartilages may stiffen and reduce or restrict rib motion, requiring greater effort to effect the same degree of chest wall motion.[4] The flattening of the diaphragm with hyperinflation reduces the mechanical advantage of that muscle, forcing it to

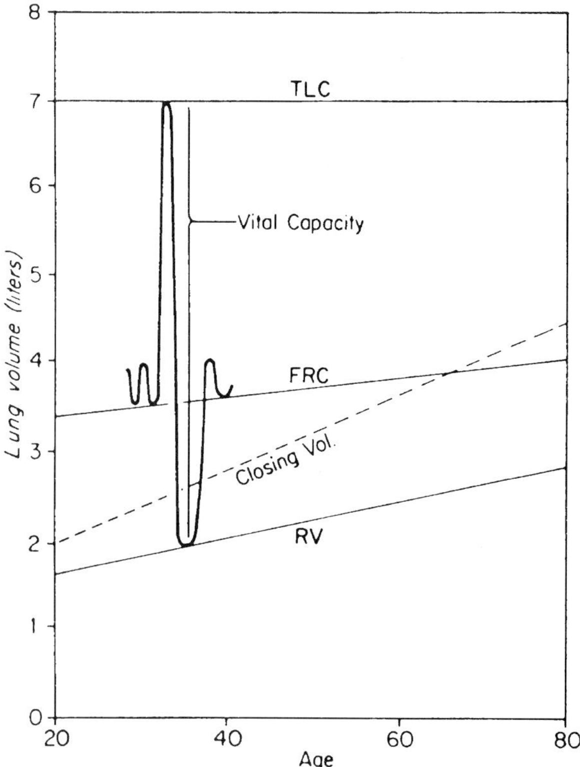

Figure 2-2 The effect of age on the subdivision of lung volume: Values shown are for men of average height; the changes with age are similar for women. TLC = total lung capacity; FRC = functional residual capacity; RV = residual volume.

work harder to achieve the same degree of negative intrathoracic pressure. These alterations in the mechanical ability of the patient are rarely important at rest but significantly decrease the reserve needed to overcome stress. The most common impairment is an inability to generate an effective cough. This places the patient at increased risk of developing atelectasis and pneumonia, particularly in the postoperative period.

Lung Parenchyma

The excised senile lung is characterized by a homogeneous enlargement of the alveolar airspace without fibrosis or destruction of the walls. Membranous bronchioles become slightly dilated and reduced in number. Studies of the functional characteristics of excised senile lungs show an increase in minimal air and a shift to the left of the elastic recoil pressure-volume curves. This is similar to, but much less pronounced than in, emphysematous lungs. (Minimal air is the volume of air remaining in an isolated lung preparation that is allowed to collapse spontaneously. It is roughly analogous to RV except that it is measured in a cadaveric lung preparation.) Maximum expiratory volumes and flows are normal. It is speculated that airspace enlargement may be responsible for changes in elasticity. The senile lung represents isolated airspace enlargement, which is a prodrome to further damage caused by emphysema. The functional abnormalities of incipient emphysema, whether centrilobular or panacinar, are identical to the functional changes associated with the senile lung. The common abnormality is an enlargement of the airspaces, which probably precedes emphysema. The enlargement of the airspaces may be responsible for the decrease in static recoil pressure and the increase in minimal air found in the senile lung. The increase in residual air is attributed to the decreases in lung elasticity. Similarly, other research indexes of lung function show similar changes. Verbeken and associates demonstrated a simultaneous increase in Lm (mean linear intercept), a decrease in Pst(1), and an increase in RV as characteristic of normal aging.[5]

Histologically, the alveolar ducts dilate, intraalveolar septa are lost, the total number of alveoli decreases, and the total lung surface area is decreased. These changes are often termed emphysematous in nature. In contrast to panacinar emphysema (PAE), senile lungs are characterized by a regular airspace enlargement, the absence of inflammatory and fibrotic lesions, and small airway disease limited to membranous bronchioles; such small airways are enlarged from the normal <0.2 mm to approximately 0.4 mm in size.[6]

The elastic fibers within the alveolar walls, which are critical for the maintenance of airway patency, are tethered to the respiratory and terminal bronchioles. Thus, they help maintain the patency of those small conducting airways at low lung volumes.[7] There is no evidence supporting a change in the length or diameter of these fibers in association with aging; instead, there is a disruption of the fiber attachments.[8] The physiological result is an increase in the compliance of the affected alveoli and a collapse of small conduction airways, producing higher closing volumes, nonuniform alveolar ventilation, and air trapping. This explains the progressive increase in RV which is taken from the VC. It also explains why closing capacity (closing volume plus RV) increases at a more rapid rate than does RV alone.

The loss of inward elastic recoil seen with increasing age, especially after age 55, is usually evenly matched by a reduction of respiratory muscle strength and increased rib stiffness, resulting in a lack of change in TLC and a minimal increase in FRC.[4]

FUNCTIONAL AND PHYSIOLOGICAL CHANGES

Clearly the lung experiences a loss of elastic recoil as a consequence of aging. This loss is much more significant at higher lung volumes and is not as noticeable at the lower lung volumes associated with resting ventilation. Conversely, maximum expiratory flow diminishes with age only at low lung volumes, suggesting that equal-pressure points (the region of the respiratory bronchiole that collapses at closing volume) are more centrally located at low lung volumes in the elderly.[3] Again, this could be surmised to be due to the loss of collagen and other structural components of the lung. Thus, the collagen fibers are associated with elastic recoil at high inflation states but with maintenance of shape and volume at low lung volumes.

The determination of "normal" aging of lung function is difficult to evaluate and distinguish from pathological disease state function. Green and coworkers[9] examined maximum expiratory flow volume (MEFV) curves by age cohort in 59 adults and noted increasing convexity to the volume axis with advancing age. Their findings were not supported by later studies, which attributed their results to poor selection of the patient population. Knudson and coworkers[3] applied strict criteria to select a "normal aging population." They were able to screen 746 patients for inclusion in their "normal" group. Inclusion required denial of all symptoms of shortness of breath (SOB), cough, and sputum production and a history negative for cardiorespiratory disease or smoking. Workup before the study included 3 years of documented ratio of forced expiratory volume one second to forced vital capacity (FEV_1/FVC) > 75%, a normal vector cardiogram, the MM phenotype for beta-antitrypsin, and a normal chest x-ray. Seventy study patients were enrolled, and 51 successfully completed the study. Eighteen were between the ages of 25 and 35 years, and another 18 were between ages 65 and 75 years. This was a very thorough, well-controlled study. The authors were able to demonstrate the anticipated progressive loss of elastic recoil and an increase in the RV/TLC with advancing age. No changes in TLC and static or dynamic compliance were noted. The loss of elastic recoil with aging is more significant at higher than at lower lung volumes. This is what prompted Knudson to conclude that "the aging effect would seem to be statistically significant and inexorable but yet not very profound."[3]

Another morphological change in the aged lung involves the decreased lymphatic drainage generally thought to be a part of the aging process. Decreasing lymphatic flow and generally decreasing serum oncotic pressure (especially serum albumin) make the elderly more susceptible to the accumulation of interstitial water and frank pulmonary edema, as predicted by the Starling equation. As a result of increasing fragmentation and depolymerization of the interstitial space hyaluronic acid gel that occurs with increasing age, lymphatic drainage is reduced further. This occurs secondary to the impairment of the ability of the interstitial space to decrease its intrinsic oncotic pressure during water accumulation by hydration of highly polymerized hyaluronic acid chains.[10] Elderly patients are therefore postulated to be more susceptible to accumulation of interstitial lung water in the face of the mild increases in hydrostatic pressure caused by the decreased compliance of the pulmonary vasculature.

The function of the lung is to exchange carbon dioxide produced by cellular metabolism for the environmental oxygen necessary to continue that metabolism. The efficiency the lung displays in accomplishing this exchange deteriorates with advancing age as a result of anatomic and physiological degradations, including cardiovascular and neurological components. Regardless of age, minute ventilation is closely tied to arterial carbon dioxide content (Pa_{CO_2}). Physiologically, elderly patients display a marked decrease in the ventilatory and cardiovascular responses to hypercarbia and hypoxemia. Compensatory increases in minute ventilation and heart rate are diminished. Comparing a population 22 to 30 years old with a population 65 to 75 years old, hypoxic ventilatory drive was decreased by 50 percent, and hypercapnic drive by 40 percent.[16] Heart rate response to hypoxia (Pa_{O_2} = 40 mmHg) was a 35 percent increase in the younger group but only a 12 percent increase in the elderly group. Similarly, heart rate increased in response to hypercapnia Pa_{CO_2}(= 55 mmHg) by 15 percent in the younger group but failed to respond to equal levels of hypercapnia in the elderly patients (Fig. 2-3). Table 2-1 summarizes these changes.[16]

Age in some way directly attenuates chemoreceptor function, although the precise defect has not been determined. Virtually all of the peripheral chemoreceptor contribution to hypercapnic ventilatory drive is lost, while considerable hypoxic ventilatory drive is retained. Similarly, it is possible that the diminished heart rate response to hypoxia in older normal men indicates a loss of both baroreceptor and chemoreceptor function with age. The diagnostic clues indicating the onset of hypoxia may be absent. Hypoxia in an elderly patient may not be signaled by either respiratory distress or tachycardia.[11] This makes monitoring the patient more difficult and means that there is less room for error, especially as these patients inherently have a reduced safety margin. Therefore, compared with young adults, elderly patients are less able to defend against acute hypoxia and hypercapnia because of reductions in their mechanical ability to ventilate and their neural drive to breathe. A consequence of this reduction in respiratory response is an increased incidence of physiologically significant but clinically inapparent hypoxemia in elderly patients, particularly in the postoperative period.

The question of how elderly patients respond to an increase in carbon dioxide production generated by exercise or by increased metabolic demands

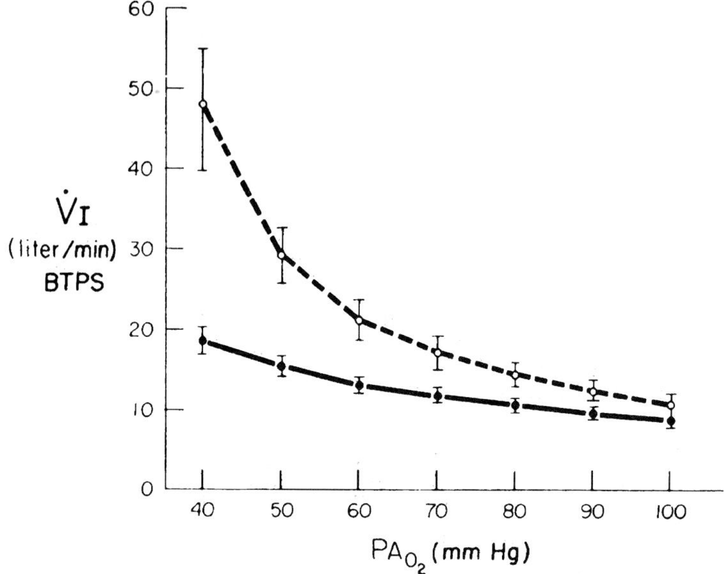

Figure 2-3 Ventilatory response to isocapnic progressive hypoxia in eight young normal men (broken line) and eight normal mean age 64–73 (solid line). Values are means ± SEM. Pa_{CO_2} = 40.9 ± 0.9 in the young men and 39.4 ± 0.7 in the old men. (*Reprinted with permission from Kronenberg RS, Drage CS: Attenuation of the ventilatory and heart rate responses to hypoxia and hypercapnia with aging in normal man. J Clin Invest 52:1812, 1973.*)

Table 2-1 Age-contrasted responses to hypoxemia and hypercapnia

Physiological stimulus	Young adults	Elderly adults
Ventilatory response		
Hypoxemia (Pa_{O_2} 40 torr)*	40 L/min	10 L/min
Hypercapnia†	3.4 L/min	2.0 L/min
Cardiac frequency increase (%)		
Hypoxemia (Pa_{O_2} 55 torr)	34.1	11.5
Hypercapnia (Pa_{CO_2} 55 torr)	15.0	−0.9

* Values given represent the mean level of minute ventilation observed in response to the hypoxic stimulus.

† Values given represent the mean increase in minute ventilation that was observed for each mmHg rise in alveolar P_{CO_2}.

SOURCE: Reprinted from Lefrak SS, Campbell EJ, Lippmann MB: Structure and function of the aging respiratory system, in Stephen CR, Assaf RAE (eds): *Geriatric Anesthesia: Principles and Practice.* Boston: Butterworth, 1986, pp 55–86. By permission of Mayo Foundation.

such as sepsis was addressed in a study designed to examine exercise responses. McConnell and coworkers[12] examined the relation between carbon dioxide sensitivity [at rest (S_R) and during exercise (S_E)] and the ventilatory response to exercise as a function of age. In younger adults during moderate exercise, minute ventilation (V_E) increases linearly with increasing carbon dioxide production (VCO_2). The gradient of this relation has been used as an index of the ventilatory response to exercise ($\Delta V_E/\Delta VCO_2$), with a steep gradient correlating with a large ventilatory response. A more youthful experimental population exhibits a strong positive correlation between $\Delta V_E/\Delta VCO_2$ and S, suggesting that in this age group S plays a role in determining the magnitude of the ventilatory response to exercise. In McConnell's experimental data, the $\Delta V_E/\Delta VCO_2$ of the elderly subjects was greater than that of the younger subjects, confirming earlier data.[13] In addition, S_R was lower for the elderly group than for the younger group. Since there was not the same correlation between $\Delta V_E/\Delta VCO_2$ and S_R, it might be concluded that the sensitivity to carbon dioxide was not a significant controlling factor in the ventilatory response to exercise. However, S_E did not differ significantly between the two groups. There was no correlation between S_E or S_R and $\Delta V_E/\Delta VCO_2$ in the elderly group, supporting the contention that there is a change in the contribution of S to the control of breathing during exercise in the elderly population and making $\Delta V_E/\Delta VCO_2$ an inappropriate index of the ventilatory response to exercise among elderly humans. This remains an area of great interest.

Even if physicians control the mechanical aspects of ventilation, as is routinely done in the operating room and the intensive care unit, the physiology of the lung affects the patient's ability to exchange carbon dioxide for oxygen. There is a progressive age-related decrease in total pulmonary diffusing capacity, usually attributed to both morphological changes (loss of surface area of the alveolar-capillary membrane) and increasing inhomogeneities in ventilation and/or blood flow.[14]

Measurements of pulmonary diffusing capacity show that the single-breath carbon monoxide diffusing capacity (DL_{CO}) increases to a maximum in the early twenties and thereafter undergoes a gradual decline with age, estimated to be approximately 0.5 percent (0.2 ml CO/min per mmHg) per year. This decline is not linear, although linear prediction regressions are used. Similarly, Pa_{CO_2} normally changes with position and age. The formula for determining the expected Pa_{CO_2} for a given inspired oxygen content (FiO_2) in the supine position on room air at sea level is Pa_{CO_2} (torr) $= 103.5 - (0.42 \times \text{age})$. Thus, a 70-year-old patient would be expected to have a Pa_{CO_2} of only 74, even in "a normal healthy state."[15]

Alterations in pulmonary circulation are also very common in the elderly and may significantly affect the gas-exchange processes that occur in the lung. Empirically, a shunt of >20 percent (normal is <5 percent) reflects respiratory failure in a healthy young adult, as this degree of shunt will result in an A-a gradient of >400 torr. In the elderly, given the normal decline in Pa_{CO_2}, a lesser degree of shunt will produce this same A-a gradient.[15]

SEX DIFFERENCES

Many physicians intrinsically expect women to have poorer lung function than do men. The preconception is that women have smaller lungs and weaker musculature than men, and thus less functional reserve is "built into the system." However, it has been determined that individual differences correlate best with height (and thus lung volume) rather than with sex per se or with implications about strength. A regression equation relating lung volume to standing height has been derived: TLC (L) $= -15.183 + [0.12233 \times \text{ht (cm)}]$. An attempt to derive an equation relating TLC (a volume measurement) to the cube of height (cm^3, a volume measurement) yielded the equation TLC $= -1.535 + (0.9342 \times 10^{-5} \times ht^3)$. This plots to a slightly curvilinear function which did not depart significantly from the linear function. Knudson and coworkers[3] postulated that "a relation may exist between lung size, or TLC, and lung recoil at given percent increments of that TLC. It is postulated that lung recoil is dependent on absolute lung size." A subset of their study population consisting of 12 subjects with a TLC between 5 and 5.5 liters showed no differences based on sex in either the ratio of TLC to height or lung elastic recoil. "When sex was excluded as a variable, multiple regression analysis revealed lung elastic recoil to be significantly related first to age and then to TLC, and, to a lesser extent, to height."[3] There do not appear to be sex differences in the bulk elastic properties of the human lung.

Some differences have been documented between males and females. Women have been found to have 10 percent lower diffusion capacity values than men of the same age and height.[14] By contrast, some authors have concluded that senescence usually affects the respiratory system of women to a lesser degree than it affects that of men.[16]

A summary of the changes in the pulmonary system that occur with aging is given in Table 2-2.

DISEASE PROCESSES IN THE ELDERLY

Finding an elderly patient in the operating room who has aged "successfully" is not the rule but the exception. Usually, an elderly patient suffers from a variety of minor or even major organ system derangements. Common pulmonary problems are found with increasing frequency in the elderly, as minor environmental or infectious insults are not handled as efficiently by the elderly lung, secondary to the decrease in functional reserve discussed above.[7] For example, the blunted inflammatory response found in the presence of infection is often a source of missed diagnosis in an aged patient.[7] Similarly, fluctuating respiratory impairment associated with seasonal change, episodic upper respiratory tract infections, and other intercurrent illness require a variety of medical and nonmedical responses to maintain the best possible respiratory status

Table 2-2 Functional divisions of the respiratory system and effects of aging

Division	Components	Function	Effect(s) of aging
Regulation of ventilation	Carotid and aortic bodies, respiratory center (pons and medulla)	Matching of ventilation to metabolic needs	Decreased responsiveness to hypercapnia and hypoxemia
Respiratory bellows	Chest wall, diaphragm, accessory muscles	Provision of mechanical forces for ventilation	Decreased chest wall compliance, decreased muscle strength and efficiency
Conducting airways	All airways from mouth to terminal bronchioles	Gas exchange between alveolar space and environment	Mural calcification, glandular hypertrophy
Lung parenchyma	Gas-exchanging airways, pulmonary capillary bed, interstitial structures	Gas exchange between alveolar space and pulmonary capillary blood	Structural changes resembling emphysema; ventilation-perfusion mismatching, decreasing arterial oxygen tension
Cardiovascular system	Heart and systemic vasculature	Tissue exchange of respiratory gases	Decreased response to hypoxemia, decreased maximal output

SOURCE: Reprinted from Lefrak SS, Campbell EJ, Lippmann MB: Structure and function of the aging respiratory system, in Stephen CR, Assaf RAE (eds): *Geriatric Anesthesia: Principles and Practice*. Boston: Butterworth, 1986, pp 55–86. By permission of Mayo Foundation.

in an elderly patient. All these factors must be evaluated and considered when one is planning anesthesia in an elderly patient.

Chronic lung diseases are frequently found in elderly patients, causing a degradation of respiratory function beyond that caused by age alone. Classic examples of lung diseases found in the elderly include interstitial lung disease, hypersensitivity pneumonitis, pulmonary vascular disease, pulmonary embolism, asthma, chronic obstructive pulmonary disease (COPD), and acute respiratory failure.

Interstitial Lung Disease

Interstitial lung diseases are a heterogeneous group of disorders characterized by inflammation (alveolitis) and destruction of the gas-exchange units (alveoli, capillaries, and small airways) and interstitial fibrosis.[17] Each of these disorders can progress to end-stage lung disease. Determination of history is important in the evaluation of interstitial disease. There are over 100 different types of interstitial lung disease. The most common disorders in the elderly are idiopathic pulmonary fibrosis, interstitial lung disease associated with collagen vascular diseases, sarcoidosis, occupational lung diseases, hypersensitivity pneumonitis, and interstitial lung disease caused by drugs and irradiation. A complete occupational history is important, as is a history of recurrent infections associated with the production of purulent sputum requiring antibiotic therapy. The earliest symptoms are usually nonspecific: fatigue, shortness of breath on exertion, a vague loss of the sense of well-being, and possibly a chronic nonproductive cough. With worsening of the disease, shortness of breath becomes more symptomatic, being noted after even minimal exercise. At the end stage, only lung transplantation is a viable long-term treatment. Patients with symptoms anywhere along this continuum may present for surgery and anesthesia for unrelated diseases or injuries. Determination of the present degree of disease is vital to an appropriate choice of anesthetic management.

Pulmonary function tests are the first step in evaluating chronic lung disease. Table 2-3 shows the effects of aging alone and the addition of interstitial disease on the results of pulmonary function tests. Interstitial lung disease is characterized by decreased lung volumes (TLC, VC, RV, and functional closing capacity), decreased DL_{CO}, and decreased Pa_{O_2}, especially with exercise. The "exercise" resulting in desaturation may simply be postoperative shivering or postoperative fever. As was discussed above, "successful aging" does not normally decrease VC or TLC; nor does Pa_{O_2} worsen with exercise, as is found in interstitial disease. Unfortunately, the patients who most need exercise testing to determine the extent of disease are generally the ones least able to tolerate the insult, while those able to perform the tests generally do not need them.

On x-ray, interstitial disease generally presents as a diffuse infiltrate that is often very nonspecific. These findings frequently correlate poorly with the results of pulmonary function tests or the degree of dyspnea. Periodic x-rays are useful when one is trying to evaluate a patient for congestive heart failure,

Table 2-3 Effect of interstitial lung diseases and aging on pulmonary functions

Pulmonary function*	Interstitial lung disease†	Aging
Lung volumes		
TLC	↓	N
VC	↓	↓
FRC	↓	↑
RV	↓	↑
Spirometry		
FEV_1	↓	↓
FVC	↓	↓
$FEF_{25–75}$	↓	↓
Diffusing capacity	↓	↓
Pa_{O_2}	↓	↓

*TLC, total lung capacity; VC, vital capacity; FRC, functional residual capacity; RV, residual volume; FEV_1, forced expiratory volume in 1 s; FVC, forced vital capacity; $FEF_{25–75}$, forced expiratory flow between 25 and 75 percent of vital capacity; Pa_{O_2} partial pressure of oxygen in arterial blood.

†N = normal; ↓ = decreased; ↑ = increased. Data from normal populations allow an age adjustment on the predicted values for individual patients.

SOURCE: Reprinted with permission from Zehr BP, Hunninghake GW: Interstitial lung disease, hypersensitivity pneumonitis, and pulmonary vascular disease in the elderly, in Hazzard WR, Andes R, Bierman EL, Blass JP (eds): *Principles of Geriatric Medicine and Gerontology*, 2d ed. New York: McGraw-Hill, 1990, pp 538–548.

pleural effusion, or parenchymal infiltrates, which may or may not be related to the underlying interstitial disease. Bronchoalveolar lavage and gallium 67 lung scans, if available, may be useful in further evaluating lung function.

Rheumatoid arthritis is highly associated with interstitial lung disease progression in elderly patients. Airway compromise secondary to involvement of the temporomandibular joint, the arytenoid cartilages, and/or the cervical spine must always be evaluated. Although it is frequently mild in nature, requiring little therapy, rheumatoid arthritis may present as a malignant disease requiring steroid and cytotoxic therapy.[17] Even without another inflammatory disease, chronic therapy for interstitial lung disease often consists of steroid and/or cytotoxic therapy, which must be considered in the formulation of the anesthetic plan. Stress steroid coverage may be required. Additionally, the effects of the cytotoxic agents on other organ systems, particularly the cardiac and renal systems, must be evaluated preoperatively. Corticosteroids administered for interstitial lung disease may significantly aggravate or accelerate the cardiovascular, renal, or joint diseases that coexist in a significant portion of elderly patients. Thus, dyspnea in an elderly patient with a history of interstitial lung disease should not elicit a random initiation of steroid therapy.

Idiopathic pulmonary fibrosis is a diagnosis of exclusion for a chronic lung disease of unknown etiology. The diagnosis often requires open lung biopsy, and treatment consists of corticosteroids.[17]

Table 2-4 Examples of hypersensitivity pneumonitis

Disease	Source of antigen	Antigen
Farmer's lung	Contaminated hay, grain, silage	Thermophilic actinomyces*
Bird-fancier's or pigeon-breeder's lung	Avian excreta	Parrot, pigeon, parakeet, chicken, dove proteins
Bagassosis	Contaminated bagasse (sugar cane)	Thermophilic actinomyces
Mushroom-worker's lung	Mushroom compost	Thermophilic actinomyces, other
Humidifier or air conditioner lung	Contaminated water from humidifiers and air conditioners	Thermophilic antinomyces, *Aureobasidium pullulans*, amoeba, others
Woodworker's lung	Pine and spruce pulp; oak, cedar, mahogany dusts	Wood dust, alternaria
Sauna-taker's lung	Contaminated sauna steam	*A. pullulans*, other
Malt-worker's lung	Moldy barley	*Aspergillus fumigatus*, *Aspergillus clavatus*
Sequoiosis	Redwood sawdust	*Aureobasidium*, *Graphium*
Maple bark-stripper's disease	Maple bark	*Cryptostroma corticale*
Miller's lung	Infested wheat flour	*Sitophilas granarius* (wheat weevil)
Coffee worker's lung	Coffee beans	Coffee bean dust

*Thermophilic actinomyces include *Thermoactinomyces vulgaris*, *T. saccharri*, *T. viridis*, *T. candidus*, and *Micropolyspora faeni*.

SOURCE: Reprinted with permission from Zehr BP, Hunninghake GW: Interstitial lung disease, hypersensitivity pneumonitis, and pulmonary vascular disease in the elderly, in Hazzard WR, Andes R, Bierman EL, Blass JP (eds): *Principles of Geriatric Medicine and Gerontology*, 2d ed. New York: McGraw-Hill, 1990, pp 538–548.

Hypersensitivity Pneumonitis

Hypersensitivity pneumonitis most likely results when a type IV cell-mediated reaction is triggered by small (1–3 μ) organic antigens inhaled into and deposited in the terminal bronchioles or alveoli. It may exist as an acute or a chronic disease but most frequently is characterized as a hypersensitivity response to repeated exposures. The offending agents may be bacteria, fungi, or proteins and may have been first encountered years earlier during occupational exposures or may have resulted more recently from heating or air-conditioning equipment or a pet (especially bird) source. Table 2-4 describes examples of hypersensitivity pneumonitis. In the acute form of the disease, symptoms develop within 4 to 6 h of exposure and consist of dyspnea, cough, fevers, chills, malaise, and myalgia. Removal of the offending agent usually leads to resolution of the symptoms within a day. Elderly patients rarely have this acute form of the disease. The chronic presentation is much more common in geriatric patients and is difficult to distinguish from other forms of interstitial lung disease. Pulmonary function tests (PFTs) will show a classic restrictive lung disease pattern, and chest x-ray will confirm a diffuse interstitial process. Only a careful history allows the differentiation from idiopathic fibrosis. Although precipitating antibodies are present in the vast majority of cases, serological studies have a very low degree of specificity, as a very high false-positive rate exists. Appropriate history, positive serology, characteristic PFTs, and x-rays are combined to make the diagnosis. Severe attacks may require prednisone as well as avoidance of the offending agent. Elective surgery may be best delayed to allow resolution of the acute symptoms. Preoperative inhaled bronchodilator therapy may be useful if surgery is urgent rather than elective.

Pulmonary Vascular Disease

Pulmonary hypertension and pulmonary embolus are two common disease entities that result in pulmonary vascular abnormalities in a significant proportion of the elderly population.

Pulmonary hypertension results from abnormal resistance in the pulmonary vascular tree. Normally, the pulmonary tree autoregulates to maintain systemic pressures below 30 mmHg across a wide variety of cardiac output states by recruiting extra segments of the lung during high-flow states or shutting down underventilated portions of the lung during low-flow states. A number of etiologies may result in a pathological increase in pulmonary artery pressure, broadly classified into congenital cardiac, venous drainage, vascular obliteration, and pathological vascular constriction etiologies. Congenital cardiac causes such as a large ventricular septal defect (VSD), associated with left-to-right shunts and excess pulmonary flow, usually result in pulmonary hypertension at a younger age and will not be discussed further here. Pulmonary venous drainage obstruction historically was associated with mitral stenosis secondary to rheumatic disease but currently is most often a result of left ventricular failure and volume overload. The pulmonary vasculature tree may be reduced in size by embolism, vasculitis, interstitial lung disease, emphysema, or infection (ARDS). Pulmonary artery vasoconstriction may also result in pulmonary hypertension. Hypoxemia is the most clinically relevant, especially in sleep apnea and Pickwickian patients. Clinically, patients present with dyspnea on exertion, angina, hemoptysis or infiltrates, and occasionally hoarseness from recurrent laryngeal nerve damage. Symptoms of right ventricular hypertrophy, dilation, and failure may be present in severe or long-term hypertension. The electrocardiogram (EKG) may show right axis deviation and right ventricular hypertrophy. Right-sided heart catheterization with direct pressure measurements is definitive. As with all medicine, treatment should be directed at the underlying causes, with treatment of symptoms reserved for diagnostic dilemmas.

The most efficacious pulmonary vasodilator is oxygen, which should be applied in any case of hypoxemia. Oxygen therapy has been shown to improve neuropsychiatric symptoms and improve long-term survival.[17] Other pulmonary vasodilators are almost always compromised in their effect by systemic vasodilation. Perhaps inhaled nitric oxide (NO) will be a future pulmonary-specific vasodilator.

Pulmonary Embolism

Pulmonary embolism is another major cause of morbidity and mortality in the geriatric age group, with the failure to consider the diagnosis contributing significantly to the damage. If a patient survives the first hour after a pulmonary embolism and appropriate therapy is instituted, the mortality rate is about 8 percent.[17] In undiagnosed embolus, the mortality rate may approach 30 percent. Three conditions predispose patients to developing venous thrombosis leading to embolism: venous stasis, vascular endothelial injury, and hypercoagulability states. The geriatric age group has a higher incidence of venous stasis because of higher incidences of congestive heart failure, chronic venous insufficiency, and immobility associated with various underlying diseases. Prophylaxis in the geriatric group is therefore more appropriate. While a sudden onset of shortness of breath, anxiety, and pleuritic pain and the presence of a pleural rub are classic presentations of embolism, they occur in only about 20 percent of cases. The most common presentation is unexplained tachypnea and/or shortness of breath. The presentation is nonspecific and may be confused with the symptoms of congestive heart failure, acute myocardial infarction, pneumonia, or atelectasis, making a certain diagnosis very difficult. The only way to eliminate the consideration of a pulmonary embolus is to obtain a negative lung perfusion scan. However, elderly people often have baseline abnormalities of lung perfusion which confuse the issue. A concurrent ventilation scan will show areas of dead space ventilation (ventilation in areas of no perfusion); this is characteristic of an embolus in over 85 percent of angiographically proven pulmonary emboli and frequently is sufficient for instituting therapy. Angiography remains the gold standard for diagnosing pulmonary emboli, especially in cases of recurrent pulmonary emboli or when the risks of empiric therapy are excessive. Therapy usually consists of heparin followed by oral anticoagulation. The newer use of low-molecular-weight heparin may decrease the risks of therapy, especially among the elderly, who are more likely to have medical conditions associated with anticoagulation complications, such as sigmoid polyps. Vena caval occlusion devices (Kimray-Greenfield filter) may be required in patients with recurrent emboli. Patients with massive emboli associated with ventricular failure may require emergent pulmonary embolectomy. The mortality associated with this operation is very high, especially in elderly debilitated patients with little cardiovascular or pulmonary reserve. Therefore, the most cost-effective method is early and effective prophylactic therapy to prevent thromboembolism.

Asthma

Asthma is a disease of smaller airways that is manifested by an increased responsiveness of the bronchiolar smooth muscle layer to environmental stimuli. The reaction may be reversed either spontaneously or with drug therapy. This reactivity is primarily under cholinergic control. Diagnosis depends on the documentation of reversible obstruction that results in air trapping and hyperinflation. Unlike adolescent asthmatics, elderly asthmatics rarely have a specific external stimulus responsible for the disease; thus, the physician is required to rely on drug therapy to increase intracellular levels of cyclic AMP. Beta-sympathomimetic drugs, especially those administered by the inhalational route, represent the vast majority of drug therapeutic regimes, since they have the greatest therapeutic safety margin. Particularly in an elderly patient, the minimal cardiac beta-agonistic side effect of the inhaled drug is important to consider. Inhaled anticholinergics and inhaled steroids usually represent the next level of therapy. Xanthine drugs and systemic steroids are added in difficult cases, although long-term steroid use in elderly patients should be avoided whenever possible because of the possible complications, including accelerated osteoporosis, cataract formation, diabetes, and congestive heart failure.

Chronic Obstructive Pulmonary Disease

Historically, chronic obstructive pulmonary disease (COPD) was used to describe both emphysema and chronic bronchitis, which may present either singly or, more commonly, in combination. Both are caused primarily by prolonged exposure to cigarette smoke and, thus, usually present in late middle age or old age. Smoking contributes to long-term airway disease, as has been clearly shown in a large body of epidemiological research. Smoking is a habit which is usually initiated in the patients' youth, when people don't know better and consider themselves immortal. The "payment" for this foolishness is extracted only after many years in the elderly phase of the patient's life, when the cumulative damage becomes manifest. Heavy smokers almost invariably have a heavy chronic productive cough. A subset population of smokers progresses to anatomic degradation of airway anatomy, resulting in chronic airway obstruction. These patients demonstrate an early decline in the FEV_1 on pulmonary function testing. The loss of function is irreversible, though both the chronic cough and the rate of loss of function usually improve with the cessation of smoking. "It is clear that almost all of those who develop irreversible airway obstruction have been cigarette smokers."[18] The diagnosis of COPD is generally historical, relying on clinical symptoms, characteristic radiographic findings, and appropriately deteriorated pulmonary function test results. COPD is most often a slowly progressive, disabling disease that severely limits the quality of life. Approximately 10 percent of the population of the United States suffers from some degree of COPD. In 1985, approximately 4 million persons had COPD; it was the fifth leading cause of death in the United States and was responsible for 75,000 deaths. Chronic bronchitis is more prevalent but less disabling than emphysema. The ease with which this condition can be detected by spirometry and the observation of slowing of ventilatory deterioration after the cessation of smoking strongly support the clinical recommendation that older smokers be routinely evaluated with this test.[7]

Simple chronic bronchitis is the mildest form of COPD and may be relatively benign, although patients with chronic bronchitis seem to be more susceptible to upper airway infections and exacerbations from environmental exposures. There is no evidence that cough alone is predictive of obstructive disease or early mortality. Airway obstruction may occur to varying degrees as chronic bronchitis progresses, generally presenting with wheezing and dyspnea, especially during acute exacerbations of the disease. Dyspnea is usually first present when the FEV_1 falls to approximately 1.5 liters. Airway narrowing is caused by hypertrophy of the smooth muscle layer and hyperplasia of the mucus-producing glands. When this is added to the normal loss of elastic recoil caused by the aging process, air trapping and V/Q mismatch occur. Blunting of the hypoxic and hypercarbic responses that occur with aging further exacerbates hypoventilation, contributing to the development of hypoxemia, polycythemia, and occasionally cor pulmonale of a primary lung etiology. The loss of elastic recoil and the resultant hyperinflation of the chest make the mechanical work of breathing greater. The respiratory muscles must generate greater negative intrathoracic pressures from a chest wall resting anatomy that is already expanded, destroying most of the mechanical advantage built into the normal anatomic configuration of the chest wall and rib.

Emphysema is a form of COPD associated with destruction of lung acinar units distal to the terminal bronchioles. It frequently copresents with bronchitis. Airway trapping is always present on spirometry, along with increased compliance represented as an increased FRC and RV. Dyspnea is frequently present and may be disabling. If hypoxemia is present, the lowest supplemental oxygen that provides an Sa_{O_2} of 90 (Pa_{O_2} of 65) should be employed to avoid blunting of the hypoxic ventilatory drive.

Respiratory Failure

Acute respiratory failure is defined as a failure of ventilation (elimination of carbon dioxide) or oxygenation. The common causes of acute hypercapnic respiratory failure are listed in Table 2-5. Respiratory failure is more prevalent in the elderly population, which has less of a reserve margin to overcome the degradation in function caused by pneumonia, sepsis, or pulmonary edema. The combination of decreased functional lung reserve and decreases in other organ system functions, particularly cardiac and renal, may make therapeutic interventions more difficult. It is more difficult to drive the oxygen delivery in a septic patient who has COPD, a poor right ventricular ejection fraction, and chronic renal -insufficiency. This is why pneumonia remains a leading cause of death among the elderly population, accounting for nearly 100,000 deaths per year in the United States. However, several studies have shown that contrary to expectations, age alone cannot be documented as being predictive of a poor outcome in critically ill patients and should not be used as a justification for withholding treatment.[18–22]

Table 2-5 Common causes of hypercapnic respiratory failure

1. Factors affecting respiratory control
   a. Primary intracranial disease (tumor, vascular)
   b. Trauma and raised intracranial pressure
   c. Drugs, poisons, and toxins
   d. Central hypoventilation
   e. Excess oxygen administration in hypercapnic patient
2. Neurological and neuromuscular diseases
   a. Spinal cord lesions (trauma, degenerative, vascular)
   b. Acute polyneuritis
   c. Myasthenia gravis
   d. Polymyositis
3. Metabolic derangements
   a. Severe acidosis
   b. Severe alkalosis
   c. Hypokalemia
   d. Hypophosphatemia
   e. Hypomagnesemia
4. Lungs and airway disease
   a. Upper-airway disease (fixed, variable, or sleep-dependent)
   b. Lower-airway disease (COPD, asthma)
5. Musculoskeletal abnormalities
   a. Kyphoscoliosis
   b. Ankylosing spondylitis (rare)
6. Obesity-hypoventilation syndrome

SOURCE: Reprinted with permission from Terry PB: Chronic airways obstruction and respiratory failure, in Hazzard WR, Andes R, Bierman EL, Blass JP (eds): *Principles of Geriatric Medicine and Gerontology*, 2d ed. New York: McGraw-Hill, 1990, pp 526–537.

Elderly patients frequently have chronic neuromuscular conditions, such as parkinsonism, which make them much more likely to suffer acute respiratory failure from an otherwise minor illness or insult. Between the degraded pulmonary function associated with aging and the degraded function accounted for by other pathological conditions, an elderly patient may have little or no margin to overcome an acute insult and may deteriorate rapidly. Severe hypothyroidism, which is often associated with clinical depression and subsequent malnutrition, is a classic example of the kind of subtle disease process which may predispose an elderly patient to an "unexpectedly" rapid collapse from an otherwise relatively benign viral pneumonia. Severe kyphoscoliosis from postmenopausal osteoporosis and vertebral body collapse is another example in which an elderly patient should be expected to have severely compromised lung function and should be subject to rapid pulmonary collapse. These patients may be very difficult to extubate after any general anesthetic.

SUMMARY

Elderly patients frequently present for anesthesia for a variety of reasons. It should be recognized that even under the best possible conditions, when a patient may not have any symptomology of respiratory dysfunction during his or her daily routine, the functional reserve of that patient's pulmonary system has diminished with advancing age. This makes elderly patients more susceptible to respiratory compromise and complications, especially in the postoperative period. More commonly, geriatric patients have concurrent lung pathology that further degrades the function of the pulmonary tree, especially if a significant smoking history is present. These deteriorations in lung function must be considered and monitored during the perioperative period.

REFERENCES

1. Owens WD: *Maturation and the Perioperative Period*, presented at Anesthesia and the Geriatric Patient, Department of Anesthesiology, Washington University School of Medicine, St. Louis, Nov. 13, 1992.
2. Dockery DW, Ware JH, Ferris BG Jr, et al: Distribution of forced expiratory volume in one second and forced vital capacity in healthy, white adult never-smokers in six U.S. cities. *Am Rev Respir Dis* 131:511, 1985.
3. Knudson RJ, Clark DF, Kennedy TC, et al: Effect of aging alone on mechanical properties of the normal adult lung. *J Appl Physiol* 43:1054, 1977.
4. Turner JM, Mead J, Wohl ME: Elasticity of human lungs in relation to age. *J Appl Physiol* 25:664, 1968.
5. Verbeken EK, Cauberghs M, Mertens I, et al: The senile lung: Comparison with normal and enphasematous lungs: I. Structural aspects. *Chest* 101:793, 1992.
6. Verbeken EK, Cauberghs M, Mertens I, et al: The senile lung: Comparison with normal and emphysematous lungs: II. Functional aspects. *Chest* 101:800, 1992.

7. Tockman MS: Aging of the respiratory system, in Hazzard WR, Andes R, Bierman EL, Blass JP (eds): *Principles of Geriatric Medicine and Gerontology*, 2d ed. New York: McGraw-Hill, 1990, pp 499–508.
8. Petty TL, Silvers GW, Stanford RE: Mild emphysema is associated with reduced elastic recoil and increased lung size but not with air-flow limitation. *Am Rev Respir Dis* 136:867, 1987.
9. Green M, Mead J, Hoppin F, Wohl ME: Analysis of the forced expiratory maneuver. *Chest* 36:335, 1973.
10. Demling RH, LaLonde C, Ikegami K: Pulmonary edema: Pathophysiology, methods of measurement, and clinical importance in acute respiratory failure. *New Horizons* 1:371, 1993.
11. Kronenberg RS, Drage CS: Attenuation of the ventilatory and heart rate responses to hypoxia and hypercapnia with aging in normal man. *J Clin Invest* 52:1812, 1973.
12. McConnell KA, Semple EGS, Davies CTM: Ventilatory responses to exercise and carbon dioxide in elderly and younger humans. *Eur J Appl Physiol* 66:332, 1993.
13. Brischetto MJ, Millman RP, Petersen DD, et al: Effect of ageing on ventilatory response to exercise and CO_2. *J Appl Physiol* 56:1143, 1984.
14. Murray JF: *Normal Lung*, 2d ed. Philadelphia: Saunders, 1986, pp 339–360.
15. Demling RH, Knox JB: Basic concepts of lung function and dysfunction: Oxygenation, ventilation and mechanics. *New Horizons* 1:362, 1993.
16. Lefrak SS, Campbell EJ, Lippmann MB: Structure and function of the aging respiratory system, in Stephen CR, Assaf RAE (eds): *Geriatric Anesthesia: Principles and Practice*. Boston: Butterworth, 1986, pp 55–86.
17. Zehr BP, Hunninghake GW: Interstitial lung disease, hypersensitivity pneumonitis, and pulmonary vascular disease in the elderly, in Hazzard WR, Andes R, Bierman EL, Blass JP (eds): *Principles of Geriatric Medicine and Gerontology*, 2d ed. New York: McGraw-Hill, 1990, pp 538–548.
18. Terry PB: Chronic airways obstruction and respiratory failure, in Hazzard WR, Andes R, Bierman EL, Blass JP (eds): *Principles of Geriatric Medicine and Gerontology*, 2d ed. New York: McGraw-Hill, 1990, pp 526–537.
19. Chelluri L, Pinsky MR, Donahoe MP, Grenvik A: Long-term outcome of critically ill patients requiring intensive care. *JAMA* 269:3119, 1993.
20. Cohen IL, Lambrinos J, Fein JA: Mechanical ventilation for the elderly patient in intensive care: Incremental charges and benefits. *JAMA* 269:1025, 1993.
21. Hyers TM: Prediction of survival and mortality in patients with adult respiratory distress syndrome. *New Horizons* 1:466, 1993.
22. Pesau B, Falger S, Berger E, et al.: Influence of age on outcome of mechanically ventilated patients in an intensive care unit. *Crit Care Med* 20:489, 1992.

CHAPTER 3

Physiological Changes in the Cardiovascular System with Advancing Age

Dale E. Solomon

INTRODUCTION

The cardiovascular system faces two sets of challenges as a result of aging. First, the structural and physiological changes seen in the majority of healthy elderly persons result in biological alterations that are considered a normal consequence of aging. In most cases, these changes limit the reserve of the cardiovascular system but allow for adequate function in the nonstressed condition. Second, cardiovascular *diseases* become more prevalent in the elderly population so that it becomes difficult to differentiate the normal process of aging from the pathophysiology associated with anatomic, physiological, or biochemical disease. For instance, at least in western society, elevations in systolic blood pressure (BP) are considered a normal part of aging. At the same time, hypertension, when defined as a disease (i.e., BP > 160/95), becomes much more prevalent in the elderly. At least some of that elevation must be due to the aging process. In fact, because the cardiovascular changes found in young hypertensive patients are so similar to those found in normotensive elderly subjects, the effect of aging on the cardiovascular system has been described as "muted hypertension."[1] Thus, the boundary between normal aging and disease can be indistinct.

Because elderly individuals are affected to different degrees by the aging process and because disease strikes the population focally, patients of advanced age form a very heterogeneous group with regard to basal function, cardiovascular reserve, and disease prevalence. Thus, an individual may range from being "healthy and old," to being an asymptomatic person with occult disease, to being relatively young with significant functional impairment. The clinician's challenge is to determine where on the spectrum an individual patient lies.

In this chapter, alterations in cardiovascular function that appear to be the unavoidable result of the acquisition of years are examined first. Next, the incidence, prevalence, and consequences of acquired cardiovascular disease in the elderly are reviewed.

PHYSIOLOGICAL CHANGES IN NORMAL AGING

The Myocardium

Structural Changes

Aging is associated with an increase in left ventricular (LV) wall thickness, which histologically is seen as myocardial cell hypertrophy and an increase in fibrous tissue, collagen, and lipid deposition between myocytes.[2–4] This ventricular hypertrophy can be seen echocardiographically, with a 30 percent increase in LV wall thickness being demonstrated from the second to the seventh decades of life[5] (Fig. 3-1). Interventricular septal wall thickness increases to a greater degree than does LV free wall thickness.[6] An increase in myocyte size is the major contributor to LV wall thickening; the total number of myocytes is diminished.[7] The great majority of elderly hearts have diffuse fibrosis in the myocardial inter-

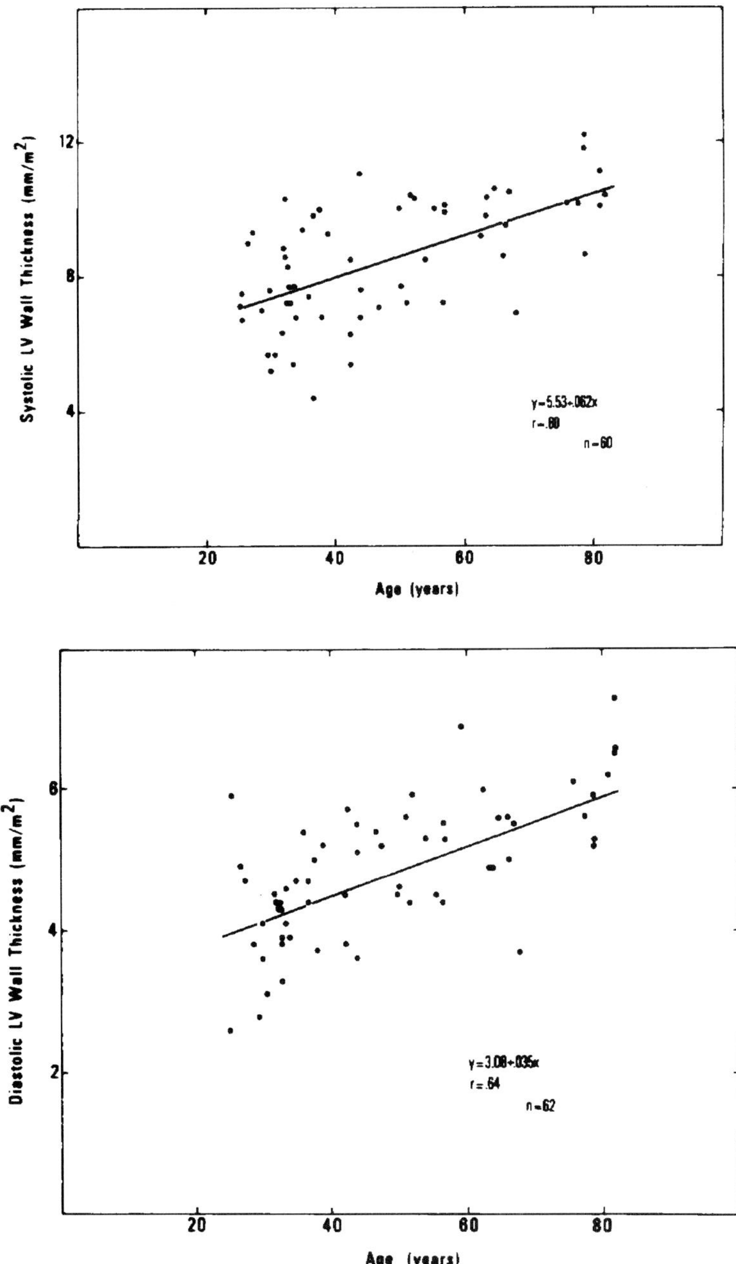

Figure 3-1 The effect of age on left ventricular (LV) posterior wall thickness in systole (*top*) and diastole (*bottom*), normalized for body surface area. (*Reprinted with permission from Gerstenblith G et al: Echocardiographic assessment of a normal adult aging population. Circulation 56:273, 1977.*)

stitium, which microscopically appears to widen the spaces between myocytes.[8] While amyloid deposition occurs in the hearts of nearly half of patients beyond age 70 years,[9] increases in ventricular wall thickness appear to result primarily from myocardial cell hypertrophy in response to systolic hypertension, not from fibrosis, collagen formation, or amyloid deposition.[10,11] Lipofuscin, a granular pigment that is considered to represent oxidized lipid pigments derived from peroxidized mitochondrial membranes, tends to accumulate in the cytoplasm of aging myocytes.[3] This can be seen grossly as "brown atrophy" in aged organs. Ventricular intracavitary end-diastolic and end-systolic volumes are little changed or increased slightly with age.[12,13] The weight of the heart increases 1 to 1.5 g per year between ages 30 and 90, although the hearts of very old persons tend to be of decreased mass either because of the extremely sedentary lifestyle of very old individuals or because an increase in heart mass does not occur in individuals who live to a very old age.[12] In longitudinal studies, the heart size, as determined by chest radiography, increases past age 60; however, a cardiothoracic ratio greater than 0.5 signifies disease. As discussed below, left atrial size increases, probably in response to decreased LV compliance.

Myocardial Function

Diastolic and Systolic Function

Ventricular hypertrophy and interstitial fibrosis result in a loss of diastolic compliance and cause impedance to passive filling of the ventricle during the relaxation phase of the cardiac cycle. In addition, senescent hearts demonstrate a prolongation of the action potential duration and a prolonged isovolumic relaxation time (the time between aortic valve closure and mitral valve opening) that delays diastolic filling (Fig. 3-2). Thus, LV relaxation is slowed and delayed.[14] Diastolic relaxation depends on transport of calcium from the cytoplasm into the sarcoplasmic reticulum and is the most oxygen-consumptive part of the cardiac cycle. Myocardial relaxation may be hindered in the elderly by (1) age-associated decreases in the ability of the sarcoplasmic reticulum to remove cytoplasmic calcium during diastole,[3,15,16] (2) inadequate oxygen delivery caused by decreases in myocardial capillary density and vascular reserve, or (3) impaired oxygen utilization at the mitochondrial level.[3] As a result of these changes, ventricular filling during early diastole declines by approximately 50 percent in the aged, but compensation during later diastole results from an increase in the contribution of atrial contraction to ventricular filling.[16,17] In fact, the contribution of synchronized atrial contraction to total cardiac output may increase from 10 percent in the young to 30 percent or more in the elderly (Fig. 3-3).

Impaired ventricular compliance and altered diastolic relaxation result in elevations in left ventricular end-diastolic pressure (LVEDP) both at rest and during exercise. The aged heart is said to exhibit diastolic dysfunction, a term used to describe a heart which, as opposed to output failure, has "input failure," requiring higher end-diastolic pressures to achieve the same end-diastolic volume and

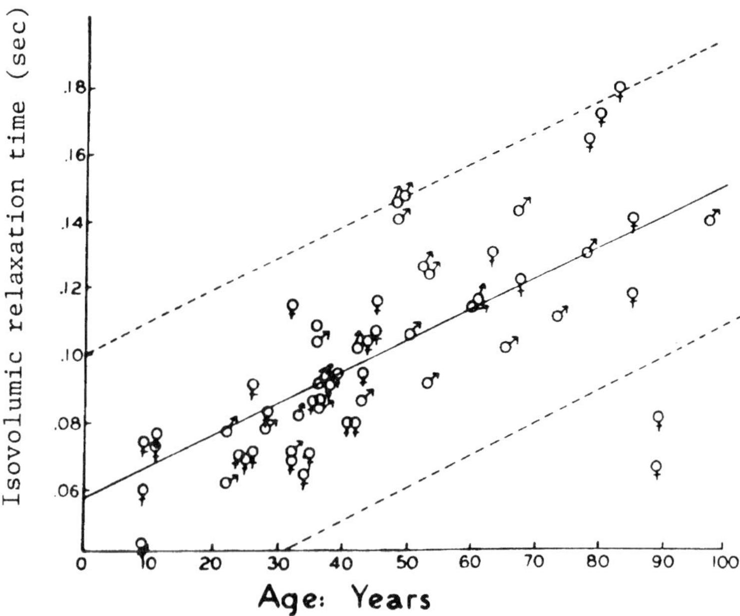

Figure 3-2 The effect of aging on the isovolumic relaxation time of the left ventricle, as measured by kinetocardiographic techniques. (*Reprinted with permission from Harrison TR et al: The relation of age to the duration of contraction, ejection, and relaxation of the normal human heart. Am Heart J 67:189, 1964.*)

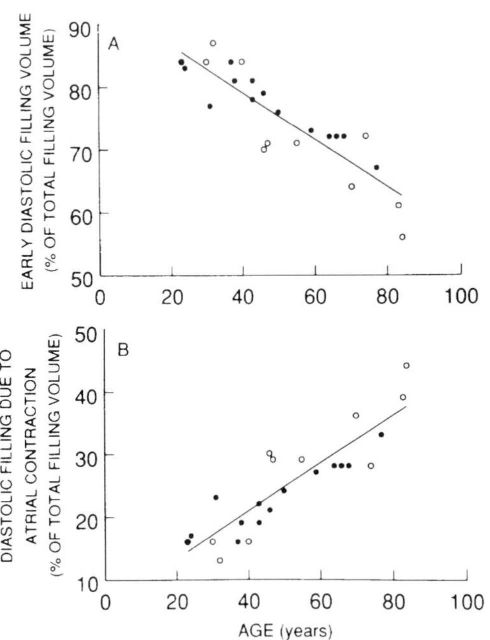

Figure 3-3 The relative contribution of early diastolic filling (*top*) and atrial contraction (*bottom*) to left ventricular filling, as assessed by echocardiographic Doppler technique in healthy men (*solid circles*) and women (*open circles*) ranging from 20 to 80 years of age. (*Reprinted with permission from Geokas MC et al: The aging process. Ann Intern Med 113:455, 1990.*)

stroke volume. Thus, the aged heart is sensitive to increases or decreases in preload; if the LVEDP is too low, the ventricle does not fill optimally and stroke volume is impaired; if it is too high, increases in the pulmonary capillary hydrostatic pressure occur. Diastolic filling is further impaired and cardiac output may fall when diastolic times become shorter as a result of tachycardia. In addition, tachycardia necessitates that left atrial and pulmonary capillary pressures increase to maintain cardiac filling. The impaired ventricular filling and the dependence on synchronized atrial contraction have caused authors to liken the hemodynamics of the aged heart to that of a patient with mitral stenosis.[18] Endurance training,[19] calcium channel blockers,[20] and beta-blockers[21] have been found to enhance the diastolic filling of the left ventricle in the elderly.

In the absence of disease, systolic ventricular function is maintained or only slightly impaired in the elderly.[11,12] The left ventricular stroke work index, the product of stroke volume and mean arterial pressure, is increased in elderly men.[12] Maximal generation of tension is maintained in isolated myocardial tissue.[4] Aging does not appear to alter contractility when measured as the ratio of end-systolic pressure to end-systolic volume, an index of preload/afterload-independent contractility.[12] Some studies have found that decreases in left ventricular ejection fraction (LVEF) and increases in left ventricular end-systolic volume (LVESV) are associated with aging, but these results may be due to the vascular changes associated with aging rather than to a decrease in systolic contractile function.[2] At rest, pulmonary artery pressures and pulmonary capillary wedge pressures are unchanged or slightly elevated in the healthy old.[13,22]

Cardiac Output

While isolated cardiac muscle shows no age-associated decrement in function,[4] many human clinical studies have reported a steady decline in cardiac output (CO) from the third decade of life onward.[23–26] For example, in 1955 the Evan blue dye dilution technique was used to measure resting CO in 67 male subjects between the ages of 19 and 86 years. These subjects were screened for cardiac disease by clinical history, physical examination, electrocardiogram (ECG), chest radiograph, and measurement of venous pressure. The resting CO was found to decline about 1 percent per year past the age of 30 years.[27] In a more recent study, the sample population was screened for the presence of occult cardiac disease by thallium exercise stress testing; resting CO was found to be maintained in elderly patients.[28] The current consensus is that resting CO tends to decrease slightly with age,[3] but this decline is due to factors other than decline in pump function, such as changes in preload, afterload, metabolic demand, and neurohumoral regulation.[29]

Exercise Response

The CO response to exercise in the elderly is generally thought to be diminished compared with that in the younger population,[3,23–25] although some studies indicate that CO is maintained in older individuals who are screened for occult cardiac disease.[28] In response to the increased demand imposed by exercise, the maximum heart rate in an 80-year-old is reduced about 30 percent compared to that in a 20-year-old. To increase CO in response to exercise, the stroke volume in the elderly is enhanced by increases in end-diastolic volume, while end-systolic volume increases to a lesser degree, resulting in an increase in stroke volume and ejection fraction (Fig. 3-4). The resultant increase in ejection fraction is less than that in the younger population[2] (Fig. 3-5). For example, during exercise,

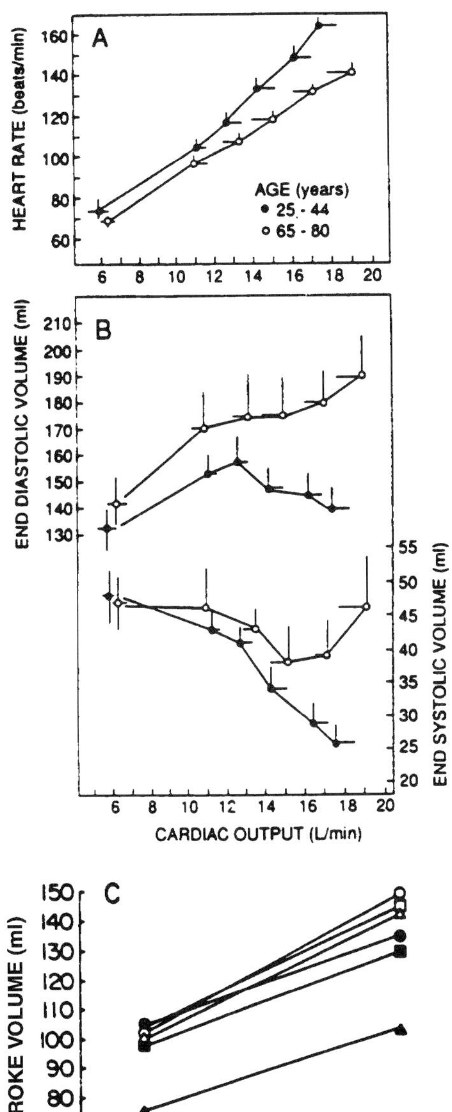

Figure 3-4 The effect of graded exercise on heart rate response (A) and end-diastolic volume/end-systolic volume relations (B) in young (*closed circles*) and elderly (*open circles*) volunteers. During exercise, stroke volume increases to a greater extent in elderly compared with young subjects (C). This is accomplished by an increase in end-diastolic volume, which increases stroke volume through the Frank-Starling mechanism. [*Reprinted with permission from Lakatta EG: Heart and circulation, in Finch C, Schneider E (eds): Handbook of the Biology of Aging, 2d ed. New York, Van Nostrand Reinhold, 1985, p 197; Rodeheffer RJ et al: Exercise cardiac output is maintained with advancing age in healthy human subjects: Cardiac dilatation and increased stroke volume compensate for a diminished heart rate. Circulation 69:203, 1984.*]

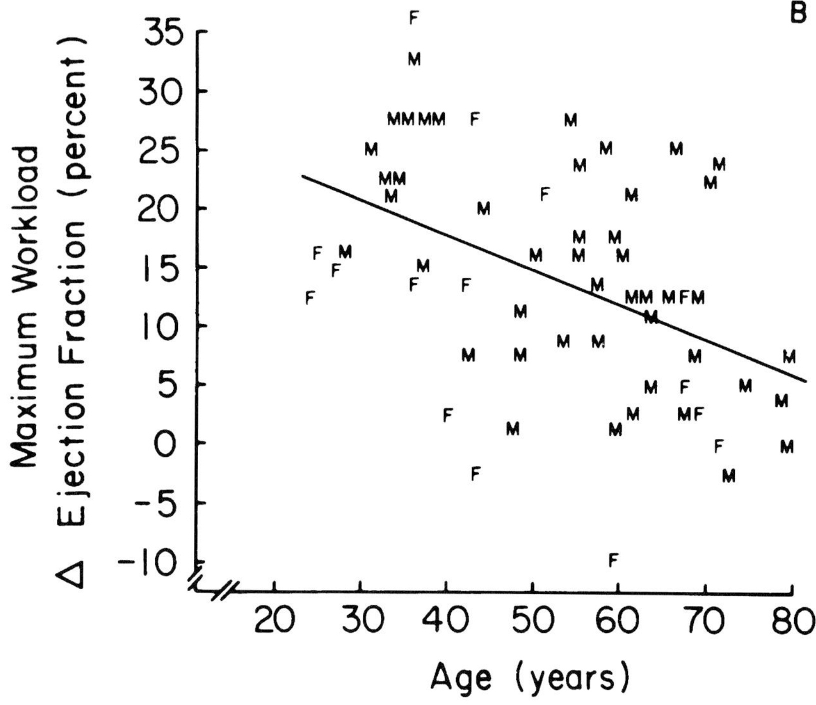

Figure 3-5 Effect of age on the change in ejection fraction from rest to maximum exercise workload. Increases in ejection fraction with exercise diminish with age. (*Reprinted with permission from Rodeheffer RJ et al: Exercise cardiac output is maintained with advancing age in healthy human subjects: Cardiac dilatation and increased stroke volume compensate for a diminished heart rate. Circulation 69:203, 1984.*)

a CO of 15 liters/min is achieved at a heart rate of 135 beats per minute (bpm) and a stroke volume of 115 ml in the young and by a heart rate of 115 bpm and a stroke volume of 135 ml in the elderly.[31] Thus, exercise-induced increases in CO rely more on the Frank-Starling mechanism than on catecholamine-induced increases in heart rate and contractility, as seen in the young.[32]

Maximal oxygen consumption (VO_2) during exercise is reduced in the elderly by about 10 percent per decade between ages 30 and 70. This may be partly due to increases in LVEDP that result in exercise-induced dyspnea at a relatively low workload but also may be caused by age-related decreases in limb/trunk muscle mass, since VO_2 occurs almost exclusively in those muscles during exercise.[2,33] Most of the diminution in VO_2 seen in the elderly can be traced to diminished muscle mass. However, some of the decreased VO_2 may be due to the fact that the elderly have a reduction in the maximal arteriovenous oxygen difference during exercise. Intensive physical training in elderly persons can enhance left ventricular performance and VO_2 max during exercise.[34] Exercise-induced increases in LVEF in trained elderly persons can approach those found in the younger population.

Cardiovascular Homeostatic Mechanisms

Part of the diminished cardiac response to exercise in the elderly appears to result from a down regulation of the cardiovascular response to catecholamines.[35,36] Young persons whose beta-adrenergic receptors are pharmacologically blocked demonstrate cardiovascular responses to exercise very similar to those seen in the elderly.[12] However, compared with the young, elderly persons have elevated serum concentrations of circulating epinephrine and norepinephrine both at rest and with exercise; thus, the slower exercise heart rate and reduced contractility in the elderly imply decreased responsiveness to catecholamines.[37] Indeed, decreased responses in heart rate and contractility to isoproterenol, terbutaline, and norepinephrine have been reported in the senescent heart[4,31,38] (Fig. 3-6). Interestingly, pacemaker-induced heart rates are not decreased in the elderly.

The exact biochemical mechanism responsible for decreased beta-adrenergic sensitivity in the elderly remains elusive. Beta-adrenergic receptor density appears to be maintained, while affinity for agonists has been reported to decline.[12,35] Decreased beta-adrenergic responsiveness might also be explained by a defect distal to protein kinase activation in the pathway to intracellular calcium release.[12] The contractile response of isolated cardiac muscle to increases in cytoplasmic calcium is well maintained.[39]

Even though serum catecholamine concentrations are elevated in the elderly, reduced beta-adrenergic responsiveness prevents an age-related increase in the resting heart rate. In fact, some studies have demonstrated a progressive decline in the resting rate with aging.[40] The intrinsic heart rate—the spontaneous rate of the sinoatrial (SA) node in the presence of autonomic blockade—is slower in the elderly, being reduced from 104 bpm at age 20 to 92 bpm by the fifth decade of life.

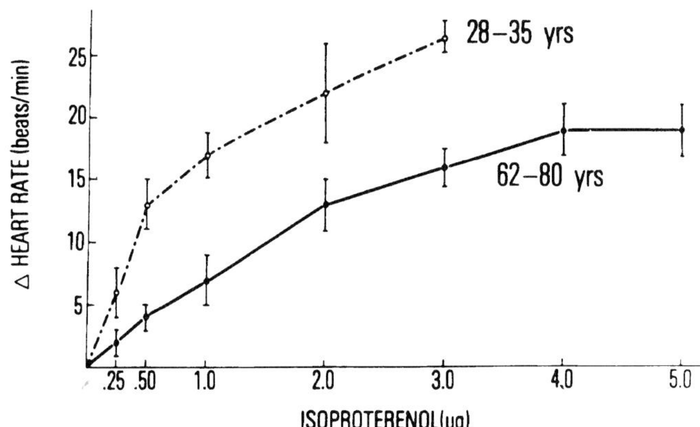

Figure 3-6 The effect of isoproterenol on heart rate in young (*open circles*) and elderly (*closed circles*) subjects. (*Reprinted with permission from Lakatta EG: Alterations in the cardiovascular system that occur in advanced age. Fed Proc 38:163, 1979.*)

Perhaps partially as a result of decreased beta-adrenergic sensitivity, cardiovascular autonomic reflexes are impaired in the elderly. For instance, baroreceptor reflex function declines despite the demonstration of maintained vascular responsiveness to alpha-adrenergic stimulation and increased serum concentrations of norepinephrine in response to a postural challenge.[31,41,42] Reduced baroreflex function entails a diminished cardiovascular response to hypotension, and postural hypotension is common among the elderly.[43] Cardiovascular homeostatic responses to hypotensive drugs are also blunted.[31] For instance, there is less tachycardia in response to the hypotension created by sodium nitroprusside, and cardiodepressant anesthetic drugs produce a greater hypotensive effect in the elderly. Interestingly, there appears to be a decreased incidence of presyncopal episodes resulting from experimentally induced postural tilt, perhaps because of diminished parasympathetic tone in the elderly.[44]

Activation of the renin-angiotensin system in response to posture and hypovolemia is diminished in the elderly,[45] who are more sensitive to increases or decreases in total body sodium. The cardiovascular response to hypoxia and hypercarbia is diminished. Finally, vagal control of the heart is also lessened. There is a dampened response to the Valsalva maneuver and less prominent sinus arrhythmia associated with normal respiration. The effect of more loosely regulated cardiovascular homeostasis is that an aged person responds more slowly and less effectively to perturbations caused by changes in body position, blood volume, venous return, afterload, and pharmacologic agents.

The Cardiac Conduction System

The aging heart is prone to senescent changes that cause alterations in cardiac rate and rhythm. The conduction system is prone to primary degeneration, ischemic injury, calcification, and fibrosis.[46] The sinus node loses 80 percent of its pacing cells by age 75 and becomes infiltrated with fat and/or collagen. Similarly, the atrioventricular node is prone to cell loss and replacement fibrosis. In the area of the division of the bundle of His into the left and right bundle branches, extensive degeneration and fibrosis have been described. This may lead to a leftward axis deviation in old age and the eventual development of left bundle branch block. The density of distal conducting fibers decreases with age.[3] Changes in the conduction system are reflected on the ECG in the form of PR interval prolongation, decreased QRS and T wave amplitude, leftward axis of the QRS, prolonged QT intervals, and ST-T wave changes.[2] The diminution of QRS voltage probably represents lung hyperinflation and thoracic spinal kyphosis.

The Vascular System

Arterial changes associated with aging become evident by the third decade of life, although atherosclerosis is demonstrable in the western population much earlier. As most arterial changes start proximally, the aorta is the first to be affected by the changes of aging. By the third decade of life, elastic fibers in the aorta begin decreasing in number and changing in histological appearance, becoming fragmented, split, and frayed.[47] Extensive calcific deposits become apparent. The collagen fiber content increases, while muscle fiber content in the tunica media diminishes. Proliferation of ground substance (acid mucopolysaccharide) replaces lost elastic fibers and degenerated smooth muscle cells. As a consequence of a loss of elastic fibers and smooth muscle and an increase in ground substance, collagen, and calcium, the aorta becomes less distensible. It becomes unable to absorb and store the energy of the volume of blood ejected by the left ventricle, a function that normally diminishes systolic arterial pressure and ventricular impedance while maintaining diastolic blood pressure. Aortic dilatation occurs along with lengthening of the aorta; the internal radius of the aorta increases by 9 percent per decade from age 20 to age 60.[48] Further increases in ventricular impedance occur as a consequence of aortic enlargement, since the mass of blood in the aorta is increased. Systolic hypertension among the elderly is thought to result from these aortic changes, which serve as an impedance to ventricular ejection.[2] The increased impedance to ejection increases LV wall tension and leads to ventricular hypertrophy, which tends to lower wall tension according to the formula of Laplace. Table 3-1 summarizes structural and physiological changes in aging arterial vasculature. Figure 3-7 demonstrates the effect of arterial changes on cardiac function.

Age-related changes in small vessels may also contribute to hypertension in the elderly. Within the media of small vessels, hyaline degeneration occurs with a resultant decrease in the overall cross-sectional area of the lumen. Total peripheral vascular resistance consequently increases.[49] In addition, an increase in ground substance in small capillaries may form a barrier to oxygen diffusion from blood to metabolic tissue, diminishing oxygen consumption at the same level of oxygen delivery.[50]

Decreased beta-receptor responsiveness in the peripheral circulation contributes to increases in systemic vascular resistance because beta-mediated vasodilation is diminished. The following seemingly compensatory mechanisms fail to normalize blood pressure in the elderly: (1) depressed renin-angiotensin

Table 3-1 Arterial changes associated with aging

Structural
Dilatation of aorta and large arteries
Increased arterial wall thickness
Increased collagen and calcium
Decreased smooth muscle
Functional
Increased arterial stiffness and wall tension
Increased left ventricular impedance and total peripheral vascular resistance
Increased systolic and mean arterial pressure
Increased systolic pressure-time index

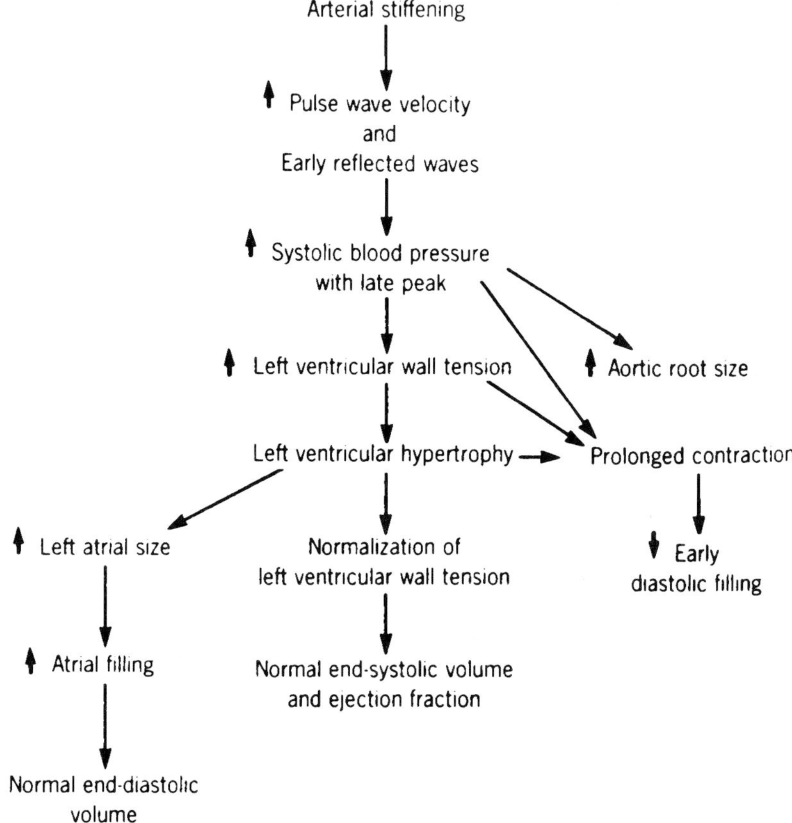

Figure 3-7 The relations of arterial vascular changes and adaptive cardiovascular responses in the healthy old. (***Reprinted with permission from Lakatta EG: Normal changes in aging. Merck Man Geriatr 28:310, 1990.***)

activity, (2) diminished levels of vasopressin, (3) increased levels of atrial natriuretic hormone,[51] and (4) decreased beta-adrenergic sensitivity. Despite the assertion that systolic hypertension is a natural consequence of aging, some primitive societies do not demonstrate this change, and it has been argued that systolic hypertension in western society is due to dietary factors, particularly a high sodium load.[1]

Loss of arterial compliance causes the elderly to be susceptible to hypovolemia: Decreases in preload and thus stroke volume lead to hypotension. In fact, splanchnic pooling of blood after a large meal can cause hypotension and syncope in the elderly. Table 3-2 presents a synopsis of the cardiovascular changes associated with normal aging.

To summarize the cardiovascular changes normally associated with aging: (1) Aortic vascular changes cause systolic hypertension and LV hypertrophy, (2) myocardial senescence, LV hypertrophy, and changes in the biochemistry of excitation-contraction-relaxation cause reduced ventricular compliance and

Table 3-2 Summary of functional cardiovascular changes in the elderly compared with the young

Parameter	Change
Resting heart rate	No change or decreased
Intrinsic heart rate (autonomic blockade)	Decreased
Maximum heart rate	Decreased
Resting cardiac index	No change or decreased
Maximum cardiac index	Decreased
LVEF (resting)	No change or decreased
LVEF (exercise)	Decreased
Stroke volume (resting)	No change or decreased
Stroke volume (exercise)	Increased
Impedance to LV ejection	Increased
Peripheral vascular resistance	Increased
Systolic blood pressure	Increased
Diastolic blood pressure	No change

impaired diastolic filling of the heart, (3) resting cardiac output is maintained or slightly decreased while exercise-induced increases in CO are diminished compared with young persons, (4) increases in CO depend more on Frank-Starling mechanics rather than on catecholamine-induced increases in heart rate or contractility, (5) cardiac and vascular responses to beta-adrenergic stimulation are decreased, (6) the resting heart rate is unchanged or decreased, (7) maximal oxygen consumption is reduced, and (8) cardiovascular homeostatic mechanisms are impaired.

CARDIOVASCULAR DISEASE IN THE ELDERLY

Disease processes that affect the cardiovascular system are more prevalent and severe in the aged population. Some diseases occur so frequently that it becomes difficult to distinguish disease from normal aging. For instance, atherosclerosis of the proximal arterial system is so prevalent that it might be considered a normal consequence of aging, yet atherosclerosis is certainly the cause of the majority of cardiovascular morbidity and mortality among the elderly. Also, it is important to delineate the effect of lifestyle and risk factors on the genesis of cardiovascular disease. For example, hypertension, elevated blood lipids, male sex, glucose intolerance, smoking history, abdominal obesity, and a sedentary lifestyle may all contribute to the accelerated development of coronary artery disease. Also, cardiovascular deconditioning may limit the response to hemodynamic stressors. In this section, the prevalence and clinical consequences of the major cardiovascular diseases found in the elderly are examined.

Coronary Artery Disease

Autopsy studies have revealed that about 60 percent of all men have a 75 to 100 percent stenosis of at least one major coronary artery by the sixth decade of life[7] (Fig. 3-8). In at least half these individuals, the disease is occult and silent ischemia appears to account for up to 90 percent of all episodes of myocardial ischemia.[52] The elderly appear to have a greater incidence of silent myocardial ischemia than do the young, perhaps as a result of altered pain transmission or perception, making diagnosis by history more difficult.[53–56] At the same time, patients with silent ischemia appear to be at higher risk for adverse cardiovascular events than are those without it.[57] While men are traditionally thought to be at higher risk for coronary artery disease (CAD), the incidence of myocardial infarction equalizes between men and women by age 70.[58]

The identification of CAD in a surgical patient is important because the presence of perioperative myocardial ischemia can predict adverse perioperative cardiovascular events. Ischemic heart disease resulting from CAD manifests as angina pectoris, myocardial infarction, congestive heart failure, valvular dysfunction, and cardiac arrhythmias. The mortality rate from any of these sequelae is higher for the elderly.[59]

Treatment of CAD and ischemic heart disease in the elderly is essentially the same as in the younger population: (1) modification of risk factors, including hypertension, blood lipids, smoking, and sedentary lifestyle, (2) nitrates, (3) beta-adrenergic blockade, (4) calcium-entry blocking agents, (5) antiplatelet agents (aspirin), and (6) invasive intervention (angioplasty, coronary artery bypass grafting).

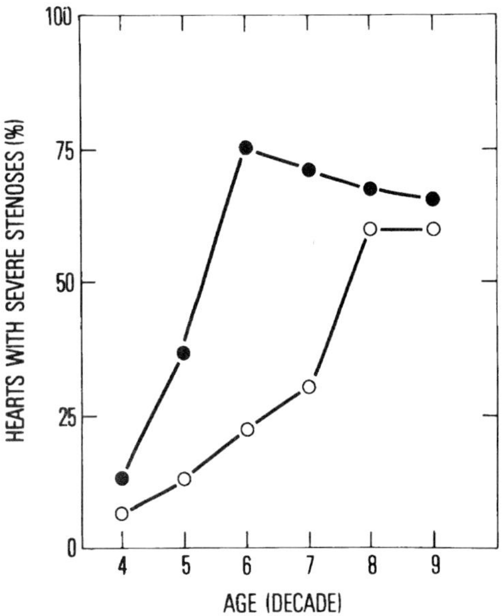

Figure 3-8 **The age-associated prevalence of significant coronary artery disease in men (*closed circles*) and women (*open circles*). By age 70, the prevalence of severe CAD in women equalizes that in men. (*Reprinted with permission from Fleg JL: Alterations in cardiovascular structure and function with advancing age. Am J Cardiol 57:33C, 1986.*)**

Hypertension

As was mentioned above, hypertension develops in the elderly because of (1) reduced aortic compliance, allowing a steeper pressure rise per unit of stroke volume, (2) an increase in peripheral vascular resistance, (3) loss of beta-mediated vasodilation with maintenance of alpha-mediated vasoconstriction, (4) decreased baroreceptor sensitivity, and (5) elevated serum catecholamines.

About 30 percent of the elderly have hypertension, defined as a BP > 160/95, and another 10 to 15 percent have isolated systolic hypertension, with a systolic BP > 160 and a diastolic BP < 90. Isolated systolic hypertension (ISH) accounts for at least 50 percent of the hypertension diagnosed after age 65 and continues to account for a greater percentage of the total into the ninth decade of life.[59] Both types of hypertension pose a risk for the development of ischemic heart disease, congestive heart failure, stroke, aortic disease, and (in association with LVH) arrhythmias and sudden death. BP reduction in hypertensive patients lowers the incidence of these complications.[60] BP reduction in patients with ISH has also recently been found to reduce the cardiovascular complication rate.[61,62] Nonfatal stroke, myocardial infarction, and congestive heart failure are reduced by active treatment of isolated systolic hypertension. The current recommendation of the Joint National Committee on Detection, Evaluation and Treatment of high blood pressure is that ISH in the elderly be treated.[39] Treatment of hypertension in the elderly may consist of (1) nonpharmacologic therapy, including salt restriction, weight loss, exercise, and decreased alcohol intake, or (2) drug therapy, including diuretics, beta blockers, angiotensin-converting enzyme (ACE) inhibitors, Ca^{2+}-entry blockers, central alpha-adrenergic agents, and nitrates. Since the SHEP trial demonstrated decreased cardiovascular morbidity when isolated systolic hypertension was treated with diuretics, diuretics remain the first line choice for ISH.[63] As the negative effects of diuretics on the lipid profile become better elucidated and with knowledge of the relative insensitivity of the aged heart to beta stimulation, vasodilating antihypertensive drugs are gaining favor over both diuretics and beta blockers for the treatment of hypertension.[39]

Congestive Heart Failure

About 8 in 1000 men age 65 to 74 develop congestive heart failure (CHF), a rate four times that in the previous decade of life. CHF is the most frequent hospital discharge diagnosis for patients over age 65; about 2 percent of the elderly population is hospitalized each year for CHF. About 10 percent of patients over age 75 demonstrate significant impairment of LV function.[65] After the diagnosis of CHF is made, about a 50 percent 5-year survival can be predicted.[66]

The normal process of aging predisposes elderly patients to CHF as a consequence of diastolic dysfunction, the result of reduced LV compliance and diastolic relaxation.[67] About one-half of all episodes of CHF in patients above 80 years old occur in those with normal or nearly normal systolic function.[68] In addition, systolic ventricular dysfunction can result from ischemic heart disease, hypertension, valvular heart disease, or cardiomyopathy. Overt CHF almost always occurs in the presence of hypertensive and/or ischemic heart disease or as a result of abnormal physiological stressors and cannot be said to be a normal consequence of aging.

CHF is difficult to diagnosis in the elderly: Ankle edema, pulmonary rales, enlarged heart size, and exercise intolerance may all be due to the normal process of aging, failure of other organ systems, or drug effects.[59] Differentiation of diastolic from systolic dysfunction is important because the therapy is different. With systolic dysfunction, the onset of symptoms is gradual with a progressive rate of decline. Enlargement of the heart occurs with decreases in systolic function demonstrated by echocardiography, MUGA, or cardiac catheterization. In contrast, diastolic dysfunction often presents abruptly with a rapid rate of decline caused by (1) increased CO demand (fever, surgery, trauma, thyrotoxicosis), (2) increased blood volume (fluid, sodium, blood transfusion), or (3) the impairment of diastolic filling (tachycardia, ischemia). Ventricular dilatation and peripheral edema are rare in CHF caused by diastolic dysfunction, and estimates of ventricular contractility are normal or nearly normal.[3] Doppler two-dimensional echocardiography can quantitate the decreased peak mitral valve flow velocity associated with diastolic dysfunction.

Diuretics, digitalis, vasodilators, and inotropic agents remain the therapy of choice for CHF caused by systolic dysfunction. For diastolic dysfunction, however, therapy is aimed at maintaining preload while enhancing ventricular relaxation and diastolic filling. To this end, beta blockers, calcium channel blockers, and ACE inhibitors are indicated. Because some symptoms of dyspnea may result from elevated right-sided heart pressures, judicious volume contraction may sometimes be beneficial. In addition, because of the reliance of ventricular filling on synchronized atrial contraction, atrial fibrillation should be treated aggressively. Table 3-3 summarizes the differentiation and management of CHF caused by systolic versus diastolic ventricular dysfunction.

Cardiac Arrhythmias

With aging, there is a progressive loss of functional cells in the sinus and atrioventricular (AV) nodes as well as cellular degeneration and fibrosis in the bundle branches and the more distal conducting system. Increased circulating serum levels of norepinephrine in the elderly may contribute to arrhythmogenesis.[66] In addition, a variety of disease states contribute to the genesis of arrhythmias, such as (1) ischemic heart disease, including myocardial infarction, (2) congestive heart failure, especially dilated cardiomyopathy, (3) left ventricular hypertrophy associated with hypertension or valvular heart disease, (4) electrolyte abnormalities resulting from renal disease or drug effects, (5) atrial enlargement caused by pulmonary disease or decreased ventricular compliance, (6) anemia, and (7) thyroid disease.[69]

Table 3-3 Differentiation and management of heart failure in the elderly

	Diastolic dysfunction	Systolic dysfunction
Onset	Abrupt	Gradual
Peripheral edema	Uncommon	Frequent
Third heart sound	Uncommon	Present
Enlarged left ventricle	Rare	Frequent
Measured ejection fraction	Normal or slightly decreased	Decreased
Treatment		
Digoxin	No	OK
Diuretics	Low dose	Higher dose
ACE inhibitors	Maybe	Yes
Calcium blockers	Probably	No
Beta blockers	Maybe	No
Nitrates	To treat ischemia	To decrease preload

Numerous studies have documented an increased incidence of arrhythmias and conduction defects in the elderly. For example, while ambulatory ECG monitoring has documented ventricular arrhythmias in about 50 percent of all adults, this prevalence increases to 80 percent in normal elderly persons age 60 to 85 years. Only about 5 percent of normal individuals, however, have frequent or complex ventricular arrhythmias.[70] The incidence of asymptomatic ventricular tachycardia during exercise testing in asymptomatic volunteers over age 65 has been reported to be 4 percent.[71] Five to 10 percent of men over 70 years old have chronic or paroxysmal atrial fibrillation, atrial flutter, or multifocal atrial tachycardia, and one study reported a 17 percent incidence of atrial fibrillation by age 80.[72]

Bundle branch block occurs in about 5 to 10 percent of the elderly, and is usually due to fibrosis of the conduction system rather than to ischemic heart disease.[46] Right bundle branch block does not appear to affect cardiovascular prognosis, while the presence of left bundle branch block carries some excess risk of mortality. First-degree heart block is common in the healthy elderly, with a reported prevalence of 44 percent after age 90, but higher degrees of AV block are uncommon in the absence of disease.[73]

The elderly are more susceptible to the adverse effects of cardiac arrhythmias because (1) diastolic dysfunction causes more severe impairment of CO with tachycardia, (2) altered autoregulation causes more organ dysfunction with arrythmia-induced hypotension, and (3) concomitant disease (e.g., CAD) exacerbates the effects of decreased perfusion.

In deciding to treat cardiac arrhythmias, the clinician must first determine the clinical significance of the arrhythmia. This is difficult because the aged are prone to dizziness and syncope resulting from causes other than cardiac arrhythmias (e.g., postural hypotension, vertebrobasilar insufficiency) and are less compliant in completing their diary cards during 24-h ambulatory monitoring. Next, the prognostic significance of the particular arrhythmia must be ascertained. Ventricular fibrillation, sustained ventricular tachycardia, torsades de pointes, and ventricular arrhythmias associated with myocardial infarction or dilated cardiomyopathy cause high mortality rates. Still, ventricular arrhythmias must be associated with symptoms before antiarrhythmic therapy is initiated,[70] since drug therapy may cause an increase in mortality among certain groups of patients.[74] When an elderly patient is symptomatic because of an arrhythmia that has prognostic significance, therapy is initiated with the same drugs used in the general population. Attention must be paid to altered hepatic and renal metabolism of these drugs in the elderly.[75]

Valvular Heart Disease

Fibrosis and calcification of the aortic valve occur commonly with aging, with aortic sclerosis having a prevalence of 20 percent in patients older than 65 years. The mitral valve is less commonly affected, and the tricuspid and pulmonary valves are rarely affected. Fibrosis and calcification lead eventually to aortic stenosis (most commonly), and/or aortic regurgitation. The recognition of aortic stenosis in the elderly is important because it is associated with increased perioperative cardiovascular morbidity and, in cases of critical aortic stenosis, with a 50 percent 1-year mortality.[76] At the same time, the development of aortic stenosis is more rapid and less easily clinically detected in the elderly.[39] Aortic valve repair can be carried out in the elderly with an acceptable risk-benefit ratio.[77] Chronic aortic regurgitation is most often managed medically in the elderly population.[59]

Calcification of the mitral valve anulus occurs in 30 to 50 percent of patients older than 90 years of age.[9] Since the circumference of the mitral valve anulus normally diminishes during ventricular systole, calcification and hardening of the anulus prevent the leaflets from achieving normal opposition, allowing regurgitation to occur during systolic contraction. In addition, the posterior valve may become fused to the adjacent ventricular wall. Ischemic heart disease may lead to acute mitral regurgitation by causing papillary muscle dysfunction. Atrial fibrillation is a frequent accompaniment of mitral regurgitation and can cause severe impairment of cardiac function in the presence of ventricular diastolic dysfunction. Medical management, including treatment of CHF, afterload reduction, and management of atrial fibrillation, is indicated initially. An elderly patient who fails on optimal medical management may require surgical repair or replacement of the mitral valve, but perioperative mortality rates are higher for mitral valve surgery than they are for aortic valve surgery.[59] Mitral stenosis is most commonly a result of rheumatic heart disease but also may result from extensive calcification of the valve apparatus.

Other Cardiovascular Diseases

A multiplicity of other cardiovascular diseases are more frequently diagnosed and cause greater compromise in the elderly. These include infective endocarditis, pulmonary embolism, amyloidosis, hemochromatosis, cor pulmonale, and metastatic heart tumors; only 5 percent of primary heart tumors occur in patients older than 65 years.

SUMMARY

The elderly encounter many hemodynamic challenges during the perioperative period. Because of altered age-related physiology, the healthy old are susceptible to complications associated with those challenges because of (1) altered cardiac diastolic function, (2) depressed cardiac reserve, (3) altered autonomic reflexes and homeostatic mechanisms, and (4) conduction system defects. In addition, an elderly patient is more likely to have cardiovascular disease, which further limits cardiac reserve and increases the cardiovascular complication rate. With knowledge of age-associated cardiovascular changes and with identification of optimized treatment modalities for cardiovascular disease, that complication rate can be minimized.

REFERENCES

1. Lakatta EG: Mechanisms of hypertension in the elderly. *J Am Geriatr Soc* 37:780, 1989.
2. Wenger NK: Cardiovascular disease in the elderly. *Curr Probl Cardiol* 17:609, 1992.
3. Wei JY: Age and the cardiovascular system. *N Engl J Med* 327:1735, 1992.
4. Lakatta EG, Yin FC: Myocardial aging: Functional alterations and related cellular mechanisms. *Am J Physiol* 242:H927, 1982.
5. Gerstenblith G, Fredericksen J, Yin FC, et al: Echocardiographic assessment of a normal adult aging population. *Circulation* 56:273, 1977.
6. Kitzman DW, Scholz DG, Hagen PT, et al: Age-related changes in normal human hearts during the first 10 decades of life: II (Maturity). A quantitative anatomic study of 765 specimens from subjects 20 to 99 years old. *Mayo Clin Proc* 63:137, 1988.
7. Lakatta EG: Heart and circulation, in Rowe JW (ed): *Handbook of the Biology of Aging*, 3d ed. San Diego: Academic Press, 1990, pp 181–216.
8. Klima M, Klima T: Cardiovascular pathology in old age, in Luchi RJ (ed): *Clinical Geriatric Cardiology*. Edinburgh: Churchill Livingstone 1989, pp 27–53.
9. Lie JT, Hammond PI: Pathology of the senescent heart: Anatomic observations on 237 autopsy studies of patients 90 to 105 years old. *Mayo Clin Proc* 63:552, 1988.
10. Virmani R, Roberts WC: Sudden cardiac death. *Hum Pathol* 18:485, 1987.
11. Lernfelt B, Wikstrand J, Svanborg A, Landahl S: Aging and left ventricular function in elderly healthy people. *Am J Cardiol* 68:547, 1991.
12. Lakatta EG: Cardiovascular regulatory mechanisms in advanced age. *Physiol Rev* 73:413, 1993.
13. Kitzmann DW, Sheikh KH, Beere PA, et al: Age-related alterations of Doppler left ventricular filling indexes in normal subjects are independent of left ventricular

mass, heart rate, contractility and loading conditions. *J Am Coll Cardiol* 18:1243, 1991.
14. Schulman SP, Lakatta EG, Fleg JL, et al: Age-related decline in left ventricular filling at rest and exercise. *Am J Physiol* 263:H1932, 1992.
15. Spurgeon HA, Steinbach MF, Lakatta EG: Chronic exercise prevents characteristic age-related changes in rat cardiac contraction. *Am J Physiol* 244:H513, 1983.
16. Lakatta EG: Changes in cardiovascular function with aging. *Eur Heart J* 11:C22, 1990.
17. Bryg RJ, Williams GA, Labovitz HA: Effect of aging on left ventricular diastolic filling in normal subjects. *Am J Cardiol* 59:971, 1987.
18. Wikstrand J: New concepts in the treatment of elderly hypertensive patients. *Am Heart J* 116:296, 1988.
19. Forman DE, Manning WJ, Hauser R, et al: Enhanced left ventricular diastolic filling associated with long-term endurance training. *J Gerontol* 47:M56, 1992.
20. Manning MJ, Shannon RP, Santinga JA, et al: Reversal or changes in left ventricular diastolic filling associated with normal aging using diltiazem. *Am J Cardiol* 67:894, 1991.
21. Wikstrand J, Berglund G, Tuomilehto J: Beta-blockade in the primary prevention of coronary heart disease in hypertensive patients: Review of present evidence. *Circulation* 84:VI93, 1991.
22. Fleg JL: Alterations in cardiovascular structure and function with advancing age. *Am J Cardiol* 57:33C, 1986.
23. Kuikka JT, Lansimies E: Effect of age on cardiac index, stroke index, and left ventricular ejection fraction at rest and during exercise as studied by radiocardiography. *Acta Physiol Scand* 114:339, 1982.
24. Granath A, Jonsson B, Strandell T: Circulation in healthy old men, studied by right heart catheterization at rest and during exercise in supine and sitting position. *Acta Med Scand* 176:425, 1964.
25. Strandell T: Circulatory studies on healthy old men. *Act Med Scand* 175:1, 1964.
26. Geokas MC, Lakatta EG, Makinodan T, Timiras PS: The aging process. *Ann Intern Med* 113:455, 1990.
27. Brandfonbrener M, Landowne M, Shock NW: Changes in cardiac output with age. *Circulation* 12:557, 1955.
28. Rodeheffer RJ, Gerstenblith G, Becker LC, et al: Exercise cardiac output is maintained with advancing age in healthy human subjects: Cardiac dilatation and increased stroke volume compensate for a diminished heart rate. *Circulation* 69:203, 1984.
29. Gerstenblith G, Lakatta EG, Weisfeldt ML: Age changes in myocardial function and exercise response. *Prog Cardiovasc Dis* 19:1, 1976.
30. Thomas SG, Paterson DH, Cunningham DA, et al: Cardiac output and left ventricular function in response to exercise in older men. *Can J Physiol Pharmacol* 71:136, 1993.
31. Docherty JR: Cardiovascular responses in ageing: A review. *Pharmacol Rev* 42:103, 1990.
32. Abrass IB: The biology and physiology of aging. *West J Med* 153:641, 1990.
33. Fleg JL, Lakatta EG: Role of muscle loss in the age-associated reduction in V02 max. *J Appl Physiol* 65:1147, 1988.
34. Ehsani AA, Ogawa T, Miller TR, et al: Exercise training improves left ventricular systolic function in older men. *Circulation* 83:96, 1991.
35. Xiao R, Lakatta EG: Deterioration of β-adrenergic modulation of cardiovascular function with aging. *Ann NY Acad Sci* 673:293, 1992.

36. Lakatta EG: Deficient neuroendocrine regulation of the cardiovascular system with advancing age in healthy humans. *Circulation* 87:631, 1993.
37. Ziegler MG, Lake CR, Copin IJ: Plasma noradrenalin increases with age. *Nature* 261:333, 1976.
38. Vestal RE, Wood AJ, Shand DG: Reduced β-adrenocepter sensitivity in the elderly. *Clin Pharmacol Ther* 26:181, 1979.
39. Weisfeldt ML, Lakatta EG, Gerstenblith G: Aging and the heart, in Braunwald E (ed): *Heart Disease*. Philadelphia: Saunders, 1992, pp 1656–1669.
40. Arora RR, Machac J, Goldman ME, et al: Atrial kinetics and left ventricular diastolic filling in the healthy elderly. *J Am Coll Cardiol* 9:1255, 1987.
41. Sowers JR, Rubenstein LZ, Stern N: Plasma norepinephrine responses to posture and isometric exercise increase with age in the absence of obesity. *J Gerontol* 38:315, 1983.
42. Shimada K, Kitazumi T, Sadakane N, et al: Age related changes of baroreflex function, plasma norepinephrine, and blood pressure. *Hypertension* 7:113, 1985.
43. Ferrari AU: Age-related modifications to neuro-cardiovascular control. *Aging* 4:183, 1992.
44. Lipsitz LA, Marks ER, Koestner J, et al: Reduced susceptibility to syncope during postural tilt in old age: Is beta-blockade protective? *Arch Intern Med* 149:2702, 1989.
45. Stern N, Tuck M: Homeostatic fragility in the elderly. *Cardiol Clin* 4:201, 1986.
46. Davies MJ: Pathology, in Martin A and Camm AJ (eds): *Heart Disease in the Elderly*. Chichester: Wiley, 1984, pp 37–57.
47. Lofland GK, Wechsler AS: Diseases of the aorta, in Luchi RJ (ed): *Clinical Geriatric Cardiology*. Edinburgh: Churchill Livingstone, 1989, pp 275–303.
48. Nichols WW, O'Rourke MF, Avolio AP, et al: Effects of age on ventricular-vascular coupling. *Am J Cardiol* 55:1179, 1985.
49. Williams BO: Cardiovascular physiology, in Luchi RJ (ed): *Clinical Geriatric Cardiology*. Edinburgh: Churchill Livingstone, 1989, pp 57–67.
50. O'Leary CE, Comporesi EM: Geriatric trauma patients, in Grande CM (ed): *Textbook of Trauma Anesthesia and Intensive Care*. St. Louis: Mosby, 1993, pp 606–618.
51. Holler BGD, Zeust H, Shaw S, et al: Effects of posture and aging on circulating atrial natriuretic peptide levels in man. *J Hypertens* 5:551, 1987.
52. Nademanee R, Intarachot V, Josephson M, et al: Prognostic significance of silent ischemia in patients with unstable angina. *J Am Coll Cardiol* 10:1, 1987.
53. Limacher MC: Clinical features of coronary heart disease in elderly. *Cardiovasc Clin* 22:63, 1992.
54. Miller PS, Sheps DS, Bragdon EE, et al: Aging and pain perception in ischemic heart disease. *Am Heart J* 120:22, 1990.
55. Stern S, Cohn PF, Pepine CJ: Silent myocardial ischemia. *Curr Probl Cardiol* 18:301, 1993.
56. Fleg JL, Gerstenblith G, Zonderman AB, et al: Prevalence and prognostic significance of exercise-induced silent myocardial ischemia detected by thallium scintigraphy and electrocardiography in asymptomatic volunteers. *Circulation* 81:428, 1990.
57. Aranow WS, Epstein S: Usefulness of silent myocardial ischemia detected by ambulatory electrocardiographic monitoring in predicting new coronary events in elderly patients. *Am J Cardiol* 62:1295, 1988.

58. Latting CA, Silverman ME: Acute myocardial infarction in hospitalized patients who are aged 70. *Am Heart J* 100:311, 1980.
59. Wenger NK: The elderly patient with cardiovascular disease, in Chatterjee K, Cheitlin M, Karliner J, et al (eds): *Cardiology: An Illustrated Text/Reference*. Philadelphia, New York: Lippincott, Gower, 1991, pp 13.28–13.41.
60. Stassen J, Fagard R, Lijnen P, et al: Review of the major hypertension trials in the elderly. *Cardiovasc Drugs Ther* 4:1237, 1990.
61. O'Malley K, Cox JP, O'Brien E: Further learnings from the European working party on high blood pressure in the elderly study. Focus on systolic hypertension. *Cardiovasc Drugs Ther* 4:1249, 1990.
62. SHEP Cooperative Research Group: Prevention of stroke by anti-hypertensive drug treatment in older persons with isolated systolic hypertension. *JAMA* 265:3255, 1991.
63. Furmaga EM, Murphy CN, Carter BL: Isolated systolic hypertension in older patients. *Clin Pharm* 12:347, 1993.
64. Tighe D, Brest N: Congestive heart failure in the elderly. *Cardiovasc Clin* 22:127, 1992.
65. Smythe CM: Congestive heart failure. *Tex Med* 89:52, 1993.
66. Leibovitch ER: Congestive heart failure: A current overview (review). *Geriatrics* 46:43, 1991.
67. Wong WF, Gold S, Fukuyama O, Blanchette PL: Diastolic dysfunction in elderly patients with congestive heart failure. *Am J Cardiol* 63:1526, 1989.
68. Luchi RJ, Snow E, Luchi JM, et al: Left ventricular function in hospitalized geriatric patients. *J Am Geriatr Soc* 30:700, 1982.
69. Fleg JL: Ventricular arrhythmias in the elderly: Prevalence, mechanisms, and therapeutic implications. *Geriatrics* 43:23, 1988.
70. Hessen SE: Clinical evaluation of the patient with ventricular arrhythmia (review). *Geriatrics* 47:63, 1992.
71. Fleg JL, Lakatta EG: Prevalence and prognosis of exercise-induced nonsustained ventricular tachycardia in apparently healthy volunteers. *Am J Cardiol* 54:762, 1984.
72. Martin A, Benbow LJ, Butrous GS, et al: Five-year follow-up of 101 elderly subjects by means of long-term ambulatory cardiac monitoring. *Eur Heart J* 5:592, 1984.
73. Bowers D: Electrocardiogram of nonagenarians. *Geriatrics* 24:89, 1969.
74. Greene HL, Roden DM, Katz RJ, et al: The cardiac arrhythmia suppression trial: First CAST ... then CAST-II. *J Am Coll Cardiol* 19:894, 1992.
75. Lynch RA, Horowitz LN: Managing geriatric arrhythmias: II. Drug selection and use [published erratum appears in *Geriatrics* 46(6):10, 1991] (review). *Geriatrics* 46:41, 1991.
76. Turina J, Hess O, Sepulcri F, Krayenbuehl HP: Spontaneous course of aortic valve disease. *Eur Heart J* 8:471, 1987.
77. Levinson JR, Akins CW, Buckley MJ, et al: Octogenarians with aortic stenosis: Outcome after aortic valve replacement. *Circulation* 80:149, 1989.

CHAPTER 4

Physiological Changes with Aging in the Endocrine System

Rahmawati Sih
John E. Morley

INTRODUCTION

Disorders of the endocrine system consist of a spectrum of emminently treatable conditions that are commonly present among older persons. However, one of the difficult aspects of geriatric endocrinology is distinguishing the effects of endocrinologic disease from the changes of aging. As a person ages, it becomes increasingly difficult to separate wellness and disease.

A loss of functional reserve associated with aging occurs in many organs, manifesting as conditions of hormonal deficiency such as hypothyroidism, diabetes mellitus, and hypogonadism. Both the decline in suppressor T cell activity and the increase in autoantibodies observed with aging lead to the increased prevalence of endocrine diseases and the tendency for more than one endocrine disorder to occur in the same person. Older persons also have a higher prevalence of neoplasms, and ectopic hormone production from nonendocrine malignancies can mimic classic endocrine diseases.

Atypical or nonspecific presentations are common features in the elderly and may result in delays in seeking medical attention, delays in making correct diagnoses, and misdiagnoses. Apathetic thyrotoxicosis is a well-recognized example of an atypical presentation, and the nonspecific symptoms of fatigue, delirium, weight loss, and dementia can be seen in hypothyroidism and hypoadrenalism.

Another complicating factor that must be recognized in treating the geriatric population is that most normal laboratory values have been derived from young, healthy individuals so that abnormal results may reflect the aging process. This is further confounded by the presence of other concurrent diseases that can alter basal and stimulated hormonal values. Table 4-1 summarizes the effects of aging on the endocrine system.

This chapter provides basic information necessary for the appropriate interpretation of endocrine tests and the recognition and treatment of endocrine diseases in an older person. Specific endocrine issues important to the care of geriatric patients during the perioperative period also are addressed.

AGING AND THE POSTERIOR PITUITARY

Arginine vasopressin (AVP)/antidiuretic hormone (ADH) is one of the principal hormones influencing salt and water balance. Synthesized in the supraoptic nucleus and, to a lesser extent, the paraventricular nucleus, AVP is stored in the posterior pituitary and released under hypothalamic control. The changes in the homeostasis of this system that occur with age are important because of an older person's increased tendency to develop both hypo- and hypernatremia. While it is well recognized that older persons have a decrease in the thirst response to osmotic changes compared with younger individuals,[1] the changes in osmoregulation of AVP are more controversial. Older persons may have impaired responses to both dehydration, through water deprivation or heat

Table 4-1 Effect of aging on hormones

Hormone	Effect of aging on serum level	Effect of aging on receptor and postreceptor functions
Arginine vasopressin	↑	↓
Atrial naturetic peptide	↑	↓
Growth hormone	↓	nc
Insulin-like growth factor-1	↓	nc
Prolactin	Mild ↑	nc
Thyrotropin	nc	nc
Thyroxine	nc	nc
Triiodothyronine	Mild ↓	nc
ACTH	nc	Mild ↓
Cortisol	nc	nc
Pregnenolone	↓	?
DHEA/DHEA-sulfate	↓	?
Renin	↓	nc
Aldosterone	↓	nc
Luteinizing hormone, male	nc	↓
Luteinizing hormone, female	↑	nc
Follicle stimulating hormone, male	↑	?
Follicle stimulating hormone, female	↑	?
Estradiol, male	nc	nc
Estradiol, female	↓	nc
Testosterone, male*	↓	↓
Insulin	↑	↓
Glucagon	nc	nc
Norepinephrine	↑	↓
Epinephrine	nc with ↑ >80 years	Mild ↓

*Greater decrease in "free" and "bioavailable" testosterone.

↑ = increase; ↓ = decrease; nc = no change.

stress, and overhydration. The sensitivity of AVP secretion in response to a rise in plasma osmolality is variably reported to increase with age[2] or to be lower than in the young.[3–6] Baseline levels of circulating AVP also have been variably reported to be higher,[7] lower,[8] or nonsignificantly different[9] in older age groups compared with younger age groups. Studies of nonosmotic stimulation of AVP by postural changes have shown an age-related blunting.[10,11]

Many older persons complain of polyuria and nocturia, which, in addition to a decrease in glomerular filtration rate and urologic problems, may be due to a deficiency of AVP[8] and a loss of the nocturnal increase in AVP seen in younger persons.[12] The aged with Alzheimer's disease may be at increased risk of dehydration during periods of fluid restriction as a result of the loss of the normal physiological response to thirst and AVP secretion. Vasopressin is under direct cholinergic control, and one of the main neuropathological correlates of Alzheimer's disease is a dropout of cholinergic neurons within the central nervous system. In older patients with Alzheimer's disease, studies have shown lower vasopressin levels and lower cerebrospinal fluid levels of vasopressin-associated human neurophysin, a vasopressin transporter peptide.[13] Patients with Alzheimer's disease also become more dehydrated in response to fluid restriction and exhibit diminished thirst as measured by water ingested during 1 h of ad lib water intake after a period of dehydration.[14]

The syndrome of inappropriate ADH (SIADH) can occur in association with cerebral and cerebellar tumors, strokes, subdural hematoma or head trauma, congestive heart failure, chest infections, diabetes mellitus, hypothyroidism, and hypoadrenalism. Ectopic ADH or ADH-like hormone may be produced by carcinomas. The hypotheses of chlorpropamide-induced SIADH and hyponatremia include the stimulation of ADH release from the posterior pituitary, ADH-like action of chlorpropamide, and the potentiation of the antidiuretic effect of ADH at the renal tubule. In older diabetic patients, the use of chlorpropamide has been associated with diminished mental function in up to 15 percent of older persons.[15]

Because of the propensity to develop abnormalities in sodium and water balance in an older person, the use of intravenous fluids during the perioperative period should be judicious. Physical examination, serum electrolytes, urine output, and specific gravity require careful evaluation, and particular attention must be paid to older persons with Alzheimer's disease to avoid dehydration. Hyponatremia with normal glucose and normal lipids in the face of euvolemia warrants further investigation for secondary causes.

DIABETES MELLITUS

Diabetes mellitus (DM) is a common and costly problem in the older population. Extrapolating from the National Health and Nutrition Examination Survey (NHANES) II findings on the prevalence of DM, it has been estimated that more than 8 million people in the United States have diabetes or hyperglycemia and that approximately half have not been diagnosed. The older population constitutes the largest proportion of those with DM, which affects approximately 18 percent of those 65 to 74 years of age.[16] Accounting for lost productivity resulting from disability and death, in 1986 the costs of non-insulin-dependent diabetes mellitus (NIDDM) were estimated at over $9.4 billion for those over age 65 years.[17] DM is also costly in terms of morbidity and mortality. Mortality rates for diabetic patients increase with age,[18–20] as does prevalence of diabetic complications.[21] Diabetic patients are also at a greater risk of institutionalization than are nondiabetics.

Mild glucose intolerance occurs with advancing age. Over the age of 50 there is a 1 to 2 mg/dl increase in fasting blood glucose per decade. The postprandial increase in glucose with age is even more marked, with a rise of 5 to 10 mg/dl for every decade beyond 50 years.[22] The World Health Organization criteria for

DM include a fasting blood glucose of 140 mg/dl or greater or a plasma glucose concentration of 200 mg/dl or greater 2 h after a 75-g oral glucose load.[23]

Insulin resistance associated with aging is the primary cause of diabetes in older persons. Multiple factors are implicated in the pathophysiology of NIDDM. Poor diet,[24] decreased physical activity,[25,26] and changes in body composition[27,28] with a tendency toward obesity[29] contribute to poor carbohydrate tolerance.

Insulin action appears to be abnormal, as evidenced by a failure of the normal suppression of plasma free fatty acids with an increase in hepatic glucose output[30] and impaired glucose uptake by peripheral muscle and fat. Changes in insulin receptors and a defect in postreceptor signaling and response mechanisms can cause impairments in glucose uptake and utilization.[31,32]

Insulin secretion is also abnormal in patients with NIDDM. The responsiveness of insulin secretion to glucose stimulation is blunted, and pancreatic responses to an elevation in glucose levels exhibit a lag.[33] There is also a loss in the pulsatile nature of insulin secretion,[34] and there may be a defect in the conversion of proinsulin to insulin in the pancreas or reduced cellular stores of insulin.[35,36] A decrease in insulin breakdown and removal[37] and elevated levels of circulating glucagon[38] also contribute to the pathophysiology of diabetes in older adults (Table 4-2).

Hyperosmolar nonketotic coma is a significant complication of DM in older persons, particularly affecting those with renal disease and those who are institutionalized and demented.[30] Medications such as propranolol, cimetidine, phenytoin, and particularly diuretics contribute to the development of hyperosmolar coma.[39] Both ketoacidosis and lactic acidosis can be present in older persons with diabetic coma and can contribute to the elevated mortality rate seen in older diabetic patients.[40]

An older individual with diabetes is also at a greater risk for hypoglycemia,[41] and a disproportionate percentage of patients who develop hypoglycemia on oral agents are older. Chlorpropamide, which has a long half-life, produces

Table 4-2 Mechanisms of hyperglycemia in NIDDM

Mechanisms
Abnormalities in insulin secretion
Impaired pulsatile secretion
Impaired beta cell response
Fewer pancreatic stores
Decreased insulin synthesis
Increased proinsulin release
Altered hepatic insulin extraction
Abnormalities in insulin action
Decreased suppression of hepatic glucose output
Impaired glucose uptake by muscle and fat
Receptor defects
Postreceptor defects

twice as many episodes of hypoglycemia in older diabetic patients than do other oral agents.[42,43] Other factors that can increase the risk of developing hypoglycemia include difficulties with food purchase, preparation, and consumption; irregularly timed meals with respect to medication administration; cognitive and psychiatric impairments; and mistakes in medication doses. When drawing up insulin, an older diabetic patient may make errors between 10 to 20 percent.[44]

Soft tissue foot infections with or without underlying osteomyelitis are a leading source of morbidity in older persons with diabetes. Approximately 50 percent of older men and 80 percent of older women who are diagnosed with gangrene have diabetes.[45] Thus, vigilance on the part of the physician and the patient regarding foot care is paramount. Visual difficulties in an older individual with diabetes can be a result of retinopathy, glaucoma, or cataracts. In those aged 50 to 69 years, the risk of developing cataracts is three times higher in diabetic patients compared with nondiabetics and is modestly increased in diabetic patients over age 70 years.[46] Among all diabetic patients who are blind secondary to retinopathy, 40 percent are over age 70 years. The increase in the prevalence of retinopathy in older diabetic patients is not completely due to the status of the disease (i.e., duration of diabetes, degree of glucose control) but may result from an interaction with age-related changes.[21] Some degree of blue-green color blindness can be an early manifestation of diabetic retinopathy.[47]

Certain diabetic complications are more or less unique to older persons.[48] Sudden paralysis of cranial nerve III or, less frequently, cranial nerves IV or VI that spontaneously resolves within 6 weeks to 3 months is not uncommon. *Pseudomonas aeruginosa* can cause malignant otitis externa, a necrotizing infection of the external auditory canal. Malignant otitis externa occurs almost exclusively in the older diabetic population. The diagnosis of renal papillary necrosis must be considered in an older diabetic patient who presents with sudden renal failure, as approximately half of those with papillary necrosis are over age 60 years. An older diabetic patient is also three times more likely to suffer from choledochal diseases than is a younger diabetic patient.[44]

Both peripheral and central nervous system disorders are frequently diagnosed in older diabetic patients. Asymmetric, progressive, and painful weakness of the muscles of the pelvic girdle and thigh, with mild sensory changes, may be the presenting symptoms of DM, particularly in older men. Spontaneous resolution of this condition—diabetic amyotrophy—can be expected within 12 months. Diabetic neuropathic cachexia is a severe form of diabetic amyotrophy with clinical findings of anorexia and marked weight loss. Older persons also appear to be more susceptible to developing diabetic neuropathy.

Central nervous system complications in diabetes are generally a result of vascular disease. Cerebrovascular accidents are more frequently seen in those with hyperglycemia, and the outcome is usually poorer.[49] Modest cognitive dysfunction, in the absence of strokes and transient ischemic attacks, occurs in diabetic patients with hyperglycemia compared with age-matched controls[50,51] and may interfere with medication compliance. Normalization of blood sugar in patients with NIDDM has been shown to improve aspects of learning and memory.[52] Even highly functional older people with NIDDM who perceive themselves as being in good health are likely to manifest greater deficits than are the healthy aged in processing complex verbal or nonverbal material.[53] Depression occurs commonly in older persons and is significant in adults with long-standing diabetes.[54] Depression can create difficulties with compliance and is strongly correlated with mortality in older diabetic individuals.

Unless a person is grossly overweight, dietary manipulations do not play a major role in the treatment of diabetic patients over 70 years of age. A study performed in a chronic-care facility comparing a regular diet and a diabetic diet found an increase of only 0.6 mmol/liter (11 mg/dl) in fasting blood glucose during the regular-diet period. There were no detrimental effects on glycosylated hemoglobin, plasma triglycerides, and cholesterol.[55] The older population, in particular, is at risk for developing deficiencies of trace elements,[56] and diabetic patients are more likely to have hyperzincuria and poor zinc absorption,[57] hypomagnesemia, and a chromium deficiency.[58] Zinc replacement in patients with NIDDM and zinc depletion improved T cell function as measured by the T lymphocyte response to phytohemagglutinin.[59] Zinc replacement also plays a role in wound healing, increasing the rate of healing of leg ulcers in zinc-deficient older persons.[60] In the perioperative setting, for an older diabetic patient who requires intravenous feeding, the use of total parenteral nutrition formulas should be looked at in light of the likelihood of deficiencies of trace elements.

For ideal management of an older diabetic patient, treatments must be individualized. In a frail institutionalized older person, blood glucose levels should be maintained between 100 and 200 mg/dl. In a healthy older person, blood sugars should be kept at or below 150 mg/dl. Normalization of blood sugars can improve polyuria, neuropathic pain, healing, lens opacity with resultant visual difficulties, and red blood cell rigidity. Because of these benefits of good blood glucose control, consideration should be given to postponement of elective surgery in a poorly controlled older diabetic patient.

Oral hypoglycemic agents should be used with caution in older diabetic patients, particularly during the perioperative period. Second-generation oral hypoglycemic agents such as glipizide and glyburide should be held on the day of surgery, when patients are likely to be nil peros (NPO). Small doses of regular insulin may be used to cover a patient who develops hyperglycemia rebound withdrawal from an oral agent. Because of the decreased renal excretion and extended half-lives of the first-generation sulfonylureas acetohexamide and chlorpropamide, these agents should be avoided in older persons. Chlorpropamide not only produces prolonged hypoglycemia in older persons but also is associated with hyponatremia. If an older diabetic patient has been previously managed with these medications, they should be discontinued several days before surgery.

Insulin need not be withheld before surgery. Rather, in a patient who requires insulin for glucose control, either a low-dose intravenous insulin infusion or half to two-thirds of the usual insulin dose in the form of an intermediate-acting insulin may be given the morning of surgery. Intravenous fluids containing 5 percent dextrose should be instituted in patients who are receiving insulin. It is imperative that every older diabetic patient have careful blood glucose monitoring throughout the perioperative period.

Persons with diabetes are at increased risk of having a myocardial infarction. In older persons, the classic signs and symptoms may present atypically or not at all. The presenting features of myocardial infarction in older persons may include dyspnea, acute onset of confusion, and syncope.

THYROID DISEASES

The diagnosis of hyper- or hypothyroidism in an older person is often missed because the subtle and nonspecific presentation can mimic many of the physiological changes associated with aging. The prevalence of hyperthyroidism is seven times higher in persons older than 60 years compared with the general population, and more than 4 percent of those over 60 years old are hypothyroid.[61]

With age, the thyroid gland becomes increasingly fibrotic, with infiltration by lymphocytes.[62] The prevalence of nodules increases markedly with age, affecting approximately 5 percent of those older than 60 years,[63] and the overall size of the thyroid has been variably reported to increase, decrease, or remain unchanged with advancing age.[64] Despite these changes in structure, most older persons have an adequate amount of thyroid hormone, and there is no correlation between these anatomic changes and thyroid function tests.

Serum thyroxine levels have been reported to increase,[65] decrease,[66] or remain unchanged with advancing age.[67] Both the production and the clearance of thyroid hormones are reduced. When thyroxine (T_4) is metabolized, it is converted either into triiodothyronine (T_3), the active thyroid hormone, or into a biologically inactive hormone called reverse T_3. The total serum T_3 concentration may be modestly decreased in normal, healthy older persons.[68] In patients with severe nonthyroidal illnesses, T_3 concentrations are reduced and reverse T_3 concentrations are increased. T_3 concentration in hospitalized older individuals is generally reduced 40 to 50 percent.[69] These changes can be seen with various illnesses and with nutritional changes such as fasting. Table 4-3 summarizes thyroid function tests in the euthyroid sick syndrome, primary hypothyroidism, and aging.

Thyroid stimulating hormone (TSH) concentrations have been variably reported to remain unchanged with age,[70] while other studies have shown a higher concentration of TSH in older men[71] and a progressive increase in older women.[72] The thyrotropin releasing hormone (TRH) stimulation test can be used to measure the reserve of pituitary TSH. With age, the TSH response to TRH has been found to remain unaffected or to decrease, particularly in men.[73–76] Medications (i.e., steroids) and concurrent illnesses (depression, malnutrition, uremia, nonthyroidal illness) can result in a blunted TSH response to

Table 4-3 Thyroid function tests in euthyroid sick syndrome, primary hypothyroidism, and aging

	Euthyroid sick syndrome	Primary hypothyroidism	Age
TSH	nl/↓	↑	nl
T_4	nl/↓	↓	nl
T_3RU	nl/↑/↓	↓	nl
FT_4I	nl/↓	↓	nl
T_3	↓	↓	nl

nl = normal; ↑ = increased; ↓ = decreased.

TRH;[77] thus, a normal response in an older person can exclude the diagnosis of hyperthyroidism, but a blunted response is nondiagnostic.

Epidemiological studies on the prevalence of hypothyroidism have been variable because of ethnicity and the availability of environmental iodine. Data from the original cohort of the Framingham study showed a prevalence of hypothyroidism of 5.9 percent of women and 2.3 percent of men over age 60 years.[78] It is clear from the multitude of epidemiological studies that the prevalence of thyroid failure is higher in the older population than in younger persons.

Hypothyroidism can be easily missed because of its slow and insidious progression, often developing over a period of 30 years, and the subtle and atypical presentations. Fatigue, lethargy, poor ability to concentrate, weight loss, depression, dry skin, constipation, weakness, and cold intolerance are common symptoms in the older population and may be mistaken for symptoms of "normal aging." Unusual manifestations of hypothyroidism include elevated creatine phosphokinase (CPK) levels, hyponatremia, anemia, myopathy, hemorrhagic diatheses, pericardial effusion, and psychotic symptoms of hallucinations and delusions.[79]

The most common cause of hypothyroidism in the older population is autoimmune thyroid disease (Hashimoto's thyroiditis). Past thyroid surgery and radioactive iodine therapy for Graves' disease are also frequent causes of hypothyroidism. Subclinical hypothyroidism is a condition characterized by an increased thyrotropin level with normal concentrations of T_4 and T_3 and few clinical symptoms. Overt primary hypothyroidism can develop in a significant number of those with subclinical hypothyroidism, and iodine exposure, amiodarone, and lithium may predispose a patient to the development of overt hypothyroidism.[80]

Up to 20 percent of older persons have elevated titers of thyroglobulin and microsomal antibodies.[64] High-titer antimicrosomal antibodies (<1:1600) combined with modestly elevated TSH levels or TSH levels greater than 20 mU/liter are highly predictive of progression to thyroid failure in patients with subclinical hypothyroidism.[81] These patients may have subtle symptoms that may improve with thyroid replacement therapy.[82] In euthyroid older persons with TSH concentrations elevated above 10 μU/ml and positive antimicrosomal antibodies, close follow-up or initiation of thyroid replacement therapy is indicated.

The treatment of hypothyroidism is done with synthetic levothyroxine sodium. In general, the required replacement dose of thyroid hormone is lower in an older patient[83] because of the reduction in the T_4 plasma clearance rate with aging.[84] Replacement doses should start at 0.025 mg/day and be titrated upward in increments of 0.025 mg every 3 weeks while TSH levels are monitored. Usually no more than 0.1 mg/day of levothyroxine sodium is required. Some studies have indicated that certain generic products may have less hormone compared with brand-name levothyroxine.[85] Thyroxine replacement may aggravate angina in some patients, particularly in the early phase of therapy. The concomitant use of verapamil in severely hypothyroid patients may improve the left ventricular ejection fraction at rest and with exertion during the first 2 months of thyroid hormone replacement.[86] In older hypothyroid persons with hypertension, thyroid hormone replacement often leads to normalization of blood pressure.

Myxedema coma is a rare but morbid and often fatal complication of hypothyroidism resulting from a loss of physiological compensations to thyroid failure. The diagnostic features of myxedema coma include altered mental status, defective thermoregulation, hypothermia, and a precipitating illness or event such as an infection; inappropriate doses of a diuretic, digoxin, or a sedative; surgery; hypothermia; and hypoglycemia. The marked peripheral vasoconstriction mediated by the relatively unopposed alpha-adrenergic stimulation leads to a decrease in total circulating volume, bradycardia, reduced cardiac output, and diastolic hypertension. Most drugs are metabolized at a reduced rate in patients with hypothyroidism. Treatment of myxedema coma includes correction of the effects of the precipitating event, supportive endotracheal intubation and mechanical ventilation in cases of carbon dioxide retention and hypoxia, diuretics and afterload-reducing agents for the treatment of congestive heart failure, and blood transfusions for the relative or absolute hypotension that occurs as a result of the decrease in blood volume. External warming of a hypothermic patient may lead to cardiovascular shock by causing peripheral vasodilation. Hydrocortisone 100 mg every 12 hr intravenously should be given until the possibility of coexisting adrenal insufficiency has been ruled out. A single dose of 0.5 mg of levothyroxine sodium intravenously is recommended for patients believed to have myxedema coma.[87,88] Despite myxedema ileus and variable oral absorption, the clinical response to oral levothyroxine sodium is rapid and effective.[89]

Hyperthyroidism occurs in 0.5 to 2 percent of older individuals, and in one study, approximately 12 percent of hyperthyroid patients were found to be age 60 years or older.[90] As in the younger population, Graves' disease is the most frequent cause of hyperthyroidism seen with aging. Plummer's disease (multinodular goiter) and single-nodule thyrotoxicosis are more commonly seen in the older population. Older persons with thyrotoxicosis present less frequently with the typical symptoms of restlessness, nervousness, heat intolerance, eye findings, and goiter.[91] Apathetic hyperthyroidism occurs almost exclusively in older patients with predominant symptoms of fatigue, lassitude, and disinterest. Weight loss and anorexia, muscle weakness, palpitations, and dyspnea are also common symptoms in older thyrotoxic persons. Atrial fibrillation occurs in up to 5 percent of individuals with thyrotoxicosis and appears to be more common as a presenting feature in older persons. Tachycardia occurs less frequently, but angina and congestive heart failure may be involved in many cases.[90,92]

The diagnosis of hyperthyroidism is confirmed by thyroid function tests. Usually there are elevations of both T_3 and T_4, although an isolated increase of either one is possible. T_3 thyrotoxicosis can be seen in patients with a solitary adenoma or in early toxic multinodular goiter. High doses of beta blockers may artificially raise T_4 levels.[93] With the advent of "supersensitive" TSH assays, a subnormal TSH may facilitate the diagnosis of hyperthyroidism; however, these assays are not sufficiently sensitive or specific in sick older persons to recommend their use as the sole means of diagnosis.[94] Autoantibodies may artificially raise TSH levels, producing false-negative test results.[45] Hyperthyroidism causes a suppressed TSH response to TRH. Because illness and/or aging may result in a blunted TSH response, only the presence of a normal TSH response is useful, as it effectively rules out hyperthyroidism.

The treatment of thyrotoxicosis in an older person depends on its etiology. Graves' disease is usually treated with radioactive iodine ablation of the thyroid gland. Short-term antithyroid drugs should be given for 2 to 3 months to deplete the gland of preformed thyroid hormone so that post-^{131}I thyroiditis will not cause the release of large amounts of thyroid hormone and exacerbation of the hyperthyroid state. Beta-adrenergic blockers may be used for symptomatic tachyarrhythmias, restlessness, and tremor. Multinodular goiter is similarly managed but requires larger and repeated doses of radioactive iodine because of variable uptake by the nodules. Surgery is an alternative therapy provided that the patient has a low cardiovascular risk and a euthyroid state is achieved preoperatively.[95] After radioactive iodine therapy, thyroid function tests should be monitored regularly.

ADRENAL DISORDERS

With aging, there is only a minimal decline in adrenal weight, but the adrenal cortex undergoes degenerative changes with the development of fibrosis, accumulation of lipofuscin, loss of steroid-containing lipids, hemorrhage, and mitochondrial fragmentation.[96] There is also a tendency to develop nodular hypoplasia.[39] There is a decrease in the cortisol production and clearance rates with advancing age; thus, the aging changes tend to balance out, and there is no change in serum cortisol levels. More recent data reveal a trend toward decreased plasma cortisol with age.[97,98]

There is minimal change in the cortisol response to adrenocorticotropic hormone (ACTH)[99,100] in older persons. The cortisol response to insulin-induced hypoglycemia is similar in healthy older and younger persons.[101,102] The ACTH response to corticotropin-releasing factor (CRF) is not altered with aging; however, older persons may have higher cortisol levels in response to perioperative stress[103] and when depressed.[104,105] Older persons tend to excrete larger amounts of cortisol and ACTH. In addition, cortisol remains elevated for longer periods, suggesting a diminished sensitivity of ACTH to negative feedback by glucocorticoids.[106]

Fewer than 10 percent of patients with Addison's disease are over age 60,[107] and adrenal insufficiency is easily missed in an older person because of its nonspecific presentation. Symptoms of fatigue, hyponatremia, hyperkalemia, hypotension, or relative hypotension and a propensity toward hypoglycemia should raise the index of suspicion for the possibility of adrenal insufficiency. Eosinophilia is commonly present in persons with adrenocortical insufficiency. The causes of adrenocortical insufficiency in older persons include Addison's disease (autoimmune etiology), tuberculosis, adrenal hemorrhage (particularly in those on anticoagulants), and invasive cancer. The diagnosis usually can be made by utilizing the cosyntropin (synthetic ACTH) stimulatory test, and the treatment is with glucocorticoid and/or mineralocorticoid replacement. Because of interference with sleep, steroid administration should be avoided in the late afternoon and evening.

Cushing's syndrome is relatively uncommon in the older population. Approximately 8 percent of patients with adrenocortical carcinoma are over 60 years of age.[108] The concurrence of hypertension, hypokalemia, diabetes, and osteoporosis should prompt consideration of Cushing's syndrome. The most common cause of Cushing's syndrome is iatrogenic; thus, steroids should be administered with care. Because of the diminished cortisol clearance with age, steroid doses for replacement therapy should be lower in an older patient. Older persons may fail to show normal cortisol suppression after an overnight dexamethasone suppression test,[109,110] particularly in the presence of depression, dementia, obesity, alcoholism, or phenytoin.

The syndrome of ectopic ACTH secretion is also more commonly seen in the older population, affecting more men than women. Clinical symptoms include cachexia, proximal muscle weakness, hypertension, hypokalemic alkalosis, increased pigmentation, and changes in mental status. Evaluation of patients with this syndrome may reveal an extremely high plasma ACTH level (>200 pg/ml), nonsuppression by high-dose dexamethasone testing, and a primary tumor on chest x-ray in 50 percent of cases.

The secretion, clearance, urinary excretion, and concentration of plasma aldosterone all decrease with age. Renin concentrations are also lower in older adults. Clinically, this predisposes older persons, particularly those with diabetes and creatinine levels between 2 to 3 mg/dl, to having hyperkalemia secondary to hyporeninemic hypoaldosteronism. Beta blockers and nonsteroidal anti-inflammatory agents can precipitate hyperkalemia.

The changes in adrenal androgen production with age are more evident than those seen in the glucocorticoids. There is a progressive decline in plasma and urinary 17-ketosteroids with advancing age. Dehydroepiandrosterone (DHEA) secretion declines linearly from 20 to 96 years,[111] and DHEA-sulfate and androsterone fall similarly. In animals, DHEA administration appears to increase life span. It may cause weight loss without altering food intake.[112] DHEA and its metabolites exert a protective effect on the development of tumors, certain immune diseases, and diabetes in experimental animals[113,114] and appears to be inversely related to cardiovascular mortality.[115] In a study of nursing home residents, low DHEA levels predicted poor functional status.[116] In animal studies, DHEA appears to play a role in cognition.[117]

Pregnenolone is another steroid hormone produced by the adrenal gland whose level declines with age.[118] Pregnenolone and its sulfate have recently become a subject of interest because of their roles as neurosteroids,[119] with the suggestion that they may regulate behavior, mood, anxiety, learning, and sleep. Within the brain of animals, regional alterations in the concentration of pregnenolone sulfate have been observed to be associated with different physiological states. Pregnenolone and pregnenolone sulfate have been found to interact with the $GABA_A$ (gamma-aminobutyric $acid_A$)[120] and NMDA (*N*-methyl D-aspartate) receptors, antagonizing GABA[121,122] and augmenting NMDA.[123,124] GABA is a major inhibitory neurotransmitter in the central nervous system, and modulation of its activity affects behavior and memory. NMDA receptors are believed to play a role in learning, hypoxic neuronal damage, and epilepsy.[125,126] Animals given pregnenolone and pregnenolone sulfate have shown some of these behavioral and memory effects,[127,128] although effects in humans have not been extensively studied.[129]

With advancing age, there is an increase in norepinephrine levels but no change in the levels of epinephrine; when an individual becomes extremely elderly, epinephrine levels also rise. The increased norepinephrine levels in geriatric patients appear to be due to both an increase in norepinephrine appearance in the plasma and a decrease in the norepinephrine clearance rate.[130–132] Body fat percentage plays an important independent role in the norepinephrine appearance rate.[133] With aging, there is a decrease in beta-adrenergic responsiveness caused mainly by a decline in receptor affinity[134] and a decrease in the activity of the catalytic unit of adenylate cyclase.[135] The changes in alpha-adrenergic receptor function associated with aging are controversial.

PARATHYROID DISEASES AND DISORDERS OF CALCIUM

Multiple changes in parathyroid hormone (PTH) physiology and calcium metabolism occur with aging. Total serum calcium declines progressively with age in men but appears not to be affected in women.[136] Lower levels of 25 (OH) vitamin D are found in some older persons[137] and may reflect less sun exposure (sometimes as a result of the use of sunblock to prevent skin cancer) as well as the decreased ability of older skin to synthesize vitamin D. While nephrogenous synthesis of $1{,}25(OH)_2$ vitamin D is not generally impaired in older adults, institutionalized elders may be at particular risk for low 1,25$(OH)_2$ vitamin D, which can result in decreased calcium absorption from the intestine.[137–139] There is an age-related rise in PTH that is attributed to reduced renal function,[140] reduced intestinal calcium absorption, and some target organ resistance to PTH action.[141] As suggested by a study of institutionalized older persons, among whom 90 percent had low 1,25$(OH)_2$ vitamin D and many had increased PTH and normal osteocalcin (a marker of osteoblast activity), there may be an inadequate osteoblast response to PTH.[139] A reduced response of the target organ to PTH may also be explained by the decreased number of intact cells rather than a decreased response of individual cells to PTH.[142]

Osteopenia is a significant cause of morbidity and mortality in the older population. It is estimated that 25 to 40 percent of women over age 70 suffer vertebral crush fractures and that approximately one-third of women have fractured a femur by age 90. Loss of skeletal mass begins during the fourth decade of life,[143,144] with an acceleration during menopause in women.[145] Hypogonadal men are also at risk of osteopenia.[146] The postmenopausal women who are likely to develop osteoporosis are White or Asian, thin, sedentary, and tobacco smoking and have a positive family history and a lifelong poor calcium intake.[143,147]

Secondary causes of osteoporosis include malignancies (particularly breast, lung, and multiple myeloma),[147] thyrotoxicosis,[148] hyperparathyroidism,[149] hypercortisolism,[150] and certain medications, such as phenytoin.[151] Primary osteoporosis has been divided into two forms[152] (Table 4-4). Type I occurs in postmenopausal women and is thought to result from the withdrawal of estrogens. Treatment with estrogen replacement is indicated. Type I osteoporosis primarily affects trabecular bone; thus, wrist and vertebral fractures are more common. Type II osteoporosis occurs in men and women over age 75 years as a result of an impaired osteoblast response to growth factors and secondary hypoparathyroidism.[153] Type II may be treated with calcium and vitamin D or calcitonin. Other modalities include the use of cyclic diphosphonates[154] and thiazide diuretics.[155] In addition to modification of risk factors such as cigarette, alcohol, and caffeine use, environmental risk factors such as loose rugs, poor lighting, and unsafe bathrooms must be addressed to prevent falls.

Table 4-4 Type I versus type II osteoporosis

	Type I	Type II
Bone type	Trabecular bone Wrist Vertebrae	Cortical bone, hip
At risk	Postmenopausal women	Men and women $>$ 75 years
Etiology	Withdrawal of estrogens	Impaired osteoblast response to growth factors, secondary hypoparathyroidism
Treatment	Estrogen replacement	Calcium, vitamin D, calcitonin

The differential diagnosis of hypercalcemia includes hyperparathyroidism, familial hypocalciuric hypercalcemia, immobilization with decreased bone formation and increased bone resorption,[156] malignancy-related hypercalcemia, granulomatous disease, and vitamin A and D supplements. Primary hyperparathyroidism generally affects those between 50 and 70 years old and affects women twice as often as men.[157] Most patients are asymptomatic, but neuromuscular and psychiatric symptoms are more common in the older than in the younger patients.[158] The diagnosis of hyperparathyroidism is made by the findings of repeatedly elevated serum calcium or ionized calcium and elevated radioimmunoassay of PTH. C-terminal assays are usually adequate, but N-terminal assays should be requested in those with renal insufficiency. The recommended treatment for those with symptomatic hypercalcemia is parathyroid surgery unless the patient is a poor surgical candidate. For those unable or unwilling to undergo surgery, medical therapy with estrogens may be an alternative.[159]

The etiology of hypoparathyroidism and hypocalcemia includes damage from neck irradiation, total thyroidectomy, and autoimmune disease as part of the syndrome of multiple endocrine gland failure.[160,161] Currently, data examining the clinical course of hypoparathyroidism in older versus younger patients are sparse. In older persons excessive use of phosphosoda enemas has been associated with hypocalcemia.

GROWTH HORMONE

Growth hormone (GH) stimulates muscular and skeletal growth as well as increasing hepatic, splenic, and renal size. GH also enhances immune function.[162] Most of the actions of GH are mediated by the release of somatomedin C [insulin-like growth factor-I (IGF-I)] in the liver and kidneys. With aging, IGF-I levels have been demonstrated to decrease,[39] but the effects of age on GH itself are less clear. Basal GH concentration declines in aging women and appears to be related to the decline in estrogen that occurs with menopause.[163,164] Basal GH levels do not appear to change in men.[165] GH is secreted primarily during the first few hours of sleep. With age, there is a reduction in GH night peaks, but the frequency and nadir of GH secretion remain unchanged.[166]

The response of GH to growth hormone releasing hormone (GHRH) has been variably reported to be markedly decreased or to remain unchanged with advancing age.[167,168] The response to insulin-induced hypoglycemia has similarly been reported to decrease or remain unchanged.[169,102] Tissue sensitivity to somatomedin C does not appear to be affected by age, as evidenced by normal receptor binding and mitogenic response of fibroblasts from aged subjects to somatomedin C.[170]

GH administration may play a role in the treatment of malnourished elderly individuals by causing an increase in weight and urinary nitrogen retention.[171]

GH has also been demonstrated to increase potassium and phosphorus balance in patients receiving total parenteral nutrition.[172] Fluid retention and hyperglycemia must be monitored while patients are receiving GH.[173]

Many of the age-related changes in body composition resemble those associated with GH deficiency, and multiple studies have examined the role of GH administration in older persons. In one study, GH administration acutely increased nitrogen retention, activated bone remodeling, and chronically increased lean mass in men with little effect on bone mass.[174] In another study, after 6 months of GH administration, lean body mass, skin thickness, and lumbar vertebral bone density increased while adipose tissue mass decreased.[175] However, in one long-term study, by 1 year many of the subjects had withdrawn because of the development of carpal tunnel syndrome, gynecomastia, or hyperglycemia. Issues such as the effects of GH on gait and balance have not been examined, and its utility as a treatment for frailty in older individuals has not been elucidated.

MENOPAUSE

Menopause occurs at an average age of 51 in the United States, with a range of 41 to 59 years.[176] In premenopausal women, estradiol and estrone are produced by the ovarian follicles and aromatization of ovarian and adrenal steroid precursors. Estrogen receptors are found in the reproductive organs, central nervous system, liver, skin, heart, pancreas, adrenal glands, kidney, and bone. Estrogen is important for the hepatic production of proteins that bind hormones and ions, angiotensinogen, certain factors of coagulation, and high-density lipoprotein (HDL) and very low density lipoprotein (VLDL) apoproteins. Estrogen increases calcium absorption and inhibits bone resorption and deposition.[39]

Between the ages of 35 and 45, women may experience variations in menstrual cycles. During the perimenopausal period, the number of ova and follicles decreases and ovarian secretion of estrogens diminishes. There is a gradual rise in follicle stimulating hormone (FSH) and luteinizing hormone (LH), and estrone becomes the predominant estrogen produced by the aromatization of adrenal androstenedione in peripheral adipose tissue.[177]

Menopausal symptoms are due largely to estrogen deprivation and include vasomotor symptoms, urogenital atrophy, and osteoporosis. The "hot flash" is the most common postmenopausal complaint that affects the majority of women for 1 to 5 years but has been reported to occur as long as 16 years after menopause.[178] Flashes are closely associated with LH pulses.[179]

Estrogen loss can lead to vaginal, vulvar, and urethral atrophy. Thinning of vaginal epithelium, a decrease in lubrication, and an increase in pH can result in burning, dryness, pruritus, bleeding, and dyspareunia. Atrophy of the urethral mucosa results in dysuria and susceptibility to urinary tract infections.

Estrogen replacement is the most effective treatment for vasomotor symptoms, and it is becoming clear that long-term use can help prevent osteoporosis and cardiovascular disease. Oral estrogens are metabolized through the liver before being made available to other tissues. The hypercoagulability and hypertension seen with oral estrogen administration are related to the production of hepatic proteins (clotting factors, angiotensinogen, hormone- and ion-binding proteins) in response to estrogen stimulation. Topical and transdermal estrogens bypass the portal circulation and produce much less stimulation of the hepatic proteins.[180] Transdermal estradiol patches can decrease vasomotor symptoms but still require concomitant cycling with a progestational agent in a woman with an intact uterus. These patches do not, however, confer the benefit of increasing HDL cholesterol. Topical estrogens are helpful for the local treatment of urogenital symptoms but, because they are well absorbed, should be avoided in women with contraindications to estrogen therapy. Estrogens are not recommended for women with breast or endometrial cancers and women who are at risk for the development of thrombosis. Their use should be considered in the care of those with hypertension and atherosclerosis. In women who cannot take estrogen, clonidine and medroxyprogesterone can alleviate hot flashes.[181] Patients should have their blood pressure monitored and have breast, abdominal, and pelvic exams. Mammograms should be obtained annually.

HYPOGONADISM

Testosterone is produced by the Leydig's cells in the testes in response to the pulsatile release of LH. Testosterone in turn, through feedback inhibition, decreases the production of LH and gonadotropin releasing hormone (GnRH). With advancing age there are changes in the hypothalamic-pituitary-testicular axis. The number of Leydig's cells decreases with age,[182] and plasma testosterone levels decrease, although they may be maintained in very healthy older men.[183] The normal diurnal peak of testosterone secretion in the early morning hours is also diminished in older men.[184] As is consistent with primary testicular failure, this leads to an increase in LH and FSH.[185] In many older men, testosterone levels are low without a rise in gonadotropins, suggesting defects at the levels of the pituitary or hypothalamus.[186,187] The effects of FSH occur primarily in the seminiferous tubules. The rise in FSH reflects the degeneration in the seminiferous tubules and spermatids. Although actual sperm counts do not decrease markedly with age, the motility and morphology may become abnormal.

Testosterone and dihydrotestosterone (DHT) are bound to sex hormone-binding globulin (SHBG) and weakly bound to albumin in the circulation. With age, there is an increase in the plasma binding of circulating testosterone, resulting in a decrease in bioavailable testosterone (non-SHBG-bound testosterone).[188] Testosterone can exert its effects directly on its target tissue, be converted to DHT by 5 α-reductase in reproductive tissue and skin, or be aromatized to estradiol by adipose tissue and some brain neurons. Testosterone is clearly important for the maintenance of libido. The role of testosterone in maintaining potency is controversial and appears to be minor. Androgens are also important in bone metabolism. Hypogonadism can lead to increased osteoclastic activity and ultimately bone demineralization and osteopenia. In frail older men, low testosterone has been associated with minimal-trauma hip fracture. Testosterone replacement may inhibit bone resorption by increasing calcitonin secretion,[189] and its effects may be vitamin D-dependent.[190] Through direct effects on muscle, testosterone can increase muscle mass. In older hypogonadal men, a 3-month trial of testosterone was demonstrated to increase upper extremity muscle strength.[191] Further studies are needed to confirm this finding and demonstrate whether this effect is maintained over longer periods. Testosterone also can stimulate hematopoiesis, although data are variable regarding whether this is effected through erythropoietin.[192,193]

Testosterone administration has some associated side effects, including prostatic tissue enlargement, fluid retention, gynecomastia (because of its aromatization to estrogens), and liver function test abnormalities. Men who receive testosterone should have frequent monitoring of the prostate, prostate-specific antigen, blood pressures, hematocrit, and liver function tests. Currently, in the United States, only testosterone injections and patches are recommended because oral forms are associated with hepatotoxicity. While testosterone is recommended for the treatment of hypogonadism, it may also play a role in the treatment of frailty in older men.

SUMMARY

Diseases of the endocrine systems are common among older patients because of the loss of functional reserve associated with aging. Atypical or nonspecific presentations are common features of these diseases and may delay an appropriate diagnosis. While reports are conflicting regarding levels of arginine vasopressin secretion with age, older persons have an increased tendency to develop hypo- and hypernatremia and have a blunted thirst response to osmotic changes. Diabetes mellitus is a significant problem in older adults primarily because of the insulin resistance associated with aging. Older patients are also susceptible to the diabetic complications of soft tissue infections, visual difficulties, mononeuropathies, amyotrophy, strokes, and cognitive dysfunction. Treatment is best individualized, although dietary manipulations and long-acting hypoglycemics should be avoided. The most common cause of hypothyroidism in older persons is Hashimoto's thyroiditis, and treatment involves replacement with levothyroxine sodium. Graves' disease and multinodular goiter are frequent causes of hyperthyroidism in older adults and can be treated with radioactive iodine. Addison's disease presents with nonspecific symptoms, and the etiology of Cushing's disease is usually iatrogenic. The treatment and diagnosis of these adrenal disorders are similar in young and old patients. With age, vitamin D decreases, PTH rises secondary to reduced renal function, and osteoporosis becomes an increasingly significant problem in older women and men. Levels of GH and insulin-like growth factor-I decline with age, and GH administration has been noted to improve lean body mass and vertebral bone density. Sex hormones decline with age in both women and men. Menopausal symptoms are generally treated with estrogens and may prevent type I osteoporosis. Testosterone replacement in older hypogonadal men can improve libido, blood counts, upper body strength, and possibly bone density.

REFERENCES

1. Phillips PA, Ledingham JGG, Rolls B, et al: Reduced thirst perception after water deprivation in a healthy elderly man. *N Engl J Med* 311:7536, 1984.
2. Helderman JH, Vestal RE, Rowe JW, et al: The response of arginine vasopressin to intravenous ethanol and hypertonic saline in man: The impact of aging. *J Gerontol* 33:39, 1978.
3. Phillips PA, Bretherton M, Risvanis J, et al: Effects of drinking on thirst and vasopressin in dehydrated elderly men. *Am J Physiol* 264:R877, 1993.
4. Phillips PA, Bretherton M, Johnston CI, Gray L: Reduced osmotic thirst in healthy elderly men. *Am J Physiol* 261:R166, 1991.
5. McLean KA, O'Neill PA, Davies I, Catania J: Changes in the response to a saline load with age. *Clin Sci* 81:6P, 1991.
6. Duggan J, Catania J, O'Neill PA, Davies I: Response to dehydration in long term care elderly patients. *Clin Sci* 82:27P, 1992.
7. Helderman JH: The impact of normal aging on the hypothalamic-neurohypophyseal-renal axis, in Korenman SG (ed): *Endocrine Aspects of Aging*. New York: Elsevier Biomedical, 1982, pp 9–32.
8. Faull CM, Holmes C, Baylis PH: Water balance in elderly people: Is there a deficiency of vasopressin? *Age Ageing* 22:114, 1993.
9. Bursztyn M, Bresnahan M, Gavras I, Bavras H: Effect of aging on vasopressin, catecholamines and alpha 2-adrenergic receptors. *J Am Geriatr Soc* 38:628, 1990.
10. Rowe JW, Minaker KL, Sparrow D, Robertson GL: Age related failure of volume-pressure mediated vasopressin release. *J Clin Endocrinol Metab* 54:661, 1982.
11. Segar WE, Moore WW: The regulation of ADH release in man: Effects of change in position and ambient temperature on blood ADH levels. *J Clin Invest* 17:2143, 1968.
12. Aspund R, Aberg H: Diurnal variation in the levels of antidiuretic hormone in the elderly. *J Intern Med* 229:131, 1991.
13. North WG, Harbaught R, Reeder T: An evaluation of human neurophysin production in Alzheimer's Disease: Preliminary observations. *Neurobiol Aging* 13:261, 1992.
14. Albert SG, Nakra BR, Grossberg GT, Caminal ER: Vasopressin response to dehydration in Alzheimer's disease. *J Am Geriatr Soc* 37:843, 1989.
15. Sloan RW, Kreider RM, Luderer JR: The effect of chlorpropamide hyponatremia on mental status in a nursing home population. *J Fam Pract* 16:937, 1983.
16. Harris MI, Hadden WC, Knowler WC, Bennett PH: Prevalence of diabetes and impaired glucose tolerance and plasma glucose levels in the US population aged 20 to 74 years. *Diabetes* 36:523, 1987.

17. Huse DM, Oster G, Killen AR, et al: The economic costs of NIDDM. *JAMA* 262:2708, 1989.
18. Trends in diabetes mellitus mortality, in Gregg MP (ed): *MMWR* Morbidity and Mortality Weekly Report, Atlanta, Centers for Disease Control, 37:769, 1988.
19. Panzram G, Zabel-Langhennig R: Prognosis of diabetes mellitus in a geographically defined population. *Diabetologia* 20:587, 1981.
20. Fitzgerald MG: Diabetes, in Brocklehurst JC (ed): *Textbook of Geriatric Medicine and Gerontology*. Edinburgh: Churchill-Livingstone, 1973, pp 458–75.
21. Naliboff BD, Rosenthal M: Effects of age on complications in adult onset diabetes. *J Am Geriatr Soc* 37:838, 1989.
22. Bennett PH: *Report of Work Group on Epidemiology* (USDHEW Publication No. NIH 76-1021), vol 3, pt 1. Washington, DC: National Commission on Diabetes, 1976, pp 63–133.
23. WHO Expert Committee on Diabetes Mellitus: *Second Report*. Geneva: WHO, 1980. World Health Organization Tech Rep Ser 646:1–80.
24. Chen M, Bergman RN, Parte D Jr: Insulin resistance and beta cell dysfunction in aging: The importance of dietary carbohydrate. *J Clin Endocrinol Metab* 67:951, 1988.
25. Tonino RP: Effect of physical training on the insulin resistance of aging. *Am J Physiol* 256:E352, 1989.
26. Hollenbeck CB, Haskell W, Rosenthal M, Reaven GM: Effect of habitual physical activity on regulation of insulin-stimulated glucose disposal in older males. *J Am Geriatr Soc* 33:273, 1984.
27. Sparrow D, Borkan GA, Gerzof SG, et al: Relationship of fat distribution to glucose tolerance: Results of computed tomography in male participants of the normative aging study. *Diabetes* 35:411, 1986.
28. Supiano MA, Hogikyan RV, Morrow LA, et al: Aging and insulin sensitivity: Role of blood pressure and sympathetic nervous system activity. *J Gerontol* 48:M237, 1993.
29. Pacini G, Baleria A, Beccara F, et al: Insulin sensitivity and beta cell responsivity are not decreased in elderly subjects with normal OGTT. *J Am Geriatr Soc* 36:317, 1988.
30. Reaven GM: Role of insulin resistance in human disease. *Diabetes* 37:1595, 1988.
31. Morley JE, Mooradian AD, Rosenthal MJ, Kaiser FE: Diabetes mellitus in the elderly. Is it different? *Am J Med* 83:533, 1987.
32. Yki-Jarvinen H, Kubo K, Zawadzki J, et al: Dissociation of in vitro sensitivities of glucose transport and antilipolysis to insulin in NIDDM. *Am J Physiol* 253 (Endocrine Metab 16):E300, 1987.
33. Chen M, Bergman RN, Pacini G, Porte D Jr: Pathogenesis of age-related glucose intolerance in man: Insulin resistance and decreased beta cell function. *J Clin Endocrinol Metab* 60:13, 1985.
34. O'Rahilly S, Turner RC, Matthews D: Impaired pulsatile secretion of insulin in relatives of patients with NIDDM. *N Engl J Med* 318:1225, 1984.
35. Duckworth WC, Kitabchi AW: Direct measurement of plasma proinsulin in normal and diabetic subjects. *Am J Med* 53:418, 1972.
36. Duckworth WC, Kitabchi AW: The effect of age on plasma proinsulin in response to oral glucose. *J Lab Clin Med* 8:359, 1976.
37. Minaker KL, Rowe JW, Tonino R: Influence of age on clearance of insulin in man. *Diabetes* 31:851, 1982.
38. Davidson MB: The effect of aging on carbohydrate metabolism: A comprehensive review and a practical approach to the clinical problem, in Korenman SG (ed): *Endocrine Aspects of Aging*. New York: Elsevier Biomedical, 1982, pp 231–267.

39. Mooradian AD, Morley JE, Korenman SG: Endocrinology in aging. *Dis Mon* July 1988, p 398.
40. Carroll P, Matz R: Uncontrolled diabetes mellitus in adults: Experience in treatment of diabetic ketoacidosis and hyperosmolar nonketotic coma with low dose insulin and uniform treatment regimen. *Diabetes Care* 6:579, 1983.
41. Morley JE, Perry HM: The management of diabetes mellitus in older individual. *Drugs* 41:548, 1991.
42. Kadowaki T, Hagura R, Kajinuma H, et al: Chlorpropamide-induced hyponatremia: Incidence and risk factors. *Diabetes Care* 6:468, 1983.
43. Feldman JM: Review of glyburide after one year on the market. *Am J Med* 79:102, 1985.
44. Puxty JAM, Hunter DM, Burr WA: Accuracy of insulin injection in elderly patients. *Br Med J* 287:1762, 1983.
45. Kaiser FE, Morley JE: Endocrine changes in the elderly, in Katlic MR (ed): *Geriatric Surgery: Comprehensive Care of the Elderly Patient.* Baltimore-Munich: Urban and Schwarzenberg, 1990, pp 115–127.
46. Leske MC, Sperduto RD: The epidemiology of senile cataracts: A review. *Am J Epidemiol* 118:152, 1983.
47. Bresnick GH, Groo A, Palta M, North K: Urinary glucose testing inaccuracies among diabetic patients: Effect of acquired color-vision deficiency caused by diabetic retinopathy. *Arch Ophthalmol* 102:1489, 1984.
48. Tattersall RB: Diabetes in the elderly—a neglected area? *Diabetologia* 27:167, 1984.
49. Pulsinelli WA, Levy DE, Sigsbee B, et al: Increased damage after ischemic stroke in patients with hyperglycemia with or without established diabetes mellitus. *Am J Med* 74:540, 1983.
50. Morley JE, Flood JF: Psychosocial aspects of diabetes mellitus in the older person. *J Am Geriatr Soc* 38:605, 1990.
51. Perlmuter LC, Hakami MK, Hodgson-Harrington C, et al: Decreased cognitive function in aged non insulin-dependent diabetic patients. *Am J Med* 77:1043, 1984.
52. Gradman TJ, Laws A, Thompson LW, Reaven GM: Verbal learning and/or memory improves with glycemic control in older subjects with noninsulin diabetes mellitus. *J Am Geriatr Soc* 41:1305, 1993.
53. Reaven GM, Thompson LW, Nahum D, Haskins E: Relationship between hyperglycemia and cognitive function in older NIDDM patients. *Diabetes Care* 13:16, 1990.
54. Murawski BJ, Chazan BI, Balodimos MC, Ryan JR: Personality patterns in patients with diabetes mellitus of long duration. *Diabetes* 19:259, 1970.
55. Coulston AM, Mandelbaum D, Reaven GM: Dietary management of nursing home residents with non-insulin-dependent diabetes mellitus. *Am J Clin Nutr* 51:67, 1990.
56. Morley JE: Impotence. *Am J Med* 80:897, 1986.
57. Kinlaw WB, Levine AS, Morley JE, et al: Abnormal zinc metabolism in type II diabetes mellitus. *Am J Med* 75:273, 1983.
58. Mooradian AD, Morley JE: Micronutrient status in diabetes mellitus. *Am J Clin Nutr* 45:877, 1987.
59. Niewoehner CB, Allen JI, Boosalis M, et al: The role of zinc supplementation in type II diabetes mellitus. *Am J Med* 81:63, 1986.
60. Hallbook T, Lanner E: Serum zinc and healing of venous leg ulcers. *Lancet* 2:780, 1972.
61. Gregerman RI: Thyroid diseases, in Hazzard WR, Andres R, Bierman EL, Blass JP

(eds): *Principles of Geriatric Medicine and Gerontology.* New York, McGraw-Hill, 1990, pp 719–738.
62. Denham MJ, Wills EJ: A clinico-pathological survey of the thyroid gland in old age. *Gerontology* 36:160, 1980.
63. Maxon HR, Thomas SR, Saenger EL, et al: Ionizing irradiation and the induction of clinically significant disease in the human thyroid gland. *Am J Med* 63:967, 1977.
64. Levy EG: Thyroid disease in the elderly. *Med Clin North Am* 75:151, 1991.
65. Britton KE, Quinn V, Ellis SM, et al: Is "T4 toxicosis" a normal biochemical finding in elderly women? *Lancet* 2:141, 1975.
66. Harman, SM, Wehman RE, Blackman MR: Pituitary-thyroid hormone economy in healthy aging men: Basal indices of thyroid function and thyrotropin response to constant infusions of thyrotropin-releasing hormone. *J Clin Endocrinol Metab* 58:320, 1984.
67. Melmed S, Hershman JM: The thyroid and aging, in Korenman SG (ed): *Endocrine Aspects of Aging.* New York: Elsevier Biomedical, 1982, pp 33–54.
68. Robuschi G, Safran M, Braverman LE, et al: Hypothyroidism in the elderly. *Endocr Rev* 8:142, 1987.
69. Wartofsky L, Burman KD: Alterations in thyroid functions in patients with systemic illness: The euthyroid sick syndrome. *Endocr Rev* 3:164, 1982.
70. Ordene KW, Pan C, Barzel US, Surks MI: Variable thyrotropin response to thyrotropin releasing hormone after small decreases in plasma thyroid hormone concentration in patients of advanced age. *Metabolism* 32:881, 1983.
71. Harman SM, Wehmann RE, Blackman MR: Pituitary-thyroid hormone economy in healthy aging men: Basal indices of thyroid function and TSH responses to constant infusion of TSH. *J Clin Endocrinol Metab* 58:320, 1984.
72. Tunbridge WMG, Evered O, Hall R, et al: The spectrum of thyroid disease in a community: The Whickham survey. *Clin Endocrinol (Oxf)* 7:481, 1977.
73. Kaiser FE: Variability of responses to TRH in normal elderly. *Age Ageing* 16:345, 1987.
74. Jacques C, Schlienger JL, Kissel C, et al: TRH-induced TSH and prolactin responses in the elderly. *Age Ageing* 16:181, 1987.
75. Snyder PJ, Utiger RD: Thyrotropin response to thyrotropin releasing hormone in normal females over forty. *J Clin Endocrinol Metab* 34:1096, 1972.
76. Snyder PJ, Utiger RD: Response to thyrotropin releasing hormone (TRH) in normal man. *J Clin Endocrinol Metab* 34:380, 1972.
77. Morley JE: Neuroendocrine control of thyrotropin secretion. *Endocr Rev* 2:396, 1981.
78. Sawin CT, Castelli WP, Hershman JM, et al: The aging thyroid: Thyroid deficiency in the Framingham study. *Arch Intern Med* 145:1386, 1985.
79. Kavorian GD, Wong NCW, Mooradian AD: Unusual manifestations of hypothyroidism in an elderly patient. *Geriatr Med Today* 6:28, 1987.
80. Kabadi UM: "Subclinical hypothyroidism": Natural course of the syndrome during a prolonged follow up study. *Arch Intern Med* 153:957, 1993.
81. Rosenthal MJ, Hunt WC, Garre PJ, Goodwin JS: Thyroid failure in the elderly: Microsomal antibodies as discriminant for therapy. *JAMA* 258:209, 1987.
82. Cooper DS, Halpern R, Wood LC, et al: L-thyroxine therapy in subclinical hypothyroidism: A double blind, placebo-controlled trial. *Ann Intern Med* 101:18, 1984.
83. Rosenbaum RL, Barzeli US: Levothyroxine replacement dose for primary hypothyroidism decreases with age. *Ann Intern Med* 96:53, 1962.
84. Gregerman RI, Gaffney GW, Shock NW: Thyroxine turnover in euthyroid man with special reference to changes with age. *J Clin Invest* 41:2065, 1962.

85. Rees-Jones RW, Rolla AR, Larsen PR: Hormonal content of thyroid replacement preparations. *JAMA* 243:549, 1980.
86. Bernstein R, Muller C, Midtbo K, et al: Cardiac left ventricular function before and during early thyroxine treatment in severe hypothyroidism. *J Intern Med* 230:493, 1991.
87. Nicoloff JT: Thyroid storm and myxedema coma. *Med Clin North Am* 69:1005, 1985.
88. Nicoloff JT, Lo Presti JS: Myxedema coma: A form of decompensated hypothyroidism. *Endocrinol Metab Clin North Am* 22:279, 1993.
89. Arlot S, Debussche X, Lalau JD, et al: Myxedema coma: Response of thyroid hormones with other oral and intravenous high-dose L-thyroxine treatment. *Intensive Care Med* 17:16, 1991.
90. Bartels EC, Kingsley JWJ: Hyperthyroidism in patients over 65. *Geriatrics* 4:333, 1949.
91. Davis PJ, Davis FB: Hyperthyroidism in patients over the age of 60 years. *Medicine (Baltimore)* 53:161, 1974.
92. Tibaldi JM, Barzel US, Albin J, Surks M: Thyrotoxicosis in the very old. *Am J Med* 81:619, 1986.
93. Mooradian A, Morley JE, Simon G, Shafer RB: Propranolol-induced hyperthyroxinemia. *Arch Intern Med* 143:2193, 1983.
94. Seth J, Kellett HA, Caldwell G, et al: Sensitive immunoradiometric assay for serum thyroid stimulating hormone: A replacement for the thyrotropin-releasing hormone test? *Br Med J* 289:1334, 1984.
95. Griffin MA, Solomon DH: Hyperthyroidism in the elderly. *J Am Geriatr Soc* 34:887, 1986.
96. Wolfsen AR: Aging and the adrenals, in Korenman SG (ed): *Endocrine Aspects of Aging*. New York: Elsevier-North Holland, 1982, pp 55–74.
97. Drafta D, Schindler AE, Stroe E, Neacsu E: Age-related changes of plasma steroids in normal adult males. *J Steroid Biochem* 17:683, 1982.
98. Serman B, Wysham C, Pfohl B: Age-related changes in the circadian rhythm of plasma cortisol in man. *J Clin Endocrinol Metab* 61:439, 1985.
99. West CD, Brown H, Simons EL, et al: Adrenocortical function and cortisol metabolism in old age. *J Clin Endocrinol Metab* 21:1197, 1961.
100. Blichert-Toft M, Blichert-Toft B, Jensen HK: Pituitary-adrenocortical stimulation in the aged as reflected in levels of plasma cortisol and compounds. *Acta Chir Scand* 136:665, 1970.
101. Cartlidge NE, Black MM, Hall MR, Hall R: Pituitary function in the elderly. *Gerontol Clin* 12:65, 1970.
102. Muggeo M, Fedele D, Tiengo A, et al: Human growth hormone and cortisol response to insulin stimulation in aging. *J Gerontol* 30:546, 1975.
103. Blichert-Toft M: Secretion of corticotrophin and somatotophin by the senescent adenohypophysis in man. *Acta Endocrinol (Copenh)* 78(suppl):115, 1975.
104. Greden JF, Flegel P, Haskett R, et al: Age effects in serial hypothalamic-pituitary-adrenal monitoring. *Psychoneuroendocrinology* 11:195, 1986.
105. Asnis GM, Sachar EJ, Halbreich U, et al: Cortisol secretion in relation to age in major depression. *Psychosom Med* 43:235, 1981.
106. Pavlov EP, Harman SM, Chrousos GP, et al: Responses of plasma adrenocorticotropin, cortisol, and dehydroepiandrosterone to ovine corticotropin releasing hormone in healthy aging men. *J Clin Endocrinol Metab* 62:767, 1986.
107. Irvine WJ, Barnes EW: Addison's disease, ovarian failure and hypoparathyroidism. *Clin Endocrinol Metab* 4:379, 1975.

108. Hutter AM, Kayhoe DE: Adrenal cortical carcinoma: Clinical features of 138 patients. *Am J Med* 41:572, 1966.
109. Davis KL, Davis BM, Mathe AA, et al: Age and the dexamethasone suppression test in depression. *Am J Psych* 141:872, 1984.
110. Nelson WH, Orr WW Jr, Shane SR, Stevenson JM: Hypothalamic-pituitary-adrenal axis activity and age in major depression. *J Clin Psychiatry* 45:120, 1984.
111. Parker LN, Odell WD: Decline of adrenal androgen production as measured by radioimmunoassay of urinary conjugated dehydroepiandrosterone. *J Clin Endocrinol Metab* 47:600, 1978.
112. Morley JE, Flood JF: An investigation of tolerance to the actions of leptogenic and anorexigenic drugs in mice. *Life Sci* 41:2157, 1987.
113. Coleman DL, Leiter EM, Applezweig N: Therapeutic effects of dehydroepiandrosterone metabolites in diabetic mutant mice (C57 GL/KsJ-db/db). *Endocrinology* 115:239, 1984.
114. Pashko LL, Schwartz AG: Effect of food restriction, dehydroepiandrosterone or obesity on the binding of 3H-7, 12 dimethylbenz(a) anthracene to mouse skin DNA. *J Gerontol* 38:8, 1983.
115. Barrett-Connor E, Khaw KT, Yen SSC: A prospective study of dehydroepiandrosterone sulfate, mortality, and cardiovascular disease. *N Engl J Med* 315:1519, 1986.
116. Rudman D, Shetty KR, Mattson DE: Plasma dehydroepiandrosterone sulfate in nursing home men. *J Am Geriatr Soc* 38:421, 1990.
117. Flood JF, Roberts E: Dehydroepiandrosterone sulfate improves memory in aging mice. *Brain Res* 448:178, 1988.
118. Morley JE, Kaiser FE: Personal communication, 1994.
119. Akwa Y, Young J, Kabbadi K, et al: Neurosteroids: Biosynthesis, metabolism and function of pregnenolone and dehydroepiandrosterone in the brain. *J Steroid Biochem Molec Biol* 40:71, 1991.
120. Majewska ME, Demirgoren S, Ondon ED: Binding of pregnenolone sulfate to rat brain membranes suggests multiple sites of steroid action at the $GABA_A$ receptor. *Eur J Pharmacol* 189:307, 1990.
121. Majewska MD, Mienville JM, Vicini S: Neurosteroid pregnenolone sulfate antagonizes electrophysiological responses to GABA in neurons. *Neurosci Lett* 90:279, 1988.
122. Majewska MD, Schwartz RD: Pregnenolone-sulfate: An endogenous antagonist of the gamma-aminobutyric acid receptor complex in brain? *Brain Res* 404:355, 1987.
123. Irwin RP, Maragakis NJ, Rogawski MA, et al: Pregnenolone sulfate augments NMDA receptor mediated increases in intracellular CA^{2+} in cultured rat hippocampal neurons. *Neurosci Lett* 141:30, 1992.
124. Wu FS, Gibbs TT, Farb DH: Pregnenolone sulfate: A positive allosteric modulator at the N-methyl-D-aspartate receptor. *Mol Pharmacol* 40:333, 1991.
125. Morris RGM, Anderson E, Lynch GS, Baudry M: Selective impairment of learning and blockade of long-term potentiation by an N-methyl-D-aspartate receptor antagonist, AP5. *Nature* 319:774, 1986.
126. Rothman SM, Olney JW: Excitotoxicity and the NMDA receptor. *Trends Neurosci* 10:299, 1987.
127. Flood JF, Morley JE, Roberts E: Memory-enhancing effects in male mice of pregnenolone and steroids metabolically derived from it. *Proc Natl Acad Sci USA* 89:1567, 1992.

128. Mayo W, Dellu F, Robel, et al: Infusion of neurosteroids into the nucleus basalis magnocellularis affects cognitive processes in the rat. *Brain Res* 607:324, 1993.
129. Steiger A, Trachsel L, Guldner J, et al: Neurosteroid pregnenolone induces sleep-EEG changes in man compatible with inverse agonistic $GABA_A$-receptor modulation. *Brain Res* 615:267, 1993.
130. Esler M, Jackman G, Bobik A, et al: Determination of norepinephrine apparent release rate and clearance in humans. *Life Sci* 25:1461, 1979.
131. Hoeldtke RD, Cilmi KM: Effects of aging on catecholamine metabolism. *J Clin Endocrinol Metab* 60:479, 1985.
132. Veith RC, Featherstone JA, Linares OA, Halter JB: Age differences in plasma norepinephrine kinetics in humans. *J Gerontol* 41:319, 1986.
133. Schwartz RS, Jaeger LF, Veith RC: The importance of body composition to the increase in plasma norepinephrine appearance rate in elderly men. *J Gerontol* 42:546, 1987.
134. Feldman RD, Limbird LE, Nadeau J, et al: Alterations in leukocyte beta-receptor affinity with aging: A potential explanation for altered beta-adrenergic sensitivity in the elderly. *N Engl J Med* 310:815, 1984.
135. Abrass IB, Scarpace PJ: Catalytic unit of adenylate cyclase: Reduced activity in aged human lymphocytes. *J Clin Endocrinol Metab* 55:1026, 1982.
136. Keating FR, Jones JD, Elveback LR, Randall RV: The relation of age and sex to distribution of values in healthy adults of serum calcium, inorganic phosphorus, magnesium, alkaline phosphatase, total proteins, albumin, and blood urea. *J Lab Clin Med* 73:825, 1969.
137. Aksnes L, Rodland O, Odegaard OR, et al: Serum levels of vitamin D metabolites in the elderly. *Acta Endocrinol (Copenh)* 121:27, 1989.
138. Riggs BL, Gallagher JC, DeLuca HF, et al: A syndrome of osteoporosis, increased serum immunoreactive parathyroid hormone and inappropriately low 1,25 dihydroxyvitamin D. *Mayo Clin Proc* 53:701, 1978.
139. Dandona P, Menon RK, Shenoy R, et al: Low 1,25 dihydroxyvitamin D, secondary hyperparathyroidism, and normal osteocalcin in elderly subjects. *J Clin Endocrinol Metab* 63:459, 1986.
140. Turner G, Brown RC, Silver A, et al: Renal insufficiency and secondary hyperparathyroidism in elderly patients. *Ann Clin Biochem* 28:321, 1991.
141. Compston JE, Silver AC, Croucher PI, et al: Elevated serum intact parathyroid hormone levels in elderly patients with hip fracture. *Clin Endocrinol (Oxf)* 31:667, 1989.
142. Morimoto S, Takamoto S, Imanaka S, et al: Comparison of the production of cyclic AMP in response to parathyroid hormone in fibroblasts from aged subjects and young subjects: Lack of an age-dependent decrease. *Gerontology* 36:249, 1990.
143. Riggs BL, Melton LJ III: Involutional osteoporosis. *N Eng J Med* 314:1676, 1986.
144. Riggs BL, Wahner HW, Dunn WL, et al: Differential changes in bone mineral density of the appendicular and axial skeleton with aging: Relationship to spinal osteoporosis. *J Clin Invest* 67:328, 1981.
145. Lindsay R, Hart DM, Forrest C, Baird C: Prevention of spinal osteoporosis in oophorectomized women. *Lancet* 2:1151, 1980.
146. Francis RM, Peacock M, Aaron JE: Osteoporosis in hypogonadal men: Role of decreased plasma 1,25 dihydroxyvitamin D, calcium malabsorption and low bone formation. *Bone* 7:261, 1986.
147. Morley JE, Gorkin MJ, Mooradian AD, et al: UCLA geriatric grand rounds: Osteoporosis. *J Am Geriatr Soc* 36:845, 1988.

148. Perry HM III: Thyroid hormones and bone mass, in Peck WE (ed): *Annual Review of Bone and Mineral Research,* 6:113–139, 1989.
149. Heath H III, Hodgson SF, Kennedy MA: Primary hyperparathyroidism incidence, morbidity and potential economic impact in a community. *N Engl J Med* 302:189, 1980.
150. Beylink DJ: Glucocorticoid induced osteoporosis. *N Engl J Med* 309:306, 1983.
151. Kleerekoper M, Avioli LV: Evaluation and treatment of postmenopausal osteoporosis, in Favus MJ (ed): *Primer on the Metabolic Bone Diseases and Disorders of Mineral Metabolism.* Richmond, VA: William Byrd Press, 1990, pp 223–229.
152. Melton LJ, Riggs BL: Epidemiology of age-related fractures, in Alvioli LV (ed): *The Osteoporotic Syndrome: Detection and Prevention.* New York: Grune & Stratton, 1983, pp 45–72.
153. Delmas PD, Stenner D, Wahner HW, et al: Increase in serum bone gamma-carboxyglutamic acid protein with aging in women: Implications for the mechanism of age-related bone loss. *J Clin Invest* 71:1316, 1983.
154. Storm T, Thamsborg G, Steinichi T, et al: Effect of intermittent cyclic etidronate therapy on bone mass and fracture rate in women with postmenopausal osteoporosis. *N Engl J Med* 322:1265, 1990.
155. Wasnich RD, Ross PD, Heilbrun LK, et al: Differential effects of thiazide and estrogen upon bone mineral content and fracture prevalence. *Obstet Gynecol* 67:457, 1986.
156. Minaire P, Neuneir P, Edouard C: Quantitative histological data on disuse osteoporosis: Comparison with biological data. *Calcif Tissue Res* 17:57, 1974.
157. Heath H, Hodgson S, Kennedy M: Primary hyperparathyroidism: Incidence, morbidity, and potential economic impact in a community. *N Engl J Med* 302:189, 1980.
158. Sier HC, Hartnell J, Morley JE, et al: Primary hyperparathyroidism and delirium in the elderly. *J Am Geriatr Soc* 36:157, 1988.
159. Selby PL, Peacock M: Ethinyl estradiol and norethindrone in the treatment of primary hyperparathyroidism in postmenopausal women. *N Engl J Med* 314:1481, 1986.
160. Salti IS, Mouradian A, Amiri Z, Khalil A: Hypopituitarism in a patient with idiopathic hypoparathyroidism. *Can Med Assoc J* 126:942, 1982.
161. Trence DL, Morley JE, Handwerger BS: Polyglandular autoimmune syndromes. *Am J Med* 77:107, 1984.
162. Weidermann CJ, Niedermuhlbichler M, Beimpold H, Braunsteiner H: In vitro activation of neutrophils of the aged by recombinant human growth hormone. *J Infect Dis* 164:1017, 1991.
163. Wiedemann E, Schwartz E, Frantz AG: Acute and chronic estrogen effects upon serum somatomedin activity, growth hormone, and prolactin in man. *J Clin Endocrinol Metab* 42:942, 1976.
164. Frantz AG, Rabkin MT: Effects of estrogen and sex difference on secretion of human growth hormone. *J Clin Endocrinol Metab* 25:1470, 1965.
165. Prinz PN, Weitzman ED, Cunningham GR, Karacan I: Plasma growth hormone during sleep in young and aged men. *J Gerontol* 38:519, 1983.
166. Vermeulen A: Nyctohemeral growth hormone profiles in young and aged men: Correlation with somatomedin-C levels. *J Clin Endocrinol Metab* 645:884, 1987.
167. Shibasaki T, Shizume K, Nakahara M, et al: Age-related changes in plasma growth

hormone response to growth hormone releasing factor in man. *J Clin Endocrinol Metab* 58:212, 1984.
168. Pavlov EP, Harman SM, Merriam GR, et al: Responses of growth hormone (GH) and somatomedin C to GH releasing hormone in healthy aging men. *J Clin Endocrinol Metab* 62:595, 1986.
169. Laron Z, Doron M, Amikam B: Plasma growth hormone in old age. *Harefuah* 73:375, 1967.
170. Conover CA, Dollar LA, Rosenfeld RG, Hintz RL: Somatomedin C binding and actions in fibroblasts from aged and progeric subjects. *J Clin Endocrinol Metab* 60:685, 1985.
171. Kaiser FE, Silver AJ, Morley JE: The effect of recombinant human growth hormone on malnourished older individuals. *J Am Geriatr Soc* 39:235, 1991.
172. Ziegler TR, Rombeau JL, Young LS, et al: Recombinant human growth hormone enhances the metabolic efficacy of parenteral nutrition: A double-blind, randomized controlled study. *J Clin Endocrinol Metab* 74:865, 1992.
173. Lehmann S, Cerra FB: Growth hormone and nutritional support: Adverse metabolic effects. *Nutr Clin Pract* 7:27, 1992.
174. Marcus R, Holloway L, Butterfield G: Clinical uses of growth hormone in older people. *J Reprod Fertil* 46:115, 1993.
175. Rudman D, Feller AG, Nagraj HS, et al: Effects of human growth hormone in men over 60 years old. *N Engl J Med* 323:1, 1990.
176. Kaiser FE, Morley JE: The menopause and beyond, in Cassel CR, Reisenberg D (eds): *Geriatric Medicine.* New York: Springer-Verlag, 1990, pp 279–290.
177. Judd HL, Shamonki IM, Frumar AM, Lagasse LD: Origin of serum estradiol in postmenopausal women. *Obstet Gynecol* 59:680, 1982.
178. Feldman BM, Voda A, Gronseth E: The prevalence of hot flash and associated variables among perimenopausal women. *Res Nurs Health* 8:261, 1985.
179. Casper RF, Yen SSC, Wilkes MM: Menopausal flushes: A neuroendocrine link with pulsatile luteinizing hormone secretion. *Science* 205:823, 1979.
180. Chetkowski RJ, Meldrum DR, Steingold KA, et al: Biologic effects of transdermal estradiol. *N Engl J Med* 314:1615, 1986.
181. Schiff I, Tulchinsky D, Cramer D, Ryan KJ: Oral medroxyprogesterone in the treatment of postmenopausal symptoms. *JAMA* 244:1443, 1980.
182. Tillenger K: Testicular morphology. *Acta Endocrinol (Copenh)* 24(suppl):1, 1957.
183. Swerdloff RS, Heber D: Effects of aging on male reproductive function, in Korenman SG (ed): *Endocrine Aspects of Aging.* New York: Elsevier Biomedical, 1982, pp 119–135.
184. Bremner WJ, Vitiello MV, Prinz PN: Loss of circadian rhythmicity in blood testosterone levels with aging in normal men. *J Clin Endocrinol Metab* 56:1278, 1983.
185. Deslypere JP, Verneulen A: Leydig cell function in normal men: Effect of age, life style, residence, diet and activity. *J Clin Endocrinol Metab* 59:955, 1986.
186. Slag MF, Morley JE, Elson MK, et al: Impotence in medical clinic outpatients *JAMA* 249:1736, 1983.
187. Morley JE, Kaiser FE: Hypogonadism in the elderly male. *Adv Endocrinol* 4:241–262, 1993.
188. Nankin HR, Calkins JH: Decreased bioavailable testosterone in aging normal and impotent men. *J Clin Endocrinol Metab* 63:1418, 1986.
189. Foresta C, Scanelli G, Zanatta GP, et al: Reduced calcitonin reserve in young hypogonadic osteoporotic men. *Horm Metab Res* 19:275, 1987.

190. Somjen D, Kaye AM, Harell A, Weisman Y: Modulation by vitamin D status of the responsiveness of rat bone to gonadal steroids. *Endocrinology* 125:1870, 1989.
191. Morley JE, Perry HM III, Kaiser FE, et al: Effects of testosterone replacement therapy in older hypogonadal males: A preliminary study. *J Am Geriatr Soc* 41:149, 1992.
192. Alexanian R: Erythropoietin and erythropoiesis in anemic man following androgens. *Blood* 33:564, 1969.
193. Weber JP, Walsh PC, Peters CA, Spivak JL: Effect of reversible androgen deprivation on hemoglobin and serum immunoreactive erythropoietin in men. *Am J Hematol* 36:190, 1991.

CHAPTER 5

Physiological Changes with Aging in the Kidney and Liver

Mary Ann Gurkowski

INTRODUCTION

This chapter examines the biological effects of aging on the renal and hepatic systems. Much literature has been published regarding the effects of aging on these two organ systems. The changes that accompany aging are both functional and structural. Anesthesiologists need to be familiar with these alterations, which can affect the methods, dosages, and dosing intervals of drug therapy in the elderly.

The wealth of available data on aging and the renal and hepatic systems precludes a detailed examination of the subject here. Thus, this chapter addresses the major changes in function with senescence in order to lay a foundation for understanding drug and fluid therapy.

RENAL SYSTEM

Anatomy of the Aging Kidney

Size

The first descriptions of anatomic alterations in the aging human kidney were published over 60 years ago.[1] A gradual decline in kidney size was the earliest renal anatomic change to be described. The kidneys decrease in size after age 30 such that an approximate 20 percent drop in weight occurs by age 70. Therefore, a kidney weighing 250 g at age 30 will weigh only 200 g by age 70. The renal mass that is lost is a combination of both cortical and parenchymal tissue, with the majority coming from the renal cortex.[2] Within the cortex, this loss is shared equally by both the glomerular and the tubular areas, and the relative relation between these two areas appears to remain constant.[3] The renal parenchyma decreases about 10 percent per decade of increasing age in both sexes.[4]

Microscopic examination of the glomeruli shows a variety of changes with aging. The number of tubular and glomerular cells decreases significantly, as does the number of glomerular tufts per unit area. Conversely, the size of the glomerular tufts and nuclei of the glomerular and tubular cells increases with advancing age.[3] Clinically, the most important histological change is the steady increase in the number of sclerotic glomeruli after age 40.[5] In fact, although fewer than 1 percent of glomeruli are sclerotic in young adults, this proportion rises to 10 to 30 percent by age 80.[6] This age-related sclerosis is not evenly distributed throughout the kidney. As was already mentioned, the loss of outer renal cortex is greater than the loss of juxtamedullary units.

Renal Tubules

The renal tubules, in particular the proximal tubules, also experience change with aging, appearing to decrease in length, number, and thickness.[3] This decrease in proximal tubule length has been found to occur in a fashion that parallels the decrease in the number of glomerular tufts.[7] This relation could explain the parallel decline in glomerular and tubular function in the senescent kidney. Diverticula of the distal and collecting tubules are also more prominent[7] and may be predecessors to the renal retention cysts often seen in the elderly.[8]

Renal Vasculature

The renal vasculature also experiences structural changes with aging. Two general patterns of change have been described in the glomerular and afferent-efferent arteriolar vascular structures.[9–10] These two patterns of change have been termed the "cortical" pattern and the "juxtamedullary" pattern. In the cortical pattern of vascular changes, the afferent arteriolar lumen becomes obliterated and blood flow ceases as glomerular myelinization and sclerosis progress. These changes can progress to complete death of the nephron. In the juxtamedullary pattern, the atrophy is asymmetric such that progressive glomerular sclerosis is not accompanied by loss of blood flow. Efferent arterioles are larger than those in the cortical areas, and alterations in afferent arteriolar and glomerular flow lead to the development of anatomic shunts between the afferent-efferent arterioles without glomerular filtration. The result is a reduction in cortical blood flow and a paradoxical increase in juxtamedullary flow. This increased medullary flow may interfere with the capacity of the countercurrent system to generate hypertonicity. These changes in medullary flow, in conjunction with the selective loss of juxtamedullary nephrons and an anatomic alteration in the renal tubules, tend to compromise an elderly patient's urinary concentrating mechanism.[7,10] In total effect, renal blood flow declines slightly while the glomerular filtration rate (GFR) and concentrating ability decline to a greater degree. For a summary of these changes, see Table 5-1.

Renal Functional Changes

Renal Blood Flow

There is a fall in total renal blood flow (RBF) of approximately 10 percent per decade after age 20. This means that RBF in a septuagenarian is only one-half

Table 5-1 Anatomic changes in the aging kidney

Decreased kidney size (cortex > medulla)
Glomerular sclerosis
Tubular loss
Renal tubular changes
Increased tubular diverticula
Decreased length, number, and thickness
Increased interstitial tissue
Renal vascular changes
Altered arteriole-glomerular flow
Atherosclerotic damage
Altered vascular pattern

(300 ml/min) of that in a young adult (600 ml/min). It is known that the major decrement in RBF is from the cortex, which appears to be secondary to the anatomic changes described above. Hollenberg and colleagues,[11] using a xenon washout technique, demonstrated that in the cortex there is a progressive decline in RBF per renal mass with age, suggesting that the decreased RBF is not secondary to tissue loss but is most likely the primary cause of parenchymal atrophy.

Glomerular Filtration Rate

It is not unexpected that the (GFR) progressively declines with age, since a fall in total RBF and a decrease in the number of glomeruli occur. It is well known that the GFR is stable after adolescence and through age 35 and then declines at a rate of approximately 10 ml/min per 1.73 m^2 per decade. This drop in GFR is only partially due to age; most of the decline is due to other factors.

Serum creatinine concentrations in the elderly cannot be extrapolated from normal values in the young. A serum creatinine level of 1 mg/dl has a different meaning for a 30-year-old than for a 75-year-old. Remember that a 75-year-old man will have a GFR that is 40 to 50 percent lower than that of a 30-year-old man of the same size. It is known that creatinine production is reduced in older patients because body muscle mass is less.

Several authors have developed nomograms, or formulas, for calculating the creatinine clearance in an elderly person. Cockroft and Gault[12] developed a formula for the rapid calculation of true creatinine clearance that is based on a patient's weight, age, and serum creatinine level:

$$\text{Creatinine clearance (ml/min)} = \frac{(140 - \text{age in years}) \times \text{lean body weight in kg}}{72 \times \text{serum creatinine in men}}$$

For women, multiply the formula by 0.85

It is important to note that the patient must be without significant increases in extracellular fluid volume and does not have severe muscle wasting for this formula to be used. One of the more commonly used nomograms for determining creatinine clearance is shown in Figure 5-1. There have also been data that indicate that a small number of older subjects have shown no decrease in their creatinine clearances when studied serially at 12- to-18 month intervals, and some of these patients (1.6 percent) actually had increases in creatinine clearance of between 1 and 6 ml/min per year.[13] This only serves to add to the confusion involved in calculating creatinine clearance, but it is always safer to assume a decrease in clearance when one is dosing medications in the elderly. Otherwise, urine and blood samples have to be taken to determine an exact clearance value.

Sodium Metabolism

Despite the critical role of the kidney in maintaining sodium balance, relatively little is known about how this function is influenced by age. Elderly

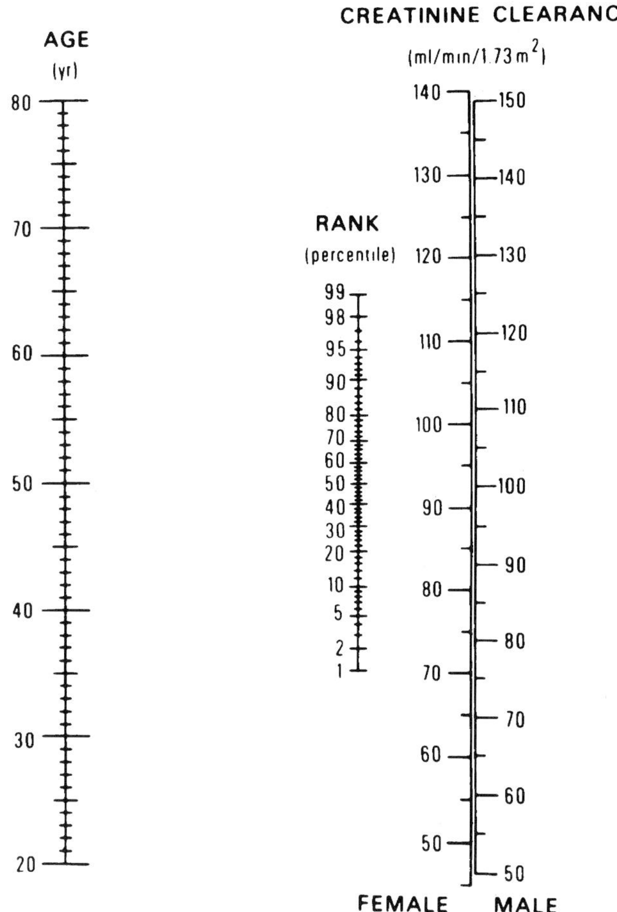

Figure 5-1 **Nomogram for ascertaining age-adjusted percentile rank in creatinine clearance.** (*Reproduced with permission from Rowe JW et al: Ann Intern Med 84:567, 1976.*)

persons, like younger persons, are able to conserve sodium when sodium-restricted, but their recovery from this deprivation is much slower. Epstein and Hollenberg[14] found that the half-time for reduction of sodium excretion after a patient was placed on a very low sodium diet was 17.6 h in a younger person (under age 30) compared with 31 h in an elderly individual (over age 60). The elderly required a much longer time to achieve equilibrium and had significantly greater urinary losses of sodium before this state could be achieved. It is believed that this delay in sodium correction may reflect abnormalities in the renin-aldosterone axis. Even though baseline renin levels are normal or only minimally diminished in the elderly, provocative maneuvers such as a low-sodium diet and furosemide administration produce lesser rises in both renin and aldosterone serum levels in the elderly compared with the young.[15]

The elderly also have a diminished ability to handle acute sodium loads.

Some studies[16,17] have reported higher levels of circulating atrial natriuretic peptide (ANP) in an elderly patient than in a young patient on the same sodium intake. In addition, the metabolic clearance of ANP is prolonged in the elderly, and it has been hypothesized that the cellular response to this peptide is also diminished.[17] The physiological importance of these changes is uncertain.

Potassium Homeostasis

Just as it has been stated in the literature that potassium balance is impaired in the elderly[18] and that the elderly are more prone to hyper- and hypokalemia, other studies have suggested that potassium homeostasis is normal on standard dietary intakes.[19] Although multiple factors (blunted renin-aldosterone axis, decreased GFR, decreased tubular mass) predict that protection against hyperkalemia in the face of increased potassium loads may be impaired, such potassium-loading studies have not been reported.[20] There also have not been any human studies to evaluate the conservation capacity of the kidney in the environment of decreased intake or of nonrenal potassium loss.

Acid-Base Metabolism

The elderly can maintain acid-base balance under normal physiological conditions but show a diminished capacity to respond when placed under stressful conditions. Several authors[21,22] have found that elderly individuals have a diminished acid excretory ability and that this decline cannot be explained by the drop in GFR. When given an ammonium chloride load, despite an equivalent fall in plasma bicarbonate concentration, older men had significantly less urinary acid excretion compared with younger men. Therefore, the altered excretion of acid appears to be due primarily to a reduction in ammonium clearance. Schück and colleagues[23] demonstrated that the diminished capacity of older subjects to increase titratable acid excretion after an acute ammonium chloride load is due to an insufficient decrease in the tubular reabsorption of phosphates. Renal capacity for adequate reduction of the urine pH after this load was unimpaired.

Water Homeostasis

It is a well-established fact that total body water decreases with age. The percentage of body mass made up by water falls progressively with age. This decrease is greater in women than in men, primarily because of a female's proportionately decreased lean body mass and increased body fat. Gains and losses of water in women therefore create more pronounced changes in body fluid osmolality.

The ability of the aged kidney to respond to both water deprivation and water loading has been shown to be impaired.[24] Lindeman and associates[25] gave an oral water load (20 ml/kg) to three different age groups of men and reported that the minimal urine osmolality after this load was 52 mosm/kg in the younger group (mean age, 31), 74 mosm/kg in the middle group (mean age, 60), and 92 mosm/kg in the elderly group (mean age, 84). Free water clearance was also lower in the older group, although when factored for GFR, the values were not different. This suggests that the higher minimal urinary osmolality in the elderly is due to an increased solute load per nephron. Crowe and coworkers[26] agreed that there is a decrease in diluting capacity with age that is explained by the known fall in GFR. Also, the serum arginine vasopressin (AVP) levels were measured and found to be equally depressed after a water load in both young and elderly subjects. This suggests that the decreased water excretion was not due to inappropriate AVP release. In fact, it is believed that the AVP secretory capacity is not impaired in the elderly.

The effects of water deprivation and renal concentrating abilities has also been studied. Exposing elderly men to 24 h of water deprivation resulted in a lower urine specific gravity (1.023) at age 90 compared with age 40 (1.030).[27] These scientists calculated an approximately 5 percent drop in maximal concentrating capacity for each decade after age 50. Rowe and colleagues[28] found that the elderly have an impaired ability to decrease urine flow rate, increase urine osmolality, or decrease osmolar clearance after 12 h of water deprivation. They estimated a 10 percent decline in the renal concentrating capacity between ages 33 and 68 (Table 5-2). This decrease in urinary osmolality did not correlate with the level of creatinine clearance, which also falls with aging.

There is no single explanation for these changes in the renal response to water deprivation. One belief is that the decline in the ability of the kidney to concentrate urine is due to a change in the functional status of the hypothalamic-pituitary-renal axis. Studies have shown[25, 28a] that the kidney's response to the administration of exogenous AVP is blunted but that the basal secretory rates and the response to changes in osmolality are greater in the aged. There are other studies that have shown baseline levels of circulating AVP to be lower[28b] or insignificantly different.[28c]

Helderman and associates[29] measured endogenous vasopressin release in response to plasma osmolality changes and discovered that the elderly showed a greater sensitivity to changes in osmolality. The serum vasopressin levels rose faster and achieved higher levels (4 to 5 times) than those in younger subjects. At a serum osmolality of 298 mosm/kg, the vasopressin levels were 60 percent higher in the older subjects. This clearly shows that the sensitivity of the hypothalamic pituitary osmoreceptors is exaggerated rather than inhibited in the elderly.

It is not understood why the renal age-related decrease in collecting tubule responsiveness to AVP exists. This lack of responsiveness may be due to an altered medullary solute gradient, a defective medullary circulation, or a defect in tubular cellular response to AVP.[30] Rowe[31] suggested two hypotheses. The first states that the decreased concentrating ability of the kidney is secondary to the redistribution of blood flow away from the renal cortex and toward the medulla. This would alter the renal medullary osmotic gradient. The second hypothesis holds that the primary event that occurs is an increased release of AVP with aging. This "resetting" of osmoreceptor-stimulated AVP secretion

Table 5-2 The effect of age on urine flow, urine osmolality, solute excretion, and osmolar clearance during fluid restriction, by age groups

	Mean age, years	Urine osmolality, mosm/kg*		Urine flow, ml/min*		Solute excretion, mosm/min†		Osmolar clearance, ml/min†	
		Period 1	Period 3	Period 1	Period 3	Period 1	Period 3	Period 1	Period 3
Young, 20–39 ($n = 31$)	33	969 ± 41	1,109 ± 22	1.02 ± 0.10	0.49 ± 0.03	0.988 ± 0.069	0.543 ± 0.036	3.40 ± 0.24	1.87 ± 0.12
Middle, 40–59 ($n = 48$)	49	949 ± 39	1,051 ± 19	0.99 ± 0.10	0.63 ± 0.03	0.940 ± 0.103	0.662 ± 0.033	3.23 ± 0.35	2.27 ± 0.11
Old, 60–79 ($n = 18$)	68	852 ± 64	882 ± 49	1.05 ± 0.15	1.03 ± 0.13	0.895 ± 0.143	0.908 ± 0.130	3.06 ± 0.48	3.11 ± 0.45

Values indicate mean 1 SEM.

* $p<0.05$ for young versus middle, middle versus old, and young versus old for period 3.

† $p<0.01$ for young versus old, $p<0.02$ for young versus middle for period 3.

SOURCE: Reproduced with permission from Rowe JW, Shock NW, DeFronzo RA: *Nephron* 17:270, 1976, S. Karger AG, Basel.

may occur in response to diminished baroreceptor sensitivity. Chronically high levels of AVP may then create a secondary down regulation of the renal response to AVP, which in turn leads to a decreased concentrating ability.[32] This decline in concentrating ability should not be clinically important unless thirst is impaired, access to water is prevented, or the water loss is severe. Interestingly, Phillips and associates[33] evaluated the renal and pituitary response, as well as the thirst response, to 24 h of water deprivation in the young (26 to 31) versus the elderly (67 to 75). They showed that thirst was significantly blunted in the elderly and that even when given free access to water, the elderly men drank less water and took hours longer to correct their water deficit.

For a summary of the functional changes in the kidney with aging, see Table 5-3.

Clinical Consequences of Physiological Changes

The anatomic and functional effects of aging on the kidneys do not by themselves result in clinical disease or disability, but these changes make older patients much more susceptible to a variety of disease-associated, environmentally induced, and drug-related stresses. For example, the depressed thirst mechanism of a centenarian can lead to a state of hypernatremia and coma if the patient also has diarrhea. Another example is the documented decline in GFR that occurs with aging. While this decline is not great enough to cause symptomatic retention of nitrogenous wastes, the low GFR is much closer to the "uremic threshold." Any illness or environmental exposure that further depresses the GFR can lead to symptomatic renal failure with amazing rapidity in an elderly person. A third example involves an elderly male who is iatrogenically fluid overloaded after transurethral resection of the prostate (TURP). This patient, because of an impaired urine-diluting capacity, will take longer to correct his hyponatremia.

It is very important to understand the renal changes with aging when one is giving renally excreted anesthetic drugs and antibiotics to the elderly. The clearance of many of these drugs is dependent on glomerular filtration, and the risk of toxicity or kidney injury is significantly increased in normal elderly patients unless judicious dosage reduction is applied.

Table 5-3 Funtional changes of aging in the kidney

Renal characteristics	Effects of healthy aging
RBF	Decreased
GFR	Decreased
Potassium homeostasis	Normal to impaired response
Acid-base metabolism	Normal
Water deprivation	Impaired response
Water loading	Probably impaired

HEPATIC SYSTEM

Anatomy of the Aging Liver

Size

In a healthy adult male, the liver makes up approximately 2.5 percent of total body weight until about age 50. The liver then slowly becomes smaller so that by age 90 it represents about 1.5 percent of total body weight.[34] The morphological changes in the liver that occur because of aging are felt to be minimal. Postmortem findings note both absolute and relative weight losses. They report a 25 percent fall in liver weight between ages 20 and 70 years, with the relative weight of the human liver dropping from 4 percent in newborn infants to 2 percent in aged persons.[35] In vivo studies confirm this fall, describing a 28 percent fall in liver volume and a 33 percent fall in liver blood flow in healthy elderly patients (> age 65) compared with patients under age 40.[36] This decline in liver weight is equally distributed throughout the lobules.

Color

Grossly, the liver is characterized by brown atrophy. This color change is caused by the accumulation of lipofuscin granules (aging pigment) in lysosomes. It has been hypothesized that these lipofuscin granules are due to food contaminants that cannot be cleared by the hepatocytes. Brown atrophy is not limited to the elderly but also can be found in younger persons who suffer from malnutrition. There is also an increase in extrahepatocytic space (parenchymal fibrosis) and intralobular collagen with aging. Even though collagen synthesis is reduced, it appears that no functional problem results.

Histological

There seem to be only minor histological alterations in the liver with aging. One of the few changes noted, although it is without known clinical importance, is an enlargement of the hepatocytes in people over age 60 years and an increase in the number of cells with large nuclei (elevated DNA). There is also a decrease in the number of mitochondria but an increase in volume. It has been suggested that these histological changes in aging liver cells may represent a hyperfunctioning state, possibly to compensate for the decline in absolute cell number.

Hepatic Functional Changes

Liver Blood Flow

As was stated earlier, there is approximately a 33 percent fall in total liver blood flow in healthy elderly patients. This change has been shown to occur in animals also. Varga and Fischer[37] found that in rats the reduction in total liver blood flow is primarily a decline in portal blood flow with essentially no change in hepatic arterial blood flow. Wynne and associates[38] looked at the effects of age on liver blood flow in healthy men, using plasma clearance of indocyanine green. They found that there was a significant negative correlation between age and liver blood flow as well as between age and liver blood flow per unit volume of liver (liver perfusion). The significance of these changes has not yet been proved, but it has been hypothesized that this could be one of the contributing factors to the decline in the clearance of many drugs undergoing liver metabolism that has been noted to occur with aging.

Liver Function Tests

The conventional liver function tests (alkaline phosphatase, serum bilirubin, and transaminase levels) do not appear to be affected by increasing age, nor are serum transferrin levels.[39] Even though serum albumin levels may be slightly decreased, this is not due to poor protein nutrition. Therefore, when liver blood chemistries are abnormal, liver disease must be seriously suspected.

Static serum blood levels do not accurately measure the true variety of liver functions. Therefore, the effect of age on some of the dynamic functions must be addressed.

Bromosulphthalein (BSP) administered intravenously (IV) is extracted from the blood by the liver, then stored by liver cells, and finally excreted unchanged in the bile. It has been shown by several researchers that with age, the amount of BSP retained in the blood after an IV dose increases, indicating that the liver's ability to extract it from the blood decreases. Thompson and Williams[40] verified that liver storage capacity decreases with age but that the secretory transport abilities do not. In 1980, Nakanishi and colleagues[41] showed that liver cells with enlarged nuclei store less BSP. The importance of this event in relation to other hepatic storage or uptake functions is unknown.

CONJUGATION Studies performed by Farah and associates[42] and Triggs and colleagues[43] addressed the issue of two major liver functions: acetylation and glucuronidation. Farah looked at acetylation using isoniazid, and Triggs looked at glucuronidation using acetaminophen. It appears that there are no major alterations in these two conjugation reactions with aging. This has also been shown to be true for hepatic metabolism via glucuronidation of lorazepam.

EXTRACTION To evaluate the ability and effectiveness of the liver in "extracting" drugs from the blood, it is important to look at drugs that normally undergo high hepatic first-pass metabolism. There are several possible mechanisms by which decreased liver function could lead to a higher plasma concentration of highly extracted drugs:[44]

1. There could be diminished first-pass extraction.
2. Decreased hepatic blood flow could cause a rise in the plasma concentrations of IV drugs.
3. The rate of drug metabolism, once extracted, could be impaired.

There are conflicting data regarding the plasma half-life ($t_{1/2}$) and clearance (Cl) of drugs with a high first-pass metabolism. After oral propranolol, the $t_{1/2}$ and Cl were unchanged even though there were higher plasma levels in older subjects compared with younger subjects. After IV propanolol, the $t_{1/2}$ was prolonged and the Cl was lower in the elderly subjects.[45] By contrast, oral lidocaine, which is also a drug with a high first-pass metabolism, was found to have a prolonged $t_{1/2}$ and an unchanged Cl.[46] In an attempt to explain these findings, it has been suggested that impaired hepatic extraction from portal blood accounted for higher plasma levels after oral administration, whereas impaired hepatic blood flow may explain the lower clearance after IV administration.[45]

MICROSOMAL HYDROXYLATION and OXIDATION Antipyrine is the model compound for comparing changes in microsomal hydroxylation and oxidation with the effects of aging. It has been noted that caffeine, cigarette smoking, and nutrition (low plasma ascorbic acid and folate levels) can impair antipyrine clearance in the elderly. But when each of these factors is controlled, it appears that antipyrine clearance is normal to only slightly decreased in aging subjects. This would imply that both microsomal oxidation and hydroxylation are not impaired. It also appears that nonmicrosomal oxidation is not impaired. Vestal and associates[47] looked at ethanol metabolism in both the young and the elderly and found that ethanol elimination was not affected by age. They did have to make the assumption that IV ethanol is cleared primarily by the nonmicrosomal alcohol dehydrogenase and not by the microsomal ethanol-oxidizing enzymes to arrive at the initial statement above.

DEMETHYLATION The model drug for demethylation is aminopyrine. The aminopyrine breath test measures the rate of demethylation of aminopyrine by the liver and estimates hepatic microsomal capacity. It has been reported that the demethylation capacity for aminopyrine is inversely related to age in humans.[48] The metabolism of the benzodiazepines is complicated, but the principal initial degradation step is *N*-demethylation. Studies have demonstrated that not only is there an increase in the free fraction of diazepam from approximately 1 percent to 3 percent with increasing age (18 to 91 years), there also is a halving in plasma clearance.[49] This helps explain the prolonged effects of benzodiazepines seen in the elderly.

PROTEIN SYNTHESIS Young and associates[50] determined that total body protein synthesis is 37 percent lower in subjects 69 to 91 years old than in subjects 20 to 23 years old. Presumably, much of this reduction in protein synthesis occurs in the liver. It is more commonly believed that the synthesis of some proteins is increased in old age, while that of others is reduced. The molecular explanations for these changes are still being studied, but evidence points to the fact that aging may reduce the breakdown and the fidelity of translation of some mRNA.[51] Although liver enzyme concentrations may not be lessened, a reduction in activity suggests that some enzymes may be present in the form of altered, or "junk," proteins.[52] This could conceivably explain phenomena such as impaired binding of drugs to albumin with increasing age. The albumin may be of a normal or only slightly decreased quantity, but its quality (binding fidelity) is affected. There is also an increase in the cholesterol-phospholipid molar ratio of liver mitochondrial membranes as aging occurs. This could potentially impair substrate access to metabolizing enzymes.[53]

Clinical Consequences of Physiological Changes

Just as with the renal system, the anatomic and functional effects of aging on the liver do not by themselves result in clinical disease and disability. However, these changes do make the individual more susceptible to the stresses of disease, environmental changes, and drug therapy. The greatest concern for the anesthesiologist is how well an elderly person metabolizes the drugs administered to him or her. The metabolism of a given drug depends on the hepatic mechanism by which that drug is metabolized. In the operating room, the best rule of thumb is to initially titrate a drug first to the desired effect rather than giving a predetermined mg/kg dose. Then, the physician should observe the clinical signs and symptoms exhibited by the patient to determine the dosing interval required.

For a summary of the effects of aging on hepatic physiology, see Table 5-4.

SUMMARY

There are many alterations in both the renal and hepatic systems with aging. A normal healthy aged individual can handle the administration of a single drug quite well. The problems begin when the patient receives multiple drugs, as in the surgical setting. It therefore becomes important to dose anesthetic drugs according to the clinical response desired. The dosing of chronically administered drugs must take into consideration the patient's renal and hepatic function. Whenever possible, drug levels must be followed to avoid toxicity. Also,

Table 5-4 Summary of the effects of aging on hepatic physiology

Liver characteristic	Effect of healthy aging
Size	Decreased
Color	Brown atrophy
Routine liver chemistries	Normal
Hepatic blood flow	Decreased
Mitochondria	↓ Quantity, ↑ size
BSP, galactose elimination	Decreased
Conjugation (glucuronidation and acetylation)	No change
Hepatic extraction (first-pass metabolism)	Probably impaired
Microsomal hydroxylation and oxydation	Normal to decreased
Demethylation	Decreased
Protein synthesis	Variable
Serum albumin	Slightly decreased

depending on the drug administered, baseline and repetitive renal or hepatic functions need to be obtained to avoid organ injury. The clinical effect of these systems on drug administration will be addressed in Chap. 6.

REFERENCES

1. Roessle R, Roulet F (eds): Mass und zahl, in *Der Patholgie*. Berlin: Springer, 1932.
2. Dunnill MS, Halley W: Some observations on the quantitative anatomy of the kidney. *J Pathol* 110:113, 1973.
3. Goyal VR: Changes with age in the human kidney. *Exp Gerontol* 17:321, 1982.
4. Gourtsoyiannis N, Prassopoulos P, Cavouras D, Pantelidis N: The thickness of the renal parenchyma decreases with age: A CT study of 360 patients. *AJR* 155:541, 1990.
5. Kaplan C, Pasternack B, Shah H, et al: Age related incidence of sclerotic glomerule in the human kidneys. *Am J Pathol* 80:227, 1975.
6. Kappel B, Olsen S: Cortical interstitial tissue and sclerosed glomeruli in the normal human kidney, related to age and sex. *Virchows Arch A Pathol Anat Histopathol* 387:271, 1980.
7. Darmady EM: The parameters of the aging kidney. *J Pathol* 109:195, 1973.
8. Baert L, Steg A: Is the diverticulum of the distal and collecting tubules a preliminary stage of the simple cyst in the adult? *J Urol* 118:707, 1977.
9. Ljungqyist A, Lagerggen C: Normal intrarenal arterial pattern in adult and aging human kidney. *J Anat* 96:285, 1962.
10. Takazakura E, Sawabu N, Handa A, et al: Intrarenal vascular changes with age and disease. *Kidney Int* 2:224, 1972.
11. Hollenberg NK, Adams DF, Solomon HS, et al: Senescence and the renal vasculature in normal man. *Circ Res* 34:309, 1974.
12. Cockroft DW, Gault MH: Prediction of creatinine clearance from serum creatinine. *Nephron* 16:31, 1976.
13. Lindeman RD, Tobin J, Shock NW: Longitudinal studies on the rate of decline in renal function with age. *J Am Geriatr Soc* 33:278, 1985.
14. Epstein M, Hollenberg NN: Age as a determinant of renal sodium conservation in normal man. *J Lab Clin Med* 87:411, 1976.
15. Weidmann P, DeMyttenaere-Bursztein S, Maxwell MH, Delima J: Effect of aging in plasma renin and aldosterone in normal man. *Kidney Int* 8:325, 1975.
16. Haller BG, Zust H, Shaw S, et al: Effects of posture and aging in circulating atrial nutriuretic peptide levels in man. *J Hypertens* 5:551, 1987.
17. Ohashi M, Fujio N, Nawata H, et al: Pharmacokinetics of synthetic alpha human atrial natriuretic polypeptide in normal man: Effects of aging. *Regul Pept* 19:265, 1987.
18. Stern N, Tuck ML: Homeostatic fragility in the elderly. *Cardiol Clin* 4:20, 1986.
19. Fulop T, Worum I, Ocsongor J, et al: Body composition in the elderly patient. *Gerontology* 31:6, 1985.
20. Beck LH, Burkhart JM: Aging changes in renal function, in Hazzard WR, Andres R, Bierman EL, Blass JP (eds): *Principles of Geriatric Medicine and Gerontology*, 2d ed. New York: McGraw-Hill, 1990, chap 55, pp 555–564.
21. Adter S, Lindeman RD, Yiengst MJ, et al: Effect of acute acid loading on urinary acid excretion by the aging human kidney. *J Lab Clin Med* 72:278, 1968.

22. Agarwal BN, Cabebe FG: Renal acidification in elderly subjects. *Nephron* 26:391, 1980.
23. Schück O, Nadvornikova H, Teplan V: Acidification capacity of the kidneys and aging. *Physiol Bohemoslov* 38(2):117, 1989.
24. Nunez JFM, Iglesias CG, Roman AB: Renal handling of sodium in old people: A functional study. *Age Ageing* 7:178, 1978.
25. Lindeman RD, Lee TD Jr, Yiengst MJ, Shock NW: Influence of age, renal disease, hypertension, diuretics, and calcium on the antidiuretic responses to suboptimal infusion of vasopressin. *J Lab Clin Med* 68:206, 1966.
26. Crowe MJ, Forsling ML, Rolls BJ, et al: Altered water excretion in healthy elderly men. *Age Ageing* 16:285, 1987.
27. Lewis WH, Alving AS: Changes with age in renal function in adult men. *Am J Physiol* 123:300, 1938.
28. Rowe JW, Shock NW, DeFrenzo RA: The influence of age on the renal response to water deprivation in man. *Nephron* 17:270, 1976.
28a. Helderman JH: The impact of normal aging on the hypothalamic-neurophyseal-renal axis, in Korenman SG (ed): *Endocrine Aspects of Aging*. New York: Elsevier Biomedical, 1982.
28b. Faull CM, Holmes C, Baylis PH: Water balance in elderly people: Is there a deficiency of vasopressin? *Age Ageing* 22: 114, 1993.
28c. Bursztyn M, Bresnahan M, Gavras I, Bavras H: Effect of aging on vasopressin, catecholamines and alpha ∂–adrenergic receptors. *J Am Geriatr Soc* 38:628, 1990.
29. Helderman JH, Vestal RE, Rowe J, et al: The response of arginine vasopressin to intravenous ethanol and hypertonic saline in man: The impact of age. *J Gerontol* 33:39, 1978.
30. Beck LH, Burkart JM: The renal system and urinary tract, in Hazzard WR, Andres R, Bierman EL, Blass JP (eds): *Principles of Geriatric Medicine and Gerontology*, 2d ed. New York: McGraw-Hill, 1990, pp 555–563.
31. Rowe JW: Aging and renal function, in Arieff AI, Defranzo RA (eds): *Fluid, Electrolyte and Acid-Base Disorders*. New York: Livingstone, 1985, pp 1231–1246.
32. Miller M: Increased vasopressin secretion: An early manifestation of aging in the rat. *J Gerontol* 42:3, 1987.
33. Phillips PA, Rolls BJ, Ledingham JG, et al: Reduced thirst after water deprivation in healthy elderly men. *N Engl J Med* 311:753, 1984.
34. Calloway NO, Foley CF, Lagerbloom P: Uncertainties in geriatric data: II. Organize. *J Am Geriatr S* 13:20, 1965.
35. Wynne HA, Copel H, Mutch E, Rawlens MD, et al: The effect of age upon liver volume and apparent liver blood flow in healthy man. *Hepatology* 9:297, 1989.
36. Wynne HA, James OFW: The aging liver. *Age Ageing* 19:1, 1990.
37. Varga F, Fischer E: Age dependent changes in blood supply of the liver and the biliary excretion of eosine in rats, in Kitani K (ed): *Liver and Aging*. North Holland Elsevier, 1978, pp 327–339.
38. Wynne HA, Cope LH, Mutch E, et al: The effect of age upon liver volume and apparent liver blood flow in healthy man. *Hepatology* 9:297, 1989.
39. McEvoy AW, James OF: Anthropathetic indices in normal elderly individuals. *Age Ageing* 11:97, 1982.
40. Thompson EN, Williams R: Effect of age on liver function with particular reference to bromsulphthalein excretion. *Gut* 6:266, 1965.
41. Nakanishi K, Fukuda M, Fujita S: Decline of BSP storage capacity in polyploid hepatocytes demonstrated by cytofluorimetry. *Exp Gerontol* 15:103, 1980.

42. Farah F, Taylor W, Rawlins MD, James O: Hepatic drug acetylation and oxidation—effects in man. *Br Med J* 2(6080):155, 1977.
43. Triggs EJ, Nation RL, Long A, Ashley JJ: Pharmacokinetics in the elderly. *Eur J Clin Pharmacol* 8:55, 1975.
44. James OFW: Drugs and the aging liver, in Evans JH, Caird FI (eds): *Advanced Geriatric Medicine.* London: Pitman, 1982, pp 100–110.
45. Castleden CM, George C: The effect of aging on hepatic clearance of propranolol. *Br J Clin Pharmacol* 7:49, 1979.
46. Nation RL, Triggs EJ, Selig M: Lignocaine kinetics in cardiac patients and aged subjects. *Br J Pharmacol* 4:439, 1977.
47. Vestal RE, McGuire EA, Tobin JD, et al: Aging and ethanol metabolism. *Clin Pharmacol Ther* 21:343, 1977.
48. Pirotte J, El Allaf D: Effect of age and sex on the N-demethylation rate ^{14}C-aminopyrine, studied by the breath test. *Digestion* 28:210, 1983.
49. Macklon AF, Barton M, James O, Rawlins MD: The effect of age on the pharmacokinetics of diazepam. *Clin Sci* 59:479, 1980.
50. Young VR, Steffee WP, Pencharz PB, et al: Total human body protein synthesis in relation to protein requirements at various ages. *Nature* 253:192, 1975.
51. Van Bezooijen CFA, Horbach GJMJ: Albumin synthesis in aging, in *Aging in Liver and Gastrointestinal Tract,* Falk Foundation Symposium No. 47. Lancaster, MTP Press, 1988, pp 199–208.
52. Schmucker DL, Wang RK: Qualitative changes in rat liver microsomal NADPH cytochrome c (P450) reductase during aging. *Age* 5:105, 1982.
53. Grinna LS: Age related changes in the lipids of the microsomal and the mitochondrial membranes of rat liver and kidney. *Mech Ageing Dev* 6:197, 1977.

CHAPTER 6

Pharmacokinetics and Pharmacodynamics in Elderly Patients

David J. Jones
David W. Glasser

INTRODUCTION

As a result of the continuous increase in the age of the general population and the requirement for safe and efficacious drug therapy, an awareness of age-induced alterations in pharmacokinetics is needed (i.e., the absorption, distribution, metabolism, and elimination of drugs). In addition, pharmacodynamic changes caused by age can occur, resulting in a reduced cellular response to a given dose of a drug. Thus, alterations in receptor characteristics and second messenger or signal transduction mechanisms as well as cellular responses can add to these changes in pharmacokinetics and influence the overall response to drugs. This chapter reviews these factors and the influence of age on both quantitative and qualitative responses to therapeutic agents. This chapter adds to the substantial literature on age-induced alterations in pharmacokinetics and pharmacodynamics that has appeared in reviews over the past 10 years.[1–28]

PHARMACOKINETICS

Typically, pharmacokinetic factors describe the disposition of a drug in the body, including absorption, distribution, metabolism, and elimination. As shown in Fig. 6-1, a compartmental analysis of these events reveals a number of factors that can both quantitatively and qualitatively alter the total drug appearing in each compartment.

Adding to the complexity of the various processes that influence "free drug" and thus action at effector sites, products formed from metabolism by the liver of a parent drug can also contribute to the overall drug response. In considering these processes, it is clear that both the function of the various organs involved in drug kinetics and the composition of the body (lean body mass, total body

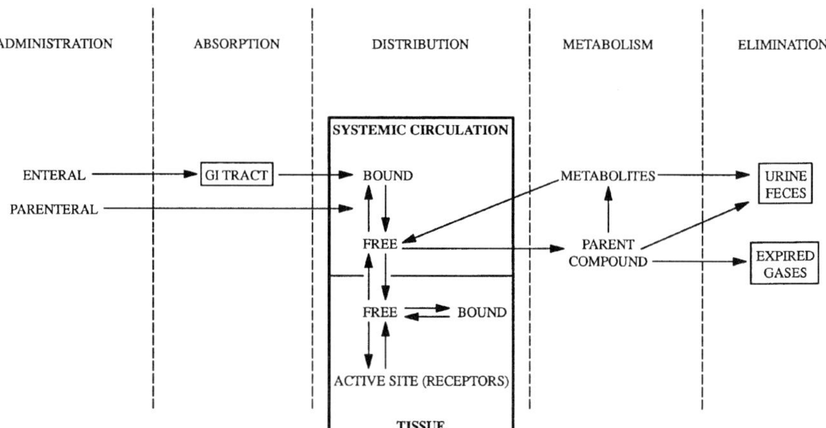

Figure 6-1 Schematic of the possible sites for pharmacokinetic and/or pharmacodynamic alterations in drug response.

water, etc.) can influence drug action. In the following section, the age-related changes that involve organs responsible for drug kinetics are reviewed, along with the changes in body composition that influence the compartmental disposition of drugs.

Absorption

Absorption of drugs into the systemic circulation via the enteral (oral) route is accompanied by much greater variability in an aged patient compared with parenteral administration. Assuming that dissolution of the drug formulation occurs, absorption across the gastrointestinal tract membranes into the systemic circulation can be influenced by a number of factors. Early studies by Bender[1] reviewed factors that influence intestinal absorption, including gastric emptying, intestinal motility, organ blood flow, the digestion process, and the "status of cellular transport mechanisms [of absorbing cells] and the epithelial membrane." While the bulk of studies suggested a delay and/or a reduction in the absorption of drugs with increased age, few hard data were available. This generally remains the case today. However, reduced gastric acid output,[29] a decrease in intestinal blood flow,[30] a decrease in the number of absorbing cells,[31] and reduced gastrointestinal mobility and thus an increase in transit time[32] have all been described in elderly subjects and could contribute to a reduction in the gastric absorption of drugs.

It is important to remember that the extent to which the absorption of drugs from the gastrointestinal tract is affected by aging depends largely on the drug being studied. For example, increased gastric pH, as might occur as a result of decreased acid production in aging persons, would favor ionization of weakly acidic drugs such as barbiturates. Thus, less drug would be absorbed into the systemic circulation. Moreover, with drugs such as diazepam, which are absorbed into the proximal small intestine, age-induced decreases in gastric emptying could potentially result in slower and probably less complete absorption. Most drugs are, however, absorbed by passive diffusion, and the majority of studies have failed to demonstrate significant alterations in drug absorption in aged patients. The fact that most drugs are administered parenterally in the surgical setting further reduces the importance to anesthesiologists of age-induced alterations in oral drug absorption.

Distribution

Drug distribution is altered by age-related changes in physiology. After absorption from the gastrointestinal tract or after parenteral administration, drugs are distributed throughout the systemic circulation. The volume of distribution (Vd) best describes the volume of the compartment into which the drug is distributed and represents an estimate at a single point in time of the amount of drug in the body as a whole relative to the amount in plasma. Vd can be calculated by dividing the total amount of drug by the drug concentration (in plasma water), allowing sufficient time for distribution and equilibration. From such a calculation, it is known that the Vd of water-soluble versus lipid-soluble drugs varies depending on factors such as lean body mass, total body water, and protein binding.

Studies have demonstrated a decrease in lean body mass with aging,[33,34] along with a loss of body water.[33,35] When this is combined with an increase in body fat[33,36] with increased age, the Vd can be altered for a large number of agents, potentially altering directly the drug response through changes in the concentration of the drug at the active site or sites. For example, the Vd of relatively water-soluble agents such as ethanol[37] and antipyrine[38] is decreased in aging persons, leading to an increase in the agent at active sites. Conversely, because of the increased fat stores that accompany aging, lipid-soluble compounds such as thiopental sodium[39] are observed to have a greater Vd, leading to less drug at the active site. Thiopental would therefore be predicted to accumulate more and cause more postoperative residual sedation in an elderly patient.

Binding of drugs to plasma proteins (albumin and alpha$_1$ acid glycoprotein) influences the total free drug in the body and hence the Vd. Alterations in total plasma proteins in aging persons have to be considered potential contributors to the concentration of drug at active sites. While a decrease in total protein is not found in aging, previous studies by Greenblat demonstrated a selective decrease in the serum albumin concentration,[40] potentially leading to an increase in free drugs, especially weak acids that bind to albumin.[41] Drugs that are weak acids and are highly bound to plasma proteins are a major concern in elderly patients. For example, phenylbutazone is bound approximately 96 percent to plasma proteins, but this total is decreased to 94 percent in aged patients,[41] resulting in 50 percent more free drug being available in the systemic circulation to produce both a therapeutic response and an increased level of toxicity. This also appears to be the case for phenytoin, where a 20 percent decrease in plasma protein binding was demonstrated in older geriatric patients.[42] It is difficult to predict whether the binding of a drug is altered in aged patients, since a number of other factors, especially disease, can markedly alter protein binding of drugs independently of advanced age.

Metabolism

A recent review by Durnas and colleagues[9,14] points out the many factors that can contribute to alterations in hepatic drug metabolism during aging. As the authors state, "Age-related changes in drug metabolism are a complicated interplay between genetics, aging, disease, and environment."[14] In general, the hepatic metabolism or clearance of many drugs is reduced in an aged individual. Both anatomic and physiological alterations play a role in this reduction.

Liver Volume

There is a decrease in liver size and volume of up to 30 percent with aging.[41,43] While other factors can contribute, studies by Bach's group[44] indicated that such a reduction in liver volume can reduce the clearance of drugs such as phenytoin. Given the difficulty in managing therapeutic levels of phenytoin, reduced clearance in aging patients potentially can lead to a longer duration of action with accumulation and enhanced side (toxic) effects. This is especially dangerous in an elderly patient in whom confusion and sedation can markedly alter daily activities.

Liver Blood Flow

The hepatic clearance of a drug depends on delivery of the free form to the liver and the functional capacity of the hepatic enzymes responsible for drug metabolism. Liver blood flow is a crucial determinant of the hepatic clearance of a drug, especially with drugs whose metabolism can be classified as flow-dependent. The rate at which the liver metabolizes a drug depends completely on the amount of drug delivered to the liver under flow-dependent conditions. The metabolism of these drugs when administered orally exhibits a "first-pass effect" kinetic profile. This implies that significant metabolism occurs before it reaches the systemic circulation. The metabolism of compounds with a high extraction ratio (0.7 or greater), in which clearance is proportional to hepatic blood flow, thus follows changes in blood flow. According to studies by Wynn and coworkers,[43] between the ages of 24 and 91 years there is a 24 to 47 percent reduction in liver blood flow. In the elderly, this reduction appears to follow from an overall reduction in cardiac output.[30] The implications of this observation are that drugs with a high extraction ratio and/or drugs converted for intravenous administration may have a reduced hepatic clearance in an aged individual. For example, the hepatic clearances of propranolol (45 percent decrease),[45] morphine (35 percent decrease),[46] and lidocaine[47] are all reduced in old versus young subjects. It is clear that independent of other factors, age-related reductions in liver blood flow can markedly alter the blood levels of a drug, leading to potential cumulative effects and toxicity.

Metabolizing Enzymes

Typically, the pathways involved in the hepatic biotransformation of agents are separated into two phases: phase 1 reactions (oxidation, reduction, hydrolysis) and phase 2 reactions (synthesis, conjugation). Phase 1 reactions convert compounds to a more water-soluble product for renal excretion and/or add a reactive site. Phase 2 reactions add glucuronides and methyl, sulfur, acyl, and other groups to this reactive site.

While there is considerable variation, most studies suggest an age-related decline in the clearance of drugs that are metabolized via phase 1 reactions.[48] Early studies by O'Malley and colleagues[49] measured phase 1 oxidative metabolism by examining antipyrine clearance and demonstrated a 45 percent increase in the half-life of this agent with aging. Antipyrine is used in studies to evaluate hepatic oxidative metabolism, since it is rapidly distributed, demonstrates low protein binding, and is extensively metabolized by microsomal oxidative enzymes and because clearance does not appear to be influenced by changes in hepatic blood flow. Although other studies have confirmed this observation, it is clear that factors other than age contribute to the prolongation of clearance of drugs metabolized via phase 1 oxidative pathways. In fact, Vestal and coworkers[38] observed that only 3 percent of the variance in the clearance of antipyrine could be attributed to aging. Twelve percent was due to smoking, and the other 85 percent was unexplained, probably being caused by genetic and environmental factors.

Greenblat and colleagues[48] reviewed data on the metabolism of drugs via oxidative pathways. An age-related decrease in clearance was noted for compounds such as diazepam, chlordiazepoxide, theophylline, propranolol, alprazolam, quinidine, and some of the diazepam metabolites. Interestingly, the clearance of desmethyldiazepam, a major active metabolite of diazepam, was reduced in elderly males but not in females.[50] Because propranolol is one of the top 25 drugs used in elderly patients[51] and can, by virtue of lowering cardiac output, further decrease liver blood flow in elderly patients who typically present with already reduced liver blood flow, it is critical to adjust the dose regimen of metabolized drugs to maintain safe blood levels.

Synthetic hepatic biotransformation reactions (phase 2) appear to change less with age. The lack of descriptions of such changes may well be related to the few studies in the literature on phase 2 biotransformation processes and aging. Conjugation with glucuronic acid, sulfuric acid, and cysteine accounts for the primary mechanism of phase 2 biotransformation of acetaminophen. Two studies have indicated a small reduction in acetaminophen clearance in aging patients. It is not clear what pathway of hepatic metabolism might account for this reduction, although sulfation was selectively reduced in one study.[54]

In addition to age-induced alterations in the capacity of phase 1 and phase 2 biotransformation processes to metabolize drugs, one has to consider age-related changes in the ability to induce or inhibit hepatic drug metabolism. Although early studies by Salem's group[55] demonstrated that the ability to induce an increase in antipyrine clearance is reduced in elderly versus young subjects, more recent studies indicate that the degree of exposure to other, more common, inducers of hepatic mixed-function oxidases is the determining factor. For example, cigarette smoke contains nicotine and polycyclic hydrocarbons, both of which induce hepatic enzymes. Smoking was associated with increased clearance of antipyrine in young but not in older subjects,[38,56] and exposure to cigarette smoke appears to quantitatively regulate hepatic mixed-function oxidases. This was shown clearly in studies of elderly subjects among whom a 40 percent higher clearance of theophylline was demonstrated in smokers compared with nonsmokers.[57] The fact that a 55 percent higher clearance was observed in young smokers versus nonsmokers suggests that less induction occurs in the elderly group. Reduced cigarette smoking or exposure to environmental inducers may well influence drug response in the older population.

The inhibition of the hepatic enzyme systems responsible for drug metabolism appears to be similar in young and elderly subjects. When either cimetidine[57,58] or ethanol[59] was used to inhibit drug metabolism, clearance of various drugs was similar in both young and aged subject groups. In contrast to smoking and the induction of liver enzymes, the inhibition of theophylline clearance by cimetidine was not different in smokers, either young or old.[60]

Excretion

The primary mechanism for the elimination of the water-soluble parent drug and its metabolites from the body is the kidney. Renal function is a primary determinant of drug elimination and involves glomerular filtration of free drug, tubular secretion, and tubular reabsorption. Early studies by Davies and Shock[61] used inulin clearance to demonstrate an age-dependent fall in glomerular filtration rate. Their calculations predicted a fall of 30 percent in inulin clearance from age 20 to age 60. Using a nomogram for creatinine clearance, Siersbaek-Nielsen and coworkers[62] demonstrated that for a 70-kg male subject at 25 years of age with a serum creatinine of 1 mg/100 ml, the creatinine clearance would be 105 ml/min. When the same values are used for an 80-year-old male, the creatinine clearance would be only 60 ml/min, a 43 percent reduction. A number of other studies have confirmed decreases of 30 to 45 percent in glomerular filtration rate with aging.[63]

The extent to which age affects drug elimination through a reduction in glomerular filtration rate depends on the percentage of total drug that is eliminated by the kidney. For example, gentamicin, an aminoglycoside antibiotic, is eliminated virtually 100 percent by glomerular filtration, and in patients from an average age of 48 to 76 years there is a 45 percent decrease in clearance.[64] This appears to be related completely to age-related differences in renal function, since when renal function is normal, no age-related differences are detected.[65] Based on these and many other observations, it is clear that one has to monitor aminoglycoside antibiotic levels and/or adjust the dosing regimen in elderly patients to avoid accumulation and potential toxicity. A review by Bennett and colleagues[66] provides dosing guidelines for the aminoglycosides and many other drugs, based on creatinine clearance.

It should be mentioned that clearance of the free drug is different from clearance of the total drug. For drugs that are highly bound to plasma proteins, age-related alterations in binding and hence the free fraction may lead to a biased interpretation of total drug clearance. For example, the measurement of no change in total drug clearance may be misleading when in fact an age-related increase in the free fraction (resulting from decreased plasma protein binding) is balanced by a clinically significant decrease in the clearance of free drug.[67]

A reduction in glomerular filtration has the capacity to also reduce the tubular secretion of substances. Early studies by Leikola and Vartia[68] demonstrated that for drugs, such as penicillin, that are actively secreted, the half-life is 0.55 h in young subjects (average, 25 years) and 1 h in elderly subjects (average, 77 years). Since absorption was the same with both groups, the investigators attributed the decrease in the elderly group to a decrease in active tubular secretion.

PHARMACODYNAMICS

Unlike pharmacokinetic alterations that influence drug delivery and removal from the active site, pharmacodynamic alterations involve a change in end-organ sensitivity. Both an increase and a decrease in sensitivity can occur. These alterations in tissue response can be mediated by changes in the number of receptors with which the drug interacts or alterations in signal transduction mechanisms that couple the receptor signal to intracellular mediators and organ response.

The changes in end-organ sensitivity with aging are represented in an altered quantitative response to drugs that interact directly with organs in which receptor systems are located. Drug action can also be modified indirectly by age-related alterations in a secondary organ response; this change is also independent of alterations in pharmacokinetics. For example, the reduction of dopamine in the corpus striatum caused by aging increases not only the therapeutic effect but also the side effects of certain neuroleptic agents.[15] This reduction also appears to be a contributing mechanism in tardive dyskinesia with metoclopramide administration in the elderly.[69] A change in the response of a secondary organ also plays a role in the exaggerated responses of older patients to antihypertensive agents.[70,71] The baroreceptor reflexes are less sensitive in older patients, producing greater sensitivity to these agents.

In general, pharmacodynamic alterations in drug action in various elderly patients reflect greater sensitivity to the effects of drugs. This is especially true with agents that affect the central nervous system (CNS). While alterations in the pharmacokinetics of benzodiazepines have been more rigorously studied as a cause of enhanced responsiveness in the elderly, greater deficits in psychomotor performance have been demonstrated to be independent of total or free drug differences between old and young test subjects when drugs are administered orally on a chronic basis.[72–74] Greater sensitivity in the elderly also appears to be the case with diazepam administered as premedication.[75,76]

It is unclear what accounts for the alteration in tissue sensitivity. Animal studies have demonstrated that neither benzodiazepine receptor number nor affinity is altered in aging.[77,78] Thus, it may be the case that coupling of the receptor to second messenger systems may be altered or that chloride channel function is somehow enhanced. It is interesting to note that the chronic administration of benzodiazepines seems to produce the same degree of pharmacodynamic tolerance to oral doses despite a longer half-life in the elderly.[79] These observations indicate that adaptive responses of the benzodiazepine receptor system in aging may involve a number of different mechanisms.

Other CNS-active agents also appear to demonstrate greater activity in the elderly. The minimal alveolar concentration for anesthetic agents such as halothane is reduced in an age-dependent fashion from newborns to those over 70 years of age.[80] In addition, much greater analgesia and sedation is evident in elderly patients with the administration of narcotic analgesics.[81–83] Finally, barbiturates also demonstrate an increased response in elderly patients.[84]

Pharmacodynamic alterations play a role in the age-dependent reduction in the dose requirement for warfarin.[85,86] Because there is no difference in the pharmacokinetics of warfarin between young and aged patients,[86,87] the mechanism appears to be increased sensitivity of the synthetic pathway of vitamin K^+–dependent clotting factors to warfarin. The obvious clinical outcome is an increased clotting time with a greater risk for hemorrhage.

In contrast to the above studies noting enhanced responsiveness in the elderly, age-related alterations in beta receptor responsiveness mediate a decrease in organ response. An early study by Vestal and coworkers[88] demonstrated a reduction in the chronotropic response to isoproterenol in elderly patients. This apparent reduction in the sensitivity of beta receptor-dependent mechanisms was consistent with a reduction in the efficacy of propranolol in blocking beta receptor responses in elderly patients.[89] Two other studies also demonstrated that in the elderly there is a reduction in the effectiveness of cardiac beta-adrenergic receptor mechanisms in mediating a response to exercise-induced stress in humans.[90,91]

The mechanisms of age-dependent alterations in beta receptor-mediated events have been studied by measuring the characteristics of both receptor binding and second messenger systems in various tissues.[92,93] An age-related reduction in beta receptor number has been demonstrated in brain tissues,[94] erythrocytes,[95] and fat cells.[96] While a decrease in lymphocyte beta receptor number was originally reported,[97] this observation has not been confirmed,[98,99] although it was reviewed recently by Rutledge and Steinberg.[100]

A number of other studies have also demonstrated decreases in beta-adrenergic receptors in various tissues.[101] The data indicate that beta-adrenergic receptors are decreased in most areas of the brain, with the exception of the cortex. Less consistency in the alterations in peripheral organ beta receptors caused by aging may be related to alterations in the affinity of beta agonists for the receptor rather than to the total number. For example, while the number of beta receptors is unaltered, decreased affinity of agonists for the beta receptor has been demonstrated in the senescent rat lung.[102] Interestingly, diet restriction retards this loss.[103] Alterations in receptor site affinity may well be related to an age-related inability to form the high-affinity state of the receptor. Guanine nucleotide-dependent binding proteins regulate this state of the receptor, and data suggest that the shift from low- to high-affinity binding may be impaired in aging.

The coupling of this event to adenylate cyclase may be impaired, along with adenylate cyclase activity. Total adenylate cyclase activity has been demonstrated to be decreased in the aging heart.[104] Moreover, activation of adenylate cyclase by sodium fluoride or forskolin (colforsin) occurs beyond the receptor-guanine nucleotide binding step and is also depressed in aging.[105] However, recent studies in rat brain have failed to demonstrate age-related changes in sodium fluoride activation of adenylate cyclase.[106] The inconsistency in organ and mechanistic alterations in beta-adrenergic receptors and second messengers demonstrates the complexity of age-related alterations in beta receptor systems.

Most of the available data suggest an age-related reduction in alpha-adrenergic receptor activity.[102,107] This occurs primarily in alpha$_2$ receptors as demonstrated by a reduced receptor number in platelets,[108] guinea pig ileum,[109] and brain.[110] Transduction mechanisms coupled to alpha$_2$ receptor activation also appear to change with aging, since guanosine triphosphate (GTP) binding and/or coupling activity of inhibitory as well as stimulatory GTP-binding regulatory protein to catalytic units is decreased in brains from aged rats.[111]

The cholinergic nervous system also appears to exhibit reduced activity in certain tissues during aging.[112] Studies have demonstrated an age-related decrease in presynaptic cholinergic activity in the hippocampus[113] and striatum[114] of rat brain. In addition, there is a reduction in presynaptic choline uptake in aged animals,[115] suggesting that overall presynaptic cholinergic neuron activity is reduced in the aged brain. Postsynaptic acetylcholine receptor systems also appear to be reduced as measured by [^{3}H]-pirenzepine binding to muscarinic M1 receptors.[116] This reduction is reflected in reduced phosphatidylinositol turnover, which is an essential second messenger system coupled to M1 receptors. As with a number of other observations of age-related alterations in receptor activity, diet restriction can reverse the effect of aging on the reduction of phosphatidylinositol turnover.[117] Much of the work on age-related alterations in the cholinergic system has focused on the role of this system in Alzheimer's disease, since it appears to mediate aspects of learning and memory.[118]

SUMMARY

Although it is unclear what clinical significance is associated with age-related alterations in the pharmacokinetics and pharmacodynamics of drugs, some important clinical strategies follow from these studies. These strategies include altering the dosing frequency of benzodiazepines and reducing the inspired concentration of anesthetics in the elderly. The body of knowledge concerning the clinical relevance of alterations in drug response is growing, to the benefit of the elderly patient population. Through consideration of age as a factor in determining patients' response to drugs, therapeutic agents can be more effectively and safely administered to elderly patients.

REFERENCES

1. Bender AD: A pharmacodynamic basis for changes in drug activity associated with aging in the adult. *Exp Gerontol* 1:237, 1965.
2. Bender AD: The effect of age on intestinal absorption: Implications for drug absorption in the elderly. *J Am Geriatr Soc* 16:1331, 1968.
3. Vestal RE: Drug use in the elderly: A review of problems and special considerations. *Drugs* 16:358, 1978.
4. Pucino F, Beck CL, Seifert RL: Pharmacogeriatrics. *Pharmacotherapy* 5:314, 1985.

5. Mitenko PA: Drug monitoring in the elderly. *Clin Biochem* 19:145, 1986.
6. Hershey LA: Avoiding adverse drug reactions in the elderly. *Mt Sinai J Med (NY)* 55:244, 1988.
7. Buechler JR, Malloy MS: Drug therapy in the elderly: How to achieve optimum results. *Postgrad Med* 85:87, 1989.
8. Cadieux TJ: Drug interactions in the elderly: How multiple drug use increases risk exponentially. *Postgrad Med* 86:179, 1989.
9. Cherry KE, Morton MR: Drug sensitivity in older adults: The role of physiologic and pharmacokinetic factors. *Int J Aging Hum Dev* 28:159, 1989.
10. Harper CM, Newton PA, Walsh JR: Drug induced illness in the elderly. *Postgrad Med* 86:245, 1989.
11. Schwertz DW, Buschmann MBT: Pharmacogeriatrics. *Crit Care Nurs Q* 12:26 1989.
12. Tsujimoto G, Hashimoto K, Hoffman BB: Pharmacokinetic and pharmacodynamic principles of drug therapy in old age: Part 1. *Int J Clin Pharmacol Ther Toxicol* 27:13, 1989.
13. Tsujimoto G, Hashimoto K, Hoffman BB: Pharmacokinetic and pharmacodynamic principles of drug therapy in old age: Part 2. *Int J Clin Pharmacol Ther Toxicol* 27:102, 1989.
14. Durnas C, Loi CM, Cusack B: Hepatic drug metabolism and aging. *Clin Pharamacokinet* 19:359, 1990.
15. Feely J, Coakley D: Altered pharmacodynamics in the elderly. *Clin Geriatr Med* 6:269, 1990.
16. Swift CG: Pharmacodynamics: Changes in homeostatic mechanisms, receptor and target organ sensitivity in the elderly. *Br Med Bull* 46:35, 1990.
17. Tregaskis BF, Stevenson IH: Pharmacokinetics in old age. *Br Med Bull* 46:9, 1990.
18. Woodhouse KW, James OFW: Hepatic drug metabolism and ageing. *Br Med Bull* 46:22, 1990.
19. Yuen GJ: Altered pharmacokinetics in the elderly. *Clin Geriatr Med* 6:257, 1990.
20. Birubaum LS: Pharmacokinetic basics of age-related changes in sensitivity to toxicants. *Annu Rev Pharmacol* 31:101, 1991.
21. Gurwitz JH, Avorn J: The ambiguous relation between aging and adverse drug reactions. *Ann Intern Med* 114:956, 1991.
22. Wright G: Geropharmacology: An individualized approach. *J Am Acad Nurs Pract* 3:85, 1991.
23. Potempa KM, Folta A: Drug use and effects in older adults in the United States. *Int J Nurs Stud* 29:17, 1992.
24. Sloan RW: Principles of drug therapy in geriatric patients. *Am Fam Physician* 45:2709, 1992.
25. Tomaselli CE: Pharmacotherapy in the geriatric population. *Spec Care Dent* 12:107, 1992.
26. Tumer N, Scarpace PJ, Lowenthal DT: Geriatric pharmacology: Basic and clinical considerations. *Annu Rev Pharmacol Toxicol* 32:271, 1992.
27. Williams L, Lowenthal DT: Drug therapy in the elderly. *South Med J* 85:127, 1992.
28. Ritschel WA: Identification of populations at risk in drug testing and therapy: Application to elderly patients. *Eur J Drug Metab Pharmacokinet* 18:101, 1993.
29. Baron JH: Studies of basal peak acid output with an augmented histamine test. *Gut* 4:136, 1963.
30. Bender AD: The effect of increasing age on the distribution of peripheral blood flow in man. *J Am Geriatr Soc* 13:192, 1965.

31. Fikry ME, Aboul Wafa MH: Intestinal absorption in the old. *Gerontol Clin* 7:171, 1965.
32. Geokar MC, Haverback BJ: The aging gastrointestinal tract. *Am J Surg* 117:881, 1969.
33. Shock NW, Natkin DM, Yiengst BS, et al: Age differences in water content of the body as related to basal oxygen consumption in males. *J Gerontol* 18:1, 1963.
34. Forbes GB, Reina JC: Adult lean body mass declines with age: Some longitudinal observations. *Metabolism* 19:653, 1978.
35. Edelman IS, Leibman J: Anatomy of body water and electrolytes. *Am J Med* 27:256, 1959.
36. Novak LP: Aging, total potassium, fat free mass and cell mass in males and females between the ages of 18 and 85 years. *J Gerontol* 27:438, 1972.
37. Vestal RE, McGuire EA, Tobin JD, et al: Aging and ethanol metabolism. *Clin Pharmacol* 21:343, 1977.
38. Vestal RE, Norris AH, Tobin JD, et al: Antipyrine metabolism in man: Influence of age, alcohol, and caffeine and smoking. *Clin Pharmacol* 18:425, 1975.
39. Christensen JH, Anderson S, Jansen JA: Pharmacokinetics and pharmacodynamics of thiopentone. *Anaesthesia* 37:398, 1982.
40. Greenblat DJ: Reduced serum albumin concentration in the elderly: A report from the Boston Collaborative Drug Surveillance Program. *J Am Geriatr Soc* 27:20, 1979.
41. Wallace S, Whiting B, Runcie J: Factors affecting drug binding in plasma of the elderly. *Br J Clin Pharmacol* 3:327, 1976.
42. Hayes MJ, Langman MJS, Short AH: Changes in drug metabolism with increasing age: Phenytoin clearance and protein binding. *Br J Clin Pharmacol* 2:73, 1975.
43. Wynne HA, Cope CH, James OFW, et al: The effect of age upon liver volume and apparent liver blood flow in healthy man. *Hepatology* 9:297, 1989.
44. Bach B, Hansen JM, Kampmann JP, et al: Disposition of antipyrine and phenytoin correlated with age and liver volume in man. *Clin Pharmacokinet* 6:389, 1981.
45. Castleden CM, George CF: The effect of aging on the hepatic clearance of propranolol. *Br J Clin Pharmacol* 7:49, 1979.
46. Ballie SP, Bateman DN, Coater PE, et al: Age and the pharmacokinetics of morphine. *Age Ageing* 18:258, 1989.
47. Aisak B, Kelly JG, Lavan J, et al: Pharmacokinetics of lidocaine in the elderly. *Br J Clin Pharmacol* 9:293, 1980.
48. Greenblat DJ, Sellers EM, Shaden RI: Drug disposition in old age. *N Engl J Med* 306:1081, 1982.
49. O'Malley K, Crooke J, Duke E, et al: Effect of age and sex on human drug metabolism. *Br Med J* 3:607, 1971.
50. Allen MD, Greenblat DJ, Harmatz JS, et al: Desmethyl-diazepam kinetics in the elderly after oral prazepam. *Clin Pharmacol Ther* 18:196, 1980.
51. Ritschel WA: Drug disposition in the elderly: Gerontokinetics. *Methods Find Exp Clin Pharmacol* 14:555, 1992.
52. Diroll M, Abernethy DR, Ameer B, et al: Acetaminophen kinetics in the elderly. *Clin Pharmacol Ther* 31:151, 1982.
53. Briant RH, Dorrington RE, Cleal J, et al: The rate of acetaminophen metabolism in the elderly and the young. *J Am Geriatr Soc* 8:359, 1976.
54. Miners JD, Penhall R, Robson RA, et al: Comparison of paracetamol metabolism in young adult and elderly males. *Eur J Clin Pharmacol* 35:157, 1988.
55. Salem SAM, Rajgayabun P, Shepard AMM, et al: Reduced induction of drug metabolism in the elderly. *Age Ageing* 7:68, 1978.

56. Wood AJ, Vestal RE, Wilkinson GR, et al: The effects of aging and cigarette smoking on the elimination of antipyrine and indocyanine green. *Clin Pharmacol Ther* 26:16, 1979.
57. Feely J, Pereira L, Guy E, et al: Factors affecting the response to inhibition of drug metabolism to cimetidine: Dose response and sensitivity of elderly and induced subjects. *Br J Clin Pharmacol* 17:77, 1981.
58. Divoll N, Greenblat D, Abernathy D, et al: Cimetidine impairs clearance of antipyrine and desmethyl-diazepam in the elderly. *J Am Geriatr Soc* 30:684, 1982.
59. Wynne HA, Mutch E, Williams FM, et al: The relation of age to the acute effects of ethanol on acetanilide disposition. *Age Aging* 18:123, 1989.
60. Vetal RE, Cusack BJ, Mercer GD, et al: Aging and drug interactions: I. Effect of cimetidine and smoking on oxidation of theophylline and cortisol in healthy men. *J Pharmacol Exp Ther* 241:488, 1987.
61. Davies DF, Shock NW: Age changes glomerular filtration rate, effective renal plasma flow, and tubular excretory capacity in adult males. *J Clin Invest* 29:496, 1950.
62. Siersbaek-Nielsen K, Hansen JM, Kampmann J, et al: Rapid evaluation of creatinine clearance. *Lancet* 1:1133, 1971.
63. Rowe JW, Andres R, Tobin JD, et al: The effect of age on creatinine clearance in men: A cross-sectional and longitudinal study. *J Gerontol* 31:155, 1976.
64. Matzke GR, Jameson JJ, Halstenson CE: Gentamicin disposition in young and elderly patients with various degrees of renal function. *J Clin Pharmacol* 27:216, 1987.
65. Bauer LA, Blouin RA: Influence of age on amikacin pharmacokinetics in patients without renal disease: A comparison with gentamicin and tobramicin. *Eur J Clin Pharmacol* 24:639, 1983.
66. Bennett WM, Aranoff GR, Morrison G, et al: Drug prescribing in renal failure: Dosing guidelines for adults. *Am J Kidney Dis* 3:155, 1983.
67. Greenblat DJ, Allen MD, Harmatz JS, et al: Diazepam disposition determinants. *Clin Pharmacol Ther* 27:301, 1980.
68. Leikola E, Vartia KO: On penicillin levels in young and geriatric subjects. *J Gerontol* 12:48, 1957.
69. Orme ML'E, Tallis RC: Metoclopramide and tardive dyskinesia in the elderly. *Br Med J* 289:397, 1984.
70. Caird FI, Andrews GR, Kennedy RD: Effect of posture on blood pressure in the elderly. *Br Heart J* 35:527, 1973.
71. Gribbin B, Pickering TG, Sleight P: The effect of age and high blood pressure sensitivity in man. *Circ Res* 29:424, 1971.
72. Swift CG, Swift MR, Ankier SI, et al: Single dose pharmacokinetics and pharmacodynamics of oral loprazolam in the elderly. *Br J Clin Pharmacol* 20:119, 1985.
73. Greenblat DJ, Allen MD, Shader RI: Toxicity of high dose flurazepam in the elderly. *Clin Pharmacol Ther* 21:355, 1977.
74. Castleden CM, George CF, Marcer D, et al: Increased sensitivity to nitrazepam in old age. *Br Med J* 1:10, 1977.
75. Reidenberg M, Levy M, Warner H, et al: Relationship between diazepam dose, plasma level, age and central nervous system depression. *Clin Pharmacol Ther* 23:371, 1978.
76. Giles HG, Mac Loed SM, Wright JR, et al: Influence of age and previous use on diazepam dosage required for endoscopy. *Can Med Assoc J* 118:513, 1978.
77. Tsang CC, Speeg KV, Wilkinson GR: Age and benzodiazepine binding in the rat cerebral cortex. *Life Sci* 30:343, 1982.

78. Pedigo NW, Shoemaker H, Morselli M: Benzodiazepine receptor binding in young, mature, and senescent rat brain and kidney. *Neurobiol Aging* 2:83, 1981.
79. Flanagan R, James IM: Diazepam tolerance: Effect of age, regular sedation and alcohol. *Br Med J* 289:351, 1984.
80. Gregory GA, Eger EI, Munson ES: The relationship between age and halothane requirement in man. *Anesthesiology* 30:488, 1969.
81. Belville JW, Forrest WH, Miller E, et al: Influence of age on pain relief from analgesics: A study of postoperative patients. *JAMA* 217:1835, 1971.
82. Kaiko RF: Age and morphine analgesia in cancer patients with postoperative pain. *Clin Pharmacol Ther* 28:823, 1980.
83. Scott JC, Ponganis KN, Stanski DR: EEG quantitation of narcotic effect: The comparative pharmacodynamics of fentanyl and alfentanil. *Anesthesiology* 62:234, 1985.
84. Bender AD: Pharmacologic aspects of aging: A survey of the effect of increasing age on drug activity in adults. *J Am Geriatr Soc* 12:114, 1964.
85. O'Malley K, Stevenson IH, Ward CA, et al: Determination of anticoagulant control in patients receiving warfarin. *Br J Clin Pharmacol* 4:309, 1977.
86. Routledge PA, Chapman PH, Davies DM, et al: Factors affecting warfarin requirements. *Eur J Clin Pharmacol* 15:319, 1979.
87. Shepherd AMM, Hewick DS, Moreland TA, et al: Age as a determinate of sensitivity to warfarin. *Br J Clin Pharmacol* 4:315, 1977.
88. Vestal RE, Wood AH, Shand DG: Reduced beta adrenoceptor sensitivity in the elderly. *Clin Pharmacol Ther* 26:181, 1979.
89. Bertal O, Buhler FR, Kiowski W, et al: Decreased beta adrenoceptor responsiveness as related to age, blood pressure and plasma catecholamines in patients with essential hypertension. *Hypertension* 2:130, 1980.
90. Lakatta EG, Gerstenblith G, Angeli CS, et al: Diminished inotropic response of aged myocardium to catecholamines. *Circ Res* 36:262, 1975.
91. Rodeheffer RJ, Gerstenblith G, Beeker LC, et al: Exercise cardiac output is maintained with advanced age in healthy human subjects: Cardiac dilation and increased stroke volume compensate for a diminished heart rate. *Circulation* 69:203, 1984.
92. Scarpace PJ, Turner N, Muder SL: Beta adrenergic function in aging: Basic mechanisms and clinical implications. *Drugs Aging* 1:116, 1991.
93. Colangelo PM, Blouiss RA, Steinmetz RA, et al: Age and beta adrenergic sensitivity to S(-)-and R, S(+/−)-propranolol in humans. *Clin Pharmacol Ther* 51:549, 1992.
94. Greenberg LH, Dix RK, Weiss B: Age related changes in the binding of ^{3}H-dihydroalprenolol in rat brain, in Roberts J, Adelman R, Cristolfado VJ (eds): *Pharmacological Intervention in the Aging Process.* New York: Plenum, 1978, pp 245–249.
95. Bylund DM, Tellez-Inon MH, Hollenberg MD: Age related parallel decline in beta adrenergic receptors, adenylate cyclase and phosphodiesterase activity in rat erythrocytic membranes. *Life Sci* 21:403, 1977.
96. Gindicelli Y, Pecquery R: Beta-adrenergic receptors and catecholamine sensitive adenylate cyclase in rat fat cell membranes: Influence of growth, cell size, and ageing. *Eur J Biochem* 90:413, 1970.
97. Schocken D, Roth G: Reduced beta adrenergic receptor concentrations in ageing. *Nature* 267:856, 1977.
98. Doyle VM, O'Malley K, Kelly JG: Human lymphocyte beta-adrenoceptor density in relation to age and hypertension. *J Cardiovasc Pharmacol* 4:738, 1982.

99. Feldman RD, Limbird LE, Nadeau JL: Alterations in leukocyte beta-receptor affinity with ageing: A potential explanation for altered beta-adrenergic sensitivity in the elderly. *N Engl J Med* 310:815, 1984.
100. Rutledge DR, Steinberg JD: Effect of age on beta-2-adrenergic responsiveness. *DICP* 25:532, 1991.
101. Scarpace AJ, Abrass IB: Alpha- and beta-adrenergic receptor function in the brain during senescence. *Neurobiol Aging* 9:53, 1988.
102. Scarpace AJ, Abrass IB: Decreased beta-adrenergic agonist affinity and adenylate cyclase activity in senescent rat lung. *J Gerontol* 38:143, 1983.
103. Scarpace AJ, Yu BP: Diet restriction retards the age-related loss of beta-adrenergic receptors and adenylate cyclase activity in rat lung. *J Gerontol* 42:442, 1987.
104. Bohn M, Dorner H, Htun P, et al: The effects of exercise on myocardial adenylate cyclase and G*i* alpha expression in aging. *Am J Physiol* 264:H805, 1993.
105. Mooradian AD, Scarpace AJ: 3,5,3^9-L triiodothyronine regulation of beta-adrenergic receptor density and adenylyl cyclase activity in synaptosomal membranes of aged rats. *Neurosci Lett* 161:101, 1993.
106. Mooradian AD, Scarpace AJ: Beta-adrenergic receptor of cerebral microvessels is reduced in aged rats. *Neurochem Res* 16:447, 1991.
107. Docherty JR: Aging and the cardiovascular system. *J Auton Pharmacol* 6:77, 1986.
108. Buckley C, Curtin D, Walsh T, et al: Ageing and platelet alpha$_2$ adrenoceptors. *Br J Clin Pharmacol* 21:721, 1986.
109. Takayanagi I, Malda O, Koike K: Effect of aging on presynaptic alpha$_2$ adrenoceptor function in guinea pig ileum. *Comp Biochem Physiol* 92:419, 1989.
110. Mollace U, Donato Di Paolo E, Gratteri S, et al: Age-related alterations in cardiovascular responsiveness to clonidine infused into the nucleus tractus solitatti in rats. *Neuropharmacology* 28:37, 1989.
111. Nomura Y, Kitamura Y, Kawai M, Segawa T: Alpha$_2$-adrenoceptor-GTP binding regulatory protein-adenylate cyclase system in cerebral cortical membranes of adult and senescent rats. *Brain Res* 379:118, 1986.
112. Muller WE, Stoli L, Schubert T, et al: Central cholinergic functioning and aging. *Acta Psychiatr Scand* 366:34, 1991.
113. Springer JE, Tayrein MW, Loy R: Regional analysis of age-related changes in the cholinergic system of the hippocampal formation and basal forebrain of the rat. *Brain Res* 407:180, 1987.
114. Consolo S, Wang JX, Florentini F, et al: In-vivo and in-vitro studies on the regulation of cholinergic neurotransmission in striatum, hippocampus and cortex of aged rats. *Brain* Res 374:212, 1986.
115. Forloni G, Angeretti N: Decreased [^{3}H]hemicholinium binding to high-affinity choline sites in aged rat brain. *Brain Res* 570:354, 1992.
116. Ohnuki T, Nomura: M1 acetylcholine receptor-mediated phosphatidylinositol turnover in adult and senescent rat brain slices. *Jpn J Pharmacol* 57:483, 1991.
117. Undie AS, Friedman E: Diet restriction prevents aging-induced deficits in brain phosphoinositide metabolism. *J Gerontol* 48:B62, 1993.
118. Joseph JA, Cutler R, Roth GS: Changes in G-protein-mediated signal transduction in aging and Alzheimer's disease. *Ann NY Acad Sci* 695:42, 1993.

CHAPTER 7

Influence of Aging on Inhalation and Intravenous Agents

Amy C. Benedikt
Lois L. Bready

INTRODUCTION

As was described in the preceding chapters, many organ functions of geriatric patients are significantly impaired. These differences, in comparison to younger patients, may lead to altered reactions and increased durations of inhaled and intravenous anesthetic agents. While past reports suggest that the elderly are more likely to suffer from deterioration of mental function after anesthesia and surgery,[1,2] more recent studies of age-related cognitive recovery after general anesthesia indicate that postoperative mental deterioration is not greater in elderly patients than in younger ones.[3,4] A probable factor in the decline of reports of postoperative delirium in elderly patients is improved knowledge and understanding of the effects of altered respiratory, cardiac, and renal functions. This enables an anesthesiologist to make well-informed decisions pertaining to the selection of anesthetic drugs and the calculation of appropriate doses and concentrations.

A question that often arises is whether regional anesthesia for elderly patients may result in less postoperative delirium compared with general anesthesia. In a recent study comparing cognitive and psychosocial functioning in elderly patients undergoing knee arthroplasty, no differences were found at 3 months postoperatively compared with preoperative function levels.[5]

ALTERATIONS IN ORGAN FUNCTION: IMPACT ON INHALATIONAL AGENTS

Effects of Altered Respiratory Function

The effects of altered respiratory function in the elderly include the following: reduced ventilatory volumes, impaired pulmonary gas exchange, decreased basal ventilation requirements because of a decreased basal metabolic rate, decreased ventilatory muscle strength, decreased lung elastance, and increased residual volumes (Table 7-1).

Other changes include loss of vital capacity, an increased closing capacity that leads to air trapping and ventilation-perfusion mismatching, increased work of breathing, and decreased maximum breathing capacity. There is an impaired response to hypoxia and hypercarbia.

Clinical Importance

These changes, along with a decreased minimum alveolar concentration (MAC) and an increased percentage of body fat, cause *rapid inhalational induction* and *prolonged emergence* from general anesthesia.

Effects of Altered Cardiac Function

The specific changes in cardiac and circulatory physiology of the elderly have been described elsewhere. Briefly stated, these changes include reduced cardiac output, conduction abnormalities, slowed circulation time, and silent myocardial ischemia (Table 7-2).

Clinical Importance

Reduced cardiac output and slowed circulation time lead to a more rapid inhalational induction of anesthesia in elderly patients. Because of depressed

Table 7-1 Changes in respiratory function with advanced age

Chest wall compliance decreases
Work of breathing increases
Lung elastance decreases
Ventilatory volumes and capacities
Total lung capacity decreases
Vital capacity decreases
Maximum voluntary minute ventilation decreases
Residual volumes increase
Closing capacity increases
Ventilatory muscle strength decreases
Efficiency of gas exchange decreases
Basal ventilation requirements decrease as a result of decreased basal metabolic rate
Response to hypoxia and hypercapnia is impaired

Table 7-2 Changes in cardiovascular function with advanced age

Cardiac output decreases
Conduction abnormalities
Heart rate response to catecholamines decreases
Dysrhythmias are more common
Need for pacemaker?
Chronotropic response to drugs decreases
Circulation time slows
Silent myocardial ischemia
Arterial calcification
Systemic vascular resistance increases
Hypertension is more prevalent

cardiac function, such a patient may be more sensitive to the cardiac depressant effects of inhalation agents.

Effects of Altered Renal Function

With aging, there is a progressive loss of functioning glomerulotubular units, leading to decreases in the glomerular filtration rate and tubular function. The renal blood flow and glomerular filtration rate decrease by 1 to 2 percent per year after age 25 years (Table 7-3). This phenomenon is manifested as decreased creatinine clearance.

Clinical Importance

The kidneys of elderly patients are less effective in handling increased fluid loads or dehydration, and renal failure is a common cause of death in elderly patients after major vascular surgery. Impaired renal function leads to a prolongation of the effects of renally excreted drugs and metabolites. These considerations could affect the choice of a specific inhalational agent, for example, the avoidance of an agent, such as enflurane, whose metabolites are potentially nephrotoxic.

Table 7-3 Changes in renal function with advanced age

Functioning glomerulotubular units decrease
Glomerular filtration rate decreases
Renal blood flow decreases
Creatinine clearance decreases
Tubular function decreases
Fluid load is tolerated poorly

Table 7-4 Changes in central and peripheral nervous system with advanced age

Progressive loss of neuronal mass
Lessened ability to cooperate
Risk of postoperative confusion increases
Decrease in respiratory response to hypoxia and hypercarbia
Synthesis of neurotransmitters decreases
Sensitivity to anesthetics increases
Inhalational
Intravenous
Peripheral myelin loss
Decreases nerve conduction velocity

Effects of Altered Central Nervous System Function

Requirements for the various inhalational agents tend to decrease with increasing age. There is some controversy regarding the specific mechanisms for this increased sensitivity. Physiological function of the brain may not decrease with age in patients whose nutrition and exercise have been maintained. In all elderly patients, however, there is a progressive loss of neuronal mass, including the neurons involved in the production and reception of neurotransmitters (Table 7-4). This anesthetic sensitivity applies to inhalational agents and is manifested by a decreased MAC.

Clinical Importance

Depressant effects of the inhalational agents are enhanced in the elderly, probably secondary to an increased sensitivity. The MACs of the individual agents decrease by about 4 percent for each decade after age 40 (Table 7-5).

SPECIFIC INHALATIONAL AGENTS

Isoflurane

The young and the elderly have similar rates of washin for isoflurane.[6] Isoflurane, with its lower blood gas partition coefficient, has a faster washin than does

Table 7-5 Minimum alveolar concentration (MAC) of potent inhalational agents

Agent	MAC in 18- to 30-year-olds, %	MAC in >65-year-olds, %
Halothane	0.75	0.65
Enflurane	1.68	~1.4
Isoflurane	1.15	1.0
Desflurane	7.25	5.17
Sevoflurane	1.7–2.0	1.48

halothane in young and elderly patients.[6] The effect of isoflurane on thermoregulatory vasoconstriction during nitrous oxide–isoflurane anesthesia has been studied. The threshold is lower in elderly than in younger patients.[7] The heart rate increases seen with isoflurane appear to be less pronounced in the elderly.

Isoflurane has a lower blood gas partition coefficient and a consequent lower solubility in fat than halothane; therefore, this agent may be preferable in an older patient with a greater percentage of body fat.

Halothane

McKinney and coworkers[8] showed that in elderly patients given either halothane or isoflurane, similar degrees of cardiovascular depression, specifically systolic and diastolic hypotension, occurred. Isoflurane produced a greater decrease in both systolic and diastolic pressures in the elderly. In a study of the rate of inhalation induction with halothane in young versus elderly patients, there was no difference in the rate of rise of end-tidal halothane concentrations.[9] Equilibration of end-tidal with inspired concentration occurred more rapidly with isoflurane than with halothane in both older and younger patients.

In 1991, a follow-up study by Dwyer and associates[6] again showed that halothane washin was slower in the elderly than in the young, while the washin of isoflurane was significantly faster than that of halothane in both the young and the elderly. This latter finding would be expected on the basis of blood gas solubility coefficients.

Enflurane

The MAC of enflurane decreases with age in a manner similar to that of other potent inhalational agents. While this agent has been used for over a decade in the geriatric population, it has largely been replaced by other potent inhalational agents.

Desflurane and Sevoflurane

As with the older inhalational agents, the MACs of the newer drugs desflurane and sevoflurane decrease with age. Both agents have much lower blood gas partition coefficients: 0.45 for desflurane (comparable to nitrous oxide) and 0.65 for sevoflurane. These agents should be eliminated more rapidly from fatty tissues than are the more soluble inhalational agents. Katoh and colleagues demonstrated this concept by showing that as a patient ages, the awakening concentration (the end-tidal anesthetic concentration at eye opening in response to a verbal command) declines with decreases in MAC for both sevoflurane and isoflurane.[10,11] The more rapid egress of the inhalational agent predicts a lower concentration of agent remaining at the conclusion of the anesthetic and a correspondingly more rapid emergence. Bennett's group[2] looked at this issue and found that elderly patients *do* recover more rapidly from desflurane than from isoflurane.

EMERGENCE FROM INHALATION ANESTHESIA

Recovery from inhalation anesthesia is slower in the elderly than in the young, as demonstrated by end-tidal and mixed expired anesthetic concentrations of isoflurane, enflurane, halothane, and methoxyflurane.[13] Aging delayed elimination of the anesthetic and increased the apparent volume of distribution (Vd) at steady state.

Strum and colleagues[13] also demonstrated that the apparent Vd for volatile agents increases with age. Estimates of tissue perfusion are decreased and those of tissue volume are increased in the elderly.

FLUID COMPARTMENTS: ALTERATIONS WITH ADVANCING AGE

The elderly have an increased percentage of body fat, decreased lean body mass, and decreased intracellular water content. These changes are more pronounced in women. The implications of this increased body fat include the tendency to retain lipid-soluble agents, both inhalational and intravenous. The elderly also have decreased total body water (primarily intracellularly) and a decreased blood volume.

PROTEIN BINDING: EFFECTS OF AGE AND CONCURRENT DISEASES

Drugs are administered to elderly patients via various routes (intravenous, oral, rectal, intranasal, sublingual, transcutaneous, and topical) and once they enter the circulation are subject to protein binding. A drug that is protein-bound does not cross membranes to a clinically significant degree and thus is not pharmacologically active. Any process that interferes with protein binding is therefore likely to result in a greater fraction of the drug being available to exert its effect in the patient.

There is less protein binding in an elderly patient than in a younger patient for several reasons. Serum albumin levels decrease with age,[14] resulting in fewer binding sites for drugs. Qualitative alterations in plasma proteins may also impair binding ability.

An elderly patient is more likely than a younger patient to have one or more medical disorders. Some disorders, such as chronic renal insufficiency, malnutrition, and cardiac failure, cause further impairment of protein production and binding. Chronic medical conditions are treated with multiple medications;

Table 7-6 Drugs bound by $alpha_1$ acid glycoprotein

Drug
Quinidine
Propranolol
Lidocaine
Bupivacaine
Meperidine
Dipyridamole
Verapamil
Alfentanil

these drugs compete for binding sites with the agents given in the perioperative period. Thus, a given dose of an anesthetic agent may result in higher plasma levels of unbound drug and consequently higher tissue levels.

The major proteins in the blood to which drugs bind are albumin, $alpha_1$ acid glycoprotein (AAG), and the lipoproteins.[15] Albumin accounts for about 60 percent of the plasma proteins and binds many drugs (Table 7-6) as well as endogenous compounds.

Albumin

Albumin accounts for 60 percent of the total plasma protein concentration, providing both drug and metabolite binding and oncotic pressure. Albumin is responsible for binding many drugs, especially acidic drugs (Table 7-7).[15] In older patients, both the quantity and the quality of albumin are altered, resulting in a greater unbound and pharmacologically active portion of highly protein-bound acidic drugs, enhancing pharmacologic activity.

$Alpha_1$ Acid Glycoprotein

AAG is another major binding protein, predominantly binding alkaline drugs (Table 7-6). Surgery and trauma increase the level of AAG.[15] This protein also

Table 7-7 Drugs bound primarily by albumin

Alfentanil	Cyclosporine	Meperidine
Amantadine	Digitoxin	Methadone
Amiodarone	Diltiazem	Nicardipine
Amitriptyline	Etoposide	Nifedipine
Amphotericin B	Fentanyl	Penicillins
Benzodiazepines	Furosemide	Phenytoin
Cephalosporins	Glipizide	Prazosin
Chlorambucil	Hydralazine	Quinidine
Chlorpromazine	Lidocaine	Propranolol
Cocaine	Lorcainide	Sulfonamides

increases quantitatively with age[16] and chronic renal failure. Therefore, alkaline drugs are more highly protein-bound in the elderly.

Concurrent Disease

The elderly have an increased incidence of concurrent disease processes that can affect protein binding, including renal disease, malnutrition, and hepatic disease. The coexistence of advanced age with one or more of these concurrent diseases can lead to further impairment in protein binding, particularly in the case of albumin, with resultant increases in the amount of free drug.

ALTERATIONS IN ORGAN FUNCTIONS: IMPACT ON INTRAVENOUS AGENTS

Cardiac Function

As was described earlier in this chapter, cardiac output is decreased, conduction abnormalities are common, and there is an increased risk of silent myocardial ischemia in elderly patients.

The maximum attainable heart rate is reduced in the elderly, and there is a reduced chronotropic response to drugs. In addition, baroreceptor function decreases with age, making postural hypotension and hypotension in response to general or regional anesthesia a greater problem. Patients rendered hypotensive by the administration of generous doses of intravenous anesthetic agents may be unable to increase their cardiac output by increasing their heart rate.

Clinical Importance

Drugs administered intravenously reach receptors more slowly because of a longer circulation time and therefore have a delayed onset of pharmacologic action.

Renal Function

The elderly have a decreased glomerular filtration rate and renal tubular function, and this decreases the renal clearance of parenterally administered drugs and metabolites, especially drugs that are primarily renally excreted.

Clinical Importance

Delayed renal excretion of intravenous sedatives, narcotics, and hypnotics may contribute to undesirably prolonged effects of these agents. Careful titration of administered drugs to achieve the desired clinical effect is important in the elderly to minimize the dose administered.

Hepatic Function

With increasing age, humans have a progressive decrease in hepatic tissue and blood flow, although liver function tests may remain normal. The liver makes lipid-soluble drugs water-soluble by oxidation and conjugation. There are conflicting data regarding the function of microsomal enzyme systems in the elderly, but there is slowed drug metabolism with a delayed decrease in the plasma concentration of drugs, especially those that undergo a significant first-pass effect or effects (Table 7-8).

Clinical Importance

When alternative drugs are available, it is prudent to select those with shorter elimination half-lives or a lesser dependence on hepatic (or renal) excretion in order to avoid a prolonged effect.

Central Nervous System Function

As was described earlier in this chapter, elderly patients are more sensitive than younger patients to the effects of many anesthetic agents, including intravenous anesthetics (Table 7-4).

Clinical Importance

Titration of intravenous agents, to administer the lowest dose consistent with a desired effect is of paramount importance in the elderly. While the anesthesiologist may compensate intraoperatively for profound sedation, it is wise to select intravenous agents whose duration is not overly prolonged (e.g., midazolam versus diazepam) in order to prevent undesired persistent sedation postoperatively. Of particular note is the diminished respiratory response to hypoxia and hypercarbia; extra precautions may be necessary in the postoperative period (e.g., pulse oximetry, supplemental oxygen, and increased level of nursing care) to prevent an adverse occurrence.

Table 7-8 Changes in hepatic function with advanced age

Hepatic tissue decreases
Hepatic blood flow decreases
Liver function tests remain unchanged
Microsomal enzyme activity decreases?
Glucose utilization impaired: risk of hyperglycemia with glucose load

Metabolic Rate

There is a decline in the basal metabolic rate with aging, leading to slower metabolism and excretion of drugs.[16] While there is considerable individual patient variation, the average decrease is about 1 percent per year after age 30 years.[17] The reduction in heat production, combined with impaired thermoregulatory compensation, contributes to intraoperative and postoperative hypothermia.

Clinical Importance

Drug effects are prolonged by the slower metabolism of the elderly. In addition, attention to maintenance of body temperature is vital and can be affected by the selection of anesthetic agents. Vasodilatory agents (thiopental sodium, isoflurane) can inhibit thermoregulatory vasoconstriction of cutaneous vessels and are, therefore, more likely to contribute to intraoperative hypothermia in an elderly patient.[7] Hypothermia itself further lowers the metabolic rate and the ability of the liver to metabolize drugs.

INTRAVENOUS AGENTS

Barbiturates

As age increases, the initial volume of distribution of thiopental decreases, resulting in higher serum levels after a bolus.[18] Other studies have verified this occurrence by showing that the elderly require decreased thiopental induction doses.[18,19] In a follow-up study to their 1985 work,[18] Stanski and colleagues established the fact that the most likely mechanism for the decrease in the required induction dose of thiopental in the elderly is diminished rapid intercompartmental clearance.[20]

In the clinical setting, the administration of a test dose of 25 to 50 mg thiopental allows some estimation of an individual patient's response (sedation, sensitivity, volume status) to the drug. It is vital to remember that the slowed circulation time of an elderly patient requires not only the thoughtful selection of an induction dose but also the passage of a sufficient amount of time before more drug is administered. If adequate time for induction effects is not allowed and subsequent doses are given, it is possible to administer an "overdose" of thiopental.

Benzodiazepines

Diazepam

The beta-elimination half-life of diazepam is prolonged with increasing age, possibly because of an increase in the initial Vd.[21] The elderly are more sensitive to diazepam than are younger patients. An increased sensitivity of the elderly to diazepam premedication was demonstrated by Reidenberg and coworkers.[22] As was discussed earlier, it is prudent to select agents that have a duration of effect appropriate to the planned surgical procedure and whose metabolites, if active, do not have a prolonged effect. For these reasons, diazepam should be considered only when a long-term effect is needed (i.e., several days to a week of sedation/amnesia).

Midazolam

Midazolam may be preferable to diazepam because of its shorter elimination half-life (2–2.5 h in young patients). Elderly subjects, compared with younger subjects, had an increased elimination half-life and a decreased clearance of intravenous midazolam; the total Vd and protein binding were not different.[23] Elderly patients can be induced with low doses of midazolam, evidencing their increased sensitivity to benzodiazepines.[24] Careful titration of midazolam in small incremental doses (0.5 mg per dose) should produce an appropriate level of sedation; however, when necessary, a specific benzodiazepine antagonist, flumazenil, can be used.[25] It is important to remember that the elimination half-life of flumazenil is 0.7 to 1.3 h, which is shorter than the elimination half-lives of both midazolam and diazepam.

Etomidate

Elderly patients require a lower dose of etomidate than do younger patients to produce unconsciousness.[26] This may be due to a lower initial Vd leading to higher initial blood levels of etomidate. The elderly also showed decreased clearance with increasing age.[26] Elderly patients have decreased plasma protein binding of etomidate compared with younger patients; this may be due partially to lower albumin levels.[27]

Ketamine

Ketamine is rarely employed as a sole anesthetic agent in the geriatric population, although it is clinically useful in small doses (e.g., 25 mg) for supplementation of not quite adequate regional blocks and for positioning a hip fracture patient before the placement of a regional block. A number of medical disorders are relative contraindications to the use of ketamine, and many of these disorders are more prevalent in geriatric patients. These contraindications include preexisting hypertension, coronary artery disease, increased intraocular pressure, and elevated intracranial pressure. Emergence after ketamine is slower than with other intravenous induction agents in younger patients and may be undesirably prolonged in the elderly.

Opioids

Morphine

Elderly patients are more sensitive to the effects (sedation, respiratory depression) of narcotics. Morphine plasma levels are higher in older patients, and the rate of decline of plasma levels is inversely related to the age of the patient.[28] Thus, morphine clearance is slower in older patients than it is in younger patients.

Sufentanil

The elimination half-lives, plasma clearance, and total Vd were unchanged for sufentanil when the young were compared with the elderly.[29] The elderly have a smaller initial Vd, leading to a higher initial plasma concentration of sufentanil.[29]

Fentanyl

In a study by Singleton and colleagues,[30] there was no difference in the clearance of fentanyl in elderly versus young patients. Also, the steady-state Vd is lower in the elderly, who therefore have higher initial fentanyl concentrations.[30] Previous studies have shown that elderly patients have a reduced plasma clearance and beta-elimination half-life with resultant higher fentanyl levels for a longer period.[31] The elderly have a reduced dose requirement for fentanyl and alfentanil and are thus more sensitive to these narcotics, as demonstrated by electroencephalographic (EEG) changes.[32]

A study of plasma levels of fentanyl and midazolam in elderly patients who underwent peripheral operations with a thigh tourniquet demonstrated that clinically significant elevation of both drugs was measurable after the release of the tourniquet.[33] These authors recommended monitoring of what is appropriate duration.

Alfentanil

In the elderly, alfentanil has an unchanged Vd and a prolonged terminal beta half-life, possibly because of decreased hepatic clearance.[34] This would imply that the initial calculated dose given to an elderly patient should be the same as that for a younger patient but that the subsequent doses required would be lower.

Propofol

Both propofol and etomidate are cardiovascular depressants in elderly patients.[35] Etomidate does not blunt the cardiovascular response to intubation as effectively as does propofol.[35] Elderly patients demonstrated sensitivity to propofol; those over 60 years old required a smaller induction dose and experienced more apnea and hypotension with a bolus injection given over 20 s.[36] Patients under age 60 required 2.25 to 2.50 mg/kg for induction, while those over age 60 required only 1.50 to 1.75 mg/kg.[29] The elderly had a lower initial Vd of propofol; thus, the concentrations of propofol after injection were higher in elderly patients.[37] The clearance of propofol was also lower in the elderly.[37] Patients over age 65 years seem to have a higher risk of hypotension with a bolus of propofol.[38] When lean tissue mass was used to calculate a propofol dose, there was no difference in the propofol ED_{50} values in elderly patients compared with younger patients.[39] These data contradict previous studies; however, other studies used total body mass[36] rather than lean tissue mass to calculate propofol doses.[39]

SUMMARY

Aging is associated with a decline in organ function. Both pharmacodynamic and pharmacokinetic alterations contribute to a decreased metabolism of both inhalational and intravenous agents. The elderly also exhibit a greater sensitivity to anesthetics. Careful titration of all drugs administered to this growing segment of the population is of the utmost importance.

REFERENCES

1. Bedford TD: Adverse effects of anaesthesia in the elderly. *Lancet* 2:259, 1955.
2. Blundell E: A psychological study of the effects of surgery on eighty-six elderly patients. *Br J Soc Psychol* 6:297, 1967.
3. Ghoneim MM, Hinrichs JV, O'Hara MW, et al: Comparison of psychologic and cognitive functions after general or regional anesthesia. *Anesthesiology* 69:507, 1988.
4. Chung F, Seyone C, Dyck B, et al: Age-related cognitive recovery after general anesthesia. *Anesth Analg* 71:217, 1990.
5. Nielson WR, Gelb AW, Casey JE: Long-term cognitive and social sequelae of general versus regional anesthesia during arthroplasty in the elderly. *Anesthesiology* 73:1103, 1990.
6. Dwyer RC, Fee JPH, Howard PJ, et al: Arterial washin of halothane and isoflurane in young and elderly adult patients. *Br J Anaesth* 66:572, 1991.
7. Kurz A, Plattner O, Sessler DI, et al: The threshold for thermoregulatory vasoconstriction during nitrous oxide/isoflurane anesthesia is lower in elderly than in young patients. *Anesthesiology* 79:465, 1993.
8. McKinney MS, Fee JPH, Clarke SJ: Cardiovascular effects of isoflurane and halothane in young and elderly adult patients. *Br J Anaesth* 71:696, 1993.
9. Dwyer R, Fee JPH, Clarke SJ: End-tidal concentrations of halothane and isoflurane during induction of anaesthesia in young and elderly patients. *Br J Anaesth* 64:36, 1990.

10. Katoh T, Suguro Y, Ikeda T, et al: Influence of age on awakening concentrations of sevoflurane and isoflurane. *Anesth Analg* 76:348, 1993.
11. Nakajima R, Nakajima Y, Ikeda K: Minimum alveolar concentration of sevoflurane in elderly patients. *Br J Anaesth* 70:273, 1993.
12. Bennett JA, Lingaraju N, Horrow JC, et al: Elderly patients recover more rapidly from desflurane than from isoflurane anesthesia. *J Clin Anesth* 4:378, 1992.
13. Strum DP, Eger EI II, Unadkat JD, et al: Age affects the pharmacokinetics of inhaled anesthetics in humans. *Anesth Analg* 73:310, 1991.
14. Greenblatt DJ: Reduced serum albumin concentrations in the elderly: A report from the Boston Collaborative Drug Surveillance Program. *J Am Geriatr Soc* 27:20, 1979.
15. Wood M: Plasma drug binding: Implications for anesthesiologists. *Anesth Analg* 65:786, 1986.
16. McLeskey CH: Anesthesia for the geriatric patient, in Barash PG, Cullen BF, Stoelting RK (eds): *Clinical Anesthesia*, 2d ed. Phildelphia: Lippincott, 1992, chap 49, pp 1353–1388.
17. Janis KM: The geriatric patient, in Kirby RR, Gravenstein N (eds): *Clinical Anesthesia Practice*. Philadelphia: Saunders, 1994, chap 62, pp 1067–1081.
18. Homer TD, Stanski DR: The effect of increasing age on thiopental disposition and anesthetic requirement. *Anesthesiology* 67:714, 1985.
19. Muravchick S: Effect of age and premedication on thiopental sleep dose. *Anesthesiology* 61:333, 1984.
20. Stanski DR, Maitre PO: Population pharmacokinetics and pharmacodynamics of thiopental: The effect of age revisited. *Anesthesiology* 72:412, 1990.
21. Klotz U, Avant GR, Schenker L, et al: The effects of age and liver disease on the disposition and elimination of diazepam in adult man. *J Clin Invest* 55:347, 1975.
22. Reidenberg MM, Levy M, Warner H, et al: Relationship between diazepam dose, plasma level, age, and central nervous system depression. *Clin Pharmacol Ther* 23:371, 1978.
23. Greenblatt DJ, Abernethy DR, Locniskar A, et al: Effect of age, gender, and obesity on midazolam kinetics. *Anesthesiology* 61:27, 1984.
24. Kanto J, Aaltonen L, Himberg JJ, et al: Midazolam as an intravenous induction agent in the elderly: A clinical and pharmacokinetic study. *Anesth Analg* 65:15, 1986.
25. Katz JA, Fragen RJ, Dunn KL: Flumazenil reversal of midazolam sedation in the elderly. *Reg Anaesth* 16:247, 1991.
26. Arden JR, Holley FO, Stanski DR: Increased sensitivity to etomidate in the elderly: Initial distribution versus altered brain response. *Anesthesiology* 65:15, 1986.
27. Carlos R, Calvo R, Erill S: Plasma protein binding of etomidate in different age groups and in patients with chronic respiratory insufficiency. *Int J Clin Pharmacol Ther Toxicol* 19:171, 1981.
28. Kaiko RF, Wallenstein SL, Rogers AG, et al: Narcotics in the elderly. *Med Clin North Am* 66:1079, 1982.
29. Matteo RS, Schwartz AE, Ornstein E, et al: Pharmacokinetics of sufentanil in the elderly surgical patient. *Can J Anaesth* 37:852, 1990.
30. Singleton MA, Rosen JI, Fisher DM: Pharmacokinetics of fentanyl in the elderly. *Br J Anaesth* 60:619, 1988.
31. Bentley JB, Borel JD, Nenad RE: Influence of age on the pharmacokinetics of fentanyl. *Anesth Analg* 61:171, 1982.
32. Scott JC, Stanski DR: Decreased fentanyl and alfentanil dose requirements with age:

A simultaneous pharmacokinetic and pharmacodynamic evaluation. *J Pharmacol Exp Ther* 240:159, 1987.
33. Schmitt H, Batz G, Knoll R, et al: Plasma level changes of fentanyl and midazolam after release of a prolonged thigh tourniquet. *Acta Anaesthesiol Scand* 34:104, 1990.
34. Helmers H, Van Peer A, Woestenborghs R, et al: Alfentanil kinetics in the elderly. *Clin Pharmacol Ther* 36:239, 1984.
35. Larsen R, Rathgeber J, Bagdahn A, et al: Effects of propofol on cardiovascular dynamics and coronary blood flow in geriatric patients. *Anaesthesia* 43:25, 1988.
36. Dundee JW, Robinson FP, McCollum JSC, et al: Sensitivity to propofol in the elderly. *Anaesthesia* 41:482, 1986.
37. Kirkpatrick T, Cockshott ID, Douglas EJ, et al: Pharmacokinetics of propofol (Diprivan) in elderly patients. *Br J Anaesth* 60:146, 1988.
38. Hug CC, McLeskey CH, Nahrwold ML, et al: Hemodynamic effects of propofol: Data from over 25,000 patients. *Anesth Analg* 77:S21, 1993.
39. Leslie K, Crankshaw DP: Lean tissue mass is a useful predictor of induction dose requirements for propofol. *Anaesth Intensive Care* 19:57, 1991.

CHAPTER 8

Influence of Aging on Neuromuscular Blocking Drugs

Thomas A. Witkowski
Joseph L. Seltzer

INTRODUCTION

Neuromuscular blocking agents were introduced into the practice of anesthesia in the 1940s. Their use has increased significantly so that 10 drugs are currently available for clinical use in the United States, with more likely to be introduced in the very near future. Because the use of these drugs is so prevalent in anesthesia and because of the increasing proportion of elderly patients undergoing surgery, a discussion of age-related pharmacologic changes with these drugs is relevant.

The pharmacology of neuromuscular blocking agents can be assessed in both clinical, pharmacokinetic, and pharmacodynamic terms. The relevant clinical features are onset, duration of action, and potency. Pharmacokinetic factors are useful in understanding why a drug behaves as it does clinically. Age-related changes in factors that affect clinical behavior can be examined in general terms as a prelude to looking at the effects of aging on individual drugs. Aging causes changes in body composition that may alter the action of neuromuscular blockers. These changes include a reduction in muscle mass and total body water and an increase in fat.[1] This appears to be more pronounced in elderly men. Despite this reduction in muscle mass, there does not appear to be a decrease in the number of neuromuscular receptors with aging. Plasma albumin concentrations decrease with aging, potentially altering the concentration of free, effective drug.[2] Protein binding for muscle relaxants has been poorly characterized, and its effect on drug concentrations is unknown. Volume of distribution (Vd) is the pharmacokinetic variable affected by these changes in body composition. Increases, decreases, and/or lack of change in Vd in the elderly have all been shown compared with a younger population, with different drugs. There is no predictability in the response with aging.

PROPERTIES OF MUSCLE RELAXANTS

Pharmacokinetic Changes

Vd can be calculated at the time of the initial injection or at steady state after initial redistribution has occurred. In general, muscle relaxants tend to be large charged molecules. They are lipid-insoluble and have Vd's of 0.2 to 0.5 liter/kg at steady state. Changes in the initial volume of distribution (Vd_{cc}) can alter the speed of onset of a muscle relaxant by changing the concentration of a standard dose of relaxant within the blood. The Vd at steady state affects recovery, as decreases in this factor may reduce the redistribution of relaxants, which helps terminate their effects.

Onset

Neuromuscular blocker onset is regulated by the distribution of a drug from the intravenous site of injection to the peripheral muscles.[3] One of the major factors related to onset is cardiac output, which decreases about 1 percent per year from age 19 to age 86. Muscle blood flow as a fraction of total cardiac output is also important but does not appear to change with aging.[4] When the relaxant reaches the muscle, receptor binding must occur. Affinity of muscle for the drug and diffusion of the drug to the receptor are important for receptor binding. These factors have not been investigated but should not change significantly with advancing age.

Potency

The potency of a relaxant also affects the speed of onset, so that a more potent drug, by virtue of having more total molecules available to bind to the receptor, will have a faster onset. Differences in the potency of a muscle relaxant between the young and the old would change onset; however, no potency change with age has been shown with any relaxant to date. Larger doses of relaxant also accelerate onset. Therefore, if the initial Vd changes with aging, the increase or decrease in the concentration of a standard dose of drug may alter the onset. Generally, initial Vd's do not appear to change with aging. In conclusion, a slower onset can be seen with neuromuscular blockers in the elderly, primarily related to their decrease in cardiac output.

Recovery

Spontaneous recovery from neuromuscular blockade occurs when the relaxant concentration at the receptor falls. This occurs when the plasma concentration decreases because of redistribution and/or elimination of the drug. Previously discussed changes in body composition may alter the redistribution and delay recovery. Age-related changes in the steady-state Vd reflect the altered redistribution. The effects of aging on drug elimination may be profound. Blood flow to the liver and kidney, primary organs of elimination for most relaxants, falls with aging.[4] There is a 35 percent fall in creatinine clearance from age 20 to age 70.[5] Tubular function and glomerular filtration decline in the elderly. Antipyrine clearance, a marker for liver function, falls approximately 40 percent in the elderly.[1] Relaxant drugs requiring hepatic or renal elimination might be expected to have a prolonged effect with aging.

SPECIFIC MUSCLE RELAXANTS

Alcuronium

Alcuronium is a semisynthetic, long-acting, curare-like nondepolarizing relaxant. It was first utilized in 1961[6] and is not currently used in the United States. The effects of this largely renally eliminated drug have been investigated in the elderly. Stephens and colleagues[7] studied 10 elderly patients (age > 60), 5 undergoing procedures involving significant blood loss (1.6 liters) and 5 undergoing procedures involving minimal blood loss (300 ml). Both groups received similar doses of alcuronium for their surgery. Elimination half-life was significantly longer and clearance was significantly lower (50 percent) in the minimal-blood-loss group. Patients undergoing major surgery had pharmacokinetic values similar to those of young adult patients. No changes in Vd were noted in either group. The observed difference was related to the blood loss and associated hemodilution in the significant blood loss group. Elimination of this drug was prolonged in elderly patients undergoing more minor procedures because of the decline in renal function in the elderly. A delayed recovery of neuromuscular function could be anticipated with this drug in older patients.

Atracurium

Atracurium is an intermediate-acting benzylisoquinoline. Part of its elimination occurs through plasma breakdown (40 percent)[8] and thus does not depend totally on organ function. For this reason, this drug has been studied extensively in the elderly population. Plasma atracurium concentrations for the maintenance of a stable neuromuscular block have been evaluated in several studies.[9–11] It was found that concentrations do not differ significantly between young and elderly patients. Also, the single doses required for a given level of blockade do not differ between younger and older patients. Thus, there appears to be no difference in the sensitivity of the neuromuscular junction to this drug. Pharmacokinetic properties and clinical recovery have also been evaluated. Kitts and colleagues[11] compared old (74–76 years) and young (22–44 years) patients receiving halothane anesthesia. Patients received atracurium by infusion until twitch was depressed to 30 percent of control values. The investigators determined total clearance of atracurium and the contributions of elimination by organs and plasma to breakdown. Total clearance was similar in both groups, but clearance by organs was decreased in the elderly (1.7 ± 0.9 versus 3.1 ± 0.9 ml/kg per min). Kent and colleagues[12] performed a similar experiment under enflurane anesthesia with a bolus dose of 0.6 mg/kg of atracurium. They found no difference in total clearance of atracurium caused by age. They also found no difference in Vd, in contrast to Kitts and colleagues,[11] who calculated a larger steady-state Vd in the elderly. This is most likely due to differences in the method of calculation and the study design. Both studies found a small increase in elimination half-life ($t_{1/2\beta}$) in the older patients (3–6 min), which is related to decreased elimination by the liver and kidney. Kent and colleagues[12] also evaluated laudanosine kinetics and found that clearance of this metabolite was decreased by 35 percent and that its $t_{1/2\beta}$ was increased from 173 ± 56 to 229 ± 54 min in the elderly. The importance of laudanosine is still widely debated. D'Hollander and associates[10] evaluated recovery from stable 90 percent block under balanced anesthesia in young, middle-aged, and older individuals. There was no difference in time to recovery from 10 to 25 percent or from 25 to 75 percent of control values (first twitch) (Fig. 8-1). Although elimination half-life is slightly increased with this drug, its clinical effects are not prolonged with advanced age.

Doxacurium

Doxacurium is a newer, potent, long-acting nondepolarizing relaxant that undergoes a high degree of renal elimination. Plasma cholinesterase breakdown and hepatic elimination are responsible for only a small proportion of clearance. This drug has been evaluated in the elderly in two studies. Dresner and associates[13] examined onset time to 96 percent block in younger and older patients under isoflurane anesthesia. The onset in the elderly was increased by 3.5 min. The level of block with a 25 μg/kg dose did not differ between groups. This indicated no change in potency with aging. There was a slower and more variable clinical recovery of T1 (first twitch height) to 25 percent of control values in the older patients (Table 8-1). Koscielniak-Nielsen and colleagues[14] performed dose-response studies with doxacurium. Aging did not alter the drug's potency. There was a slower and more variable recovery of doxacurium in the elderly in this study, similar to the results of Dresner. Time for recovery of T1 from 10 to 25 percent of control values increased from 22.7±1.9 to 39.6±2.4 min with aging. Steady-state Vd with this drug was increased in the elderly, but $t_{1/2\beta}$ and clearance did not differ between groups. Clinical use of this drug in older patients will require less frequent dosing because of delayed recovery despite the similar clearances in younger and older patients.

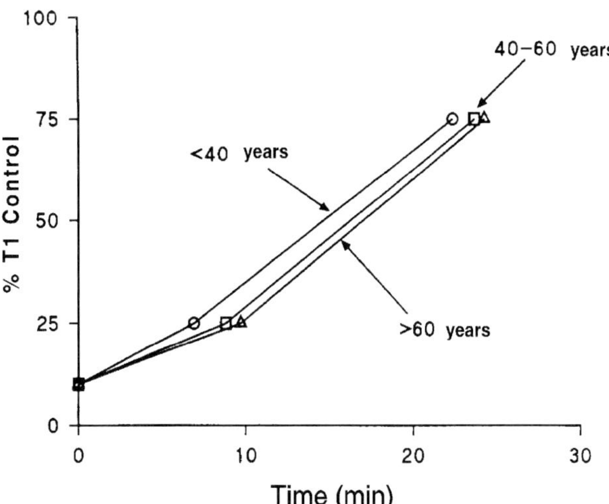

Figure 8-1 Recovery from atracurium infusion of 90 min in three age groups. (*Adapted from D'Hollander and associates.*[10])

Table 8-1 Comparison of doxacurium (25 μg/kg) in young and old patients

	Young (22–49 years) $n = 8$	Old (67–72 years) $n = 8$
Onset (min)	7.7 ± 1.0	11.2 ± 1.1*
25% recovery (min)	67.5 ± 8.2	97.1 ± 20.1*
$t_{1/2b}$ (min)	86 ± 50	96 ± 20
Clearance (ml/kg/min)	2.22 ± 1.09	2.47 ± 0.69
Vd_{ss}(ml/kg)	150 ± 40	220 ± 80.2*

*$p < 0.05$ between groups.

SOURCE: Modified from Dresner and associates.[13]

d-Tubocurarine

The effects on the elderly of this oldest muscle relaxant were initially evaluated in 1954. Based on a retrospective evaluation of dosing by clinical criteria, Dundee found no difference between older and younger patients in the amount of *d*-tubocurarine used.[15] Matteo and coworkers[16] compared patients 30 to 56 years of age with those age 70 to 87 years in terms of their responses to curare. The study was performed under N_2O-halothane anesthesia. The Vd of curare both initially and at steady state was significantly decreased in the elderly. Elimination half-life was increased from 173±38 to 268±51 min, and clearance was significantly decreased from 1.71±0.32 to 0.79±0.18 ml/kg per min in older patients. The plasma concentration needed to achieve a given level of block was not different between younger and older patients; thus, the drug's pharmacodynamics for the two groups is similar. Recovery parameters, as expected from the pharmacokinetic data, were prolonged by increased age. Time to spontaneous recovery of T1 to 50 percent and 75 percent of control values was prolonged significantly with an initial curare dose of 0.3 mg/kg. The recovery index (25–75 percent) doubled with aging (Table 8-2). Therefore, the initial dose requirements are lower with this drug as a result of the decreased Vd_{cc}, and recovery is prolonged with advancing age.

Metocurine

Metocurine and its close relative curare were evaluated by Matteo and coworkers[16] for changes seen with aging. The plasma concentration required to achieve a given level of block did not differ between young and old patients. Clearance and Vd initially and at steady state were significantly lower with metocurine in elderly subjects. These patients, as might be anticipated, had significantly prolonged $t_{1/2\beta}$ values (530±83 min versus 269±56 min for younger patients). Clinical recovery parameters were greatly slowed. Times of spontaneous recovery, using a 0.15 mg/kg dose, to 50 percent and 75 percent of T1 control values were doubled in the elderly with recovery from 25 to 75 percent

Table 8-2 Effect of age on recovery from *d*-tubocurarine and metocurine

	Age group	25–75% recovery, min
d-Tubocurarine (0.3 mg/kg)	Young (30–56 years)	48±12
	Old (73–83 years)	94±32*
Metocurine (0.15 mg/kg)	Young (30–59 years)	47±10
	Old (73–83 years)	110±35*

*$p<0.05$ between groups.

SOURCE: Modified from Matteo and colleagues.[16]

also being prolonged by a factor of 2 (Table 8-2). The behavior of this drug is much like that described for curare.

Mivacurium

No peer-reviewed information is available on the effects of aging on this new short-acting muscle relaxant. Basta and colleagues[17] reported no alteration in onset, recovery, or pharmacokinetic variables in a 1989 abstract.

Pipecuronium

Pipecuronium is a long-acting steroidal relaxant with no cardiovascular side effects that undergoes primarily renal elimination. The pharmacodynamics of this drug, that is, the dose to achieve a given level of block, does not differ between younger adults and the elderly.[18,19] Ornstein and colleagues[18] looked at onset, spontaneous recovery, and pharmacokinetic variables with a 70 μg/kg dose of this drug under balanced anesthesia in patients younger than 60 and older than 70 years of age. These patients were healthy, and all had creatinine levels below 1.5 mg/dl. Time of onset to maximal block was faster in younger patients, but these patients achieved an average 100 percent block while the older patients did not. The relatively higher dose received by the younger patients could have accelerated onset and confounds analysis. Clearance of this drug did not differ between the younger and the older patients. The steady-state Vd and the elimination half-life were not increased significantly in the elderly. Times from 10 to 25 percent recovery of T1 and recovery index (25 to 75 percent) values did not differ between these two groups. Thus, the action of this drug appears not to be prolonged in older patients without evidence of renal disease.

Pancuronium

The effects of this commonly used long-acting relaxant have been widely studied in an elderly population. McLeod and colleagues[20] evaluated the response to pancuronium (4 mg) in 19 patients ranging in age from 20 to 86 years who were undergoing balanced anesthesia. They noted a fall in pancuronium clearance with increasing age. Initial and steady-state Vd's did not appear to change with aging. Somogyi[21] evaluated plasma clearance in 38 patients ranging in age from 15 to 77 years and found no relation between age and clearance. Duvaldestin and colleagues[22] assessed pancuronium pharmacokinetics in groups of elderly (>75 years) and younger (25 to 60 years) patients under balanced anesthesia. This study found a 35 percent reduction in pancuronium clearance in the older population, while steady-state Vd was not significantly changed. Clinical recovery parameters were also assessed. Clinical duration of pancuronium (from injection to recovery of 25 percent of T1 control values) and recovery index (from 25 to 75 percent recovery) were significantly increased in the older patients (Table 8-3). In a more recent study, Rupp and colleagues[23] examined the pharmacokinetics of pancuronium in younger (30 to 57 years) and older (70 to 79 years) patients under halothane anesthesia. This study determined plasma pancuronium concentrations by mass spectrometry in contrast to spectrofluorometric determination in the older studies. Mass spectrometry detects only the parent compound, not the active metabolities of pancuronium. The patients studied were generally in good health. The investigators found no alteration in Vd with aging, similar to the other studies. Plasma clearance tended to be lower and elimination half-life higher in the elderly, but this did not achieve statistical significance. The difference in the health of subjects between studies and the method of determining pancuronium levels were thought to be responsible for the lack of statistical correlation. In spite of this, the authors concluded there was a difference between these groups. Neither Duvaldestin nor Rupp found a difference between young and old patients in regard to pancuronium pharmacodynamics. This finding is similar to that seen with other relaxants. The duration of an injected dose of pancuronium is increased with advancing age because of the reduction in clearance of this drug.

Rocuronium

Rocuronium is a new steroidal intermediate-acting muscle relaxant that has been shown to have a rapid onset. Recently, the pharmacokinetics, pharmacodynamics, and clinical behavior of this drug were compared in elderly and

Table 8-3 Recovery of T1 after pancuronium in young and old patients

	Young (25–60 years) $n = 17$	Old (>75 years) $n = 13$
25% recovery (min)	44 ± 10	73 ± 22*
25–75% recovery (min)	39 ± 13	62 ± 30*

*$p<0.01$ between groups.

SOURCE: Modified from Duvaldestin and colleagues.[22]

younger patients.[24] Patients received a bolus dose of 600 μg/kg of rocuronium under balanced anesthesia. The pharmacodynamics of this drug were not altered by aging. Time to onset did not differ between groups, but recovery from injection to 25 percent of T1 control values was prolonged by 40 percent (Table 8-4) in older patients. The recovery from 25 to 75 percent was also increased. The initial Vd did not differ with age, but that determined at steady state was decreased in the elderly. Clearance of this drug was reduced significantly, but the elimination half-life difference did not achieve statistical significance. This drug undergoes primarily hepatic metabolism, and the decrease in splanchnic blood flow and liver function may account for this phenomenon. The effect of a decreased steady-state Vd and clearance is the prolonged clinical effect seen in the older population.

Succinylcholine

Comparatively little information exists on the effect of aging on succinylcholine, which has been in clinical use since 1952. A recent study[25] assessed the onset of this drug in four groups: 1 to 3 years, 3 to 10 years, 20 to 40 years, and 60 to 80 years old. Patients received subparalyzing (0.3 mg/kg) or paralyzing doses (1.0 mg/kg) of succinylcholine under balanced anesthesia. The onset time to maximal block increased with increasing age. This effect would be correlated with changes in cardiac output and blood flow distribution with aging. No information exists on recovery with this drug. It has been reported[26] that plasma cholinesterase activity decreases 24 percent in elderly males (70–80 years) compared with young men (18–35 years). This difference was not found in women. It is not likely that this change can significantly increase the duration of action of succinylcholine.

Vecuronium

The action of this steroidal relaxant in the elderly has been widely evaluated. The dose-response relation of vecuronium is not altered with increasing age.[27–29] This finding, similar to that with other relaxants, indicates that the neuromuscular sensitivity to this drug does not change despite decreasing

Table 8-4 Effect of age on rocuronium (600 μg/kg) pharmacokinetics

	Young (27–57 years)	Old (70–78 years)
Onset (min)	4.1 ± 1.5	4.5 ± 2.4
25% recovery (min)	27.5 ± 7.1	42.4 ± 14.5*
25–75% recovery (min)	13.2 ± 6.1	21.7 ± 10.7*
Clearance (ml/kg/min)	5.03 ± 1.5	3.67 ± 1.0*
Vd_{ss} (ml/kg)	552.9 ± 279	399.4 ± 122*

*$p<0.05$ between groups.

SOURCE: Modified from Matteo and associates.[24]

muscle mass in the elderly. Koscielniak-Nielsen and colleagues[25] evaluated the onset of this drug in toddlers, children, adults, and elderly adults. Onset time with subparalyzing (0.03 μg/kg) and paralyzing doses (0.1 μg/kg) increased with aging. D'Hollander and coworkers[30] evaluated the onset of 70 μg/kg of vecuronium in patients age 18 to 85 years and found an increase in time to peak block with aging. In contrast, O'Hara and colleagues[28] compared onset times of vecuronium in subparalyzing doses (0.01–0.04 mg/kg) in young (20–40 years) and old (>70 years) patients under balanced anesthesia. They found no difference in time to maximal block. Recovery from this drug under balanced anesthesia and the infusion requirements to maintain 90 percent twitch depression were assessed by D'Hollander and colleagues[27] in patients less than 40 years, 40 to 60 years, and over 60 years old. Steady-state requirements for vecuronium were significantly decreased in patients over 60 years old. Time for recovery from 10 to 25 percent and 25 to 75 percent of T1 control values was prolonged in those over 60 years of age compared with both younger groups after a 90-min vecuronium infusion (Fig. 8-2).

Rupp and colleagues[23] compared pharmacokinetic variables for vecuronium in patients age 30 to 57 years old and 70 to 84 years old receiving N_2O-halothane anesthesia. There was a 30 percent fall in clearance and steady-state Vd in these healthy older patients. No difference in $t_{1/2\beta}$ was found. Lien and associates[31] evaluated the pharmacokinetics in young and old patients after a 0.1 mg/kg bolus of vecuronium under balanced anesthesia. They found a significant (54 percent) fall in vecuronium clearance with an increased elimination half-life. Vd's were not different between groups. These differences in Vd changes and the effects on $t_{1/2\beta}$ are probably due to differences in anesthetic

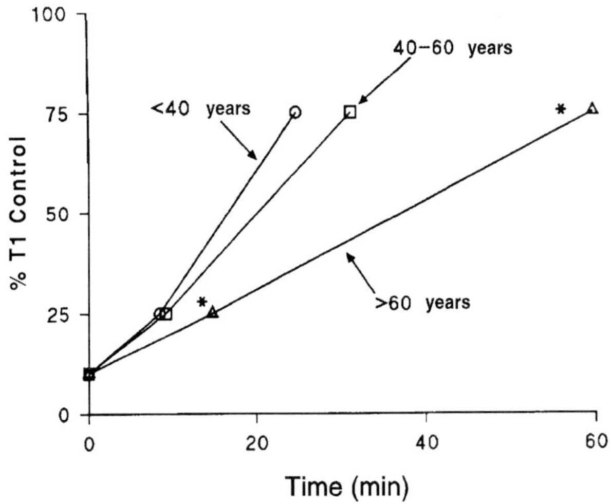

Figure 8-2 Recovery from a 90-min vecuronium infusion in three age groups. (*Modified from D'Hollander and associates.*[27])
*Significantly different ($p<0.05$) in the elderly.

conditions and vecuronium dosing between these two pharmacokinetic studies. Lien and associates[31] also reported significant prolongation of times to spontaneous recovery to 5 percent, 25 percent, 50 percent, and 75 percent of T1 control values and of the recovery index with vecuronium in the elderly (Table 8-5). Thus, vecuronium, like rocuronium, appears to have a prolonged effect in the elderly that may be related to decreased hepatic function.

REVERSAL AGENTS

Neostigmine

Neostigmine is commonly used to facilitate recovery from neuromuscular blockade. Marsh and colleagues[32] studied recovery from pancuronium under balanced anesthesia in patients 17 to 33 years and 70 to 91 years old. Reversal with neostigmine and atropine was carried out 30 min after the final dose of pancuronium, and train-of-four data were collected beginning 1 min after neostigmine. They found a slight but not significant prolongation in recovery to train-of-four >60 percent in the older population. Chmielewski and associates,[33] using a similar study design, evaluated recovery from *d*-tubocurarine. They found no difference between young and old patients in recovery of train-of-four to >0.6. Another investigation[14] examined recovery from doxacurium blockade with a dose of neostigmine given at 25 percent of T1 control values. Recovery after 10 min was evaluated. There was no difference between younger and older patients with regard to neostigmine requirements for achieving reversal at 10 min. The effects of neostigmine do not appear to be altered by aging in terms of reversing long-acting relaxants. It is important, however, that adequate spontaneous recovery be present before reversal if problems are to be avoided.

SUMMARY

Advancing age causes many physiological changes in humans. These alterations in cardiac, renal, and hepatic function have an impact on the pharmacol-

Table 8-5 Pharmacokinetics and recovery from vecuronium (0.1 mg/kg)

	Young (26–48 years) $n = 8$	Old (72–86 years) $n = 8$
$t_{1/2\beta}$ (min)	78 ± 21	125 ± 55*
Clearance (ml/kg/min)	5.6 ± 3.2	2.6 ± 0.6*
Vd_{ss} (L/kg)	0.49 ± 0.02	0.44 ± 0.01
25% recovery (min)	32.0 ± 11.6	73.8 ± 24.4*
25–75% recovery (min)	15.0 ± 8.0	49.4 ± 11.4*

*$p<0.05$ between groups.

SOURCE: Modified from Lien and associates.[31]

ogy of neuromuscular blocking drugs. In general, the required initial dose of these drugs does not change in an elderly patient, although onset to peak block may be delayed because of a decline in cardiac output with aging. The effects on pharmacokinetics are more variable. These drugs are largely metabolized and excreted through the liver and kidney. Because both of these organs undergo a decline in function with advancing age, clearance of these drugs is often reduced and the elimination half-life is frequently prolonged. The time to clinical recovery may be prolonged, and additional drug doses can be expected to be less frequent. Atracurium, because of the plasma breakdown that occurs, is least affected by advancing age. However, any of these drugs can be used safely in an elderly population with careful monitoring of neuromuscular function and redosing only when evidence of recovery is present.

REFERENCES

1. Crooks J, O'Malley K, Stevenson IH: Pharmacokinetics in the elderly. *Clin Pharmacokinet* 1:280, 1976.
2. Greenblatt D, Sellers EM, Shader RI: Drug disposition in old age. *N Engl J Med* 306:1081, 1982.
3. Donati F: Onset of action of relaxants. *Can J Anaesth* 35:S52, 1988.
4. Bender AD: Effect of age on the distribution of peripheral blood flow in man. *J Am Geriatr Soc* 13:192, 1965.
5. Rowe JW, Andres R, Tobin JD, et al: The effects of age on creatinine clearance in man: A cross-sectional and longitudinal study. *J Gerontol* 31:155, 1976.
6. Lund I, Stovner J: Experimental and clinical experiences with a new muscle relaxant R04-3816, diallyl-nor-toxiferine. *Acta Anaesthesiol Scand* 62:85, 1962.
7. Stephens ID, Ho PC, Holloway AM, et al: Pharmacokinetics of alcuronium in elderly patients undergoing total hip replacement or aortic reconstructive surgery. *Br J Anaesth* 56:465, 1984.
8. Fisher DM, Canfell PC, Fahey MR, et al: Elimination of atracurium in humans: Contribution of Hoffman elimination and ester hydrolysis versus organ based elimination. *Anesthesiology* 65:6, 1986.
9. Parker CRJ, Hunter JM, Snowdon SL: Effect of age, gender, and anaesthetic technique on the pharmacodynamics of atracurium. *Br J Anaesth* 70:38, 1993.
10. D'Hollander AA, Luyckx C, Barvais L, et al: Clinical evaluation of atracurium besylate requirements for a stable muscle relaxation during surgery: Lack of age related effects. *Anesthesiology* 59:237, 1983.
11. Kitts JB, Fisher DM, Canfell PC, et al: Pharmacokinetics and pharmacodynamics of atracurium in the elderly. *Anesthesiology* 72:272, 1990.
12. Kent AP, Parker CJR, Hunter JM: Pharmacokinetics of atracurium and laudanosine in the elderly. *Br J Anaesth* 63:661, 1989.
13. Dresner DL, Basta SJ, Au HH, et al: Pharmacokinetics and pharmacodynamics of doxacurium in young and elderly patients during isoflurane anesthesia. *Anesth Analg* 71:498, 1990.
14. Koscielniak-Nielsen ZJ, Law-Min JC, Donati F, et al: Dose response relations of doxacurium and its reversal with neostigmine in young adults and healthy elderly patients. *Anesth Analg* 74:845, 1992.

15. Dundee JW: The relationship of the dosage of d-tubocurarine chloride and laudolissin to body weight, sex, and age. *Br J Anaesth* 26:174, 1954.
16. Matteo RS, Backus WW, McDaniel DD, et al: Pharmacokinetics and pharmacodynamics of d-tubocurarine and metocurine in the elderly. *Anesth Analg* 64:23, 1985.
17. Basta SJ, Dresner DL, Shaff LP, et al: Neuromuscular effects and pharmacokinetics of mivacurium in elderly patients under isuflurane anesthesia. *Anesth Analg* 68:S18, 1989.
18. Ornstein E, Matteo RS, Schwartz AE, et al: Pharmacokinetics and pharmacodynamics of pipecuronium bromide (arduan) in elderly surgical patients. *Anesth Analg* 74:841, 1992.
19. Azad SS, Goldberg ME, Larijani GE, et al: The dose-response evaluation of pipecuronium bromide in the elderly population under balanced anesthesia. *Anesthesiology* 67:A370, 1987.
20. McLeod K, Hull CJ, Watson M: Effects of aging on the pharmacokinetics of pancuronium. *Br J Anaesth* 51:435, 1979.
21. Somogyi AA: Pancuronium plasma clearance and age. *Br J Anaesth* 52:360, 1980.
22. Duvaldestin P, Saada J, Berger JL, et al: Pharmacokinetics, pharmacodynamics and dose response relationships of pancuronium in control and elderly subjects. *Anesthesiology* 56:36, 1982.
23. Rupp SM, Castagnoli KP, Fisher DM, Miller RD: Pancuronium and vecuronium pharmacokinetics and pharmacodynamics in younger and elderly adults. *Anesthesiology* 67:45, 1987.
24. Matteo RS, Ornstein E, Schwartz AE, et al: Pharmacokinetics and pharmacodynamics of rocuronium (ORG 9426) in elderly surgical patients. *Anesth Analg* 77:1193, 1993.
25. Koscielniak-Nielsen ZJ, Bevan JC, Popovic V, et al: Onset of maximum neuromuscular block following succinylcholine or vecuronium in four age groups. *Anesthesiology* 79:229, 1993.
26. Shanor SP, Van Hees GR, Baart N, et al: The influence of age and sex on human plasma and red cell cholinesterase. *Am J Med Sci* 242:357, 1961.
27. D'Hollander AA, Massaux F, Nevelsteen M, Agoston S: Age dependent dose-response relationship of ORG NC45 in anaesthetized patients. *Br J Anaesth* 54:653, 1982.
28. O'Hara DA, Fragen RJ, Shanks CA: The effects of age on the dose-response curves for vecuronium in adults. *Anesthesiology* 63:542, 1985.
29. Bell PF, Mirakhur RK, Clarke RSJ: Dose response studies of atracurium, vecuronium, and pancuronium in the elderly. *Anaesthesia* 44:925, 1989.
30. D'Hollander AA, Nevelsteen M, Barvais L, Baurain M: Effect of age on the establishment of muscle paralysis induced in anaesthetized adult subjects by ORG NC45. *Acta Anaesthesiol Scand* 27:108, 1983.
31. Lien CA, Matteo RS, Ornstein E, et al: Distribution, elimination, and action of vecuronium in the elderly. *Anesth Analg* 73:39, 1991.
32. Marsh RHK, Chmielewski AT, Goat VA: Recovery from pancuronium: A comparison between old and young patients. *Anaesthesia* 35:1193, 1980.
33. Chmielewski AT, Pybus DA, Loach AB, et al: Recovery from neuromuscular blockade: A comparison between old and young patients. *Anaesthesia* 33:539, 1978.

CHAPTER 9

Benefits of Regional Anesthesia and Influence of Aging on the Use of Local Anesthetics

Lauri S. Nuutinen

INTRODUCTION

Aging produces changes in virtually every subcellular and tissue element. The organs most relevant to anesthetic practice include the brain and peripheral nervous system, the lungs and cardiovascular system, the hepatic and renal systems, and the sympathoadrenal mechanisms (which maintain autonomic homeostasis of hemodynamics and respiration). Age-related alterations of function or functional reserve are important to notice. It is also important to distinguish between the processes of aging and age-related diseases.[1]

The number of geriatric patients is growing in every developed country. Today in the United States, individuals more than 65 years old make up approximately 12 percent of the population. It is predicted that this number will increase to 13 percent by the year 2000.[2] In Great Britain, it has been predicted that 20 percent of the population will be over 60 years old by the year 2000.[3] As a result of increased life expectancy and advances in regional and general anesthesia and intensive care, there has been an increase in the number of elderly patients presenting for surgery and anesthesia. An understanding of the physiological consequences of the aging process is critical to the ability to administer safe anesthesia to elderly patients. Physiological changes that are associated with old age are characterized by a decreased response of the organism to stress.[1,3] In addition to age, other factors, especially associated disease processes, significantly increase the risk of mortality and morbidity in geriatric patients.[4]

The incidences of hypertension, arteriosclerosis, renal disease, chronic obstructive pulmonary disease, liver disease, and cerebrovascular abnormalities are quite high, ranging from 5 to 50 percent in these different disease groups.[5]

AGE-RELATED CHANGES RELEVANT TO REGIONAL ANESTHESIA

Nervous System

The nervous system is the target organ for local anesthetics; therefore, age-related changes in nervous system function may have implications for the anesthetic plan. The functional reserve of the nervous system is compromised by attrition of neurons and depletion of transmitters.[6] Also, the loss of peripheral, motor, sensory, and autonomic nerve fibers, with a subsequent reduction in both afferent and efferent nerve conduction velocities and a generalized deafferentation process, has an impact on the use of local anesthetics.[4] Decreasing afferentation in the form of loss of receptors and peripheral nerve fibers is not necessarily associated with a clinically significant increase in the pain threshold, with a concomitant decreased need for analgesic or local anesthetic agents.[6,7] Elderly patients may have elevated thresholds for superficial discomfort but reduced thresholds for severe or visceral pain.

Structural changes in the anatomy also affect regional anesthesia. Intervertebral spaces are narrowed in elderly patients. These individuals often have dorsal kyphosis and a tendency to flex the hips and knees because of osteoarthritic changes and cartilage calcification. These changes affect the capacity of the vertebral canal and its contained cerebrospinal fluid volume. The volume of local anesthetic agents required for epidural and spinal analgesia is consequently less for the same height of block compared with a young adult.[8,9] The decreased spinal blood flow and therefore oxygen delivery may compromise the vitality of neurons during hypotension and hypoxia, leading to an increased risk of nerve damage after relatively minor hemodynamic alterations.

Elderly patients often have impairment in all forms of perception, including vision, hearing, touch, proprioception, smell, peripheral pain, and thermoregulation.[4] Parkinson's disease and Alzheimer's disease are common nervous system disorders and reflect specific neurotransmitter deficits. The management of regional anesthesia may be difficult because of these diseases, although the majority of geriatric patients have intelligence, personality, and memory comparable to those of young adults.

The autonomic reflex responses that maintain cardiovascular homeostasis are degraded in geriatric patients.[10] Baroreflex responsiveness, the vasoconstrictor response to cold stress, and responses after postural changes are less rapid in onset, smaller in magnitude, and thus, less effective in stabilizing blood pressure. In the elderly, the neurons of the sympathoadrenal pathways undergo attrition and fibrosis as the adrenal mass decreases. Compensatory plasma levels of epinephrine and norepinephrine are 2 to 4 times higher compared with young subjects.[11] The effects of these higher levels, which would be expected to be manifested in young adults, are blunted by the marked reduction in autonomic end-organ responsiveness associated with aging.[4,10] If anesthetic techniques such as spinal and epidural anesthesia disrupt end-organ function or reduce plasma catecholamines, the occurrence of hypotension is more likely in elderly surgical patients than in young patients[4] and may require more aggressive intervention.

Cardiovascular System

It is necessary to briefly review the age-related changes in the cardiovascular system before discussing the effects of regional anesthesia techniques.[12,13] Increased systemic vascular resistance, myocardial ischemia, and arrhythmias all contribute to decreased cardiac output. About 40 percent of patients over age 65 are hypertensive (blood pressure greater than 150/100).[3] The chronotropic and inotropic effects of beta-agonist drugs are reduced significantly in elderly individuals.[14] The homeostatic baroreflex mechanisms are also diminished in effectiveness with advancing age. The number of receptors is normal, but adrenergic receptor quality is impaired.[14] The diminished elasticity and fibrotic changes of the heart muscle make the aged heart noncompliant and thus both volume-sensitive and volume-intolerant.[3] All these observations have important clinical implications for the treatment of patients undergoing regional anesthesia. Elderly patients are particularly predisposed to arterial hypotension when there is interruption of venous return, as can occur with spinal or epidural anesthesia. This is especially true in a patient with atrial fibrillation, in which the loss of atrial contribution during diastolic filling can critically compromise stroke volume and cardiac output.

Respiratory System

With advancing age, lung elastic content decreases and fibrous connective tissue increases proportionately.[15] Elderly persons have a marked reduction in the ventilatory response to imposed hypoxia and hypercapnia. They have increased periodic breathing and apnea during sleep, and this increases the tendency to develop airway obstruction in the recovery room. This obstruction may also be manifested during surgery in heavily sedated patients undergoing regional anesthesia.[16] The physiological shunting and reduced efficiency of oxygen exchange lead to a linear decrease in arterial oxygen tension with advancing age.[3] Atrophy of intercostal muscles and restrictive changes impair the capacity for the accessory muscle breathing necessitated by a high-level spinal or epidural blockade. About 15 percent of the geriatric surgical population also presents with evidence of chronic obstructive pulmonary disease.[5] The monitoring of oxygen saturation is mandatory in these patients, and the addition of oxygen may be necessary.

Renal and Hepatic System

Hepatic and renal function is reduced about 1 percent per year beyond age 30. The reduced ability of an elderly patient to excrete administered drugs and their metabolites is due to a decline in glomerular filtration rate and a reduction in renal blood flow. The renal functional reserve needed to withstand imposed water and electrolyte imbalances in elderly patients may be minimal.[17,18]

The liver shrinks with aging, perhaps to 40 to 50 percent of a young adult's hepatic size. Liver blood flow is also proportionally reduced, and this appears to play a major role in the age-related decline in rates of drug clearance for anesthetics that require hepatic biotransformation, for example, amide-type local anesthetics.[4] Oxidative metabolism is more impaired than reductive metabolism in liver tissue, and this contributes further to the delayed fall in plasma drug concentration in the elderly.[19] Ester-type local anesthetics such as 2-chloroprocaine are broken down rapidly by plasma pseudocholinesterases. The hepatic synthesis of plasma cholinesterases is, however, deficient in many elderly men. Older women seem to be better able to maintain this enzymatic function.[20]

Body Composition

The most important changes in body composition in elderly patients include a loss of skeletal muscle and an increase in the percentage of body fat.[21] The result is an increased availability of lipid storage sites and a greater reservoir for the deposition of lipid-soluble anesthetic drugs. This increases the time period required for drug elimination, resulting in a greater residual plasma concentration and prolonged anesthetic effects.

Decreasing levels of circulating serum proteins, especially albumin, reduce available protein-binding sites for a variety of anesthetic drugs.[22] Also, the binding effectiveness of the available proteins is reduced because of qualitative changes. Amide-type local anesthetics have a high affinity for plasma proteins and for proteins within the erythrocyte envelope. Alpha$_1$-acid glycoprotein (AAG) binds amide-type local anesthetics in plasma.[22] Many conditions may affect the concentration of AAG. The concentration increases after major trauma, in connection with malignancy, after myocardial infarction, and in patients with inflammatory gastrointestinal disease or rheumatoid arthritis. These offsetting mechanisms may make it difficult to predict the effects of protein binding on plasma concentrations of local anesthetics.

PHARMACOKINETICS, DOSES, AND TOXICITY OF LOCAL ANESTHETIC AGENTS

Pharmacokinetics

Regional anesthesia is a complex function of pharmacokinetics, pharmacodynamics, the physiological consequences of neural blockade, and the physiological status of the patient. Local anesthetics can gain access to a great distributional space in the body by virtue of their small molecular size and high lipid solubility.[22] In the elderly, decreased volumes of distribution, decreased liver mass and hepatic blood flow, and limitations in renal function result in reduced dose requirements, a prolonged drug effect, perhaps higher initial plasma levels, and an enhanced possibility of side effects.[1–5] Distribution of local anesthetics depends on regional blood flow, the pH and pKa of the drug, penetrance, fat and water solubility, and the protein-binding rate.[22,23] The greater the fat solubility of a drug, the more that drug is distributed to lipophylic tissues, including nerves. Bupivacaine, tetracaine, and etidocaine have the highest fat solubility rates among local anesthetics, partially explaining their potency. Protein binding and uptake by plasma and erythrocytes also have a significant influence on the distribution of local anesthetics. The protein binding of bupivacaine is 95 percent, and that of lidocaine is 65 percent. The increased AAG levels are associated with increased protein binding and a reduced free fraction of these drugs. Decreased serum albumin and decreased binding capacity may result in an increased free fraction of these drugs. In such a case, highly extracted drugs such as lidocaine might be expected to have enhanced clearance as a result of increased availability for hepatic extraction. In an elderly patient, this hepatic extraction may be reduced by the decrease in hepatic blood flow, thus minimizing this expected difference.[24,25]

The degree of neural blockade depends on the potency of the drug and the local concentration in the vicinity of the nerve fibers. An important factor determining the potency of a local anesthetic drug is its lipid solubility. The amount of drug injected and the rate of absorption into the circulation are other contributing factors. Local anesthetics are weak bases. This form of drug penetrates biological membranes. The rate of onset of block depends on the pKa of the drug. Thus, the lower the pKa of a drug, the more rapidly that drug penetrates the surrounding sheath and neurolemma and produces a block. It seems that pKa is a more important factor than lipid solubility in determining the onset of block. The pKa value for prilocaine is 8.9; for both ropivacaine and bupivacaine, 8.1; and for lidocaine, 7.7.[22,23]

Toxicity and Dosing Requirements

The rate of absorption influences the toxicity of local anesthetics. Absorption depends on the vascularity of the injection site and the drug's solubility in tissues at this site, breakdown rate, concentration, and penetrance. Both the circulatory uptake and removal of local anesthetic agents from a variety of tissues and spaces are heavily influenced by anything that alters local capillary perfusion. The absorption of local anesthetics is increased by the vasodilatation caused by local anesthetics (except cocaine). The absorption rate is decreased by mixing with vasoconstricting agents such as adrenaline, cocaine, noradrenaline, and Felypressin (octapressin).[22,23] Hypoperfusion resulting from hypovolemia or cardiovascular disease slows local anesthetic absorption after different blocks. Conversely, a hyperkinetic circulation may decrease the duration of block because of an enhanced systemic uptake of local anesthetic. For example, a decreased duration of brachial plexus block in patients with chronic renal failure can be explained by the hyperkinetic circulation often seen in those patients.[22] Acidosis also enhances absorption into the blood, because local anesthetics diffuse from tissues of high pH to those of low pH. Acidosis is not uncommon in elderly hypovolemic emergency patients. In these patients, the toxicity of local anesthetics may be increased while the potency and duration of the block are decreased.

The site of injection also affects the possibility of producing toxic blood levels of local anesthetic agents. The anesthetic drug level is highest in the blood after intercostal nerve blockade, followed in order of decreasing concentration by injection into the lumbar epidural space, brachial plexus, and subcutaneous tissue.[22] Therefore, it is very important to remember that the use of a fixed dose of a local anesthetic agent may be potentially toxic in one area of administration but not in others. The peak venous plasma level of lidocaine may reach the level of 7 μg/ml after the injection of 400 mg for intercostal block. The same dose of lidocaine used for brachial plexus block yields a maximum blood level of 3 μg/ml, which is rarely associated with toxic signs compared to the higher levels that may cause symptoms of CNS toxicity.[22] A vasoconstrictor agent, usually epinephrine in a concentration of 5 μg/ml

(1:200,000), significantly reduces the peak blood levels of lidocaine and mepivacaine, independent of the administration site. The peak blood levels of bupivacaine and etidocaine after peripheral blocks are reduced significantly by the addition of a vasoconstrictor. However, vasoconstrictors only minimally influence the absorption of these drugs after injection into the lumbar epidural space.[22,23]

Plasma concentrations of local anesthetics after epidural and other nerve blocks are poorly correlated with age and weight. Dose requirements for epidural anesthesia decrease in a linear manner after age 18.5 years. There is a trend toward more rapid absorption after epidural and caudal injections in elderly patients. Segmental dose requirements seem to change in a complex manner, reflecting reduced compliance of the epidural space. Dose requirements do not differ significantly between adult and elderly patients after the injection of small volumes of local anesthetic solutions, whereas injection of large volumes may be followed by markedly increased cephalad spread of the drug.[22] In 1969, Bromage[8] showed that the number of milliliters or the dose in milligrams of an epidurally administered local anesthetic (2% lidocaine) required to block a dermatome is decreased with age. Table 9-1 demonstrates the relation between age and the dose of lidocaine necessary to block a spinal segment.[8]

The effect of age on the systemic absorption, disposition, and pharmacodynamics of bupivacaine after epidural administration was recently studied by Veering and colleagues.[24] The results showed that the maximal height of analgesia increased with age and that the time to maximal caudal spread and the initial time of onset of motor blockade decreased with age. Age did not affect the total duration of analgesia or motor blockade, but recovery time from analgesia increased with age. These data confirmed that increasing age leads to a more extensive spread of epidural analgesia. This implies that a more extensive sympathetic blockade, with corresponding hemodynamic changes, is likely in elderly patients. The observed increased duration of analgesia may be related to gradual degeneration of the peripheral and central nervous systems with age, rendering both more sensitive to the effects of local anesthetics. The authors[24] concluded that changes in pharmacodynamics and local distribution were more important than pharmacokinetic changes. This important study

Table 9-1 Relation between age and dose of local anesthetic (2% lidocaine, ml or mg) necessary to block a spinal segment

Age, years	mg/Spinal segment	ml/Spinal segment
18	28	1.4
50	22	1.1
70	18	0.8
80	15	0.65

SOURCE: Modified from data by Bromage.[8]

implies that not only should the dose of an epidural local anesthetic be decreased in the elderly, but in addition, the onset of the block will be faster and these patients will be subjected to a more rapid onset of more severe cardiovascular side effects. Therefore, both the level of the block and the patient's blood pressure should be checked frequently in the first 15 min after injection to allow for early treatment.

After subarachnoid injection, there appears to be a slight prolongation of effect in the elderly. The effects of hypobaric spinal anesthetic solutions are less reliable in an elderly patient because of the higher average specific gravity and greater individual variation in the volume of cerebrospinal fluid.[25] Table 9-2 summarizes block- and disease-related factors that may alter the systemic disposition of local anesthetics.[22]

Systemic toxic reactions to local anesthetics involve primarily the central nervous system (CNS) and the cardiovascular system.[22,26] These reactions result from high blood levels of the drug caused by the injection of an excessive dose, accidental intravenous injection of all or part of a therapeutic dose, and/or abnormal rates of absorption and biotransformation of the drug. In an elderly patient with reduced cooperation, the symptoms and signs of mild toxic reactions may be difficult to recognize. The patient should be well instructed, and verbal contact is important, if possible. The signs of mild toxic reactions include dysarthria, light-headedness, vertigo, tinnitus, headache, apprehension, excitement, tachycardia, slight hypertension, tachypnea, a metallic taste and dryness of the mouth, occasionally nausea and vomiting, and sometimes slight twitching of muscle groups.[26] The symptoms and treatment of moderate and

Table 9-2 Systemic disposition of local anesthetic: Block- and disease-related factors

High epidural block	Hepatic blood flow ↓ Vasodilatation in legs Vasoconstriction in arms
Cardiovascular disease Heart failure	Volume of distribution ↓ Clearance ↓ Plasma concentrations ↑
Liver disease Decreased synthesis capability	Plasma pseudocholinesterases ↓ Thus procaine plasma half-life ↑ Lowered clearance of amide-type local anesthetic
Renal disease Metabolism of amide-type local anesthetics	Unaffected Procaine hydrolysis ↓
Pulmonary disease Pulmonary uptake of lidocaine slightly lowered	

severe toxic reactions are outside the scope of this review. Prevention is the best treatment in an elderly patient. Epinephrine is used to reduce the peak plasma drug level, and repeated attempts to aspirate during injection demonstrate that the bevel of the needle is not in a blood vessel.[26]

Bupivacaine has the lowest ratio of cardiac collapse to CNS toxicity. The estimated threshold plasma concentrations for CNS toxicity vary from 2 to 4 μg/ml for bupivacaine and etidocaine to 5 to 10 μg/ml for lidocaine and mepivacaine.[22] Bupivacaine, by blocking the cardiac sodium channel, depresses the maximal rise of the cardiac action potential in a dose-dependent manner. This cardiac sodium channel response lasts longer with bupivacaine than with other local anesthetic agents. The recovery from the block is always slow with bupivacaine, and the block can accumulate, resulting in reentrant phenomena.[23] This can explain the sudden onset of ventricular dysrhythmias when bupivacaine is administered intravenously in toxic doses. The combination of acidosis and hypoxia enhances the negative chronotropic and inotropic action of bupivacaine to a greater extent than is the case with lidocaine.[22] Cardiac resuscitation is always difficult and less effective in those conditions. Thus, in elderly patients, low doses of bupivacaine are recommended and the use of test doses of 3 to 5 ml is essential. The use of fractional dosing and the process of following signs of toxicity are vital aspects of good clinical practice. It is important to ask the following questions: Is bupivacaine needed in high doses? Could spinal anesthesia be selected instead of epidural or neural blockade, and could lidocaine or ropivacaine be substituted for bupivacaine? Ropivacaine is a homologue of bupivacaine and mepivacaine.[23] It is less lipid-soluble than bupivacaine. Ropivacaine appears to be less cardiotoxic and less arrythmogenic and produces fewer depressant effects on various cardiac electrophysiological and mechanical variables than does bupivacaine.[23]

The suggested maximum doses and block characteristics of the most widely used local anesthetics are listed in Table 9-3. All the doses listed assume healthy adult patients.[26] In elderly patients, the doses should be selected individually and much lower doses are often sufficient. Even small doses can produce serious or life-threatening side effects if accidentally injected into a blood vessel or in a highly vascular area. The selection of anesthetic techniques and specific drugs for elderly patients requires careful review of the patient's physical condition and analysis of the nature and severity of age-related and coexisting disease processes.[1–5]

INFLUENCE OF REGIONAL ANESTHESIA ON ENDOCRINE AND METABOLIC RESPONSE

The metabolic response to surgery is a net effect of responses to injury and to semistarvation caused by the preoperative fasting period. Anesthetic techniques can modify this response. The response to surgery has been considered to be an adaptation to the insult of injury and a homeostatic defense mecha-

Table 9-3 Maximum single dose of local anesthetics in adults*

Agent	Duration (h)	Maximum dose, mg/kg (total mg)		Comments
		Plain	With epinephrine	
Lidocaine	1–2 (3)	4 (300)	7 (500)	Rapid onset Motor block++
Mepivacaine	1.5–3 (4)	4 (300)	7 (500)	Rapid onset Motor block++
Prilocaine	1–2 (3)	7 (500)	8.5 (600)	Rapid onset Motor block++
Least toxic amide agent methemoglobinemia with > 600 mg				
Bupivacaine	1.5–6 (24)	2.5 (175)	3.5 (225)	Ventricular arrhythmias and cardiovascular collapse after rapid IV injection Motor block + (less with low concentrations)
Chloroprocaine	0.5–1	11 (800)	14 (1000)	Lowest systemic toxicity Not intrathecally

*Doses for elderly patients should be lower and should be determined individually.

nism important for the healing of tissue.[27] The intensity of the stress response is directly related to the degree of tissue trauma. Superficial surgery evokes a very transient response, whereas a major surgical procedure elicits responses that may last up to several days or weeks, especially if complications occur. The prolonged stress response may have a detrimental effect in elderly patients because of the resulting devastating nutritional consequences, leading to depletion of several essential body components. The reserves of these components in the aged may be limited, leading to increased postoperative morbidity.

The influences of spinal or epidural anesthesia on the endocrine and metabolic responses per se during surgery and postoperatively are presented in Table 9-4. Some of the results presented are still controversial and depend on the study material, the coexisting diseases, and the intensity of surgery. The metabolic and endocrine response depends on the degree of afferent and efferent neural blockade.[27] For example, the epinephrine response is mediated by afferent neural pathways combined with efferent sympathetic pathways to the adrenal medulla. The cortisol response to lower abdominal surgery can be prevented by sensory blockade from T4 to S5. The hyperglycemic response to surgery is regulated through both afferent and efferent neural pathways and is easily inhibited by neural blockade (T11–L1).[27]

A short-acting single-dose neural blockade by spinal or epidural analgesia has only a short-lasting inhibitory effect on the stress response. For major surgery, it has become popular to combine both neural blockade and general

Table 9-4 Influence of spinal/epidural anesthesia on endocrine and metabolic responses; intra- and postoperatively

Hormone/metabolic response	Blockade T9–10	Blockade T2–6	Intraoperative response	Postoperative response
P-epinephrine	→	↓	↓	↓
P-norepinephrine	→	↓	↓	↓
P-cortisol (hydrocortisone)	→	→	↓	↓
P-insulin	→	→	↘	↘
P-glucagon	→	→	→	→
P-beta-endorphin	?	?	↓	↘
P-growth hormone	→	→	↓	↓
P-renin	?	?	↓	↓
P-aldosterone	?	?	↓	↓
P-ADH	?	?	↓	↓
Beta-glucose	→	→	↓	↓
Glucose tolerance	→	↘	↑	→
P-free fatty acids	→	→	↓	→
P-ketones	→	→	↓	↗
P-lactate	→	→	↓	→
Nitrogen balance	→	→	?	↑
O_2 consumption	?	?	↘	↘

P = plasma; ? = no data; → = no effect on response; ↑ = improvement or normalization; ↗ = slight increase; ↘ = slight inhibition of response; ↓ = reduction of response.

anesthesia intraoperatively, with the possibility of continuing postoperative pain relief for longer periods. This may have benefits in terms of reducing immediate postoperative morbidity. Also, local anesthesia has been demonstrated to have beneficial metabolic effects in elderly patients. Plasma catecholamine, plasma glucose, and cardiovascular responses were studied in elderly patients undergoing cataract surgery under general or local anesthesia. The results showed the beneficial effects of local anesthesia in preventing the hormonal, metabolic, and cardiovascular changes found when cataract surgery was conducted under general anesthesia.[28]

INFLUENCE OF REGIONAL TECHNIQUES ON POSTOPERATIVE MORBIDITY: REGIONAL VERSUS GENERAL ANESTHESIA

Mortality

Morbidity and mortality have consistently been demonstrated to occur more frequently in elderly surgical patients than in younger counterparts undergoing comparable surgery. The follow-up period for comparing the rate of perioperative complications should be at least 30 days from the time of surgery. The

30-day perioperative mortality for patients 65 years of age or older varies from 5 to 10 percent.[1–5] These numbers are 3 to 5 times those for young adults. Table 9-5 shows the most important pre- and postoperative factors associated with increased mortality in elderly patients.[1–5] The preoperative physical and nutritional status of elderly patients correlates with perioperative mortality. The possibility of age-related disease also increases with the greater average age of a surgical population. The rates for perioperative morbidity and mortality are determined largely by the severity of coexisting disease. The risk for fit, healthy elderly patients is not significantly higher than that for young adults undergoing similar procedures.

The influence of spinal or epidural anesthesia on mortality after major surgery in elderly patients is shown in Table 9-6.[29–35] Only the studies of McLaren and associates[33] and McKenzie and coworkers[34] demonstrate the beneficial effect on mortality of regional anesthesia. There is evidence that regional techniques have a positive effect on early mortality after acute surgery for hip fracture; this initial difference in mortality disappears later on. The explanation for reduced initial mortality may be the lower amount of thromboembolic complications or pulmonary complications. Factors other than the choice of anesthesia may be crucial for long-term survival. The correction of a fractured upper femur is one of the most common operations in elderly patients, and reported hospital mortality has varied between 2.7 and 28 percent.[30–36]

Blood Loss

The relation between anesthetic technique and blood loss during different surgeries is variable. In patients undergoing hip fracture surgery, the effect of

Table 9-5 Pre- and postoperative factors associated with increased mortality in elderly patients

Preoperative factors
Physical status and activity
Poor nutritional status
Age, especially over 85 years
Ischemic heart disease
Cardiac failure
Arrhythmias
Dementia, cerebral dysfunction
American Society of Anesthesiology (ASA) class III or IV
Emergency operation
Operative site
Blood loss, hypotension, hypoxemia
Postoperative factors
Major organ system insult
Cerebrovascular damage
Lung infection
Renal failure

Table 9-6 Influence of regional anesthesia (spinal/epidural) on mortality after major surgery in elderly patients

Spinal/ epidural	Regional anesthesia, mortality/ total *n*	General anesthesia, mortality/ total *n*	*p*	Postoperative observation, months	Reference
Vascular surgery					
Epidural	4/49	3/51	NS	6	Christopherson et al[29]
Hip surgery					
Spinal	17/259	16/279	NS	1	Davis et al[30]
Spinal	3/64	9/68	NS		Davis and Laurenson[31]
Spinal	5/35	NS 4/35	NS	3	Racle et al[32]
Spinal	4/56	17/60	<0.05	1	McLaren et al[33]
Spinal	3/73	12/75	<0.05	1/2	McKenzie et al[34]
Spinal	17/281	24/297	NS	1	Valentin et al[35]
Total	53/817 (6.5%)	85/865 (9.8%)			

anesthetic technique is not clear, but intraoperative blood loss may be reduced with spinal anesthesia.[36] Intraoperative losses are also reduced significantly with both spinal and epidural techniques in patients undergoing total hip arthroplasty compared with general anesthesia.[36] This blood-sparing effect may be due to the emptying of dilated vessels by gravity, especially in the lateral position, and the absence of controlled (positive-pressure) ventilation.[36] If venous drainage by gravity is indeed occuring, one might postulate an increased risk of venous air embolism under such circumstances.

The reduction of blood loss has been well documented in patients undergoing retropubic[37] or transurethral prostatectomy.[38] Spinal anesthesia reduced intraoperative blood loss by 45 percent in patients undergoing hysterectomy[39] and by 51 percent in patients undergoing lower limb amputation.[40] No difference, however, could be seen in patients undergoing abdominal procedures during thoracic or lumbar epidural analgesia compared with general anesthesia. It appears that intraoperative blood loss is reduced about 30 percent during operations in the lower part of the body in patients under regional anesthesia.[27]

Thromboembolism

Earlier studies demonstrated evidence of deep venous thrombosis (DVT) in 40 to 50 percent of hip fracture patients.[31–36] The incidence of a fatal pulmonary embolism in patients without prophylaxis has been estimated to be 3 to 5 percent.[27,36] Many studies have demonstrated a reduction in DVT in surgical patients after spinal or epidural anesthesia compared to general anesthesia. Table 9-7 shows the incidence of thromboembolic complications in some pa-

Table 9-7 Incidence of thromboembolic complications in patients operated on under spinal/epidural or general anesthesia

Spinal/epidural	Regional anesthesia, comp/total	General anesthesia, comp/total	p	Reference
Hip surgery				
Spinal	17⁄37 (46%)	30⁄39 (76%)	0.05	Davis and Laurenson[31]
Epidural	3⁄30 (10%)			Modig et al[41]
Prostatectomy				
Epidural	2⁄17 (12%)	11⁄21 (52%)	0.02	Hendolin et al[37]
Vascular surgery				
Epidural	2⁄49 (+)(4%)	11⁄51 (22%)	0.01	Christopherson et al[29]

tient groups anesthetized with a spinal or epidural or with general anesthesia.[29,31,37,41] Davis and Laurenson[31] found a decrease in DVT in 132 elderly patients undergoing emergency hip surgery when comparing subarachnoid block to general anesthesia, using the 125-J-fibrinogen uptake test to document thrombotic prevalence. They suggested that regional anesthesia, by blocking or reducing the sympathetic response to surgery, may affect coagulation and/or fibrinolytic mechanisms. McKenzie and colleagues[34] used contrast venography to study 40 patients 7 to 10 days after surgery. The results demonstrated a 40 percent incidence of DVT after spinal anesthesia compared with 76.2 percent after general anesthesia.

In patients undergoing total hip arthroplasty, the published rates of venographically evident DVT range from 26 percent to 55 percent when epidural anesthesia is used.[36] The proposed predisposing factors for DVT are obesity, smoking, previous DVT, prolonged bed rest, recent stroke, congestive heart failure, underlying malignancy, and the use of cement during surgery.[42] More recent data suggest that the intraoperative management of both surgery and anesthesia influences rates of DVT. The surgical time, intraoperative blood loss, intraoperative venous stasis, and postoperative immobilization and thromboprophylaxis affect the incidence of DVT.[42] Warfarin (Coumadin), low-molecular-weight heparin, dextran, and pneumatic compression boots are used nowadays for thromboprophylaxis. It is clear that regional anesthesia should not be regarded as a substitute for effective primary antithrombotic prophylaxis.

Continuous epidural analgesia (24 h) reduced the occurrence of thromboembolism in patients undergoing retropubic prostatectomy by 77 percent.[37] In contrast, no difference has been shown between regional and general anesthesia in the incidence of DVT among patients undergoing abdominal surgery.[27]

A recent study demonstrated that regional anesthesia seems to offer some advantage over general anesthesia in patients undergoing peripheral vascular surgery.[29] One hundred patients were randomized to carefully managed regimens of either epidural anesthesia followed by epidural analgesia or general anesthesia followed by intravenous patient-controlled analgesia. The results demonstrated a significant decrease in the incidence of peripheral vascular graft thrombosis with epidural anesthesia. No statistically significant differences were found, however, in overall incidence of death, major cardiac morbidity, and myocardial ischemia.

Perioperative changes in hemostasis may explain the high frequency of DVT and pulmonary embolism after surgery. Increased plasma concentrations of coagulation factors, decreased concentrations of coagulation inhibitors, enhanced platelet reactivity, and impaired fibrinolysis have been reported postoperatively.[42,43] Rosenfeld and colleagues[43] demonstrated the prevention of postoperative inhibition of fibrinolysis in patients undergoing regional analgesia combined with epidural fentanyl. Another favorable factor in connection with regional anesthesia is a pronounced increase in blood flow to the lower extremities.[44]

Pulmonary Complications

It is well documented that regional anesthesia, like intercostal blockade and spinal/epidural analgesia, may improve several parameters of pulmonary function postoperatively by preventing postoperative pain. Continuous blockade is apparently more effective than a single short-acting blockade. Cumulative data presented by Kehlet suggest that neural blockade may reduce postoperative pulmonary infections.[27] In a study of 70 women over 75 years old undergoing hip surgery, 22.9 percent of the patients subjected to general anesthesia developed bronchopneumonia as opposed to 8.6 percent in the spinal anesthesia group.[32] In the multicenter study of Davis and colleagues,[30] 538 elderly hip surgery patients had a similar incidence of pneumonia in both the general and the spinal anesthesia groups. In an earlier study immediately after general anesthesia, the mean fall in PaO_2 in patients undergoing emergency hip surgery was 6.5 mmHg compared with the preoperative value but only 1.2 mmHg after spinal block ($p < 0.01$).[31] At 24 h postoperatively, the fall in PaO_2 was similar in both study groups. The number of patients suffering pulmonary embolism has been generally lower in regional than in general anesthesia groups. In elderly patients, the capacity of lung function may be limited and all measures that reduce pulmonary infections and atelectases are beneficial.

Circulatory Effects of Regional Anesthesia

There are some differences between spinal and epidural anesthesia in the effects on cardiac function and circulation. Spinal anesthesia usually has a more rapid cephalad spread, increased motor blockade, less patient movement during surgery, and in some studies, less urinary retention requiring catheterization.[30] The major advantage postulated for the extradural route is the threat of hypotension caused by spinal sympathetic blockade. In a study of 65 patients undergoing hip arthroplasty, epidural anesthesia was successful employing an initial dose of 15 ml of 0.5% bupivacaine, and spinal anesthesia when administering a dose of 4 ml of 0.5% isobaric bupivacaine.[45] The two techniques were similar with regard to the level of sensory blockade, degree of hypotension, and perioperative hemorrhage. To decrease the hemodynamic effects of spinal anesthesia, the use of continuous spinal anesthesia with a microcatheter has been tested in elderly patients.[46] Continuous spinal anesthesia with a low anesthetic dose produced a satisfactory quality of anesthesia, but with fewer hemodynamic effects than was the case with continuous epidural anesthesia or single-dose spinal anesthesia. However, with continuous microcatheter spinal anesthesia, some precautions to avoid local neurotoxicity must be observed.

The addition of thoracic epidural analgesia to general anesthesia may reduce cardiovascular dysfunction and signs of cardiac ischemia. However, in a recent study of patients undergoing lower extremity vascular surgery, the cardiac outcomes were similar in both the epidural and general anesthesia groups.[29] The patients had continuous electrocardiographic monitoring from the day before surgery through the third postoperative day.

Cerebral Complications

Deterioration of mental function is a major concern for elderly patients. The etiology of mental dysfunction is multifactorial and may relate to preexisting disease, perioperative complications, hospitalization, and the effect of analgesics and other medications. Anticholinergic medications have been implicated. Depression and cognitive impairment are predisposing factors. The reported incidence of postoperative delirium varies from 7 to 44 percent.[47] Some studies have demonstrated that the incidence of mental confusion is lower in patients undergoing regional anesthesia, especially during the immediate postoperative period.[48] However, most studies have not found any significant differences between regional and general anesthesia (Table 9-8).[49–52]

Postoperative confusional states are transient, as demonstrated in many studies performed 1 week to some months postoperatively.[49–52] However, the confusion significantly prolongs hospitalization. The best treatment is prevention. Good care, information, and instructions in the language most familiar to the patient are important. The avoidance of anticholinergic medications and high doses of other incrementally administered medications, along with aggressive treatment of hypoxia and hypovolemia, may prevent confusional states.

ADVANTAGES AND CONTRAINDICATIONS OF REGIONAL ANESTHESIA

Advantages of Regional/Local Techniques

There is no "best" anesthetic for elderly patients. Most randomized, controlled studies indicate a slight advantage for regional as opposed to general anesthesia. In elderly patients with a compromised physical condition, a field block,

Table 9-8 Influence of type of anesthesia on postoperative mental function

Type of operation	n	Regional vs. general anesthesia	Time to psychological assessment	Reference
Transurethral prostatic resection	44	Spinal >> general	6 h	Chung et al[48]
		Spinal > general	3 days	
Knee arthroplasty	64	Spinal = general	3 mo	Nielsen et al[49]
Femoral fracture	57	Epidural = general	7 days	Berggren et al[50]
Urologic surgery	60	Spinal = general	1 mo	Crul et al[51]
Hip arthroplasty	30	Epidural = general = epidural + general	1 wk/3 mo	Riis et al[52]

>=better than; = no difference.

local infiltration, and nerve block are probably the safest anesthetic procedures. The use of epidural and spinal anesthesia causes a pharmacologic sympathectomy that minimizes postsurgical pain and stress responses. These features may provide reductions in perioperative morbidity in some elderly patient groups. The evidence is quite convincing with regard to the reduction in blood loss and thromboembolism in elderly patients undergoing hip replacement and prostatectomy.

In the early days of anesthesia and until recently, local anesthesia and regional anesthesia were often safer for the patient because of the lack of monitoring during surgery and the poor quality of postoperative care. In general, it is clear that in the immediate postoperative period, regional anesthesia is superior with regard to mental function and mortality. However, this difference disappears later. Nevertheless, regional anesthesia is an appropriate selection for a geriatric patient undergoing transurethral resection of the prostate, a gynecologic procedure, inguinal herniorrhaphy, or repair of a fractured hip. An important prerequisite for selecting a regional technique is an alert and cooperative patient. Maintenance of consciousness during surgery provides for rapid recognition of acute disorders in cerebral function and problems such as angina.

Spinal and epidural anesthesia both have their own advantages and disadvantages. The advantages of spinal anesthesia are as follows: easier to perform in elderly patients, more objective endpoint (presence of cerebrospinal fluid in the needle), more rapid onset of anesthesia, more predictable spread of anesthesia, lower amount of local anesthetic, and less toxicity. The advantages of epidural anesthesia are as follows: duration controllable with continuous catheter technique, low gradual dosing possible, less concern over local spinal cord damage and postspinal puncture headache, and usually milder hemodynamic changes.

Additional advantages of regional techniques over general anesthesia are that the technique is familiar, simple, and easy and that the problems of a difficult airway may be avoided. Regional techniques are suitable in most emergencies or if there is suspicion of food in the stomach. The avoidance of intubation in the prone position may be beneficial. Regional techniques are well tolerated by patients with various diseases. Continuous epidural and other continuous nerve blocks are very suitable for postoperative pain treatment.

Contraindications to Regional Anesthesia

There are only a few strong contraindications to regional techniques. The most important are patient refusal, patient inability to maintain stillness during a procedure, raised intracranial pressure (spinal, epidural), true allergy, and unbalanced systemic coagulopathy, either idiopathic or intrinsic. Relative contraindications are coagulopathy, infection at the site of needle insertion, hypovolemia, lack of experience, septicemia, hysteria, poor patient cooperation, and preexisting neurological disease. Diseases such as the peripheral neuropathy of multiple sclerosis are often contraindicated by legal rather than medical considerations.

SUMMARY

In the elderly, age-related changes in nervous system function, liver and renal functional capacity, and the anatomy have an impact on regional anesthesia. The management of regional anesthesia requires the knowledge of associated disease processes and their medications, which may significantly increase the risk of mortality and morbidity in geriatric patients. The autonomic reflexes maintaining cardiovascular homeostasis and the tolerance of hypovolemia are impaired.

Age may not affect the duration of regional anesthesia or motor blockade, but in general the dose requirement decreases and the recovery time from analgesia may increase. Prevention is the best treatment for systemic toxic reactions to local anesthetics. The use of fractional dosing and carefully watching for signs of toxicity are vital.

Regional anesthesia seems to offer some advantages over general anesthesia because of diminished blood loss during surgery, a decrease in the incidence of peripheral vascular graft thrombosis, and a decrease in the incidence of thromboembolism and pulmonary complications. Surprisingly, most studies have not found any significant differences between regional and general anesthesia in terms of mental dysfunction. Regional anesthesia should be carefully examined as a potential option when anesthesia for the elderly is required.

REFERENCES

1. Muravchick S: Anesthesia for the elderly, in Miller RD (ed): *Anesthesia*, 3d ed. New York: Churchill Livingstone, 1990, chap 62, pp 1969–1983.

2. McLeskey CH: Anesthetic considerations for the geriatric patient. 1993 Annual ASA Refresher Course Lectures, p 521.
3. Waldman C: Anaesthesia for the elderly, in Kaufnan L (ed): *Anaesthesia Review 9.* Edinburgh: Churchill Livingstone, 1992, chap 11, pp 194–211.
4. Muravchick S: Anaesthesia for the aging patient. *Can J Anaesth* 40:R63, 1993.
5. Cote J, Lapointe P: Anaesthetic management for the elderly patient. *Can Anaesth Soc J* 32:188, 1985.
6. Creasey H, Rapoport SI: The aging human brain. *Ann Neurol* 17:2, 1985.
7. Dax EM: Receptors and associated membrane events in aging. *Rev Biol Res Aging* 2:315, 1985.
8. Bromage PR: Ageing and epidural dose requirements: Segmental spread and predictability of epidural analgesia in youth and extreme age. *Br J Anaesth* 41:1016, 1969.
9. Sharrock NE: Epidural anesthetic dose responses in patients 20 to 80 years old. *Anesthesiology* 49:425, 1978.
10. Collins KJ, Exton-Smith AN, James MH, Oliver DJ: Functional changes in autonomic nervous responses with ageing. *Age Ageing* 9:17, 1980.
11. Ziegler MG, Lake CR, Kopin IJ: Plasma noradrenaline increases with age. *Nature* 261:333, 1976.
12. Kennedy RD, Chaird FI: Physiology of aging of the heart. *Cardiovasc Clin* 12:1, 1981.
13. Lakatta EG: Alterations in the cardiovascular system that occur in advanced age. *Fed Proc* 38:163, 1979.
14. Lakatta EG: Diminished beta-adrenergic modulation of cardiovascular function in advanced age. *Cardiol Clin* 4:185, 1986.
15. Wahba WM: Influence of aging on lung function—clinical significance of changes from age twenty. *Anesth Analg* 62:764, 1983.
16. Kronenberg RS, Drage CW: Attenuation of the ventilatory and heart rate responses to hypoxia and hypercapnia with aging in normal men. *J Clin Invest* 52:1812, 1973.
17. MacLachlan MSF: The aging kidney. *Lancet* 2:143, 1978.
18. Epstein M: Effects of aging in the kidney. *Fed Proc* 38:168, 1979.
19. Woodhouse KW, Mutch E, Williams FM, et al: The effect of age on pathways of drug metabolism in human liver. *Age Ageing* 13:328, 1984.
20. Shanor SP, Van Hees GR, Baart N, et al: The influence of age and sex on human plasma and red cell cholinesterase. *Am J Med Sci* 242:357, 1961.
21. Fulop T Jr, Worum I, Csangor J, et al: Body composition in elderly people. *Gerontology* 31:6, 1985.
22. Tucker GT, Mather LE: Properties, absorption, and disposition of local anesthetic agents, in Cousins MJ, Bridenbaugh PO (eds): *Neural Blockade*, 2d ed. Philadelphia: Lippincott, 1988, chap 3, pp 47–110.
23. Veering BT: Local anaesthetics: an update. *Anaesth Pharmacol Rev* 1:159, 1993.
24. Veering BT, Burm AGL, Vletter AA, et al: The effect of age on the systemic absorption and systemic disposition of bupivacaine after epidural administration. *Clin Pharmacokinet* 22:75, 1992.
25. Veering BT, Burm AGL, Vletter AA, et al: The effect of age on systemic absorption and systemic disposition of bupivacaine after subarachnoid administration. *Anesthesiology* 74:250, 1992.
26. Bonica JJ, Buckley FP: Regional analgesia with local anesthetics, in Bonica JJ (ed.): *The Management of Pain*, 2d ed. Philadelphia: Lea & Febiger, 1990, chap 94, pp 1883–1896.

27. Kehlet H: Modification of responses to surgery by neural blockade: Clinical implications, in Cousins MJ, Bridenbaugh PO (eds): *Neural Blockade*, 2d ed. Philadelphia: Lippincott, 1988, chap 3, pp 145–188.
28. Barker JP, Vafidis GC, Robinson PN, Hall GM: Plasma catecholamine response to cataract surgery: A comparison between general and local anaesthesia. *Anaesthesia* 46:642, 1991.
29. Christopherson R, Beattie C, Frank SM, et al: Perioperative morbidity in patients randomized to epidural or general anesthesia for lower extremity vascular surgery. *Anesthesiology* 79:422, 1993.
30. Davis FM, Woolner DF, Frampton C, et al: Prospective, multicentre trial of mortality following general or spinal anaesthesia for hip fracture surgery in the elderly. *Br J Anaesth* 59:1080, 1987.
31. Davis FM, Laurenson VG: Spinal anaesthesia or general anaesthesia for emergency hip surgery in elderly patients. *Anaesth Intensive Care* 9:352, 1981.
32. Racle JP, Benkhadra A, Poy JY, et al: Comparative study of general and spinal anaesthesia in the elderly female patients undergoing hip surgery. *Ann Fr Anesth Reanim* 5:24, 1986.
33. McLaren AD, Stockwell MC, Reid VT: Anaesthetic techniques for surgical correction of fractured neck of femur. *Anaesthesia* 33:10, 1978.
34. McKenzie PJ, Wishart HY, Dewar KMS, et al: Comparison of the effects of spinal anaesthesia and general anaesthesia on postoperative oxygenation and perioperative mortality. *Br J Anaesth* 52:49, 1980.
35. Valentin N, Lomholt B, Jensen JS, et al: Spinal or general anaesthesia for surgery of the fractured hip? *Br J Anaesth* 58:284, 1986.
36. Covert CR, Fox GS: Anaesthesia for hip surgery in the elderly. *Can J Anaesth* 36:311, 1989.
37. Hendolin H, Mattila MAK, Poikolainen E: The effect of lumbar epidural analgesia on the development of deep vein thrombosis of the legs after open prostatectomy. *Acta Chir Scand* 147:425, 1981.
38. McGowan SW, Smith GFN: Anaesthesia for transurethral prostatectomy. *Anaesthesia* 35:847, 1980.
39. Blunnie WP, McIlroy PDA, Merrett JD, Dundee JW: Cardiovascular and biochemical evidence of stress during major surgery associated with different techniques of anaesthesia. *Br J Anaesth* 55:611, 1983.
40. Mann RAM, Bisset WIK: Anaesthesia for lower limb amputation. *Anaesthesia* 38:1185, 1983.
41. Modig J, Borg T, Karlström G, et al: Thromboembolism after total hip replacement: Role of epidural and general anesthesia. *Anesth Analg* 62:174, 1983.
42. Sharrock NE, Ranawat CS, Urquhart B, Peterson M: Factors influencing deep vein thrombosis following total hip arthroplasty under epidural anesthesia. *Anesth Analg* 76:765, 1993.
43. Rosenfeld BA, Beattie C, Christopherson R, et al: The effects of different anesthetic regimens on fibrinolysis and the development of postoperative arterial thrombosis. *Anesthesiology* 79:435, 1993.
44. Bonica JJ, Akamatsu T, Berges PU, et al: Circulatory effects of peridural block: II. Effects of epinephrine. *Anesthesiology* 34:514, 1971.
45. Davis S, Erskine R, James MFM: A comparison of spinal and epidural anaesthesia for hip arthroplasty. *Can J Anaesth* 39:551, 1992.
46. Klimscha W, Weinstabl C, Ilias W, et al: Continuous spinal anesthesia with a

microcatheter and low-dose bupivacaine decreases the hemodynamic effects or centroneuraxis blocks in elderly patients. *Anesth Analg* 77:275, 1993.

47. Buckley N: Regional vs. general anaesthesia in orthopaedics. *Can J Anaesth* 40:R104, 1993.
48. Chung F, Meier R, Lautenschlager E, et al: General or spinal anesthesia: Which is better in the elderly? *Anesthesiology* 67:422, 1987.
49. Nielson WR, Gelb AW, Casey JE, et al: Long-term cognitive and social sequelae of general versus regional anesthesia during arthroplasty in the elderly. *Anesthesiology* 73:1103, 1990.
50. Berggren D, Gustafson Y, Eriksson B, et al: Postoperative confusion after anesthesia in elderly patients with femoral neck fractures. *Anesth Analg* 66:497, 1987.
51. Crul BJ, Hulstijn W, Burger IC: Influence of the type of anaesthesia on postoperative subjective physical well-being and mental function in elderly patients. *Acta Anaesthesiol Scand* 36:615, 1992.
52. Riis J, Lomholt B, Haxholdt O, et al: Immediate and long-term mental recovery from general versus epidural anesthesia in elderly patients. *Acta Anaesthesiol Scand* 27:44, 1983.

CHAPTER 10

Preoperative Evaluation and Preoperative Medications

Edward A. Wilson

INTRODUCTION

A geriatric patient has arbitrarily been defined as a patient 65 years old or older, and the term is used interchangeably with the term *elderly patient*. Twelve percent of the population in the United States is 65 years old or older (30 million persons). This number is projected to increase to 17 percent by the year 2050, when there will be 55 million elderly persons.[1] Anesthesiologists are being asked to provide anesthesia service to an increasing number of these geriatric patients, who frequently have complex illnesses.

To care for a geriatric patient appropriately, the anesthesiologist must be aware of the physiological changes that occur with aging and the illnesses associated with aging, as well as interactions of the drugs used to treat those illnesses. The aging process normally results in a decline or deterioration in the physiological functions of the body's organ systems. Emphasis has been placed on the fact that individuals do not all "age" at the same rate. Rowe and Kahn[2] used the term *successful aging* to describe individuals who age with minimum impairment of physiological function and the term *usual aging* to describe or identify persons who have undergone normal deterioration of physiological functions. When the same concept is used, there is an alternative classification using the terms *typical aging* and *atypical aging*. Typical aging represents the process of normal deterioration of physiological function, and atypical aging may be subclassified into accelerated atypical aging and decelerated atypical aging. Accelerated atypical aging represents more rapid deterioration of the system's functions than is usually associated with aging, and decelerated atypical aging represents a reduced rate of deterioration of physiological functions. The decline in basic organ function occurs in all the major organ systems and progresses at an approximate rate of 1 percent per year. Peak function occurs during the late twenties or early thirties. The assessment of the patient's biological age becomes an important factor in the evaluation of a geriatric patient during the preoperative assessment. The patient's biological, rather than chronological, age has a greater impact on both anesthetic management and its inherent risks.

RISK STRATIFICATION

It is generally accepted that an elderly patient is at a higher risk for developing postoperative complications than is a younger patient. Coté and Lapointe[3] studied factors influencing postoperative mortality in elderly patients. They noted a significant increase in mortality related to associated diseases, increasing age, emergency surgery, operative site, and length of the operation.

Associated Diseases

Stephen[4] reviewed the incidence of preexisting diseases in elderly patients during the preoperative period in 1000 patients over 70 years old (Table 10-1). Concomitant diseases associated with the cardiovascular, pulmonary, and renal systems were most frequently observed. Preexisting hypertension was noted in 46.6 percent of the patients, and renal disease in 31.4 percent. The perioperative mortality in the total group was 5.8 percent, with 84 percent of those who died

Table 10-1 Preanesthetic complications encountered in 1000 elderly patients

Complication	Percent of patients
Hypertension	46.6
Atherosclerosis	26.9
Myocardial infarction	18.5
Cardiomegaly	13.6
Congestive heart failure	7.5
Angina	6.4
Cerebrovascular accident	5.8
Chronic obstructive pulmonary disease	14.0
Diabetes	9.2
Renal disease	31.4
Liver disease	8.5

SOURCE: Reprinted with permission from Stephen CR: The risk of anesthesia and surgery in the geriatric patient, in Krechel (ed): *Anesthesia and the Geriatric Patient.* New York: Grune & Stratton, 1984, p 231.

having had three or more preexisting diseases. Farrow and Fowkes[5] reviewed the factors affecting mortality in hospitalized patients who underwent 109,000 surgical procedures (Table 10-2). There were 2,391 postoperative deaths, with 186 (15.8 percent) deaths occurring in patients with preexistent congestive heart failure. Preoperative renal function impairment was associated with 86 postsurgical deaths (10.8 percent mortality rate). Preexisting coronary disease was associated with a 7 percent surgical mortality. The mortality in patients who had no preexisting concomitant disease in the preoperative period was 0.5 percent.

Increasing Age

Palmberg and Hinsjari[6] reviewed factors associated with postoperative mortality in 17,199 patients. The mortality among patients over 70 years old was 9.2 percent and it was 0.25 percent among those under 70 years old. The overall mortality was 2.3 percent. Patients over 70 years of age represented 20 percent of the surgical cases; however, 91 percent of the total deaths that occurred were in this age group. Denny and Denson[7] analyzed the outcome of 272 geriatric patients over 90 years old. The overall mortality was 29 percent. Pneumonia was the cause in 38 percent of the deaths, and arterial sclerotic heart disease (ASHD) and cerebrovascular accident (CVA) caused death in 31 percent and 6 percent, respectively. Denny and Denson[7] noted that the patients who were free of preoperative concomitant diseases had a mortality of 4.9 percent. Mohr[8] reviewed postoperative mortality in 34,140 surgical patients and noted mortality rates of 8.2 percent in patients over 80 years and 6.8 percent in patients 71 to 80 years old compared with 2.3 percent in patients 41 to 50 years old.

Emergency versus Elective Surgery

Palmberg and Hinsjari[6] also studied the incidence of postoperative mortality in emergency versus elective surgical procedures. In patients over 70 years old

Table 10-2 Mortality by selected preoperative condition

Condition	Deaths	Operations	Mortality, %
Cardiac failure	186	1,175	15.8
Impaired renal function	86	779	10.8
Angina, arteriosclerosis, ischemic heart disease	544	7,77	67.0
Diabetes	82	1,452	5.7
Chronic lower respiratory tract infection	408	8,060	5.1
No preoperative condition	206	43,483	0.5

SOURCE: Reprinted with permission from Farrow SC, Fowkes GR: Epidemiology in anesthesia: II. Factors affecting mortality in hospital. *Br J Anaesth* 54:811, 1982.

undergoing elective surgery, the mortality rate was 7.8 percent, while the post-operative mortality rate for emergency surgery was 36.8 percent. Pulmonary embolism was the cause of death in 33.3 percent of the patients, and pneumonia and cardiovascular incidents caused death in 20.4 percent and 11.1 percent, respectively. The use of compression devices on the lower extremities and minidose heparin has reduced the frequency of postoperative pulmonary embolism. Emergency operations remain a risk factor in predicting postsurgical complications.

Operative Site

Warner and Hoskin[9] reviewed postoperative mortality in regard to the relation between surgical site and mortality at 48 h and at 30 days in 301 procedures performed on surgical patients over 90 years old. As would be expected, a higher mortality rate was associated with more complex or invasive surgical procedures, such as vascular, biliary, and thoracic surgery. Major vascular procedures were associated with the highest mortality at 48 h (20 percent), whereas thoracic procedures were associated with the highest mortality at 30 days (37.5 percent). Major vascular, biliary, and gastrointestinal surgeries were associated with a significant mortality at 30 days: 20 percent, 26.9 percent, and 23.8 percent, respectively. Less invasive procedures, from transurethral prostatic resection (TURP) to ophthalmologic surgery, were associated with a zero mortality rate in this review.

Length of Surgery

The effect of duration of surgery on the mortality rate in 289 patients over 70 years old was reviewed by Palmberg and Hinsjari.[6] When the operative time was less than 2 h, the mortality rate was 7.5 percent. The mortality rate in operations lasting more than 2 h was 36.4 percent. Stern and Tinker[10] noted that the incidence of infarction in patients with a history of previous infarction who underwent surgery was 5.9 percent when the duration of the procedure was less than 3 h and 15.9 percent in procedures lasting more than 3 h. The mortality associated with reinfarction was 69 percent. Stern and Tinker[10] suggested that the correlation between the reinfarction rate and the length of surgery was valid only if the surgical procedure was thoracic or abdominal (i.e., the length of surgery in less invasive procedures was not associated with an increased infarction rate).

PREANESTHETIC ASSESSMENT

The preoperative assessment affords the anesthesiologist an opportunity to (1) assess the patient's physical and mental status, (2) make a judgment regarding the need for additional treatment, evaluation, or consultation, (3) formulate an anesthetic plan, and (4) discuss with the patient the proposed anesthesia, including planned techniques, risks involved, and consent required. A focused history and physical examination should be performed, with increased awareness of the normal deterioration of physiological function in the elderly and the high incidence of anticipated concomitant diseases involving the cardiovascular, pulmonary, and renal systems. Ideally, this examination should be performed before the day of surgery to allow adequate time for possible additional evaluation or laboratory studies. While performing the preanesthetic assessment of a geriatric patient, the anesthesiologist should focus on a number of key areas during the history and physical examination. Cheng and Wang-Cheng[11] (Table 10-3) have identified a number of key points to focus on during assessment of the patient's history.

History

Pulmonary

Fourteen percent of geriatric surgical patients have a history of chronic obstructive pulmonary disease (COPD).[10] Denny and Denson[7] reported that

Table 10-3 Key points in history taking

General
Nutritional habits
Alcohol and tobacco use
Medications
Cardiac
Previous myocardial infarction
Current angina
Exercise tolerance
How many stairs climbed?
How many blocks walked?
Symptoms and signs of congestive heart failure
Dyspnea
Orthopnea
Edema
Pulmonary
Chronic cough
Dyspnea
Smoking history
Recent infections
Neurological
Light-headedness or syncope
Stroke or transient ischemic attack

SOURCE: Reproduced from Cheng EY, Wang-Cheng RM: Impact of aging on preoperative evaluation. *J Clin Anesth* 3:330, 1991. By permission of Butterworth-Heinemann.

preoperative pulmonary disease was associated with a 63 percent mortality in a study of 272 surgical patients over 90 years of age. It is advisable to inquire about the patient's history of respiratory illness: Is the patient a smoker? If so, how long and how much? Does the patient have a history of a cough? If so, how frequent? When? Is the cough productive of sputum? What color is the sputum? Has he or she had any recent infections: colds, bronchitis, sore throats, or pneumonia? Has the patient ever had asthma or emphysema? If so, what treatment has he or she had, and when? Does the patient have shortness of breath at rest or with exercise? How far can the patient walk without becoming short of breath? How many flights of stairs can the patient climb without becoming short of breath? This information is basic for an adequate pulmonary history.

Cardiovascular

Stephen's[4] review of preanesthetic concomitant illness in geriatric surgical patients (Table 10-1) revealed a significant incidence of cardiovascular-related illnesses. Hypertension occurred in 46.6 percent of the patients. Atherosclerosis, myocardial infarction, and cardiomegaly/congestive heart failure (CHF) occurred in 26.9 percent, 18.5 percent, and 21.1 percent, respectively. Factors associated with an increased incidence of coronary artery disease include age, positive family history, history of smoking, hyperlipidemia, hypertension, and history of diabetes mellitus. The interviewer should focus the questions carefully on the cardiovascular history: Does the patient have a history of chest pain or angina? How often? What precipitates the chest pain? How long does it last? Has the character of the pain changed recently? What relieves the pain? What treatment is the patient receiving? Has she or he had a "heart attack"? Coronary occlusion or infarction? Does the patient experience chest pain with exercise? How much exercise? Does she or he experience chest pain at rest? Has the patient been told he or she has carotid artery disease? Has the patient experienced fainting spells, weakness, or paralysis of the arms or legs? Does he or she experience pain in the legs with exercise? Has the patient ever had heart failure? Does he or she experience swelling of the legs? Does the patient have any problem with his or her heart "skipping" or irregular beats? How often? What treatment?

Renal and Hepatic

Stephen[4] noted renal disease in 31.4 percent of presurgical geriatric patients and an incidence of diabetes mellitus and liver disease of 9.2 percent and 8.5 percent, respectively. During the early phases of these illnesses, patients may not have obvious symptoms; however, it is appropriate to attempt to elicit information regarding the function of the various systems with focused questions. It is usually best to begin with very simple questions: Has the patient ever had any kidney or bladder problems? Has the patient ever had abnormal blood glucose levels? Has the patient had any trouble with his or her liver or with yellow jaundice? If the anesthesiologist then suspects an underlying renal or hepatic disease, more focused questions should be asked.

Physical Examination

The preanesthetic examination should focus on high-risk areas: general state of health, neurological status, the cardiovascular system, and the pulmonary system (Table 10-4).[11]

Airway

Geriatric patients are susceptible to arthritic changes in the cervical spine and the temporomandibular joint and may have restricted mobility of the neck and

Table 10-4 Key points in physical examination

General
Weight
Nutritional status
Vital signs: postural blood pressure and heart rate changes
Connective tissue
Skin
Turgor
Areas of breakdown
Spine
Cervical mobility
Dorsal kyphosis
Extremities
Contractures
Venous access
Edema
Cyanosis
Cardiac
Murmurs
S_3, S_1
Arrhythmias
Pulmonary
Rales
Pleural effusion
Decreased air movement
Neurological
Carotid bruits
Mental status

SOURCE: Reprinted from Cheng EY, Wang-Cheng RM: Impact of aging on preoperative evaluation. *J Clin Anaesth* 3:331, 1991. By permission of Butterworth-Heinemann.

mandible. Any limitation in range of motion should be identified preoperatively. Geriatric patients frequently have dentures, partial plates, and chipped or loose teeth. Such abnormalities should be noted and documented on the preanesthetic record.

Nutritional Status

Geriatric patients frequently reside in nursing homes and have limited financial resources. They are socially isolated and are often emotionally depressed. As a result, they may be malnourished and have poor control of chronic medical illnesses. When assessing the nutritional and hydration status of a patient, the physician must keep in mind the usual changes associated with aging. For example, skin turgor is not a reliable indicator of hydration status in elderly patients because wrinkling of the skin and a loss of skin turgor may be associated with the normal aging process, secondary to loss of supporting subcutaneous tissue.

Neurological Status

Cerebrovascular disease is common in geriatric patients. A history of CVA has been reported in 5.8 percent of presurgical geriatric patients (Table 10-1).[4] Denny and Denson[7] reported that CVA was the cause of death in 6 percent of 272 surgical patients over 90 years old. The preoperative neurological evaluation enables the anesthesiologist to establish the patient's mental status and baseline neurofunction, identify risks of anesthesia, and form an appropriate plan for anesthetic management. For example, asymptomatic carotid bruits have been reported in 7 percent of the elderly over age 65 but are not associated with an increased rate of perioperative stroke and, therefore, do not require additional evaluation.[12,13] A patient with a symptomatic carotid bruit is at increased perioperative risk, and preoperative evaluation of the bruit is warranted.

Pulmonary Status

The chest should be examined for signs of COPD, such as increased anteroposterior diameter of the chest, flattening of the diaphragm on chest x-rays, rales, wheezing, and/or decrease in breath sounds. A patient with pulmonary disease may also have a frequent cough and dyspnea with exertion. Clubbing and cyanosis may also be evident.

Cardiovascular Status

Examination of the cardiovascular system includes assessment of peripheral pulses: carotid, femoral, and dorsalis pedis. The physician should look for signs of CHF, such as S_3 gallop, jugular venous distension, peripheral edema, rales during auscultation of the lungs, dyspnea on exertion, and paroxysmal dyspnea.

Cardiac arrhythmias are common in geriatric patients and may be secondary to underlying cardiac disease.

Musculoskeletal Systems

Geriatric patients frequently have a history of osteoporosis, osteoarthritis, or rheumatoid arthritis. These illnesses not only affect the mobility of the joints, they also result in an increased risk of injury during surgery if adequate precautions are not taken. It is important to determine the presence of restricted joint mobility of the extremities, including the head, neck, and jaw.

Laboratory Evaluation

Preoperative laboratory tests may assist an anesthesiologist in (1) determining the functional status of various organ systems, (2) identifying the need for additional treatment or evaluation, (3) determining the risk of postoperative complications, and (4) developing a plan for anesthetic management. Focused laboratory testing can be used by the anesthesiologist in optimizing the patient's condition preoperatively as well as assisting in the formulation of a plan for anesthetic management. Nonselective laboratory screening is not advisable because it results in increased cost, is not an efficient technique for detecting new disease processes, and results in increased risk to the patient. Nonselective screening results in "false-positive tests," which necessitate additional invasive testing to verify that the values are not secondary to disease processes. If laboratory abnormalities, for example, "false-positive tests," are not investigated with additional studies, the physician may be at increased medical-legal risk if there is an adverse surgical outcome. Laboratory evaluation of a surgical patient should be based on abnormalities identified by a focused history and physical examination during the preoperative assessment rather than nonselective screening for disease processes. Roizen[14] has presented current recommendations for preoperative testing of asymptomatic surgical patients (Table 10-5). Using these guidelines will minimize the risk and cost of unnecessary studies that is inherent in broad screening techniques.

CARDIAC EVALUATION

During the history and physical exam, the anesthesiologist may identify indicators that suggest underlying cardiovascular disease. Additional cardiac consultation or evaluation may then be warranted. Roizen[14] has compiled a list of risk factors and suggested an algorithm to assist in the selection of appropriate tests for a geriatric patient with possible cardiac disease (Fig. 10-1 and Table 10-6). It is the anesthesiologist's responsibility to make a judgment on the appropriateness and completeness of the preoperative evaluation. The presence of current CHF, unstable angina, or recent myocardial infarction (MI) (less than

Table 10-5 Simplified strategy for preoperative testing

Preoperative condition	HGB M	F	WBC	PT / PLT PTT	BT	Elect	Creat BUN	Blood GLUC	SGOT/Alk PT Ase	X-ray	ECG	Preg.	T/S
Procedure with blood loss	X	X											X
Procedure without blood loss													
Neonates	X	X											
Age < 40		X											
Age 40–49		X									m		
Age 50–64		X									X		
Age > 65	X	X								+	X		
Cardiovascular disease							X			X	X		
Pulmonary disease										X	X		
Malignancy	X	X	*	*						X			
Radiation therapy			X							X	X		
Hepatic disease				X					X				
Exposure to hepatitis									X				
Renal disease	X	X				X	X						
Bleeding disorder				X	X								
Diabetes						X	X	X			X		
Smoking > 20 pack–yr	X	X								X			
Possible pregnancy												X	
Diuretic use						X	X						
Digoxin use						X	X				X		
Steroid use						X		X					
Anticoagulant use	X	X		X									
CNS disease			X			X	X	X			X		

Not all diseases are included in this table. The physician's own judgment is needed regarding patients with diseases not listed.
Symbols: + = perhaps obtain: * = obtain for leukemias only; X = obtain; m = men only.
Abbreviations: HGB = hemoglobin; WBC = white blood cell count; PT = prothrombin time; PTT = partial thromboplastin time;
PLT = platelet count; BT = bleeding time; Elet = electrolytes (i.e., sodium, potassium, chloride, carbon dioxide, and proteins);
Creat/BUN = creatinine or blood urea nitrogen; SGOT/ALK PT Ase = serum glutamic-oxaloacetic transaminase and alkaline phosphatase;
T/S = blood typing and screen for unexpected antibodies.
Modified from Roizen et al, Kaplan et al, and Blery et al.
SOURCE: Reprinted with permission from Roizen MF: Preoperative patient evaluation. New Orleans Anesthesiology Comprehensive Review Course, June 1992.

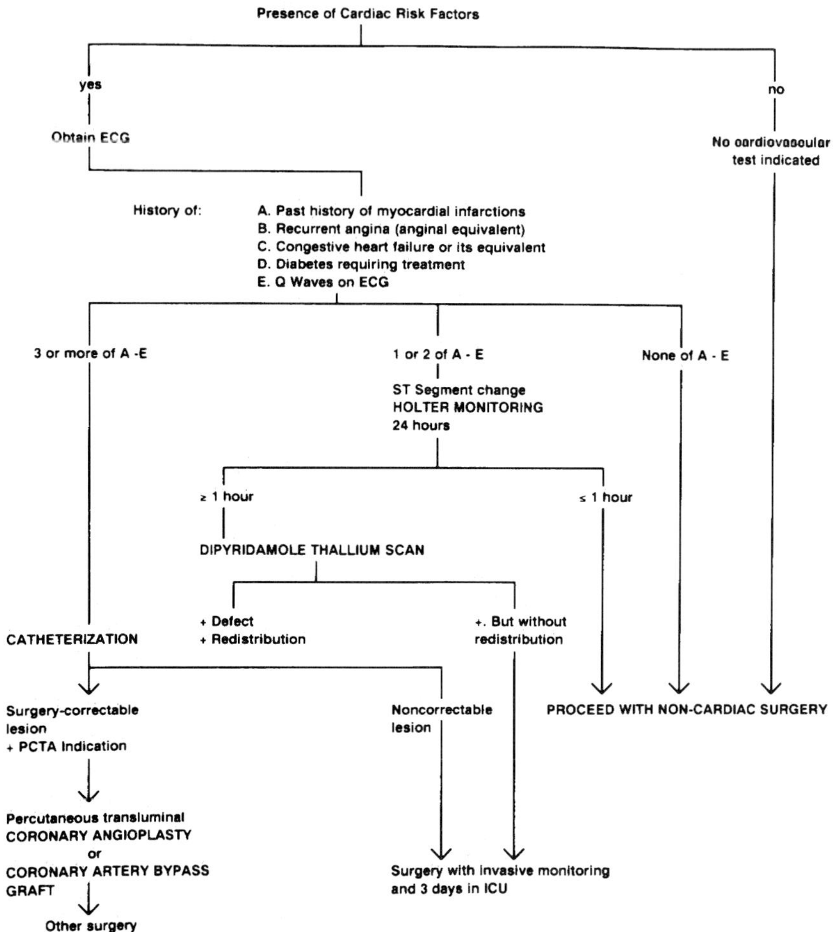

Figure 10-1 How to decide which cardiovascular laboratory test to obtain. Use history to segregate patients. *(Adapted with permission from Roizen MF: Preoperative patient evaluation. New Orleans Anesthesiology Comprehensive Review, June 1992.)*

3 months) is associated with an unacceptably high risk of postsurgical mortality. Therefore, elective surgical procedures should be delayed. Underlying cardiovascular disease is associated with a number of conditions: hypertension, diabetes mellitus, smoking, and chest pain. If one or more of these risk factors are noted, additional cardiac evaluation may be indicated. The minimum testing recommended is an electrocardiogram (ECG). If a more intensive cardiac evaluation is warranted, it is appropriate for the anesthesiologist or surgeon to request a cardiology consult. The request for a cardiology consultation should not be a "request for cardiology clearance for surgery." The anesthesiologist should identify areas of concern uncovered by the history, physical exam, or preliminary laboratory studies. Specific questions may be raised regarding additional treatment to improve the physical status of the geriatric patient,

Table 10-6 Risk factors for cardiac disease

Does the patient meet one or more of the following criteria?
1. Chest pain
2. Angina or anginal equivalents
3. Congestive heart failure symptoms or equivalents
4. History of high blood pressure
5. Diabetes
6. History of symptoms of dysrhythmia
7. History of shortness of breath
8. History of myocardial infarction
9. Age in males ≥ 40 or age in females ≥ 50
10. History of smoking
11. Patient not able to exercise without shortness of breath or chest pain
12. Patient needs vascular surgery

SOURCE: Reprinted with permission from Roizen MF: Preoperative patient evaluation. New Orleans Anesthesiology Comprehensive Review Course, June 1992.

reducing the risk of perioperative complications. It is then the responsibility of the cardiologist to implement the appropriate cardiac evaluation. The anesthesiologist should be familiar with various cardiovascular studies as well as the significance of abnormal test results.

Holter Monitoring

This technique of continuous ECG ambulatory monitoring of a patient may provide useful information. Patients are monitored for 24 h for dysrhythmias or ischemic changes. It has been demonstrated that 75 percent of cardiac ischemic events are silent (asymptomatic). Ischemic changes noted preoperatively have been associated with a 36 percent incidence of major cardiac complications during the perioperative period.[15–17] The absence of ischemic changes is associated with a lack of cardiac complications postoperatively. Holter monitoring is a useful, noninvasive, relatively inexpensive procedure that can provide information about the stability of the coronary artery disease and the risk of perioperative complications.

Thallium 201 Myocardial Imaging

The radioisotope thallium 201 is administered intravenously; it distributes to the myocardium in proportion to the regional coronary blood flow and is taken up by viable myocytes. Exercise or pharmacologic dilators (dipyridamole) may be used to enhance blood flow to areas of the myocardium served by coronary arteries, so that more thallium is then taken up in these areas. Dipyridamole is a nonspecific vasodilator used to enhance blood flow to the myocardium. It is useful for improving the sensitivity of the test in patients who are unable to exercise because of physical disabilities such as arthritis and peripheral vascular disease. A scan of the distribution of the isotope is then performed. Adequately or normally perfused areas demonstrate a homogeneous distribution of the isotope. Areas of myocardium distal to a coronary obstruction (stenosis of 70 percent or greater) appear as a defect on thallium perfusion imaging. A repeat scan 4 to 6 h later may show a "persistent defect" pattern or a homogeneous "reversible defect" pattern. A defect that disappears is indicative of hypoperfused areas of viable myocardium that are at risk for or vulnerable to infarction. A defect that does not disappear (a "persistent defect" when the scan is repeated) is indicative of scar (previous MI), that is, nonviable, nonvulnerable myocardium. The presence of a reversible defect (hypoperfused viable myocardium) represents a significant risk of perioperative ischemia or infarction in a geriatric surgical patient. An irreversible persistent defect (hypoperfused scarred myocardium) represents an area at less risk because the area has previously infarcted and healed with scar formation.

Coronary Angiography

Coronary artery catheterization and angiography remain the gold standard for the evaluation of suspected coronary artery disease. Angiography demonstrates the coronary artery anatomy but does not provide direct information regarding the physiological significance of an obstruction or stenosis of a coronary artery. This information may be obtained with thallium imaging or exercise ECG. Coronary angiography is expensive and is associated with some risk and therefore should be used with discretion.

PULMONARY EVALUATION

An increased incidence of major postoperative pulmonary complications (i.e., pneumonia, respiratory failure, atelectasis, and bronchitis) is associated with preexisting pulmonary illnesses as well as with the site of surgery. If underlying pulmonary disease is suspected, additional pulmonary evaluation is warranted. Tisi[18] has suggested indications for pulmonary function tests (Table 10-7). Pulmonary function tests may help the physician determine the extent of the patient's pulmonary disease, establishing a baseline of pulmonary function, identifying any reversible component of the disease process, and determining the risk of perioperative complications. Spirometry and arterial blood gas analysis are considered the most reliable and cost-effective means of evaluating pulmonary function.

Clinical Spirometry

Vital Capacity

Vital Capacity (VC) is one of the most commonly used measurements of lung function. It represents the maximal volume exhaled after a maximal inspiration. VC is considered abnormal if the volume measured falls below 80 percent

Table 10-7 Indications for preoperative evaluation of pulmonary function

Planned thoracic surgery
Planned upper abdominal surgery
History of heavy smoking and cough
Marked obesity
Age > 70 years
History of pulmonary disease

SOURCE: Adapted and reprinted with permission from Tisi G: Preoperative identification and evaluation of the patient with lung disease. *Med Clin North Am* 71:399, 1987.

of the predicted value. Charts are available to determine the predicted value on the basis of age and size. Reduced VC is associated with restrictive pulmonary disease (pneumonia, atelectasis, pulmonary fibrosis, and loss of pulmonary distensibility after surgery). Reduction in VC is also seen in patients with muscle disease, increased intraabdominal pressure, and postoperative respiratory splinting caused by pain.

Timed Expiratory Spirograms

This group of studies includes forced vital capacity, maximal flow rate, and maximal voluntary ventilation.

FORCED VITAL CAPACITY Forced vital capacity (FVC) is the volume exhaled with maximal force after a maximal inspiration, and the volume is related to time (liters/min). Usually 3 to 4 s are required to perform the expiration. Values are reduced by the conditions noted above that reduce VC. FEV_1 is the forced expiratory volume measured in 1 s. It may be expressed as an absolute volume or as a ratio of the total FVC (i.e., FEV_1/FVC). Normal young patients can exhale 75 to 80 percent of the FVC in 1 s and the remainder of the FVC in an additional 2 to 3 s. The FEV_1/FVC is reduced in patients with obstructive airway disease (asthma, bronchitis).

MAXIMAL FLOW RATE The measurement of peak flow rate during FVC is effort-dependent and subject to wide variations. More commonly $FEF_{200-1200}$ and $FEV_{25-75\%}$ are used because they are reported to be less effort-dependent. $FEF_{200-1200}$ is the flow in liters/min measured after expiration of the initial 200 ml. The normal value is approximately 500 liters/min, and the flow is markedly reduced by obstruction of the large airways (asthma). This study may be useful in determining a patient's response to bronchodilator therapy. Postoperative values less than 50 percent of the predicted value are associated with an increased risk of postoperative pulmonary complications. $FEV_{25-75\%}$ is the forced expiratory volume measured during the middle part of FVC. The normal flow of $FEV_{25-75\%}$ is 4.5 to 5.0 liters. Reduction in this expired volume is associated with small airway obstruction. Some researchers have suggested that the test is sensitive for the detection of early obstruction. It is less effort-dependent than some tests; however, wide variations in normal volume have been noted, and a normal value may be as low as 2 liters.

MAXIMAL VOLUNTARY VENTILATION Maximum voluntary ventilation (MVV) is a measurement of maximal breathing capacity and is the maximal volume a patient can breathe voluntarily per minute. Normal values are 150 to 175 liters/min and are reduced by increases in airway resistance (obstructive pulmonary disease). MVV is also reduced by a decrease in elasticity of the chest wall and lung, in muscle strength, and in effort. An estimated value of MVV can be obtained by multiplying the FEV_1 by 35. The MVV is a nonspecific test that may be useful in identifying gross impairment in respiratory function.

Arterial Blood Gas Analysis

Preoperative arterial blood gas (ABG) analysis may allow an anesthesiologist to establish a preoperative baseline and estimate the degree of pulmonary impairment. Aging is associated with pulmonary parenchymal changes which alter lung function. Geriatric patients experience a decrease in elasticity of the lungs that results in a progressively increased closure of the small airways, producing an increase in the closing volume of the lungs. As a result, a greater portion of the patient's tidal volume occurs at a lung volume below the closing volume, producing air trapping and V/Q mismatching that reduces the efficiency of oxygen exchange. Arterial oxygen tension in an elderly patient breathing room air declines linearly with age and may be estimated by the following formula: $Pa_{O_2} = 100 - [0.4 \times \text{age (years)}]$ mmHg.[19]

Shapiro[20] has suggested another guideline for estimating normal arterial oxygen tension in an elderly patient. Using a normal baseline of a minimum of 80 mmHg at 60 years of age, one subtracts 1 mmHg for each year of age over 60. For example, a minimum acceptable oxygen tension for a 70-year-old would be 70 mmHg; for an 80-year-old, 60 mmHg. This guideline does not apply to patients over 90 years of age, and a Pa_{O_2} of 40 mmHg or less is considered severe hypoxemia at any age. The Pa_{CO_2} is normally within 35 to 45 mmHg, with the pH from 7.35 to 7.45. In an elderly patient without pulmonary disease or any other coexisting disease, the Pa_{CO_2} and pH of the ABG are expected to be within these ranges. Variation from these values may be associated with pulmonary or metabolic abnormalities.

PREOPERATIVE MEDICATION

During the past several years there has been a trend toward a reduction in the amount of premedication given to surgical patients. The administration of medication preoperatively may be used to (1) allay anxiety, (2) prevent pain associated with planned instrumentation (arterial line, regional anesthesia, central venous access) or positioning of the patient, (3) reduce the risk of complications (aspiration, increased ICP, intubation-induced hypertension), (4) provide amnesia of the perioperative events, and (5) continue treatment of coexisting diseases (diabetes mellitus, hypertension, coronary artery disease, and endocrine disorders). The preoperative medications should be prescribed in a goal-oriented manner and should be tailored to the specific needs of the individual geriatric patient.

Routine Premedication

Most of the drugs used for routine premedication can be included within one of the following categories: anxiolytics, analgesics, anticholinergics, antacids, and H_2 antagonists.

Anxiolytics

A preoperative visit with an elderly surgical patient frequently will reduce anxiety. If sedation is required, most geriatric patients require less medication than do younger patients. Long-acting sedatives given in the preoperative period may result in an increased incidence of sedation or disorientation in the postoperative period. Benzodiazepines (diazepam, lorazepam, and midazolam) are frequently used for preoperative sedation.

Marjot and Valentine[21] studied the arterial saturation of 15 patients after premedication for cardiac surgery. The patients were premedicated with 7.5 to 15 mg of morphine intramuscularly (IM), 2 to 3 mg of lorazepam PO, and 2.5 to 5 mg of droperidol IM. Twelve (80 percent) of the patients developed hypoxemia, and 33 percent developed changes in the ECG consistent with ischemia. Marjot and Valentine[21] concluded that oxygen should be administered to patients receiving the above premedication and similar regimens.

The effect of an oral benzodiazepine premedication on arterial saturation in 80 geriatric patients scheduled for regional anesthesia was studied by Munoz and Dagnino.[22] The patients received 1 mg flunitrazepam, 1 mg lorazepam, 7.5 mg midazolam, or no premedication. The incidence of hypoxemia (arterial saturation less than 90 percent for more than 30 s) was 15 percent in the unmedicated patients. In the treated patients, the incidence of hypoxemia was 45 percent, 20 percent, and 60 percent for flunitrazepam, lorazepam, and midazolam, respectively. Munoz and Dagrino[22] concluded that the benzodiazepines may produce hypoxemia in a geriatric patient during spinal anesthesia and that monitoring the patient's arterial oxygen saturation and the administration of supplemental oxygen after premedication are mandatory. A geriatric patient has an increased sensitivity to benzodiazepines as well as an exaggerated and prolonged response. Bell and Sprickett[23] noted that a reduced dose of diazepam was required for "grip relaxation" in a geriatric patient (20 mg in a 20-year-old versus 10 mg in an 80-year-old). Reeves and Franger[24] also noted a reduced requirement of midazolam to induce sleep in an elderly patient (0.3 mg/kg was 100 percent effective in inducing sleep in patients 62 to 76 years old compared with 0.5 mg/kg being only 60 percent effective in patients 29 to 40 years old).

Diazepam continues to be widely used orally for preoperative sedation of elderly patients. Caution must be used when medicating frail and very elderly patients to avoid oversedation and hypoxemia. A regimen of 5 to 10 mg (0.1 mg/kg) administered orally 90 to 120 min before surgery is commonly used for patients who are to receive regional anesthesia (e.g., for cataract surgery). Midazolam is used more frequently than diazepam in the operating room. It is shorter-acting, has better amnesic properties, and is associated with a significantly lower incidence of thrombophlebitis when administered intravenously. Midazolam may be administered orally; however, satisfactory sedation and amnesia can be obtained by administering it in the operating room in increments of 0.5 mg intravenously and titrating to the desired level of sedation. Usually 1 to 2 mg is adequate for a geriatric patient. Benzodiazepines can cause excessive sedation, and patients who receive these drugs orally, intramuscularly, or intravenously should be monitored in regards to their levels of sedation and oxygenation. The use of a pulse oximeter (Sa_{O_2}) is recommended and has been included in the ASA monitoring standards. If intravenous sedatives or narcotics are administered in the surgical suite, the anesthesiologist must stay with the patient or ensure that another capable person monitors the patient appropriately.

Analgesics

In the past, narcotics were a major part of preoperative medications. Morphine sulfate and meperidine were the most commonly used narcotics for premedication. They were used for sedation, relief of anxiety, and pain relief during instrumentation. They were also used as anesthetics, as adjuvants, and to blunt the response of blood pressure to intubation. Opioids, however, are associated with a high incidence of side effects. The incidence of nausea with morphine and meperidine is 49 percent and 36 percent, respectively, and the incidence of vomiting is 67 percent and 51 percent, respectively. Opioids may cause a delay in gastric emptying and spasm of Oddi's sphincter. They cause a decrease in patient response to hypoxemia and hypercarbia. Over the past few years there has been a trend toward a reduced use of narcotic and sedative premedication. More frequently, the patient is given oral sedation on the ward and intravenous opioids (fentanyl or sufentanyl) or benzodiazepines are administered in the operating room. Geriatric patients are susceptible to oversedation and hypoxemia, and if opioids are to be used as a preoperative medication, the dose should be reduced. This is especially important when the opioid is combined with a sedative.

Anticholinergics

The routine use of anticholinergic premedication as a "drying agent" is less common today. Physicians more commonly use these drugs when they are specifically indicated. Anticholinergic drugs may be useful in reducing secretions in patients who receive ketamine or undergo bronchoscopy. They may be used for amnesia or for prophylaxis or treatment of bradycardias associated with the administration of succinylcholine, the administration of anticholinesterases to reverse muscle relaxants, and reflex stimulation of the oculocardiac reflex, carotid sinus stimulation, or traction on the gastrointestinal tract. The drugs commonly used are atropine, glycopyrrolate, and scopolamine.

Atropine is usually administered IM in a dose of 5 μg/kg. It is less drying and has a greater potential to increase the heart rate than does either glycopyrrolate or scopolamine. Atropine crosses the blood-brain barrier and may cause delayed emergence from anesthesia and confusion in the postoperative period, especially in an elderly patient more prone to central anticholinergic crisis.

Glycopyrrolate does not cross the blood-brain barrier and does not cause sedation. It is reported to be as effective as atropine in treating reflex bradycardias and is usually administered in doses of 2 to 5 μg/kg IM or IV.

Scopolamine crosses the blood-brain barrier and causes greater sedation amnesia and antisialagogue effects than either atropine or glycopyrrolate. It is usually given in doses of 2 to 5 μg/kg IM or IV. Its use has greatly diminished because of undesirable CNS side effects, particularly in the elderly, and the advent of superior drugs.

Anticholinergic agents cause mydriasis and may increase intraocular pressure (IOP). This may be of concern in glaucoma patients. However, because of the relatively small doses given, atropine and glycopyrrolate can be used in these patients. Scopolamine has a greater effect on IOP than do atropine and glycopyrrolate. Anticholinergic agents are reported to relax the lower esophageal sphincter; however, this has not been shown to be clinically significant.

Antacids

It is widely accepted that aspiration of gastric fluid with a pH below 2.5 is associated with extensive pulmonary damage. The administration of an oral nonparticulate antacid is highly effective in raising the pH of gastric contents above this critical pH of 2.5, and aspiration of nonparticulate antacids has not been associated with significant pulmonary injury. The aspiration of particulate antacids may result in damage to lung tissue. The prophylactic use of clear nonparticulate antacids has been recommended as an appropriate preoperative medication for surgical patients. The commonly used nonparticulate antacids are 0.3 m sodium citrate (30 ml), Bicitra (30 ml), and Alka-Seltzer (two tablets in 30 ml of water). It is recommended that the antacid be given orally 15 to 30 min before the induction of anesthesia. Increased mixing of the antacid and the gastric fluids may be achieved by rotating the patient from side to side after administration. The preoperative use of antacids is indicated especially in patients with diabetes, hiatal hernia, or a "full stomach."

Histamine Receptor Antagonists

Gastric acid secretion may be reduced by the administration of histamine receptor antagonists (cimetidine, ranitidine, or famotidine). H_2-receptor antagonists raise the pH of the gastric fluid and variably reduce the gastric fluid volume without having an effect on the gastric emptying time.

Cimetidine may be given IM on the morning of surgery; however, it is most effective when an evening dose (300 mg PO) is combined with a dose on the morning of surgery (300 mg IM PO 60 to 90 min before surgery). Weber and Hirshman[25] reported that this combination was 100 percent effective in raising the pH of the gastric fluid to a pH above 2.5. Cimetidine reduces hepatic blood flow and inhibits the metabolism of some drugs by inhibiting the cytochrome P450 system. Cimetidine may prolong the half-lives of lidocaine, bupivacaine, warfarin, theophylline, propranolol, and diazepam.

Ranitidine is effective in decreasing gastric acid secretion and has minimal effect on the hepatic metabolism of drugs. It may be given orally (50–200 mg 60 min before surgery) or intravenously (50–100 mg 60 min before surgery). Ranitidine has few side effects and is effective for 8 to 10 h; therefore, it may be preferred to cimetidine, which has a duration of 3 to 4 h.

Famotidine, like ranitidine, does not interfere with the metabolism of drugs by the liver. It has few side effects and may be administered orally (10–20 mg 60 min before surgery) or intravenously (10–20 mg 30 to 60 min before surgery). Famotidine has a duration of action of 6 to 10 h and is an acceptable alternative to ranitidine.

Mental confusion, hallucinations, and disorientation can occur with the administration of H_2-receptor antagonists. However, the incidence is low after a single dose and much lower with ranitidine and famotidine. These antagonists are useful in reducing the risk of aspiration in routine surgical patients by raising the gastric fluid pH and are especially useful in high-risk geriatric patients (patients with diabetes mellitus, hiatal hernia, or morbid obesity).

Gastrokinetic Agents

These drugs increase the motility of the stomach and are useful in reducing the volume of gastric contents, reducing the risk of aspiration. Metoclopramide is a gastrokinetic agent commonly used as a preoperative medication.

Metoclopramide is a dopamine antagonist that increases gastrointestinal motility, increases lower esophageal sphincter tone, and relaxes the pylorus and duodenum. This results in increased emptying of gastric contents. Metoclopramide also has antiemetic properties. It may be administered orally (10–20 mg 30 to 60 min before surgery) or intravenously (5–20 mg 15 to 30 min before surgery). The effect lasts 4 to 6 h. The effect on the gastrointestinal tract may be blocked by the prior administration of an anticholinergic agent. Metoclopramide is most useful in patients who are likely to have incomplete emptying of the stomach (a patient who has eaten within a few hours, a pregnant patient, and a morbidly obese patient). It is highly effective when combined with an H_2-receptor antagonist.

SPECIAL CONSIDERATIONS

A number of disease states require special consideration with regard to preoperative medication. These include (1) ischemic heart disease, (2) diabetes mellitus, (3) asthma or chronic obstructive pulmonary disease (COPD), (4) hypertension, and (5) a patient on chronic steroid therapy.

Ischemic Heart Disease

Ischemic heart disease is frequently present (18.5 percent) as a preexisting disease in geriatric surgical patients. It is especially important that the treatment of the condition be continued during the preoperative period. Medications commonly encountered include adrenergic blockers, calcium channel blockers, digitalis preparations, and anticoagulants. In general, beta blockers and calcium channel blockers should not be stopped or tapered preoperatively. Placing the patient NPO after midnight will result in the omission of the early morning medication and a potentially low serum drug level. This can result in a subtherapeutic drug concentration and withdrawal symptoms. Therefore, these medications must be ordered to be given on the morning of surgery with a sip of water. Digitalis preparations are most commonly given for treatment of CHF or control of dysrhythmias. If the digitalis is given to control rapid atrial fibrillation, it should be continued on the day of surgery to optimize the patient's condition. Rapid atrial fibrillation may be precipitated intraoperatively in a patient who had digitalis withheld on the morning of surgery, especially a patient with a marginal digitalis blood level. If the digitalis is being used to treat CHF, it may be withheld. Patients on anticoagulation therapy should have warfarin (Coumadin) discontinued in sufficient time to allow the prothrombin time to return to within 20 percent of normal. Consideration may be given for the use of low-dose heparin coverage as the Coumadin is discontinued. The Coumadin usually can be restarted on the second or third postoperative day in an uncomplicated surgical patient.

Diabetes Mellitus

Stephen[4] noted a 9.2 percent incidence of diabetes mellitus in geriatric surgical patients. Fifteen percent of type II (insulin-dependent) diabetic patients are reported to be at risk for life-threatening ketoacidosis in the absence of insulin therapy. There continues to be controversy regarding appropriate control of blood sugar in a diabetic surgical patient. Those who promote "tight control" (blood sugar in range of 100–200 mg) suggest this rationale to prevent metabolic decompensation (ketoacidosis, excessive diuresis, dehydration, hyperosmolarity, impaired CNS function, and electrolyte disturbances), reduce the incidence of perioperative sepsis, and avoid decreased surgical wound strength.

A study[26] of blood sugar levels in 430 patients who experienced a global ischemic episode after cardiac arrest revealed a mean blood glucose level of 341 mg/dl in patients who failed to awaken versus 262 mg/dl in patients who did awaken. In those persons who did awaken with persistent neurological deficits, mean blood sugar levels were 286 mg/dl versus 251 mg/dl in those who awakened without a neurological deficit. Although there are questions regarding the relation of hyperglycemia and ischemic brain damage, the current recommendation is to maintain the blood sugar below 250 mg/dl during periods of potential cerebral ischemia. The routine use of glucose-containing intravenous solutions in the operating room has been discontinued. It also seems prudent to maintain the blood sugar of a diabetic surgical patient below 250 mg/dl during the perioperative period.

Hypoglycemia should be avoided in the perioperative period. The dangers of undetected hypoglycemia intraoperatively are increased in a patient undergoing a general anesthetic. A number of regimens have been proposed for the perioperative management of diabetic patients, and it is probably more important to monitor the patient closely and treat the patient appropriately than to select a specific regimen. Roizen[27] has proposed a regimen that may be used in the perioperative period to control blood sugar in surgical patients (Tables 10-8 and 10-9).

Asthma/Chronic Obstructive Pulmonary Disease

Asthma and COPD are chronic illnesses that may have relatively symptom-free intervals interrupted by episodes of exacerbation. COPD has been reported in 14 percent of presurgical geriatric patients (Table 10-1). Information

Table 10-8 Classic nontight control regimen

Aim: To prevent hypoglycemia; to prevent ketoacidosis and hyperosmolarity

1. **The day before surgery, the patient should be given no solids for 24 h before a planned operation and nothing by mouth after midnight; a glass of apple juice should be at the bedside for emergency use.**
2. **At 6 A.M. on the day of surgery, institute intravenous fluids using plastic cannulae and a solution containing 5% dextrose, infusion at the rate of 125 ml/h per 70 kg body weight.**
3. **After intravenous infusion is instituted, give one-half the usual morning insulin dose subcutaneously.**
4. **Continue 5% dextrose solutions through the operative period, giving at least 125 ml/h/per 70 kg body weight.**
5. **In the recovery room, monitor blood glucose concentrations every 1 to 2 h and treat with a sliding scale.**

SOURCE: Reprinted with permission from Roizen M: Preoperative management of the diabetic patient. ASA 1992, Annual Refresher Course Lectures 223:1, 1992.

Table 10-9 Tight control regimen 1

Aim: To keep plasma glucose levels between 79 and 200 mg/dl; may improve wound healing and prevent wound infections

1. The evening before the operation, determine preprandial blood glucose level.
2. Through a plastic cannula, begin intravenous infusion of 5% dextrose in water at the rate of 50 ml/h per 70 kg.
3. Next "piggyback" to the dextrose infusion and infusion of regular insulin (50 units in 250 ml or 0.9% sodium chloride) and infusion pump. Before attaching this piggyback line to the dextrose infusion, flush the line with 60 ml of infusion mixture and discard the flushing solution. This approach saturates insulin-binding sites of the tubing.
4. Set the infusion rate using the following equation: Insulin (units/h) = plasma glucose (mg/dl)/150. (*Note*: This denominator should be 100 if patient is taking corticosteroids, e.g., 100 mg of prednisone a day.)
5. Repeat measurements of blood glucose levels every 2 to 4 h as needed and add just insulin appropriately to obtain blood glucose levels of 100 to 200 mg/dl.
6. On the day of surgery, intraoperative fluids and electrolytes are managed by continuing to administer nondextrose, non-lactate-containing solutions, as described in steps 3 and 4.
7. Determine plasma glucose level at the start of operation and every hour for the rest of the 24-h period. Adjust insulin dosage appropriately.

Treatment of hypoglycemia may be required (i.e., blood glucose levels less than 50 mg/dl). You should be prepared to do so with 15 ml of 50% dextrose in water (7.5 g of dextrose in a 70-kg patient raises the blood glucose level approximately 30 mg/dl). Under such circumstances, the insulin infusion would be terminated.

SOURCE: Reprinted with permission from Roizen M: Perioperative management of the diabetic patient. ASA 1992, Annual Refresher Course Lectures, 223:1, 1992.

obtained during the history and physical of a patient who is at increased risk of perioperative pulmonary complications may assist the anesthesiologist. A patient who is actively wheezing usually is not a candidate for elective surgery. Patients with a history of severe episodes of bronchospasm during the months preceding the surgical procedure are at an increased risk of exacerbation of symptoms during the postoperative period. Measures may be taken to minimize the rate of complications (Table 10-10). Discontinuation of smoking 8 weeks before surgery may allow the mucociliary transport mechanism to return to normal, reduce the production of mucous secretions, and allow a reduction in carboxyhemoglobin (COHb) levels in the blood. Discontinuing smoking as little as 24 h before surgery can also be beneficial in allowing a reduction in COHb levels and improvement in the oxygen-carrying capacity of the blood. The use of bronchodilators pre-, intra-, and postoperatively may be beneficial in patients with a reversible bronchospastic component to their disease. The performance of pulmonary function tests after bronchodilatory therapy helps identify geriatric patients who are most likely to respond to this mode of therapy. Inhalation bronchodilator therapy should be continued during the preoperative period and may be given before transporting a surgical

Table 10-10 Maneuvers to reduce risk of postoperative pulmonary complications

1. Discontinuation of smoking
2. Bronchodilator therapy
3. Treatment of pulmonary infection
4. Lung expansion procedures
   Deep breathing exercises
   Coughing exercises
   Incentive spirometry
   Early ambulation
5. Chest physiotherapy
6. Improved postsurgical pain control

patient to the operating room on the day of surgery. Preoperative instruction in deep breathing, coughing exercises, and incentive spirometry have been shown to decrease postoperative pulmonary complications.

Parasympathetic blockade may be used to alleviate bronchospasm. Patients who wheeze when exposed to cold air, under emotional stress, or when exercising may particularly benefit from pretreatment with inhaled atropine. An atropine analogue, ipatroprium bromide, is available in a metered dose inhaler. It is well tolerated, effective, and relatively free of side effects. The starting dose is two inhalations (36 μg) four times a day. The most common adverse side effects are oral dryness (2.4 percent), cough (5.9 percent), nausea (2.8 percent), dizziness (2.4 percent), and blurring of vision (1.2 percent). Postoperative pulmonary complications (atelectasis, pneumonia, bronchitis, and respiratory failure) continue to be major problems in surgical patients. Efforts to optimize the patient's pulmonary status preoperatively may reduce the incidence of these complications.

Hypertension

Preoperatively, hypertension is encountered in 46.6 percent of geriatric surgical patients (Table 10-1). A significant number of these patients are on antihypertensive medications, including diuretics. It is recommended that the diuretics be withheld on the morning of surgery unless the patient is to have placement of a Foley catheter preoperatively or has a history of recent or current CHF. Other antihypertensive agents usually are continued on the morning of surgery. Special precautions are advised when one is discontinuing clonidine in the perioperative period. The abrupt discontinuation of clonidine may result in severe rebound hypertension. If the patient will be unable to continue the clonidine in the postoperative period, it is advisable for the surgeon to convert the patient to another antihypertensive agent before surgery. The management of patients on high-dose beta blockers is controversial. It is important for the anesthesiologist to be aware that patients on high-dose beta blockers may have impaired cardiovascular response to the stress of surgery. Fifty percent of the elderly are reported to have hypertension, and 50 percent of these patients are not aware of their illness. Up to 60 percent of the patients being treated may be inadequately treated. Hypertension has been defined as a systolic pressure greater than 160 mmHg or a diastolic pressure greater than 90 mmHg. An inadequately treated hypertensive patient may have vasoconstriction of the vascular bed and is susceptible to episodes of hypotension after anesthesia induction. Perioperative hypotension or hypertension is associated with an increased risk of myocardial ischemia, dysrhythmias, CHF, myocardial infarction, and stroke. It is generally recommended that elective surgery be delayed in patients with systolic pressures greater than 190 to 195 mmHg or a diastolic pressure greater than 110 mmHg.

Glucocorticoid Deficiency

The most common cause of secondary adrenal insufficiency is associated with chronic glucocorticoid therapy. The adrenal response in a normal patient who is undergoing surgery is proportional to the degree of surgical stress. Patients with suppressed adrenal function may have cardiovascular instability in the

Table 10-11 Perioperative corticosteroid coverage

For minor surgery	The patient should take 1½ to 2 times usual glucocorticoid dosage on the morning of surgery. The following day, the patient should take the normal prednisone dose (or parenteral equivalent if gut cannot be used). The surgeon and anesthesiologist should be aware that the patient is glucocorticoid-dependent and should be prepared to administer more "steroids" if the surgery becomes prolonged or more extensive.
For moderate surgery	The patient should be given 2 times the usual glucocorticoid dosage orally (if possible) on the morning of surgery and/or 25 mg hydrocortisone IV before operation, then 75 mg hydrocortisone IV during operation, and 50 mg hydrocortisone IV after operation; then the dose should be rapidly tapered over 18 h to the usual dose—if postoperative course is uncomplicated.
For major surgery	The patient should be given 2 times the usual glucocorticoid dosage orally (if possible) on the morning of surgery and/or 50 mg hydrocortisone IV before operation, then 100 mg hydrocortisone IV during operation. After operation, 100 mg IV q 8 h for 24 h should be administered and then rapidly tapered (over 48–72 h) to the patient's usual glucocorticoid dosage—if postoperative course is uncomplicated.

SOURCE: Reprinted with permission from Brussel T, Chernow B: Perioperative management of endocrine problems: Thyroid, adrenal cortex, pituitary. ASA Refresher Courses in Anesthesia 18:48, 1990.

absence of corticosteroid supplementation when subjected to this stress. Brussel and Chernow[28] have proposed steroid coverage that is based on the degree of surgical stress (Table 10-11). Perioperative steroid therapy is used to prevent acute adrenal insufficiency while attempting to avoid the adverse effects associated with steroid therapy (infection, hyperglycemia, metabolic acidosis, and infarction). The dose recommended approximates the increase in steroid secretion in a normal patient when subjected to the stress of surgery and represents a reduction in the dose that has been recommended traditionally. Gradual reduction in the dose to the presurgical level should be started on the second postoperative day, and the reduction should continue as rapidly as the patient's condition allows.

SUMMARY

The aging process normally results in a decline or deterioration of the physiological functions of the body. A geriatric surgical patient frequently has coexisting disease (cardiovascular, pulmonary, renal, and CNS), which increases the risk of perioperative morbidity and mortality. A thorough preoperative assessment of a geriatric patient may enable the anesthesiologist to formulate and implement a plan for the anesthetic management of the patient that will result in a reduction in the risk of perioperative complications.

REFERENCES

1. U.S. Bureau of the Census: *Statistical Abstract of the United States*, 110th ed. Washington: U.S. Bureau of the Census, 1990, p 12.
2. Rowe JW, Kahn RL: Human aging: Usual and successful. *Science* 237:143, 1987.
3. Coté J, Lapointe P: Anesthetic management for the elderly. *Can Anaesth Soc J* 32:188, 1985.
4. Stephen GR: The risk of anesthesia and surgery in the geriatric patient, in Krechel S (ed): *Anesthesia and the Geriatric Patient.* New York: Grune & Stratton, 1984, p 231.
5. Farrow SC, Fowkes FG: Epidemiology in anesthesia: II. Factors affecting mortality in hospital. *Br J Anaesth* 54:811, 1982.
6. Palmberg S, Hinsjari E: Mortality in geriatric surgery. *Gerontology* 23:103, 1979.
7. Denny JH, Denson JS: Risk of surgery in patients over 90. *Geriatrics* 27:115, 1972.
8. Mohr D: Estimation of surgical risk in the elderly: A correlative review. *J Am Geriatr Soc* 31:99, 1983.
9. Warner MA, Hoskin MP: Surgical procedures among those ≥ 90 years of age. *Ann Surg* 207:380, 1988.
10. Stern P, Tinker J: Myocardial reinfarction after anesthesia and surgery. *JAMA* 239:2566, 1978.
11. Cheng EY, Wang-Cheng RM: Preoperative evaluation of the geriatric patient. *J Clin Anesth* 3:324, 1991.

12. Lefkowitz D: Asymptomatic carotid artery disease in the elderly. *Clin Geriatr Med* 7:417, 1991.
13. Ropper AH, Weshsler LR, Wilson LS: Carotid bruit and risk of stroke in elective surgery. *N Engl J Med* 307:1388, 1982.
14. Roizen MF: Preoperative patient evaluation. New Orleans Anesthesiology Comprehensive Review Course, June 1992.
15. Raby KE, Goldman L: Correlation between preoperative ischemia and major cardiac events after peripheral vascular surgery. *N Engl J Med* 321:1296, 1989.
16. Ouyang P, Jerstenblith G: Frequency and significance of early postoperative silent myocardial ischemia in patients having peripheral vascular surgery. *Am J Cardiol* 64:1113, 1989.
17. Pasternack PF, Grossi EA: The value of silent myocardial ischemia monitoring in prediction of postoperative myocardial infarction in patients undergoing peripheral vascular surgery. *J Vasc Surg* 10:617, 1989.
18. Tisi GM: Preoperative evaluation of pulmonary function: Indications and benefits. *Am Rev Respir Dis* 119:293, 1979.
19. McClesky CH: Principles of anesthetic managment of elderly patients. IARS 1989 Review Course Lectures, 1989, pp 144–149.
20. Shapiro BA, Harrison RA: *Clinical Application of Blood Gases*, 4th ed. Chicago: Year Book, 1989, chap 6, p 82.
21. Marjot R, Valentine SJ: Arterial oxygen saturation following premedication for cardiac surgery. *Br J Anaesth* 64:737, 1990.
22. Munoz HR, Dagnino JA: Benzodiazepine premedication causes hypoxemia during spinal anesthesia in geriatric patients. *Reg Anaesth* 17:139, 1992.
23. Bell GD, Sprickett GP: Intravenous midazolam for upper gastrointestinal endoscopy. *Br J Clin Pharmacol* 23:241, 1987.
24. Reeves JR, Frangen RJ: Midazolam: Pharmacology and uses. *Anesthesiology* 62:310, 1985.
25. Weber C, Hirshman CA: Cimetidine for prophylaxis of aspiration pneumonitis: Comparison of intramuscular and oral dosage schedules. *Anesth Analg* 58:426, 1979.
26. Longstreth WT, Iniu TS: High blood glucose level on hospital admission and poor neurological recovery after cardiac arrest. *Ann Neurol* 15:59, 1984.
27. Roizen M: Preoperative management of the diabetic patient. ASA 1992 Annual Refresher Course Lectures 223:1, 1992.
28. Brussel T, Chernow B: Perioperative management of endocrine problems: Thyroid, adrenal cortex, pituitary. ASA Refresher Courses in Anesthesia 18:33, 1990.

CHAPTER 11

Perioperative Fluid Therapy in Geriatric Patients

Robert F. Bossard
Girish P. Joshi
Charles W. Whitten

INTRODUCTION

Physiological changes in multiple organ systems occurring as a result of the aging process and preexisting disease alter fluid and electrolyte balance in the geriatric patient. A diminished capacity to compensate for fluid and electrolyte shifts associated with perioperative events places these patients at increased risk for perioperative morbidity and mortality. Fluid and electrolyte management in these patients requires a careful and enlightened approach.

IMPACT OF AGING AND AGE-RELATED CHANGES ON FLUID THERAPY

Aging and the Cardiovascular System

Physiological changes in the cardiovascular and autonomic nervous systems associated with aging significantly impair the ability of the elderly to respond to alterations of fluid and electrolyte status. These physiological changes have important influences on fluid and electrolyte management in the elderly. Appropriate intravascular volume repletion is of prime importance in the aged because their ability to maintain cardiac output and organ perfusion is limited.

Patients undergoing anesthesia and surgery depend on autonomic reflexes to maintain homeostasis. With advanced age, alterations of autonomic nervous system function decrease the ability to compensate for changes in volume status in the perioperative period.[1,2] In addition, patients with autonomic nervous system dysfunction are sensitive to the depression of homeostatic reflexes that occurs in the presence of anesthetics.[3,4] The compensatory responses to acute hemodilution are also reduced in this patient population. Diseases and medications that often accompany old age represent confounding factors. These mechanisms increase the incidence of perioperative hypotension and cardiovascular instability in the elderly. Simple and noninvasive tests of autonomic nervous system function (e.g., Valsalva maneuver, change in heart rate with vital capacity breathing, change in heart rate and blood pressure upon assuming the upright posture) may be of value in assessing patients in the aged population who are at risk for the development of perioperative hypotension.

As a result of decreased cardiac reserve and autonomic reflex dysfunction, the elderly are limited in the extent to which they can elicit intrinsic inotropic, chronotropic, and vasomotor reflexes. They depend on the Frank-Starling mechanism to increase their cardiac output during stress from anesthesia and surgery.[5] This implies that increased filling pressures are necessary to maintain adequate cardiac output in these patients. However, older patients have noncompliant ventricles and steep pressure-volume curves (Fig. 11-1), and increased filling pressures may lead to pulmonary edema. Poor compliance in both the heart and the vasculature of geriatric patients decreases cardiac output and increases systemic and pulmonary perfusion pressures. Therefore, careful maintenance of fluid balance is critical in the elderly.

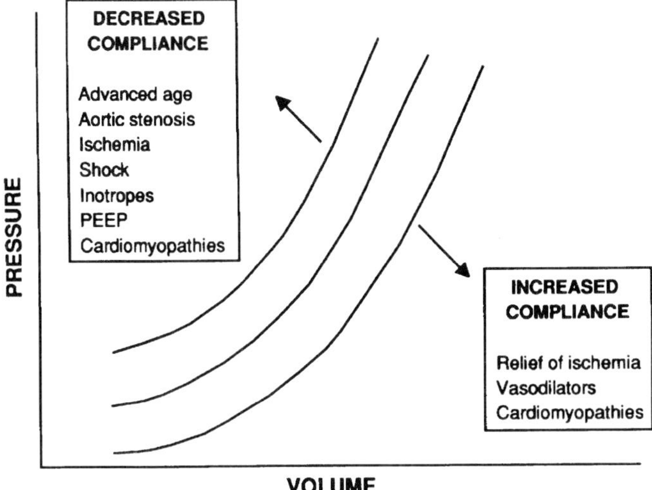

Figure 11-1 Ventricular compliance is the relation between end-diastolic pressure and volume. Increased compliance shifts the curve downward and to the right, whereas decreased compliance shifts it upward and to the left. Factors causing changes in compliance that are commonly seen in the care of geriatric patients are shown in the boxes. (*Adapted from Kaplan JA: Hemodynamic monitoring, in Kaplan JA: Cardiac Anesthesia, 2d ed. San Diego: Harcourt Brace Jovanovich, 1987.*)

Aging and the Renal System

Progressive decline of renal function with age may affect the regulation of fluid and electrolyte balance, contributing to perioperative morbidity. The changes that occur in aging kidneys are both anatomic and functional. With increasing age, renal mass and weight decrease. The number and surface area of effective glomeruli and the length of proximal tubules decrease.[6,7] Vascular changes similar to those caused by hypertension lead to an increased number of sclerotic glomeruli. These changes are particularly prominent in the renal cortex.

Glomerular filtration rate (GFR) is reduced progressively from age 30 at a rate of approximately 1 to 1.5 percent per year, falling to approximately 50 to 70 percent of the maximum value by age 80 years.[8] The decreased GFR impairs the ability of the kidneys to handle fluids and electrolytes administered in the perioperative period. The exact cause of this fall in GFR is unknown. One theory states that vascular sclerosis is responsible. Another possibility is that the reduction in GFR parallels the age-related decrease in renal blood flow, which may be a direct result of the progressive fall in cardiac output or, alternatively, may be secondary to the decrease in renal mass. The fall in renal blood flow is relatively greater in the renal cortex than in the medulla, and this may contribute to a loss of the concentrating function of the kidneys.

Although there is a decrease in creatinine clearance in the elderly, serum creatinine levels are not increased because decreased muscle mass leads to a decreased production of creatinine. Thus, renal function cannot be determined accurately by measurements of serum creatinine. Normal concentrations of serum creatinine in the elderly reflect a GFR approximately half that of younger patients, whereas elevated serum creatinine levels in the elderly indicate a severe derangement in renal function. Prerenal failure is observed more frequently in elderly than in young patients. Furthermore, age affects the prognosis of acute renal failure, which carries greater mortality in the geriatric population. Therefore, meticulous attention to fluid and electrolyte balance is necessary to prevent renal complications, especially in cardiac, aortic, and biliary tract operations, which are associated with a higher incidence of renal failure.

Changes in Body Composition with Age

The inability of the renal and thirst mechanisms to regulate the *milieu interior* in the elderly makes the aged population susceptible to altered water and electrolyte balance, which can be exaggerated by the stress of anesthesia and surgery. With aging, there is a fall in total body water that is related to a decrease in muscle mass and an increase in total body fat. The decrease in total body water is reflected mainly as a deficit within the intracellular volume.[9] There is a relative increase in the extracellular volume. Contrary to previous information that 20 to 30 percent of blood volume is lost by the age of 75 years, it is now known that blood volume is well maintained in healthy, physically active elderly persons.[10]

The exact mechanisms and factors involved in age-related alterations in electrolyte homeostasis are not well understood. Age-related changes, such as decreased basal renin activity and aldosterone secretion, occur in the renin-angiotensin-aldosterone system.[11,12] Impaired angiotensin II production, which has been noted in hypernatremic elderly patients, may be one of the mechanisms of impaired thirst.[13] A deficient thirst mechanism is generally present in the elderly and makes them highly prone to dehydration and hypernatremia.[14,15] There is a decrease in the antidiuretic hormone (ADH) response to volume stimuli but an increase in the ADH response to osmotic stimuli. Furthermore, modulation of water excretion by the kidneys in response to ADH is impaired. Inappropriate and excessive ADH release in response to stress [syndrome of inappropriate ADH release (SIADH)] is exaggerated in elderly persons and predisposes them to water intoxication.[16,17] The risk of hyponatremia is further increased in patients who are taking medications that impair water excretion or undergoing surgical procedures (e.g., transurethral prostate resection) associated with a risk of fluid overload.

The concentrating function of the kidneys is impaired, limiting the excretion and reabsorption of water, sodium, potassium, and hydrogen ions. The various mechanisms postulated for this decreased concentrating ability are (1) fall in GFR, (2) washout of medullary tonicity and impaired countercurrent mechanism caused by medullary blood flow that is relatively higher than cortical blood flow, (3) impaired sensitivity of the hypothalamic-hypophyseal-renal system, and (4) tubulointerstitial nephropathy of the elderly.[18] The propensity of geriatric patients to develop hypernatremia as well as hyponatremia severely increases perioperative morbidity.[15,19,20] Maintenance of potassium and hydrogen ion homeostasis may be impaired, increasing the risk of developing hyperkalemia and acidosis during stress.[21] Drugs such as potassium-sparing diuretics, beta-adrenergic blocking agents, and nonsteroidal anti-inflammatory drugs, because of their potential to alter potassium homeostasis, should be used with caution in the elderly.

Extravascular volume is normally regulated by the total sodium content of the body. The ability of the elderly to manage a high sodium load is limited primarily as a consequence of a progressive fall in the GFR that impairs excretion of sodium by the kidney. Similarly, there is incomplete sodium conservation in response to sodium deprivation, probably principally as a result of changes in renal hemodynamics and a diminished aldosterone response with advancing age. These factors interfere with the regulation of extravascular volume.[15,19,20]

PATHOPHYSIOLOGY OF BODY FLUIDS

Changes Secondary to Anesthesia and Surgery

The deleterious impact of the physiological changes associated with aging on fluid and electrolyte balance can be compounded by the physiological effects of anesthesia and surgery. The degree of derangement in fluid homeostasis depends on the preoperative medical condition of the patient and the type of surgery performed. Both general anesthesia and regional anesthesia are associated with vasodilatation, which results in relative hypovolemia and decreased cardiac output. In addition, general anesthetics depress myocardial contractility and sympathetic tone, further decreasing cardiac output. This may decrease renal perfusion in spite of renal afferent and efferent dilation, and decreased renal perfusion lowers GFR.[22]

Fluid requirements in the intraoperative period are also increased for other reasons, including (1) preoperative preparation, (2) dehydration from disease or impaired thirst mechanisms, (3) increased insensible skin loss, and (4) evaporative losses from the use of dry gases during artificial ventilation. Furthermore, major operations (e.g., abdominal and thoracic procedures) may cause significant evaporative loss from exposed surfaces, fluid redistribution, and blood loss.

Extensive tissue destruction from surgical trauma causes both localized and generalized edema, accumulation of fluid in the lumen and walls of the gut, and formation of ascites and pleural effusions in predisposed patients.[23] The obligatory expansion of the extracellular and in some cases intracellular spaces, commonly referred to as acute sequestered edema or the "third space," is manifested as salt and water retention in response to severe trauma.[24,25] The exact anatomic location of the third space has not been determined. The electrolyte composition and tonicity of the third space are similar to those of plasma. The third space results in a nonfunctional appendage of the interstitial fluid compartment that is relatively unavailable for mobilization into the vascular compartment. The transfer of functional extracellular fluid into the third space results in an extracellular fluid deficit, which is the most commonly observed disturbance of fluid and electrolytes in surgical patients.[26] The degree of third space loss varies considerably in proportion to the severity of the surgical trauma. This sequestered fluid is eventually returned to the vascular compartment 48 to 72 h after surgery. Because of inadequate cardiac reserve and renal function, redistribution of the sequestered fluid into the vascular compartment in the postoperative period may result in fluid overload in a geriatric patient.

Decreased intravascular volume, surgery, and anesthesia all increase concentrations of ADH, renin, aldosterone, adrenocorticotropic hormone (ACTH), and catecholamines.[27] Furthermore, ADH may indirectly increase the release of ACTH and aldosterone. These hormonal changes and the decreased GFR contribute to sodium and water retention, as well as potassium excretion, in the perioperative period. Therefore, geriatric patients, who often also take diuretics, may develop either hypokalemia or hyperkalemia, the latter of which has already been discussed.

Electrolyte Disturbances

Disturbances of electrolyte concentrations in the perioperative period can affect cerebral, neuromuscular, respiratory, and cardiac function. Drugs used during anesthesia, the stress of anesthesia and surgery, and perioperative fluid shifts influence the concentrations of various electrolytes. Abnormalities in electrolyte homeostasis in the elderly are commonly due to age-related pathophysiological mechanisms.

Sodium

Sodium is the predominant extracellular cation. Abnormal plasma sodium concentrations may occur as a result of either abnormal whole body sodium or total body water content. Hyponatremia can be caused by loss of sodium (e.g., renal, gastrointestinal, skin losses), excessive water intake, or retention of water (e.g., SIADH, renal disease, congestive heart failure, cirrhosis), and these cases are associated with low serum osmolality. In contrast, redistribution of water as a result of hyperglycemia or mannitol infusion causes hyponatremia, which is associated with high serum osmolality. Pseudohyponatremia is a different phenomenon that is characterized by a falsely decreased measurement of serum sodium concentration in the presence of hyperlipidemia and/or hyperproteinemia. This generally occurs in the presence of a normal serum osmolality.

Hyponatremia and water intoxication are particularly common in geriatric patients.[16,17] Reduction of the serum sodium concentration causes osmotically induced cellular edema. Cerebral edema increases intracranial pressure and may cause anoxic encephalopathy associated with changes in mental status, respiratory depression, and seizures. Rapid restoration of serum sodium levels may cause devastating delayed demyelinating brain lesions such as central pontine myelinolysis.[28] The clinical syndrome of central pontine myelinolysis includes quadriplegia with dysarthria, dysphagia, varying levels of consciousness, and the "locked-in" syndrome. The delayed neurological deterioration that may follow correction of hyponatremia has been described as "osmotic demyelination syndrome."[29] In one study, rapid correction of symptomatic hyponatremia to the mildly hyponatremic range did not result in clinical or anatomic evidence of neurological damage.[30] It is not known whether the neurological damage is caused by hyponatremia itself or by its rapid correction.[31]

Hypernatremia may be due to excessive sodium administration, inadequate water intake, or excessive water loss. It is associated with high serum osmolality and a relative or absolute water deficit that causes cellular dehydration. The clinical features of high serum sodium include increased thirst, weakness, lethargy, irritability, seizures, cerebral hemorrhage, hypovolemia, hypotension, and polyuria. Hypernatremia can be severe in the elderly because compensatory mechanisms such as an increase in thirst are deficient in this age group.

Lithium

Lithium ion (from exogenously administered lithium carbonate for the treatment of manic-depressive illnesses) mimics sodium ion and enters the cell during excitation. However, it depresses the excitability of the cell and may potentiate neuromuscular blockade because it is removed slowly from the cell. In addition, increased lithium levels may cause other electrolyte abnormalities, such as hypermagnesemia.

Potassium

Potassium is a vital ion at the cellular level and is regulated more tightly than any other ion. Potassium is predominantly located intracellularly, and therefore plasma concentration is a poor reflection of total body stores. Total body potassium is regulated primarily by the kidneys via aldosterone. Uptake of potassium by the cells influences extracellular concentration and is affected by insulin, sympathetic activity, and H^+ ion concentration. Even minor changes in the extracellular potassium concentration may have lethal consequences. Changes in the ratio of intracellular to extracellular concentrations are more important than the extracellular potassium concentration itself with respect to cell excitability.

Hypokalemia may alter the electrical activity of the heart, increasing susceptibility to arrhythmias, particularly in patients on digitalis. Skeletal muscle weakness may occur, potentiating the action of muscle relaxants. Gastric emptying is delayed. Hypokalemia depresses the compensatory mechanisms after the Valsalva maneuver.[32] By accentuating the autonomic nervous system dysfunction caused by aging, hypokalemia may increase the incidence of postural and perioperative hypotension. Loss of potassium as a result of either vomiting and diarrhea or renal excretion is the leading cause of hypokalemia. Patients receiving diuretics, $beta_2$-adrenergic agonists, xanthines, and steroids are highly prone to hypokalemia.

Hyperkalemia can be caused by renal failure or caused iatrogenically by intravenous fluids containing potassium, rapid massive transfusion of old blood, or drugs such as angiotensin-converting enzyme inhibitors and succinylcholine. Hyperkalemia decreases the excitability of the myocardium, causing impairment of the conduction system or asystole. It may also cause skeletal muscle weakness and increased insulin secretion.

Magnesium

Magnesium, a principal intracellular cation, is an important cofactor for several enzymatic reactions. Serum electrolyte studies in the elderly should routinely include the determination of magnesium levels. Depletion of magnesium may be associated with cardiac arrhythmias, digitalis toxicity, congestive cardiac failure, and hypertension. Hypomagnesemia commonly results from gastrointestinal or renal abnormalities. Gastrointestinal causes include decreased gastrointestinal intake, nasogastric suction, malabsorption, and diarrhea. Renal causes include diuretics, hereditary renal wasting, and postobstructive diuresis. Miscellaneous causes include antibiotics and alcoholism. Hypomagnesemia may exacerbate electrolyte abnormalities such as hyponatremia, hypokalemia, hypocalcemia, and hypophosphatemia. Potassium and magnesium are closely linked at the cellular level, and refractory potassium repletion may occur as a result of hypomagnesemia.[33] Hypomagnesemia, a frequent finding after cardiopulmonary bypass, predisposes the patient to ventricular arrhythmias and cardiac insufficiency; prophylactic magnesium administration decreases the incidence of arrhythmias and improves stroke volume and cardiac index after a postbypass.[34] Magnesium may also be useful therapeutically in response to postbypass arrhythmias and poor cardiac function when given either empirically or in response to a demonstrated decrease in serum magnesium.

Hypermagnesemia is commonly iatrogenic secondary to the administration of magnesium-containing preparations such as antacids, enemas, and intravenous infusions, especially in patients with renal dysfunction. Hypothyroidism, Addison's disease, lithium intoxication, and metabolic acidosis are rare causes of increased magnesium levels. Hypermagnesemia causes suppression of membrane excitability, resulting in muscle weakness. Other clinical manifestations include hypotension, heart block, and cardiac arrest.

Calcium

Calcium is a major intracellular messenger and is essential in muscle excitation-contraction coupling, cardiac automaticity, neuronal conduction, synaptic transmission, blood coagulation, hormone secretion, and enzyme function. Ionized calcium is the physiologically active form, and its deficiency causes increased neuromuscular irritability (e.g., seizures, tetany, laryngospasm), decreased myocardial performance (e.g., ventricular dysfunction, hypotension), and cardiac arrhythmias (e.g., digitalis insensitivity, bradycardia, prolonged S-T interval, cardiac arrest).

Hypocalcemia can occur as a result of alkalemia, chelation by citrate from blood transfusion, renal failure, hypomagnesemia, hyperphosphatemia, vitamin D and parathormone deficiency, acute pancreatitis, sepsis, and anticonvulsant therapy. Alkemia from hyperventilation during controlled ventilation is a common iatrogenic cause. Symptomatic hypocalcemia requires immediate treatment; however, the underlying cause of hypocalcemia should be identified. Measurement of serum magnesium and phosphate levels is important in patients with ionized hypocalcemia.

Hypercalcemia is caused by increased bone resorption (e.g., malignancy, sarcoidosis, tuberculosis, immobilization), vitamin D intoxication, hyperparathyroidism, adrenal insufficiency, renal failure, and drugs (e.g., thiazides, lithium, milk-alkali syndrome). The clinical sequelae of hypercalcemia include muscle weakness, renal failure (e.g., diminished glomerular function and urine-concentrating ability), and cardiovascular dysfunction (e.g., hypertension, arrhythmias).

Phosphate

Phosphate is primarily located intracellularly and is necessary for the production of cellular energy from adenosine triphosphate (ATP) and the production of 2,3-diphosphoglycerate (DPG) within red blood cells. Hypophosphatemia leads to muscle weakness, respiratory failure and inability to be weaned from mechanical ventilatory support, congestive cardiomyopathy, impaired glucose tolerance, and neurological effects (e.g., ataxia, confusion, paresthesias, seizures). Hypophosphatemia is caused by carbohydrate loading, diuretics, alkalosis, renal and gastrointestinal losses, and alcoholism. Treatment consists of correction of the underlying cause and phosphate administration.

Hyperphosphatemia may be caused by excessive intake, decreased renal excretion, parathyroid hormone deficiency, rhabdomyolysis, or cytotoxic chemotherapy for leukemia. The clinical effects of hyperphosphatemia are due to calcium and phosphate precipitation causing hypocalcemia.

Chloride

Chloride is the predominant extracellular anion. The kidneys play an important role in the maintenance of normal chloride levels. Bicarbonate secretion by the kidneys is regulated by the chloride-bicarbonate exchanger in the distal nephron.[35,36] Hypochloremia results from vomiting, gastric aspiration, diuretics, and incomplete or delayed recovery from hypercapnic acidosis. Chloride depletion most commonly leads to metabolic alkalosis and hypokalemia. Chloride depletion is invariably associated with volume contraction that stimulates aldosterone secretion, increasing renal losses of hydrogen and potassium.[36] Chloride can be supplemented as sodium chloride, potassium chloride, or ammonium chloride.

Hyperchloremia leading to metabolic acidosis is usually caused by renal dysfunction that results in loss of bicarbonate. Measurement of serum chloride is valuable in assessing metabolic acidosis with both a normal and an increased anion gap. Urine chloride levels aid in the diagnosis of metabolic alkalosis and hyperchloremic metabolic acidosis.[35]

PERIOPERATIVE FLUID REPLACEMENT

The Requirement for and Sequelae of Fluid Therapy

The purpose of intraoperative fluid administration is maintenance of homeostasis, including intravascular volume, cardiac preload, cardiac output, and tissue perfusion. These goals can be difficult in a geriatric patient, who commonly undergoes complex, stressful procedures while simultaneously presenting with compensatory mechanisms that are impaired by normal physiological aging and concurrent illnesses. For example, fluid must be titrated to avoid both inadequate intravascular volume and fluid overload, each of which may compromise cardiac performance and perfusion of tissues. The underlying pathological condition in specific pertinent organ systems, including the pulmonary, cardiac, vascular, renal, hepatic, and hematologic systems, in addition to the patient's overall function and nutritional status, must be carefully considered. The clinician must also be aware of the direct consequences of surgery and anesthesia, as discussed earlier in this chapter.

One consequence of surgical trauma potentially exacerbated by inappropriate or overzealous fluid administration is tissue edema. The relative merits of colloid versus crystalloid solutions in modifying this response have been widely debated. Although a natural result of tissue trauma, the impact of generalized edema on the patient may be deleterious.[37] Traumatic cerebral edema can be worsened and the outcome can be adversely affected by hydration with crystalloid solutions.[38] Pulmonary edema can develop or be worsened secondary to excessive fluid administration, although the choice of colloid over crystalloid solutions has no impact at normal hydrostatic pressures,[39] probably secondary to effective lymphatic drainage and the extravascular diffusion of osmotically active molecules.[40] Also, perioperative increases in extravascular lung water (EVLW) may actually be unrelated to detrimental changes in oxygenation, and increased EVLW can resolve in spite of persistently increased intrathoracic blood volume and pulmonary blood volume, as demonstrated after bypass in cardiac surgical patients.[41] Aggressive crystalloid hydration resulting in extreme normovolemic hemodilution has been shown to decrease thoracic compliance.[42] Gastrointestinal tract edema can cause ileus, inadequate enteric alimentation, systemic translocation of bacteria, sepsis, and multiorgan failure.[43,44] Generalized edema can increase the duration of ventilator dependence and prolong intensive care unit (ICU) stay.[37] While adequate crystalloid therapy is required for good renal function and may in fact be more advantageous than colloid,[45] excessive fluids can result in the need for diuretics or even dialysis.[37] Clearly, careful volume repletion with an appropriate fluid plays a crucial role in the perioperative management of geriatric patients.

Specific Fluids: Indications, Contraindications, Benefits, Risks, Complications

Crystalloids

A confusing array of fluids are available, generally classified into two groups: crystalloids and colloids. Crystalloids, also commonly referred to as balanced salt solutions, contain dissolved crystalline solids. Colloidal suspensions contain larger particles that nevertheless are too small to form a sediment secondary to gravitational forces. In the presence of a semipermeable membrane such as a capillary membrane, colloids exert oncotic pressure. Crystalloid infusion augments the entire extracellular space, whereas colloid expands the intravascular space in the absence of increased vascular permeability. Commonly utilized crystalloid and colloid solutions and their components are outlined in Tables 11-1 and 11-2.

In reality, there is little practical difference between the various isotonic crystalloid solutions, especially in the absence of electrolyte abnormalities. The essential caveat remains the infusion of sufficient quantities of fluid to replete the extracellular space and support organ function. Some nuances can arise. For example, excessive amounts of normal saline may generate a hyperchloremic-induced metabolic acidosis,[46] a condition worsened by aldosterone secretion in the presence of hypovolemia. By contrast, metabolic alkalosis may occur from Plasma-Lyte (Baxter Healthcare Corp., Deerfield, IL 60015) or Normosol (Abbott Laboratories, Abbott Park, IL 60064) secondary to hepatic metabolism of lactate, acetate, or gluconate. Nevertheless, in most clinical circumstances, the decisions involving isotonic crystalloids are quantitative rather than qualitative.

Isotonic fluids are often categorized as replacement fluids, which are used primarily to correct a loss or sequestration of body fluids. Hypotonic fluids such as 5% dextrose in water (D_5W) are often categorized as maintenance fluids and are used to replace free water loss. A consequence of excessive use of hypotonic fluid intraoperatively is severe and potentially life-threatening hy-

Table 11-1 Commonly used parenteral fluids

- Crystalloids
  - Maintenance crystalloids
    - 5% dextrose in water (D_5W)
    - D_5 0.45% normal saline
  - Replacement crystalloids
    - 0.9% sodium chloride
    - D_5 0.9% sodium chloride
    - Lactated Ringer's
    - D_5 lactated Ringer's
    - Plasma-Lyte
    - Normosol-R
  - Special purpose
    - 5% sodium chloride
- Colloids
  - Albumin (5% and 25%)
  - Plasma protein fraction
  - Hydroxyethyl starch
  - Pentastarch
  - Dextran (40 and 70 molecular weight)
  - Fresh whole blood
  - Packed red blood cells
  - Fresh frozen plasma
  - Platelets
  - Cryoprecipitate
  - Factor concentrate

Table 11-2 Composition of parenteral fluids

	Na^+, mEq/L	K^+, mEq/L	Cl^-, mEq/L	Ca^{2+}, mEq/L	Mg, mEq/L	Lactate, mEq/L	Gluconate, mEq/L	Acetate, mEq/L	Osmolality, mOsm/L	CHO, g/L	Protein, g/L
Extracellular fluid	142	4	103	5	3	5	0	0	280–310	90–110	0
0.9% sodium chloride	154	0	154	0	0	0	0	0	308	0	0
D5W	0	0	0	0	0	0	0	0	253	50	0
D5 0.9% sodium chloride	154	0	154	0	0	0	0	0	407	50	0
Lactated Ringer's	130	4	109	3	0	28	0	0	278	0	0
Plasma-Lyte	140	5	98	0	3	0	23	27	312	0	0
Normosol-R	140	5	98	0	3	0	23	27	295	0	0
Albumin	130–160	≤1	100	0	0	0	0	0	270–300	0	50
Plasma protein fraction (contains <15 mmol/L sodium citrate)	130–160	.025	100	0	0	0	0	0	270–300	0	50
Hydroxyethyl starch	154	0	154	0	0	0	0	0	310	0	0
Dextran 70	150	0	150	0	0	0	0	0	300	0	0

ponatremia.[46] As was mentioned above, hyponatremia and water intoxication are common in geriatric patients,[16] particularly perioperatively in the face of their characteristically exaggerated release of ADH and aldosterone in response to surgical stress.[17] Additionally, geriatric patients are predisposed to hyperglycemia and hyperosmolar nonketotic coma caused by aberrations in glucose homeostasis, including an increased renal threshold for glucose.[16] Glucose-containing solutions result in a poor tolerance to cerebral ischemia and a worsened neurological outcome.[47] The only indication for glucose infusion, with possible rare exceptions (e.g., acute intermittent porphyria), is in the care of a diabetic patient,[48] and D_5W in limited doses (50 to 125 ml/kg per hour) is commonly employed in diabetic patients in concert with close monitoring of serum glucose. Otherwise, given the adverse sequelae from hypotonic fluid infusion, as well as a propensity for predominantly isotonic fluid losses, isotonic fluids without glucose are the usual choice intraoperatively. Special-purpose fluids such as hypertonic saline, which is sometimes utilized for rapid resuscitation of trauma or burn victims, are also available.

Colloids

The ideal characteristics of a preferred colloidal agent include (1) maintenance of circulatory volume and a salutary effect on tissue edema via intravascular oncotic forces, (2) absence of extravascular leakage, (3) lack of side effects, and (4) reasonable cost. Table 11-3 delineates some of the purported advantages and disadvantages of colloid versus crystalloid resuscitation. Table 11-4 delineates some of the advantages, disadvantages, indications, and other pertinent information regarding various colloidal solutions. The use of these fluids is controversial. Nevertheless, they are efficient volume expanders. The usual intravascular half-life of exogenously delivered albumin is 16 h, although this may be reduced to 2

Table 11-3 Colloid versus crystalloid resuscitation: Reported advantages and disadvantages

Solution	Advantages	Disadvantages
Colloid	Smaller volume required Sustained plasma volume increase Less peripheral edema Lower intracranial pressure	Expensive Coagulopathy (dextran > HES) Impaired cross-match (dextran) Vasodilation (PPF) Pulmonary edema
Crystalloid	Inexpensive Promotes urinary flow Restores third space losses	Worsened cerebral edema Pulmonary edema Decreased chest wall compliance Peripheral edema Gastrointestinal tract dysfunction Prolonged ventilator dependence and ICU stay Transient hemodynamic effects

Table 11-4 Characteristics of various colloidal solutions

Colloid solution	Advantages	Disadvantages	Indications	Expiration	Comments
Stored whole blood ACD (adenine-citrate-phosphate)	Apparently physiological	Hepatitis, hemolytic reaction risk, high cost, low availability, requires type and cross-match, high K, low Ca, low platelets	Anemia, hemorrhage, shock, blood dyscrasias	21 days	Na = 140 mEq/L, protein 5% (5 g/100 ml)
Stored whole blood CPDA (citrate-phosphate-dextrose-adenine)	Apparently physiological	Same	Same	Can be stored up to 35 days	Contains 125% of usual concentration of glucose, adenine
Fresh whole blood	Most physiological; normal pH, electrolytes	Same as whole blood, except clotting factors normal	(?) Bleeding due to thrombocytopenia	Up to 2–3 days for platelet survival	Not easily available; given to increase platelets and clotting factors
Packed red blood cells (CPD or CPDA stored)	Permits component therapy more economically than whole blood	Same as whole blood; increased viscosity	Anemias where increased Hb level required	Up to 35 days	Na = 140 mEq/L, protein 2% (2 g/100 ml); advised for patients with heart disease, chronic and severe anemia, severe sepsis, toxemia, very old patients
Fresh frozen plasma	Contains coagulation factors	Hepatitis; high cost; requires cross-matching	Hemophilia	Used immediately after thawing	Na = 130, protein 5% (5 g/100 ml); should be administered through 170 μ filter
Human serum albumin 5%, 25%	No hepatitis, apparently physiological	High cost; in short supply	Hypoalbuminemia	Should be administered within 4 h after starting infusion	Na = 130, protein 5% (5 g/100 ml), 25% (25 g/100 ml); heat-treated, therefore no risk of hepatitis

Plasma protein fraction (Plasmanate)	No hepatitis	If given rapidly, chance of hypotension; rarely allergic reactions	Hypoalbuminemia	2 years	Na = 130, protein 5% (5 g/100 ml); hepatitis virus inactivated by 6-h pasteurization
Hydroxyethyl starch (HES) 6%, molecular weight 10,000–1,000,000	Volume expander	HES said to have few side reactions or antigenic properties	Volume expansion	Should be administered within 24 h after starting infusion	Intravascular half-life 6 h; synthetic polymer prepared from amylopectin by introduction of hydroxyethyl group in glucose residue
Dextran 70 (Macrodex), dextran 6%/0.9% NaCl, molecular weight 70,000–75,000	Inexpensive, long shelf-life; effective volume expander; no hepatitis	Interferes with typing and cross-matching; anti-platelet and antithrombic activity, therefore produces increased bleeding; prolonged storage causes some precipitation; can cause allergic phenomenon	??	10 years	Na = 150; intravenous half-life 6 h; type and cross-match patient's blood before infusing dextran; produced by Leuconostoc mesenteroides bacteria on agar sucrose plates
Dextran 40 (Rheomacrodex), dextran 10%/0.9% NaCl, molecular weight 40,000	Same; because of low molecular weight, easy flow in micro-circulation	Same; severe allergic reactions to antidextran antibodies; plugs renal tubules in shock and oligemia	?	Same	Intravenous half-life 2 h

to 4 h in pathological conditions of increased vascular permeability.[49] Hetastarch [hydroxyethyl starch (HES)] has similar volume expansion properties,[49] and the effect of HES as a volume expander persists from 3 to 24 h after infusion.[50]

Albumin, prepared from healthy human donors and heat-treated to inactive viruses, is available in 5% and 25% (salt-poor) concentrations. Since the latter is more expensive, it is ideally reserved for patients with a contracted intravascular space but an expanded interstitial volume, such as burn patients and postoperative patients. Purified protein fraction (PPF), which is composed of 80% albumin, with the remainder being alpha-, beta-, and gamma-globulins, has a vasodilatory effect, possibly secondary to prekallikrein activators, and therefore is less widely used.

HES, available as a 6% solution in normal saline, is a heterogeneous class of synthetic molecules similar to glycogen with molecular weights ranging from 10,000 to over 1 million. The kinetics of HES are complex; smaller molecules are eliminated via the kidney, while larger particles are metabolized in blood and tissues, including the reticuloendothelial system (RES). Although HES particles are retained for long periods (up to 17 weeks) in the liver, there are no known significant sequelae.[51] Manufacturer's dosing guidelines suggest an upper infusion limit of 20 ml/kg per day, but these doses have been exceeded without an adverse effect on the renal, hepatic, pulmonary, and immune systems.[51,52]

Pentastarch, a lower-molecular-weight hydroxyethyl starch, and its derivative, pentafraction, which is obtained by filtering and removing smaller molecules, may have certain advantages, including (1) more significant volume expansion,[53] (2) more effective degradation and elimination,[54] and (3) less of an effect on coagulation parameters.[55] The absence of smaller molecules decreases interstitial swelling and edema,[56] while the lack of large molecules reduces interference with coagulation.[55] Pentafraction is retained more avidly in the intravascular space, being reflected back from the interstitial compartment. Studies show that pentafraction has a sealant property, collecting at the capillary basement membrane and increasing the capillary barrier to the loss of smaller molecules, thus retaining and recruiting albumin molecules that would otherwise be lost to the interstitium.[57–59]

As of October 1994, only pentastarch has been approved for clinical use, being employed for leukapheresis. These fluids may be utilized more widely in the future as volume expanders.

Dextrans, which are colloidal suspensions of glucose polymers, have potent volume expansion properties. Dextran 70, with an average molecular weight of 70,000, is usually preferred to dextran 40, with an average molecular weight of 40,000, because of its slower excretion. As a result of adverse reactions, including anaphylactic and anaphylactoid responses, induction of hemostatic defects mediated through factor VIII, and interference with cross-matching of blood,[51] dextrans are rarely employed for volume repletion. More commonly, they are used in clinical situations where the maintenance of favorable microvascular rheology or the patency of a critical vascular anastomosis is crucial.

As was noted above, complications can occur with the use of colloids. Anaphylaxis to albumin infusion is rare, involving less than 0.011 percent of patients, and is not significantly greater with the use of HES, which has an incidence of anaphylaxis of 0.085 percent.[60] The effect of colloids on coagulation is a matter for concern. The impact of albumin is probably dilutional. However, changes in coagulation caused by HES appear to consist of more than simple dilution, and an increase in activated partial thromboplastin time, a decrease in factor VIII activity, and a decrease in both platelet count and adhesion have been described.[61,62] Nevertheless, when HES is given within recommended dosing guidelines, studies have not documented increased clinical bleeding in a variety of patient populations.[63–65] Even a larger than recommended dose of 3600 ml of HES over 24 h in trauma patients failed to create evidence of systemic coagulopathy.[52] HES has been shown to aggravate von Willebrand's disease.[66] In general, it would seem most prudent to avoid HES in patients with preexisting alterations involving hemostatic mechanisms.

Colloid versus Crystalloid Controversy

There is an ongoing, largely unresolved difference of opinion among practitioners regarding the appropriate choice between colloids and crystalloids. Clearly, tissue trauma of a significant degree results in an obligatory expansion of the extracellular volume[24] and potentially of the intracellular volume,[25] which dictates the necessity for the infusion of isotonic crystalloids. The advantages of the additional use of colloid in the resuscitation of patients continues to be debated. Evidence does not show an advantage pertaining to lung function or interstitial lung water accumulation with colloids compared with crystalloids; however, soft tissue edema may be limited by colloid resuscitation.[67] Although there is evidence that crystalloid infusion may be advantageous in preserving renal function,[45] Davidson and colleagues have demonstrated improved renal transplant survival when albumin is given intraoperatively.[68] Moss and Gould reviewed evidence comparing colloid and crystalloid resuscitation in shock states and found no benefit from the addition of colloid.[69] A metaanalysis of mortality incorporating data from numerous studies found a preference for crystalloid in the care of trauma patients, whereas mortality decreased with the use of colloid in nontrauma patients.[70]

In summary, it can be stated that there are no definitive scientific or consensus criteria for colloid therapy, and that the decision to infuse colloid continues to be a matter of individual clinical judgment and regional standards. A reasonable recommendation would be to give colloid when significant volumes of crystalloid fail to support hemodynamics or when the colloid oncotic pressure or serum protein level is less than 30 percent of normal.[71] Either HES in recommended doses or albumin would be appropriate in these situations.

One important consideration is the avoidance of hypervolemia with colloids, because unlike crystalloids, these fluids are not eliminated by simple diuresis or even dialysis. Colloids should be used cautiously with careful observation and clinical monitoring in the geriatric population because of limitations in cardiovascular compliance and reserve. In addition, the infusion of inordinate amounts of hemoglobin-free colloid may make the subsequent infusion of red cells difficult or even impossible without inducing volume overload, resulting in an anemia that is iatrogenic and difficult to treat. For example, after separating from cardiopulmonary bypass, colloids are sometimes used to rapidly expand the intravascular volume, since hypovolemia is a common cause of postbypass hypotension. Nevertheless, overzealous use of colloids can make the subsequent infusion of pump prime, which contains red cells, difficult. Therefore, some interim reliance on crystalloid solutions, in addition to judicious quantities of colloids, is advisable in such a situation.

Red Blood Cell Products and Transfusion

Although strictly speaking blood products other than albumin and protein fraction are colloidal, they are discussed separately here because they are used for different purposes. For example, the sole purpose for providing red blood cells is to increase the oxygen-carrying capacity of the patient's blood (Table 11-5). Transfusion of blood products entails an analysis of benefit versus risk and potential complications (Table 11-6). In essence, surgical trauma, hemorrhage, and appropriate resuscitation can be viewed as a dynamic hemodilution in which normovolemia is maintained and the patient's hematocrit then becomes a reasonable guide for transfusion.[72] A commonly used "transfusion trigger" is a hematocrit of 25 percent. However, the point of optimal oxygen delivery and tissue demand for oxygen, on the basis of theoretical considerations of rheological principles and cardiovascular work, respectively, occurs near a hematocrit of 30 percent (Fig. 11-2). A hematocrit even higher than this may be a reasonable goal in geriatric patients,[46] particularly patients with coexisting disease (e.g., cardiovascular or cerebrovascular disease, liver or kidney impairment, or other problems). Clearly, the decision to transfuse should be individualized and based on consideration of the patient's pathophysiology (Table 11-7). The short-term benefit of an increased oxygen-carrying capacity must be weighed against the risks of both immediate and long-term complications of transfusion. An illustration in a geriatric patient is the anticipated

Table 11-5 Oxygen delivery and blood oxygen content

$D_{O2} = Q \times Ca_{O2} \times 10$

$Ca_{O2} = Hgb \times 1.39 \times Sat + Pa_{O2} \times 0.003$

where:
- D_{O2} = oxygen delivery (ml/min/m^2)
- Q = cardiac index (L/min/m^2)
- Ca_{O2} = oxygen content of arterial blood (ml/dl)
- 10 = dl/L
- Hgb = hemoglobin (g/dl)
- 1.39 = oxygen bound to hemoglobin (ml/g)
- Sat = percent saturation of hemoglobin with oxygen
- Pa_{O2} = arterial partial pressure of oxygen (mmHg)
- 0.003 = dissolved oxygen (ml/mmHg)

Table 11-6 Complications of homologous blood transfusion

Transfusion reactions
Allergic reactions
Febrile reactions
Acute hemolytic reactions
Delayed hemolytic reactions
Metabolic abnormalities
Metabolic alkalosis
Hyperkalemia/hypokalemia
Decreased 2,3-diphosphoglycerate
Citrate intoxication/hypocalcemia
Transmission of infectious diseases
Hepatitis C (non-A, non-B hepatitis)
Hepatitis B
Cytomegalovirus
Epstein-Barr virus
Human immunodeficiency virus
Human T cell leukemia virus type 1
Microaggregate infusion
Posttransfusion pulmonary dysfunction
Immunosuppression
Graft versus host disease

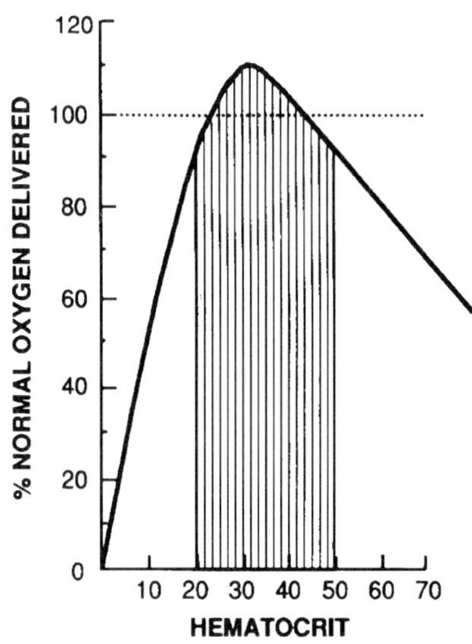

Figure 11-2 Oxygen transport varies with hematocrit level. Maximum oxygen delivery is at a hematocrit of 30 percent. "Normal" oxygen delivery relates here to oxygen delivered at a hematocrit of 45 percent. (*From LeVeen HH, Ip M, Ahmed N, et al: Lowering blood viscosity to overcome vascular resistance. Surg Gynecol Obstet 150:139–149, 1980. By permission of Surgery, Gynecology & Obstetrics.*)

Table 11-7 Patient groups at risk from anemia and/or hypovolemia

Coronary artery disease
Valvular heart disease (e.g., hemodynamically significant aortic stenosis)
Congestive heart failure
Patients at risk for cerebral ischemia
History of transient ischemic attacks
Previous thrombotic stroke
Liver/kidney disease

survival of the patient. For example, in dealing with the very old (over 85 years), it seems reasonable to transfuse to a higher hematocrit because of the limited life expectancy of these patients. Nevertheless, the limited ability of geriatric patients to compensate for anemia remains the paramount consideration.

Physiological adaptation to anemia involves two principal mechanisms (Table 11-8): (1) increased oxygen release from hemoglobin and (2) increased cardiac output. The latter is due primarily to increased stroke volume occurring secondary to increased contractility, decreased afterload, or both. The decrease in afterload occurs secondary to decreased blood viscosity and vasodilation. Vasodilation is mediated in peripheral tissues vis-à-vis local factors such as hypoxia, lactic acid, and nitric oxide.[73] If decreased ventricular function exists, an increased heart rate predominates as a compensatory mechanism. In contrast, normovolemic patients with good ventricular function do not increase their heart rate, except at more extreme levels of hemodilution. As a result of an inability to mount a cardiovascular response, whether because of normal physiological aging or a specific pathology (e.g., secondary to ischemic cardiomyopathy or aortic stenosis), advanced age is a factor that limits adaptation to anemia.

Transfusion of patients with mild anemia (hemoglobin 8–10 g/dl) may not alter myocardial oxygen demand,[74] since compensation is largely passive as a

Table 11-8 Adaptations to anemia

Increased oxygen release from hemoglobin
Increased oxygen extraction
Shift of oxyhemoglobin dissociation curve (decreased oxygen affinity) secondary to
Increased levels of 2,3-diphosphoglycerate
Bohr effect
Increased cardiac output
Decreased afterload secondary to
Vasodilation
Diminished blood viscosity
Increased contractility
Tachycardia

result of afterload reduction. Because blood viscosity bears a curvilinear relation to hematocrit (Fig. 11-3), even moderate hemodilution (hemoglobin less than 8–10 g/dl) may improve oxygen delivery in tissues, including those serviced by diseased vessels.[75,76] Patients with normal coronary patency uniformly respond to anemia with increased coronary blood flow, a crucial adaptation because of the high oxygen extraction ratio of the resting heart. Coronary artery disease can impede this increased flow. For example, one study of patients after peripheral vascular surgery demonstrated a significantly increased incidence of myocardial ischemia and cardiac morbidity in the presence of a hematocrit below 28 percent.[77] This represents a subpopulation of patients with a high probability of significant coronary artery disease who are likely to respond adversely to anemia.

One model of coronary insufficiency demonstrated tolerance of extreme hemodilution in normal controls, whereas subjects with an exhausted vasodilatory reserve capacity presented with decreased myocardial oxygenation and abnormal contractility in the presence of only moderate hemodilution (hemoglobin less than 8–10 g/dl).[78] Moderate hemodilution adversely affects myocardial work and oxygen demand. Although a given patient may be capable of increased ventricular contractility or heart rate in response to moderate anemia, this response may be undesirable in patients with coronary disease. Therefore, while some elderly patients, whether as a result of normal aging, deconditioning, or coexisting disease, cannot mount a compensatory response to anemia, others are simply unable to tolerate such a response, which manifests as increased myocardial contractility, heart rate, and myocardial oxygen demand, without developing ischemia.[74]

Another scenario pertains to a patient with active ischemia, in whom transfusion may both increase myocardial oxygen demand and decrease oxygen supply, the latter secondary to pulmonary edema. In addition, increased blood

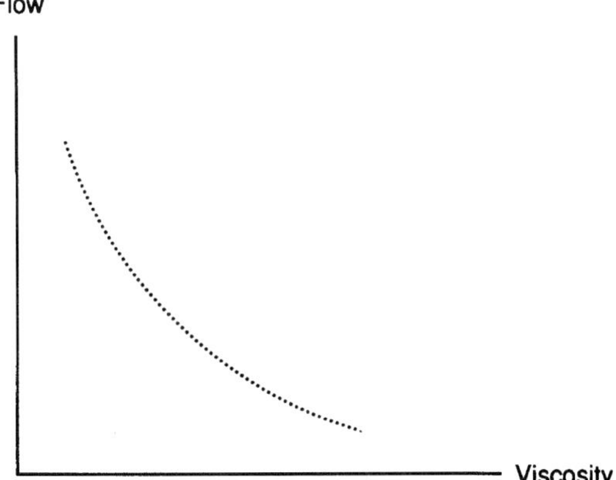

Figure 11-3 Blood flow varies in a nonlinear fashion with viscosity and increases with decreasing viscosity.

viscosity from a transfusion can further impair coronary microcirculatory flow and oxygen delivery. Such a case requires its own risk-benefit analysis with reference to the advisability of further transfusions to treat anemia.[79]

Other organ systems must be considered in the analysis, particularly in light of the depressant effects of anesthetics on cardiac function and specific organ perfusion. For example, one model of hemodilution in anesthetized subjects demonstrated adverse effects on hepatic perfusion, oxygenation, and function.[80] These results would logically have an impact on the care of a patient with hepatic cirrhosis in light of the deleterious effects of this disease process on hepatocellular oxygenation. Similar concepts may apply to coexisting renal pathology and avoidance of acute renal failure or the hepatorenal syndrome.

Numerous strategies exist to minimize homologous red cell transfusion (Table 11-9). The clinician should avoid unnecessary transfusion and recognize that transfusion of a single unit may suffice. Surgical hemostasis is obviously necessary. Significant iatrogenic anemia can be created via phlebotomy generated by unnecessary laboratory testing. The average ICU patient in one study lost 43.6 ml of blood per day as a result of laboratory testing.[81]

Because of the reduction in compensatory mechanisms and the risks inherent in decreasing perfusion and oxygen-carrying capacity simultaneously, deliberate hypotension has limited application within this age group. Supplemental oxygen therapy, by contrast, can be useful in improving oxygen delivery to tissues in anemic patients.

Antifibrinolytics are playing an expanding role, particularly in cardiac surgery, where ε-aminocaproic acid is being used successfully. Aprotinin, a serine pro-

Table 11-9 Ways to reduce homologous red cell transfusion

Ways to reduce homologous red cell transfusion
Single-unit transfusion
Meticulous surgical hemostasis
Avoidance of unnecessary phlebotomy and laboratory testing
Deliberate hypotension
Antifibrinolytics
Aprotinin
ε-aminocaproic acid
Tranexamic acid
Desmopressin
Use of supplemental oxygen therapy (increased oxygen content of blood)
Autologous blood transfusion
Preoperative collection and storage
Acute perioperative normovolemic hemodilution
Perioperative scavenging
External hemoconcentration
Recombinant human erythropoietin
Blood substitutes (investigational)

tease inhibitor used worldwide, is being investigated actively in this country.[82,83] Desmopressin, a vasopressin analogue that stimulates factor VIII–related activity, after an initial wave of enthusiasm,[84,85] now appears to have indications limited to mild factor VIII deficiency (hemophilia A), type I von Willebrand's disease, and uremia.[74,86]

Preoperative autologous donation has been applied successfully to the geriatric age group, and there are no age limits. Patients with unstable angina or critical aortic stenosis should be excluded, as should those with potential bacteremia. Standards require the hemoglobin value to be greater than 11 g/dl or the hematocrit to be over 33 percent before donation. Each patient should be considered individually. Autologous predonation has been utilized successfully in patients undergoing elective cardiac surgery, including coronary artery bypass,[87] and other procedures. Predonated units have been collected from high-risk patients in donor centers that provide careful hemodynamic monitoring.[88]

Although currently approved only for use in chronically anemic uremic patients, erythropoietin has been found to improve autologous blood predonation in coronary artery bypass patients, including an effective, lower-cost subcutaneous regimen.[89] This drug may see wider use in the future if its efficacy and cost-effectiveness can be established.

Acute normovolemic hemodilution (ANH), involving the removal of up to 2 liters of blood just before or after the induction of anesthesia and its simultaneous replacement with equal volumes of colloid or 3 times the volume with crystalloid, decreases homologous blood transfusion requirements. In fact, in a series of patients receiving retropubic prostatectomy, ANH was found to reduce the need for homologous transfusion compared to predonation, and the two techniques were judged to be medically equivalent.[90] Circumstances may arise in which both are useful. The technique has been well described in cardiac surgical patients, in whom blood can be removed before or after heparinization. In the latter case, blood can be withdrawn from the oxygenator tubing early during cardiopulmonary bypass in patients with ischemic cardiomyopathy or valvular stenosis who would otherwise be unable to tolerate such perturbations before a bypass; in this way, the cardiac lesion is obviated during harvest.[74] Interestingly, in at least one patient population (i.e., patients with known coronary artery disease undergoing abdominal aortic surgery), ANH may actually improve intraoperative hemodynamics; this is based on data demonstrating a decreased incidence of myocardial ischemia as evaluated by transesophageal echocardiographic and electrocardiographic (ECG) data during cross-clamping in hemodiluted patients compared to controls.[91] Generally, decreased tissue oxygenation caused acutely by ANH is not a concern even in a geriatric population with known coronary artery disease and stable angina because of the minimal degree of dilutional anemia that results.

Intraoperative autotransfusion using the Cell Saver (Haemonetics Corp., Braintree, MA 02184) can permit the salvage and reinfusion of up to 50 percent of shed blood.[92] Postoperative drainage from the mediastinal or pleural cavities can be reinfused. Salvaged blood has high levels of free hemoglobin, reduced or absent platelets, and few or no coagulation factors. Dilutional coagulopathy or coagulopathy for other unknown reasons is a concern,[74] and in addition, an anaphylactic-like syndrome termed "salvaged blood syndrome," which is thought to be caused by the release of leukotrienes and other mediators from white cells and platelets activated during centrifugation, has been described.[93] This appears to be of concern primarily when blood with a hematocrit below 20 percent is "salvaged."

In general, reperfusion of autologous blood is not altogether benign, and complications have been described, including cryptogenic hypotension.[94] Particularly with regard to predeposit autologous blood, clerical error may occur, resulting in inadvertent homologous transfusion. Unrecognized bacteremia or bacterial contamination may occur during collection, creating septic autologous units. Posttransfusion hypervolemia must be avoided. Cardiovascular depression can result from acute hypocalcemia secondary to the citrate anticoagulant. Hypersensitivity reactions and hypotension may occur secondary to exposure to plasticizers or sterilizing agents (e.g., ethylene oxide).

The indications for reinfusion of autologous blood, particularly with the use of ANH, can be less stringent than those for homologous transfusion, but the decision should not be made casually, and autologous transfusion should be triggered only by clinically relevant anemia.[74] In other words, because autologous blood carries less risk than does homologous blood, separate criteria may be applied to the transfusion of autologous versus homologous units. Situations may arise where the infusion of autologous, but not homologous, blood products is deemed appropriate. However, there is no applicable experimental evidence, and this recommendation is based on theoretical considerations only.[95] Furthermore, controversy exists, and some experts recommend identical or nearly identical criteria for the infusion of autologous versus homologous blood products.[96,97]

Coagulation Factors

Platelets, fresh frozen plasma (FFP), and cryoprecipitate are fractionated from donated whole blood. Platelets also can be collected from single donors by pheresis techniques, reducing the risk of disease transmission. FFP contains all coagulation factors except platelets, while cryoprecipitate is rich in factor VIII and fibrinogen. Factor VIII and factor IX concentrates are also available.

Coagulation factors should not be given prophylactically but rather to increase the level of specific clotting factors in patients with a demonstrated deficiency in the presence of microvascular bleeding. Coagulation can be monitored perioperatively with tests of clot formation rate and strength, utilizing the Thromboelastograph (Haemoscope Corp., Skokie, IL 60007) or the Sonoclot (Scienco, Inc., Morrison, CO 80465), activated coagulation time (ACT), prothrombin time (PT), activated partial thromboplastin time (aPTT), thrombin time, fibrinogen level, presence of fibrin split products or D-dimers, bleeding time, and platelet count. Massive transfusion may generate a coagulopathy, most commonly via dilutional thrombocytopenia, although disseminated intravascular coagulopathy can occur. Coagulopathy after cardiopulmonary bypass is most commonly due to a qualitative platelet defect,[74] although augmented fibrinolysis also plays a role.[98] Thrombocytopenia is the most common defect in traumatized patients.[99]

FFP is indicated for the treatment of isolated or multiple-factor deficiencies, including antithrombin III deficiency (heparin resistance), when specific component therapy is not available or is contraindicated. It is never indicated for volume expansion or as a nutritional supplement. Platelet transfusions are indicated to control bleeding caused by deficiencies of platelet number and/or function.[74] Active microvascular bleeding associated with acute thrombocytopenia ($<$50,000 to 100,000/mm^3) would be an appropriate indication for the transfusion of platelets. When questions arise, the use of the Thromboelastograph or a bleeding time may delineate whether platelet transfusion is advisable.[99]

RECOMMENDATIONS FOR FLUID MANAGEMENT

Implications of Physiological Constraints for Fluid Management

Significant changes in body composition, cardiac function, and renal function, even those which occur with normal aging, strongly affect fluid and electrolyte management of geriatric patients, dictating precision and careful clinical judgment. In terms of compositional changes secondary to aging, the clinician should recognize that although total body water is decreased, extracellular water is relatively increased. This may alter the patient's requirements for exogenous electrolytes, increasing sodium requirements and decreasing potassium needs; however, in real terms, these effects are probably minor. More significant is the maintenance of blood volume at normal levels until about age 75, after which a slight decline occurs.[10,17] This information allows the calculation of estimated blood volume and percentage of blood loss.

Normal changes in cardiac function with aging, including progressive loss of baroreceptor function, impaired diastolic filling, diminished inotropism, increased afterload, and decreased vascular compliance, impede the cardiovascular response to fluid depletion, volume overload, anesthesia-induced cardiovascular depression, and surgical stress. Coexisting coronary artery disease and acquired aortic stenosis, both of which are common in this age group, worsen the inability to compensate. Coexisting lung disease, which is also often present, can play a role via negative effects on oxygenation, thoracic compliance, cardiac filling, and pulmonary vascular resistance. Recognition of these normal physiological changes and the presence of coexisting disease is critical to successful management. As an example, a systemic diastolic blood pressure of 85 to 90 mmHg and a systolic pressure near 145 mmHg fall within the norm for these patients and may be optimal,[100] and euvolemia in conjunction with appropriate therapeutic manipulations to maintain a perfusion pressure at somewhat higher limits than for younger patients seems reasonable. Furthermore, it is also worthwhile to establish a baseline indication of normality for a particular patient that is based on previously recorded blood pressures and to use this information to help determine appropriate perioperative perfusion pressures.

As was discussed above, the progressive decline in renal blood flow, GFR, and tubular function minimizes the response to superimposed water and/or electrolyte imbalance. Renal failure can easily occur in the face of decreased cardiac output, dehydration, or sodium or water overload. Altered glomerulotubular function diminishes the response to serum electrolyte changes, and urine tends to be isosthenuric. Therefore, careful attention to electrolyte abnormalities and repletion of deficits is warranted. The clinician should also be aware that the perioperative stress response, including SIADH, contributes to electrolyte abnormalities and can be ameliorated by adequate anesthesia and postoperative analgesia.

In summary, aged-related physiological changes in the cardiovascular and renal systems and in the body composition of fluids predispose the elderly to fluid and electrolyte imbalances, including dehydration, fluid overload, hypernatremia, hyponatremia, hyperkalemia, hypokalemia, hypomagnesemia, and acidosis. It is imperative that anesthesiologists have a high degree of suspicion for these conditions in this age group and maintain accurate fluid and electrolyte replacement guided by adequate monitoring.

Fluids and Resuscitation

The severity of tissue trauma created by a given procedure dictates the amount of local and generalized edema and therefore the rate of fluid infusion. As a rough guide, procedures with minimal tissue trauma (e.g., eye surgery) require the infusion of only 1 to 2 ml/kg per hour of isotonic fluid. Procedures with severe tissue trauma (e.g., resection of pancreatic cancer) can require up to 15 ml/kg per hour. Procedures with moderate trauma are intermediate in fluid requirements. Such recommendations, however, must be utilized with extreme flexibility and must be based on a given patient's demonstrated requirements. For example, as a result of impaired thirst mechanisms, geriatric patients may be hypovolemic before surgery, leading to hypotension after anesthetic induction unless additional fluid is given. A variety of other factors also intervene and are constantly changing, including the effects of anesthesia and surgery (hormonal changes, progressive edema formation, vasodilation, cardiac depression), hemorrhage, diuresis, and variable evaporative losses through the wound or endotracheal tube.

Repletion of intravascular volume is of critical importance in the maintenance of tissue perfusion and the prevention of shock, which is defined as the absence of adequate tissue perfusion. Shock may be classified into four categories: (1) hypovolemic, (2) cardiogenic, (3) distributive (e.g., secondary to arteriovenous shunting), and (4) obstructive (e.g., tension pneumothorax). Hypovolemia is the most common primary etiology. Hypovolemia may also play a role in cardiogenic, distributive, or obstructive shock states in the form of relative (venous pooling) or absolute (increased vascular permeability) hypovolemia.

Criteria pertinent to the evaluation of the adequacy of volume repletion depend in part on the type of fluid employed. Crystalloid infusion is generally best monitored by urine output, blood pressure, and heart rate. Overzealous infusion of crystalloids leads primarily to tissue edema and diuresis rather than to increases in central venous pressure (CVP) or pulmonary artery occlusion pressure (PAOP). This is due to easy extravascular diffusion of crystalloids. Nevertheless, given the limited ability of geriatric patients to mount a significant diuresis in addition to their reduced cardiac reserve, caution should be exercised when one is infusing large quantities of crystalloids. Problems can arise not only acutely after an inappropriately large infusion of crystalloid intraoperatively but also postoperatively when patients begin to mobilize excessive fluids from the interstitium into the intravascular space, resulting in the potential for fluid overload and congestive heart failure.[101]

With the infusion of colloids, more pertinent monitors include CVP, PAOP, blood pressure, and heart rate. For a given volume, colloids tend to increase CVP and PAOP more than crystalloids. This means that central volume overload, congestive heart failure, and pulmonary edema are more likely to occur with the use of colloids. By contrast, crystalloid infusion, despite the resultant decrease in colloid oncotic pressure (COP), less commonly results in pulmonary edema. Nevertheless, some investigators, such as Rackow,[52,60,102] continue to stress the importance of COP in the prevention of pulmonary edema. Rackow recommends maintaining a COP-PAOP gradient between 8 and 16 mmHg, stating that either an increase in COP or a decrease in PAOP is likely to reduce flow of fluid into the lungs of critical patients. COP is easily measured.

Other indexes of importance include mentation, capillary filling, skin color, temperature, skin turgor, absence or presence of dry mouth, acid-base balance, lactate levels, oxygen consumption (calculated as the product of cardiac index and arteriovenous oxygen difference), oxygen delivery (Table 11-5), and mixed venous oxygen saturation.

A dynamic interaction exists between hemodynamic parameters and intravascular volume (Fig. 11-4). In a geriatric patient, the Frank-Starling mechanism plays a role of increased importance. The Frank-Starling principle states that myocardial fiber contractility improves with increased fiber length (or "preload") until a point of decompensation is reached. End-diastolic volume (EDV), which relates directly to diastolic fiber length, is determined in part by venous return to the ventricle. Preload can be manipulated to optimize cardiac output. In most patients, cardiac output increases until the PAOP reaches 15 mmHg, with further increases in PAOP either failing to increase cardiac output or actually decreasing it. However, each patient is unique.

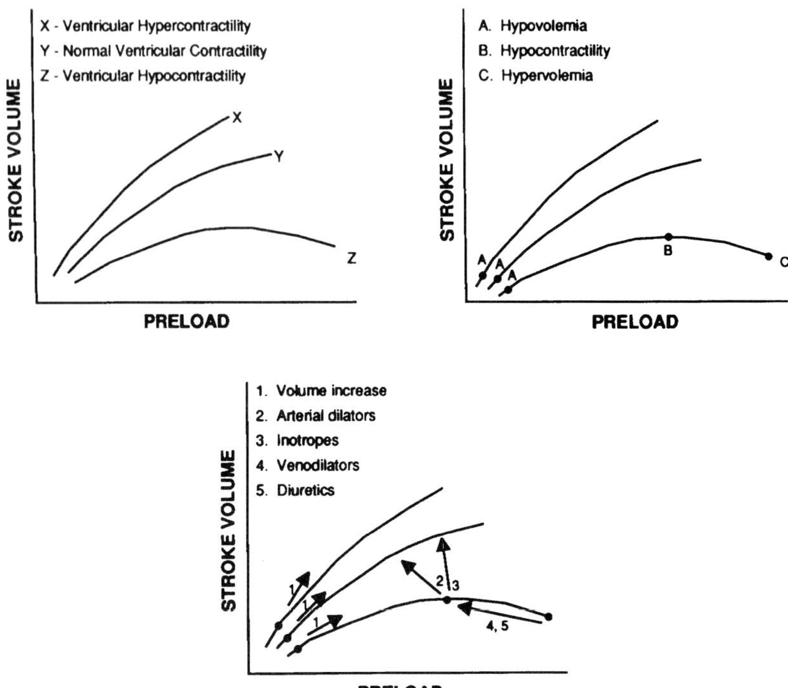

Figure 11-4 Hemodynamic parameters and intravascular volume interact to affect cardiac function and stroke volume. (A) Classic Frank-Starling relation shows how stroke volume varies with varying preload. (B) Causes of low stroke volume include hypovolemia, hypocontractility, and hypervolemia. (C) Various therapeutic maneuvers can be applied to increase stroke volume, depending on the existent ventricular contractility and the volume status of the patient.

When incremental boluses of fluid infusions are followed by measurement of PAOP and cardiac index (CI), optimal preload conditions can be determined for a patient. This can be done preoperatively, which is especially desirable before a stressful procedure such as elective aortic aneurysmectomy, which challenges the compensatory limitations of a geriatric patient. A prospective study of critical patients found that the complication rate after major vascular or general surgery was reduced significantly when the perioperative PAOP was maintained within 3 mmHg of the best preoperative value based on optimizing CI.[103] Normal CI ranges from 2.5 to 4.0 liters/min per square meter. Values under 2.2 liters/min per square meter correlate with critical tissue hypoperfusion. Therefore, reliance on determinants of preload is less appropriate than consideration of the relation between preload and cardiac output. CVP or PAOP measurements can have a variable relation to EDV, which is more directly representative of actual preload conditions. Pericardial tamponade, constrictive pericarditis, and even positive end-expiratory pressure can increase the ratio of end-diastolic pressure to EDV. Patients in myocardial failure may require high end-diastolic pressures to effectively increase stroke volume. Also, multiple causes of inaccurate CVP or PAOP readings are often present.[104]

In a patient monitored with a CVP catheter only, failure of evidence of improved tissue perfusion in spite of a rising CVP after multiple fluid boluses should prompt measurement of PAOP and CI. Pulmonary artery catheter (PAC) placement is indicated for patients with problems in four general categories: (1) pulmonary artery hypertension, (2) right ventricular dysfunction, including cor pulmonale, (3) left ventricular dysfunction, and (4) failure to reverse oliguria with a reasonable fluid challenge. Common specific examples include right or left ventricular infarction, adult respiratory distress syndrome, and shock.

Evidence of inadequate tissue perfusion, such as lactic acidosis, hypotension, and inadequate urine output, should prompt interventions to increase cardiac output. An initial response is volume infusion, with a goal for PAOP up to 18 mmHg if a PAC is present. Subsequent appropriate measures include the withdrawal of negative inotropes (e.g., volatile anesthetic agents and beta blockers), the addition of an inotropic agent such as dobutamine, and/or vasodilator therapy if mean arterial pressure and systemic vascular resistance are high. If these measures are inadequate, vasopressors such as dopamine and epinephrine may be added and titrated to maintain an appropriate mean arterial pressure (approximately 80 mmHg if possible) and CI (above 2.2 liters/min per square meter).

The concept of pathological supply dependency for oxygen consumption in shock has been promulgated recently.[105] This approach is based on the assumption that oxygen consumption is coupled to oxygen supply in some shock states,[106,107] and the use of supranormal levels of CI (>4.5 liters/min per square meter) and oxygen delivery (>670 ml/min per square meter) has been reported to treat tissue oxygen debt and optimize oxygen consumption (>166 ml/min per square meter) in shock. However, experimental evidence showing improved survival under these conditions may be flawed by the mathematical coupling of oxygen consumption and oxygen delivery equations,[108] and contradictory evidence exists.[108,109] At the present time, the concept of pathological supply dependency for oxygen consumption contradicts conventional wisdom, which suggests that survival in shock states is related to the time course of inadequate perfusion and blood lactate levels rather than to the coupling of oxygen consumption and delivery.[109]

In geriatric patients, limitations of preload augmentation and inotropic/vasodilator therapy must be determined for each patient. Increased preload can cause pulmonary edema in patients with poor ventricular compliance caused by elevated pulmonary capillary hydrostatic pressure. Also, increased preload can impair subendocardial myocardial perfusion via increased end-diastolic pressure, especially in patients with coronary artery disease and an exhausted coronary vasodilating reserve. Oxygen demands are related to heart rate, contractile state, and wall tension. Wall tension is a function of both preload and afterload. However, increases in heart rate and afterload are the principal determinants of myocardial oxygen consumption, and the heart rate–systolic pressure product estimates myocardial oxygen demand.

SUMMARY

A geriatric patient poses special challenges relative to perioperative fluid therapy. In addition to alterations in fluid and electrolyte status, which are a universal consequence of anesthesia and surgery, a geriatric patient is often affected by compensatory mechanisms that are diminished secondary to both normal aging and coexisting disease in pertinent organ systems, especially the cardiovascular, renal, and endocrine systems. Disturbances of both fluid volume and composition are common. Appropriate repletion of fluids can be critical in this patient population. In general, if hemoglobin levels are sufficient, the adequacy of fluid infusion is of greater consequence than is the type of fluid employed. Perioperative intravenous fluid therapy should be guided by the compensatory abilities of the individual patient, the degree of tissue trauma, and information derived from clinical variables and appropriate monitors.

ACKNOWLEDGMENT

The authors wish to thank the following individuals: Dr. A. H. Giesecke for his insightful recommendations during revision of this chapter, Mrs. Theresa de Guia and Ms. Debbie Bramlett for their expert and invaluable secretarial assistance, and Ms. Brenda Jackman, who was instrumental in developing the figures used in this chapter.

REFERENCES

1. Shannon DC, Carley DW, Benson H: Aging of modulation of heart rate. *Am J Physiol* 253:H874, 1987.
2. Lipsitz LA, Mietus J, Moody GB, Goldberg AL: Spectral characteristics of heart rate variability before and during postural tilt: Relations to aging and risk of syncope. *Circulation* 81:1803, 1990.
3. Latson TW, Ashmore TH, Reinhart DJ, et al: Autonomic reflex dysfunction is associated with post-induction hypotension in both diabetic and non-diabetic patients. *Anesthesiology* 80:326, 1994.
4. Latson TW: Heart rate variability and anesthesiology: Reasons for cautious optimism. (editorial). *J Cardiothorac Vasc Anesth* 6:647, 1992.
5. Tasch MD: The autonomic system and geriatric anesthesia. *Int Anesthesiol Clin* 26:143, 1988.
6. Anderson S, Brennar BM: The aging kidney: Structure, function, mechanism, and therapeutic implications. *J Am Geriatr Soc* 35:590, 1987.

7. Anderson S, Brenner BM: Effects of aging on the renal glomerulus. *Am Med J* 80:435, 1986.
8. Lindemann RD, Tobin J, Shock N: Longitudinal studies on the rate of decline in renal function with age. *J Am Geriatr Soc* 33:278, 1985.
9. Muravchick S: Current concepts: Anesthetic pharmacology in geriatric patients. *Prog Anesthesiol* 1:2, 1987.
10. Fulop T Jr, Worum I, Csonger J, et al: Body composition in elderly people: I. Determination of body composition by multiisotope method and the elimination kinetics of these isotopes in healthy elderly subjects. *Gerontology* 31:6, 1985.
11. Silver AJ: Aging and risks for dehydration. *Cleve Clin J Med* 57:341, 1990.
12. Tsunoda K, Abe K, Goto T, et al: Effect of age on the renin-angiotensin-aldosterone system in normal subjects: Simultaneous measurement of active and inactive renin, renin substrate, and aldosterone in plasma. *J Clin Endocrinol Metab* 62:384, 1986.
13. Yamamoto T, Harada H, Fukuyama J, et al: Impaired arginine-vasopressin secretion associated with hypoangiotensinemia in hypernatremic dehydrated elderly patients. *JAMA* 259:1039, 1988.
14. Phillips PA, Rolls BJ, Ledingham JGG: Reduced thirst after water deprivation in healthy elderly men. *N Engl J Med* 311:753, 1984.
15. Synder NA, Feigal DW, Arieff AI: Hypernatremia in the elderly patient. *Ann Intern Med* 107:309, 1987.
16. Watters JM: Preventive measures in the elderly surgical patient. *Can J Surg* 34:561, 1991.
17. Tucker GL: Fluid therapy before, during, and after operation in the elderly, in Stephen CR, Assaf RAE (eds): *Geriatric Anesthesia: Principles and Practice.* Stoneham, Mass.: Butterworth, 1986, pp 327–344.
18. Beck LH: Perioperative renal, fluid, and electrolyte management. *Clin Geriatr Med* 6:557, 1990.
19. Sunderam SG, Mankikar GD: Hyponatraemia in the elderly. *Age Ageing* 12:77, 1983.
20. Mahowald JM, Himmelstein DU: Hypernatremia in the elderly: Relation to infection and mortality. *J Am Geriatr Soc* 29:177, 1981.
21. Agarwal B, Cabebe FC: Renal acidification in elderly subjects. *Nephron* 26:291, 1980.
22. Myers BD, Moran SM: Hemodynamically mediated acute renal failure. *N Engl J Med* 314:97, 1986.
23. Shires T, Williams J, Brown F: Acute changes in extracellular fluids associated with major surgical procedures. *Ann Surg* 154:803, 1961.
24. Lucas CE, Ledgerwood AM, Rachwal WJ, et al: Colloid oncotic pressure and body water dynamics in septic and injured patients. *J Trauma* 31:927, 1991.
25. Bock JC, Barker BC, Clinton AG, et al: Post-traumatic changes in, and effect of colloid osmotic pressure on the distribution of body water. *Ann Surg* 210:395, 1989.
26. Giesecke AH, Egbert LD: Perioperative fluid therapy—crystalloids, in Miller R (ed): *Anesthesia*, 2d ed. London: Churchill-Livingstone, 1986, pp 1313–1328.
27. Espiner EA: The effects of stress on salt and water balance. *Clin Endocrin Med* 1:375, 1986.
28. Laureno R: Central pontine myelinolysis following rapid correction of hyponatremia. *Ann Neurol* 13:232, 1983.
29. Sterns RH, Riggs JE, Schochet SSJ: Osmotic demyelination syndrome following correction of hyponatremia. *N Engl J Med* 314:1535, 1986.

30. Ayus JC, Krothapali RK, Arieff AI: Treatment of symptomatic hyponatremia and its relation with brain damage. *N Engl J Med* 317:1190, 1987.
31. Arieff AI, Ayus JC: Treatment of symptomatic hyponatremia: Neither haste nor waste. *Crit Care Med* 19:748, 1991.
32. Weiner M, Epstein EH: Signs and symptoms of electrolyte disorders. *Yale J Biol Med* 43:76, 1970.
33. Whang R, Whang DD, Ryan MP: Refractory potassium repletion: A consequence of magnesium deficiency. *Arch Intern Med* 152:40, 1992.
34. England MR, Gordon G, Salem M, Chernow B: Magnesium administration and dysrhythmias after cardiac surgery. *JAMA* 268:241, 1992.
35. Koch SM, Taylor RW: Chloride ion in intensive care medicine. *Crit Care Med* 20:227, 1992.
36. Rosen RA, Julian BA, Dubovsky EV, et al: On the mechanism by which chloride corrects metabolic alkalosis in man. *Am J Med* 84:449, 1992.
37. Ratner LE, Smith GW: Intraoperative fluid management. *Surg Clin North Am* 73:229, 1993.
38. Vassar MJ, Perry CA, Gannaway WL, et al: 7.5% sodium chloride/dextran for resuscitation of trauma patients. *Arch Surg* 126:1065, 1991.
39. Metild LA, Shackford SR, Virgilio RW, et al: Crystalloid vs colloid in fluid resuscitation of patients with severe pulmonary insufficiency. *Surg Gynecol Obstet* 158:207, 1984.
40. Zarins CK, Rice CL, Peters RM, et al: Lymph and pulmonary response to isobaric reduction in plasma oncotic pressure. *Circ Res* 43:925, 1978.
41. Hachenberg T, Tenling A, Rothen H, et al: Thoracic intravascular and extravascular fluid volumes in cardiac surgical patients. *Anesthesiology* 79:976, 1993.
42. Brinkmeyer S, Safar P, Motoyama E: Superiority of colloid over electrolyte solution for fluid resuscitation (severe normovolemic hemodilution). *Crit Care Med* 9:369, 1981.
43. Baker JW, Deitch ED, Ma LM, et al: Hemorrhagic shock induces bacterial translocation from the gut. *J Trauma* 28:896, 1988.
44. Wilmore DW, Smith RJ, O'Dwyer ST, et al: The gut—a central organ following surgical stress. *Surgery* 104:917, 1988.
45. Siegel DC, Cochin A, Geocaris T, et al: Effects of saline and colloid resuscitation on renal function. *Ann Surg* 177:51, 1973.
46. Giesecke AH, Grande CM, Whitten CW: Fluid therapy and resuscitation of traumatic shock. *Crit Care Clin* 6:61, 1990.
47. Sieber FE, Smith DS, Traystman RJ, Wollman A: Glucose, a reevaluation of its intraoperative use. *Anesthesiology* 67:72, 1987.
48. Melakiewicz RM, Hall GM: Diabetes and anesthesia, the past decade. *Br J Anaesth* 68:198, 1992.
49. Nearman HS, Herman ML: Toxic effects of colloids in the intensive care unit. *Crit Care Clin* 7:713, 1991.
50. Carlson RW, Rattan S, Haupt MT: Fluid resuscitation in conditions of increased permeability. *Anesthesiol Rev* XVIII(III):14, 1990.
51. Griffel MJ, Kaufman BS: Pharmacology of colloids and crystalloids. *Crit Care Clin* 8:235, 1992.
52. Rackow EC, Fein IA, Siegel J: The relationship of the colloid osmotic-pulmonary artery wedge pressure gradient to pulmonary edema and mortality in critically ill patients. *Chest* 82:433, 1982.
53. Shatney CH, Deepika K, Militello PR, et al: Efficacy of hetastarch in the resuscitation of patients with multisystem trauma and shock. *Arch Surg* 118:804, 1983.

54. London MJ, Ho JS, Triedman JK, et al: A randomized clinical trial of 10% pentastarch (low molecular weight hydroxyethyl starch) versus 5% albumin for plasma volume expansion after cardiac operations. *J Thorac Cardiovasc Surg* 97:785, 1989.
55. Villauer PJ: Pentastarch may cause fewer effects on coagulation than hetastarch. *Transfusion* 28:257, 1988.
56. Morisaki H, Bloos F, Keys J, et al: Compared to crystalloid, colloid therapy slows the progression of extra-pulmonary tissue injury in sheep. *J Appl Physiol*, 1994 (in press).
57. Zikria BA, King TC, Stanford J, et al: A biophysical approach to capillary permeability. *Surgery* 105:625, 1989.
58. Zikria BA, Subbaro C, Oz MC, et al: Macromolecules reduce abnormal microvascular permeability in rat limb—reperfusion injury. *Crit Care Med* 17:1306, 1989.
59. Schell RM, Cole DJ, Osborne AHT: Pentastarch decreases blood-brain barrier permeability following temporary cerebral ischemia in rats. *Anesth Analg* 72:S235, 1991.
60. Rackow EC, Falk JL, Fein IA, et al: Fluid resuscitation in circulatory shock: A comparison of the cardiorespiratory effects of albumin, hetastarch and saline solutions in patients with hypovolemic and septic shock. *Crit Care Med* 11:839, 1983.
61. Strauss RG: Review of the effects of hydroxyethyl starch on the blood coagulation system. *Transfusion* 21:299, 1981.
62. Stump DC, Strauss RG, Henriksen RA, et al: Effects of hydroxyethyl starch on blood coagulation, particularly factor VIII. *Transfusion* 25:349, 1985.
63. Gold MS, Russo J, Tissot M, et al: Comparison of hetastarch to albumin for perioperative bleeding in patients undergoing abdominal aortic aneurysm surgery. *Ann Surg* 211:482, 1990.
64. Claes Y, Van Hemerlrijck J, Van Gerven M: Influence of hydroxyethyl starch on coagulation in patients during the perioperative period. *Anesth Analg* 75:24, 1992.
65. Kirklin JK, Lell WA, Konchoukos NT: Hydroxyethyl starch versus albumin for colloid infusion following cardiopulmonary bypass in patients undergoing myocardial revascularization. *Ann Thorac Surg* 37:40, 1984.
66. Strauss RG, Stump DC, Henriksen RA: Hydroxyethyl starch accentuates von Willebrand's disease. *Transfusion* 25:235, 1985.
67. Harms BA, Pahl AC, Radosevich DG, Starling JR: The effects of hypoproteinemia and volume expansion on lung and soft tissue transvascular fluid filtration. *Surgery* 105:605, 1989.
68. Davidson IJ, Sandor ZF, Coorpender L, et al: Intraoperative albumin administration affects the outcome of cadaver renal transplantation. *Transplantation* 53:774, 1992.
69. Moss GS, Gould SA: Plasma expanders: An update. *Am J Surg* 155:425, 1988.
70. Velanovich V: Crystalloid versus colloid fluid resuscitation: A meta-analysis of mortality. *Surgery* 105:65, 1989.
71. Giesecke AH: Personal communication, 1993.
72. Messmer K, Kreimeier V, Intaglietta M: Present state of intentional hemodilution. *Eur Surg Res* 18:254, 1986.
73. Moncada S, Higgs A: The L-arginine-nitric oxide pathway. *N Engl J Med* 329:2002, 1993.
74. Faust RJ, Bukowski E, Furman EB, et al: *Questions and Answers about Transfusion Practices*, 2d ed. Park Ridge, IL: American Society of Anesthesiologists, 1992.

75. Leone BJ, Spahn DR: Anemia, hemodilution, and oxygen delivery. *Anesth Analg* 75:651, 1992.
76. Ernst E, Mortoi A, Kollar L: Placebo-controlled, double-blind study of haemodilution in peripheral vascular disease. *Lancet* 1:1449, 1987.
77. Nelson AH, Fleisher LA, Rosenbaum SH: The relationship between postoperative anemia and cardiac morbidity in high risk vascular patients in the ICU. *Crit Care Med* 2:860, 1993.
78. Crystal GJ, Salem HR: Myocardial oxygen consumption and segmental shortening during selective coronary hemodilution in dogs. *Anesth Analg* 67:500, 1988.
79. Welch GA, Meehan KR, Goodnough LT: Prudent strategies for elective red blood cell transfusion. *Ann Intern Med* 116:393, 1992.
80. Noldge GF, Priebe HJ, Geiger K: Splanchnic hemodynamics and oxygen supply during acute normovolemic hemodilution alone and with isoflurane-induced hypotension in the anesthetized patient. *Anesth Analg* 75:660, 1992.
81. Foulke GE, Harlow DJ: Effective measures for reducing blood loss from diagnostic laboratory tests in intensive care unit patient. *Crit Care Med* 17:1143, 1989.
82. Jobes DR, Ellison N: The pharmacology of hemostasis in the surgical patient. *Anesth Analg* 75:317, 1992.
83. Alajma F, Calami G, Perna AM, et al: High dose aprotinin: Hemostatic effects in open heart operations. *Ann Thorac Surg* 48:536, 1989.
84. Rocha E, Llorens TL, Paramo JA, et al: Does desmopressin acetate reduce blood loss after surgery in patients on cardiopulmonary bypass? *Circulation* 77:1319, 1988.
85. Hackman T, Gascoyne RD, Neiman SC, et al: A trial of desmopressin (1-desamino-8-D-arginine vasopressor) to reduce blood loss in uncomplicated cardiac surgery. *N Engl J Med* 321:1437, 1989.
86. Brown MR, Swygert TH, Whitten CW, et al: Desmopressin acetate following cardiopulmonary bypass: Evaluation of coagulation parameters. *J Cardiothorac Vasc Anesth* 3:726, 1989.
87. Love TR, Hendren WG, O'Kaete D, et al: Autologous blood in elective cardiac surgery. *Ann Thorac Surg* 43:508, 1987.
88. Spiess BD, Sassett RJ, McCarthy RF, et al: Autologous blood donation: Hemodynamics in a high risk patient population. *Transfusion* 32:17, 1992.
89. Kulier AH, Gombotz H, Fuchs G, et al: Subcutaneous recombinant human erythropoietin and autologous blood donation before coronary artery bypass surgery. *Anesth Analg* 76:102, 1993.
90. Ness PM, Bourke DL, Walsh PC: A randomized trial of perioperative hemodilution versus transfusion of preoperatively deposited autologous blood in elective surgery. *Transfusion* 32:226, 1992.
91. Catoire P, Saade M, Liu N, et al: Effect of preoperative normovolemic hemodilution on left ventricular supplemental wall motion during abdominal aortic surgery. *Anesth Analg* 75:654, 1992.
92. Kruskall MS: Intraoperative autotransfusion, in Rossi EG, Simon TL (eds): *Principles of Transfusion Medicine*. Baltimore: Williams & Wilkins, 1991, pp 417–418.
93. Bull BS, Bull MH: The salvaged blood syndrome: A sequel to mechanochemical activation of platelets and leukocytes? *Blood Cells* 16:5, 1990.
94. Miller AC, Scherba-Krugliak L, Toy P: Hypotension during transfusion of autologous blood. *Anesthesiology* 74:624, 1991.
95. *Technical Manual*, 11th ed. Washington, D.C.: American Association of Blood Banks, 1993, pp 491–506.

96. Yomtovian R: Personal communication, 1993.
97. Kruskall MS, Yomtovian R, Dzik WH, et al: Health policy review: On improving the cost-effectiveness of autologous blood transfusion practices. *Transfusion* 34:259, 1994.
98. Spiess BD: The contribution of fibrinolysis to postbypass bleeding. *J Cardiothorac Vasc Anesth* 5:13, 1991.
99. Whitten CW, Allison PM: Bleeding and thrombosis problems in the postoperative trauma patient, in Grande CM (ed): *Trauma Anesthesia and Critical Care*. Philadelphia: Mosby Yearbook, 1993, pp 800–833.
100. Farnett L, Mulrow CD, Linn WD, et al: The J curve phenomenon and the treatment of hypertension. *JAMA* 265:489, 1991.
101. Gold MS: Perioperative fluid management. *Crit Care Clin* 8:409, 1992.
102. Rackow EC: Clinical significance of colloid oncotic pressure. *Anesthesiol Rev* XVII(Suppl III):6, 1990.
103. Yang SC, Puri VK: Role of preoperative hemodynamic monitoring in intraoperative fluid management. *Am Surg* 52:536, 1986.
104. Tuman KJ, Carroll GC, Ivankovich AD: Pitfalls in interpretation of pulmonary artery catheter data. *J Cardiothorac Vasc Anesth* 3:625, 1989.
105. Fleming A, Bishop M, Shoemaker W, et al: Prospective trial of supranormal values as goals of resuscitation in severe trauma. *Arch Surg* 127:1175, 1992.
106. Shoemaker WC, Appel PL, Kram HB: Tissue oxygen debt as a determinant of lethal and nonlethal postoperative organ failure. *Crit Care Med* 16:1117, 1988.
107. Shoemaker WC, Kram HB, Appel PL: Therapy of shock based on pathophysiology, monitoring, and outcome prediction. *Crit Care Med* 18:519, 1990.
108. Vermeij CG, Feenstra BWA, Bruining HA: Oxygen delivery and oxygen uptake in postoperative and septic patients. *Chest* 98:415, 1990.
109. Bakker J, Coffernils M, Leon M, et al: Blood and lactate levels are superior to oxygen-derived variables in predicting outcome in human septic shock. *Chest* 99:956, 1991.

CHAPTER 12

Anesthesia for Cancer Surgery in Geriatric Patients

Dawn P. Desiderio
Ronald A. Kross

INTRODUCTION

Over 50 percent of all cancers occur after age 65.[1] Although the probability of developing cancer is only 1 to 1.5 percent between the ages of 20 and 40 years, it increases to 17 to 23 percent between ages 65 and 85 years.[2] Cancer is primarily a disease of the elderly. People over 65 now constitute nearly 12 percent of the population of the United States and are projected to account for 20 percent by the year 2020.

Advances in cancer treatment utilizing multidisciplinary management methods (chemotherapy, radiation therapy, and surgery) have allowed less radical surgical procedures to be effective. Indeed, the development of laparoscopic and thoracoscopic surgical techniques has increased the number of patients who may benefit from surgical intervention for cancer staging and treatment by allowing those with more advanced disease and additional comorbid illnesses to undergo what is considered a less risky procedure. This, along with advances in preoperative, intraoperative, and postoperative monitoring, means that an elderly patient with cancer is no longer precluded from undergoing appropriate therapy. In addition, palliative procedures performed to improve and sustain the quality of life, while not curative, are performed more frequently. Therefore, patients who formerly were not considered surgical candidates because of age alone are no longer excluded from receiving surgical therapy.

An anesthesiologist caring for these patients must be able to manage the hematologic, metabolic, and physiological derangements that result from age, cancer, and the treatment of cancer. A Mayo Clinic study on surgical outcome in patients over 90 years of age demonstrated a 48-h morbidity of 9.4 percent and a mortality of 1.6 percent. Perioperative morbidity was related to ASA classification, emergency surgery, male gender, associated organ system deficits (renal, hepatic, CNS), and site of surgery.[3]

A geriatric cancer patient is not unlike a noncancer patient in that comorbid conditions frequently coexist and contribute to perioperative morbidity and mortality. Lewis and Khoury[4] compared morbidity and postoperative complications in two groups of patients undergoing colon resection: those 70 to 79 years of age and those over 80 years of age. After curative resection, mortality in the younger group was 2 percent versus 7 percent in the older group. For those undergoing palliative resection for tumors with local or distant spread, the mortality was 21 percent in the group 70 to 79 years old and 38 percent in the older group (Table 12-1). Benton and colleagues[5] compared two groups of

Table 12-1 Mortality after colon resection in geriatric cancer

Age, years	Curative, %	Palliative, %
70–79	2	21
80 or more	7	38

SOURCE: Lewis and Khoury.[4]

patients undergoing colon surgery for cancer: those between 75 and 80 years of age and those over 80 years of age. Mortality in those 75 to 80 years was 5 percent, and in those over 80 it was 17 percent. The authors concluded that physiological status is the major determinant of postoperative mortality. Cardiovascular and pulmonary disease are the major comorbid conditions that contribute to surgical morbidity and mortality.[6] In addition to these conditions, geriatric cancer patients present additional physiological derangements and metabolic disturbances caused by the malignancy or by the systemic effects of chemotherapy and radiation therapy.

PREOPERATIVE EVALUATION

Appropriate preoperative evaluation of a geriatric cancer patient by necessity requires an understanding of the natural history of the patient's malignancy as well as other abnormalities, such as acid-base disorders, malnutrition, infection, respiratory insufficiency, hepatic and renal dysfunction, anemia, and clotting abnormalities.[7] Although there may be a degree of urgency that limits the length of time available to correct preoperative derangements, prompt initiation of at least partial correction of the deficits should be undertaken with appropriate laboratory work, radiological diagnostic testing, and invasive preoperative monitoring in an intensive care unit (ICU), if necessary. Common diseases of the elderly such as arteriosclerotic coronary artery disease, pulmonary insufficiency resulting from chronic obstructive pulmonary disease (COPD) or pneumonia, and diabetes must be investigated, and the condition of the patient must be optimized. Unless surgery is of an emergent nature, these conditions may be evaluated and treated on an outpatient basis after appropriate consultations have been obtained. Early involvement of the anesthesiologist in the preoperative evaluation helps prevent costly delays in treating the patient's malignancy.

In addition to the presence of natural comorbid conditions, an elderly cancer patient may have previously been treated with radiation or chemotherapy. The effects of these therapies on the lungs, heart, kidney, and hematologic system are of special concern to the anesthesiologist and complicate the preoperative evaluation. For example, pulmonary toxicity is commonly associated with bleomycin chemotherapy. The typical clinical presentation of bleomycin toxicity is a nonproductive cough, dyspnea, and tachypnea.[8] The physical examination may be unremarkable except for fine inspiratory rales on auscultation. Pulmonary function tests may reveal decreased diffusion capacity and a restrictive pattern. Chest x-ray may reveal interstitial pneumonitis. Baseline arterial blood gases can be helpful in guiding subsequent management.

In addition to hypertension and coronary artery disease, causes of cardiac disease in geriatric cancer patients include tumor invasion of the pericardium, pericardial effusion, sepsis, endocarditis, previous thoracic radiation therapy, and toxicity of antineoplastic drugs such as doxorubicin.[9] It was recently demonstrated that measurements of ventricular function at rest are valuable in monitoring patients with cancer who have received potentially cardiotoxic agents. Serial radionuclide imaging techniques that allow for the calculation of ejection fraction at rest have been shown to guide therapy with doxorubicin.[10] It has also been shown that additional measurements during exercise do not add to the prognostic assessment.[11] These studies may obviate the need for older methods of assessing cardiac toxicity, such as endocardial biopsy.

The clinical manifestations of chemotherapy-induced cardiac toxicity may present acutely or chronically. Acutely, electrocardiographic changes such as nonspecific ST segment changes, arrhythmias, heart block, and low voltages may be noted. Chronic toxicity is associated with cardiomyopathy. Patients with congestive heart failure secondary to doxorubicin-induced cardiomyopathy have an increased risk of developing cardiovascular decompensation intraoperatively.[12] Invasive hemodynamic monitoring may be required in these patients.

EFFECTS OF RADIATION THERAPY

Patients who are to receive surgery after radiation therapy may present with pulmonary, cardiac, or hepatic toxicity. Patients with breast cancer, a common cancer among the elderly, may survive for many years after therapy, which commonly includes radiation to the chest or mediastinum. Patients who have received radiation to lung tissue may develop radiation pneumonitis, which may progress to pulmonary fibrosis.[13] These effects may be enhanced by a history of smoking and may be potentiated by chemotherapy.

Cardiac disease after radiation therapy has been shown to occur in anywhere from 3.4 to 9.6 percent of patients.[14] The effects of radiation therapy have been shown to enhance the cardiotoxic effects of chemotherapy with doxorubicin.[15] Both symptomatic and asymptomatic patients have shown anatomic evidence of heart disease.[16] The anesthesiologist must be aware of early and late manifestations of radiation-induced cardiotoxicity. Radiation pericarditis with or without pericardial effusion is most commonly the first manifestation of cardiotoxicity. Chest radiography and echocardiography may be diagnostic.

Patients with cardiac tamponade may present to the operating room urgently for the creation of a pericardial window. Occasionally preoperative pericardiocentesis cannot be performed, and the anesthesiologist may be presented with a patient in extremis. Induction of anesthesia should be delayed until the patient is prepped and draped and the surgeon is ready to make the incision. Preinduction invasive hemodynamic monitoring may be advisable. Induction agents with myocardial depressant or vasodilatory properties should be avoided. Once the pericardial effusion has been drained, the patient's hemodynamic state should improve markedly. If it does not, other sources of cardiac compromise (cardiomyopathy, tumor invasion) may have to be considered. A pulmonary artery catheter is a diagnostic tool that can be used as a guide in the management of these critically ill patients.

The late effects of radiation therapy include constrictive pericarditis, restrictive cardiomyopathy, coronary artery insufficiency, and valvular dysfunction. Diffuse myocardial fibrosis and vascular changes in large intrathoracic vessels such as the aorta have been described.[17]

Pelvic radiation therapy results in fibrosis of tissue and adherence of blood vessels to fascial planes. This makes surgical dissection very difficult, and the possibility of large blood loss intraoperatively must be considered. The possible intraoperative need for large amounts of typed and cross-matched blood should be addressed preoperatively with the blood bank.

METABOLIC DISTURBANCES

Hypercalcemia

A geriatric cancer patient may present with various metabolic disturbances (Table 12-2). The paraneoplastic syndromes include these metabolic derangements. Among these syndromes, hypercalcemia is the most common, occurring in 10 to 20 percent of all patients with cancer.[18] It is often encountered in patients with malignancies of the breast, head and neck, and lung.[19] Occasionally hypercalcemia can be associated with cancer of the esophagus or kidney or with hematologic malignancies such as multiple myeloma.

Tumor-induced hypercalcemia and tumor-induced osteolysis are caused by activation of osteoclasts. The most common cause of hypercalcemia of malignancy is the parathyroid hormone–like peptide (PTH-RP).[20] This peptide causes increased renal tubular resorption of calcium. Hypercalcemia is usually associated with hypophosphatemia. Other factors that can cause tumor-induced hypercalcemia include transforming growth factors, prostaglandins, colony-stimulating factors, interleukin-1, lymphotoxin, and tumor necrosis factor.[21]

Hypercalcemia results in renal vasoconstriction, the development of nephrogenic diabetes insipidus, and severe volume depletion. Clinical manifestations include dehydration, muscle weakness, changes in mental status, nausea, vomiting, ileus, polyuria, and cardiac arrhythmias. Although hypercalcemia of malignancy is resistant to conventional treatment with intravenous hydration and diuresis, volume status must be restored before consideration of surgical intervention. The type of hemodynamic monitoring utilized depends on the patient's overall status and on other comorbid conditions. Antiresorptive therapy

Table 12-2 Metabolic disturbances in cancer patients

Hypercalcemia
Hypocalcemia
Hyponatremia
Acid-base disorders

includes calcitonin, mithramycin, diphosphonates, and gallium nitrate. Hemodialysis can reduce serum calcium acutely and may be used initially in symptomatic patients with or without renal failure.

Hypocalcemia

Hypocalcemia usually occurs as a result of hypoparathyroidism after thyroid or parathyroid surgery. However, after extensive neck dissections for head and neck tumors or cervical esophageal tumors, permanent hypoparathyroidism may ensue.[22] Hypocalcemia may result in muscle spasms, psychosis, extrapyramidal system dysfunction, increased intracranial pressure, hypotension, cardiac arrhythmias, and congestive heart failure. Prompt correction of hypocalcemia by calcium and vitamin D supplements is essential before surgery.

Hyponatremia

Hyponatremia is the most common electrolyte abnormality seen in cancer patients, especially those with advanced cancers, as may be seen in the geriatric population. Hyponatremia is usually accompanied by increased total body water with peripheral edema and/or ascites.[23] Hyponatremia usually occurs whenever the effective plasma volume is reduced, as in states such as liver failure caused by invasive carcinoma, malignant ascites, hypoalbuminemia, venous obstruction by tumor, and congestive heart failure. The retention of sodium and water by the kidney as compensation, along with the administration of intravenous fluids, results in hyponatremia. Hyponatremia may also occur in volume-depleted patients as a result of gastrointestinal losses, hemorrhage, or diuretic use.

In all hyponatremic states, plasma vasopressin is elevated.[24] The syndrome of inappropriate secretion of antidiuretic hormone (SIADH) has been associated with small cell lung cancer; cancers of the pancreas, prostate, adrenal, esophagus, colon, head, and neck; carcinoid tumors; thymoma; and mesothelioma.[25] Hyponatremia has also been associated with postirradiation hypopituitarism, pulmonary infections, and CNS disorders and can be a side effect of drugs such as opiates, cyclophosphamide (Cytoxan), vincristine, barbiturates, diuretics, beta agonists, and sulfonylureas.[26] The diagnosis of SIADH is made by the presence of an elevated urinary osmolarity in the presence of hyponatremia and a decreased plasma osmolarity (less than 280 mOsm/liter). Therapy for hyponatremia is directed toward the underlying cause. Slowly occurring hyponatremia may be asymptomatic or may present as subtle mental changes. Acute hyponatremia may result in cerebral edema with asterixis, coma, and seizures. Volume depletion should be corrected with normal saline. Volume overload caused by SIADH is treated with fluid restriction and the establishment of a negative daily fluid intake. Treatment of the underlying tumor may correct hyponatremia over a period of weeks.

Acid-Base Disturbances

The presence of the acid-base disturbances of metabolic and respiratory acidosis and alkalosis are commonly seen in geriatric cancer patients. The likelihood of the presence of these disturbances is great if the patient has had prior surgery or chemotherapy or is in a state of advanced cancer.[27] The anesthesiologist must frequently evaluate such patients in preparation for urgent or emergent procedures. Cancer patients may become acidotic from excessive biliary or pancreatic drainage, ureteroenterostomy or malfunctioning ileostomy, shock, or sepsis as well as from the other common causes of metabolic acidosis. Septic patients commonly have metabolic acidosis and respiratory alkalosis. Most commonly, these patients have had previous abdominal surgery (esophagogastrectomy, pancreatectomy, hepatic resection, etc.) and return to the operating room for drainage of intraabdominal fluid collections. It would be beneficial to hemodynamically monitor these patients preoperatively in an ICU with appropriate invasive monitoring and cardiopulmonary support to optimize hemodynamics before surgery.

SPECIFIC TYPES OF CANCER

More than 60 percent of cancer deaths occur after 65 years of age. The incidence of cancer is higher in women until age 50. After age 60, there is a greater increase in the incidence among men. The types of cancer that occur in the geriatric population also differ with the patient's sex. For women, colorectal, breast, and lung cancers are most common in that order, and for men, lung, prostate, and colorectal cancers are the most common.[28] In addition, cancers of the head and neck are also discussed in this section, since patients with these cancers are usually elderly and since the nature of the disease poses a particular challenge to the anesthesiologist in regard to airway management (Table 12-3).

Colorectal Carcinoma

Carcinoma of the colon is a common geriatric cancer. Carcinomas of the right hemicolon are especially insidious and may remain asymptomatic until an advanced stage. These patients usually present with anemia, which can complicate the anesthetic management, especially in the presence of comorbid condi-

Table 12-3 Common geriatric cancers

Colorectal
Prostate
Lung
Breast
Pancreas

tions. There has been considerable discussion about whether perioperative blood transfusion has a detrimental effect on the length of survival as a result of immune suppression. Wiig[29] reviewed 14 studies on the effect of blood transfusion on the recurrence of colorectal cancer after surgery. Eight studies showed detrimental effects of transfusion, and six found no detrimental effects. Busch and colleagues[30] performed a randomized trial to investigate whether the prognosis in patients with colorectal cancer would be improved by autologous transfusion as opposed to allogeneic transfusion. They demonstrated that the use of autologous blood as opposed to allogeneic blood did not improve the prognosis in patients with colorectal cancer and that transfusion is associated with poor prognosis. This is probably due to other factors, such as the extent of tumor growth, the dissecting skill of the surgeon, and the nutritional status of the patient.[30] Clearly, this issue is far from resolved. However, there is some evidence that blood transfusion is an independent risk factor for postoperative infectious complications.[31]

Hypothermia is a common problem in patients undergoing major abdominal surgery, especially in the geriatric population, as the elderly are often frail, have a lower metabolic rate, and have little subcutaneous fat. Elderly patients have also been shown to become more hypothermic during surgery and to take longer to rewarm postoperatively. This may be due to failure to trigger thermoregulatory responses.[32]

Carcinoma of the Prostate

Adenocarcinoma of the prostate is the most common cancer in men over age 60. In the United States, radical prostatectomy is the preferred mode of therapy for localized stages.[33] The most common intraoperative problem is bleeding and rectal injury. Large-bore intravenous cannulae and appropriate invasive hemodynamic monitoring should be utilized. Either epidural or general anesthesia is acceptable, or a combination of both with postoperative epidural patient-controlled analgesia may be useful. Many studies have been performed comparing general and regional anesthesia during major surgical procedures. Yeager and colleagues[34] demonstrated a reduced incidence of postoperative complications, cardiac failure, and infectious complications in "high-risk" surgical patients when epidural anesthesia and postoperative analgesia were utilized.

These patients appear to be excellent candidates for predeposit autologous blood donation. However, it has been demonstrated that there is no difference in the rate of tumor recurrence or death after radical prostatectomy when allogeneic transfusion is compared with autologous transfusion.[35]

Head and Neck Tumors

The occurrence of carcinomas of the head and neck is directly related to the use of tobacco and alcohol, and those substances act synergistically in increasing the risk for such cancers, especially oropharyngeal and laryngeal cancers.[36]

Furthermore, elderly cancer patients with head and neck tumors are candidates for major reconstructive surgical procedures.[37] The anesthesiologist must preoperatively evaluate these patients for airway compromise and for cardiac, pulmonary, and nutritional status. These patients are commonly malnourished and dehydrated.

Surgical procedures in head and neck cancer range from panendoscopy to major resections with free flap reconstruction. An elderly patient undergoing panendoscopy is especially at risk for myocardial ischemia secondary to reflex sympathetic stimulation.[38] The anesthesiologist must prevent this from occurring through the use of adequate depth of anesthesia and other pharmacologic interventions.

The evaluation of the airway starts with a thorough history and physical examination, including indirect laryngoscopy and appropriate radiological evaluation. Dyspnea and stridor are hallmarks of severe respiratory obstruction. They may be preceded by hoarseness, dysphagia, odynophagia, and speech disturbances.[39]

Every patient with upper airway tumors or obstruction should be considered a difficult intubation. This can be compounded, however, if the patient has had previous surgery or radiation therapy. Endotracheal intubation by conventional laryngoscopy may be impossible because the fibrosis secondary to radiation results in an immobile larynx and epiglottis. Furthermore, radiation therapy can result in airway edema and trismus. One must be aware of the potential for an unrecognized difficult airway even when no tumor is currently present.

Patients with large friable tumors of the base of the tongue or larynx should be taken to the operating room, where tracheostomy can be performed with appropriate hemodynamic monitoring, oxygenation, and judicious use of sedation and local anesthetics. This procedure also requires proper lighting, sterile conditions, appropriate instruments, and proper patient positioning. Any attempt at induction of general anesthesia may result in complete airway obstruction. Furthermore, attempts at oral endotracheal intubation with a conventional laryngoscope may precipitate total loss of the airway from swelling or hemorrhage. Selected patients may be intubated awake, using a fiberoptic laryngoscope, if conditions permit. This technique is particularly suitable for patients who have already undergone surgery for head and neck tumors or have undergone radiation therapy to the head and neck, where intubation may be difficult even when the airway is not compromised. General anesthesia may be induced only after the airway has been secured and ventilation has been verified by positive end-tidal CO_2 and bilateral chest movement. Communication with the surgeon and advanced planning are essential if disaster is to be averted.

The relation between perioperative blood transfusion, infection, and tumor recurrence is currently being investigated, with the initial results being inconclusive.[40] It has been concluded, however, that the use of predonated autologous blood is a reasonable option for the majority of patients with head and neck tumors.[41]

CHEMOTHERAPY TOXICITY AND ANESTHESIA

Cancer care consists of three modalities: chemotherapy, surgery, and radiation. Surgery has made the largest advances in cancer practice based on an understanding of the aging process.[42] However, with the increasing incidence of malignancies in patients over age 65, physicians need to make decisions about chemotherapy treatment regimens for the elderly.[43] Recent studies have shown that older patients with solid cancers can be treated with chemotherapy as successfully as can younger patients. The response, remission, and survival are similar for older and younger cancer patients. This may not be true for hematologic malignancies in which intensive therapy is poorly tolerated in older patients who have a more limited ability to withstand myelosuppression and the end-organ toxicities of standard induction regimens. The use of hematopoietic growth factors may play a role in allowing the safe delivery of such treatment to elderly cancer patients.[44] This is discussed, along with other individual chemotherapy agents, in this section. It is generally felt that malignancies responsive to chemotherapy should be treated with the same regimens in elderly and younger patients, but with doses adjusted for organ function.[45] The aging process is highly individualized and cannot be defined by chronological landmarks. Therefore, there is no reason to exclude an elderly patient from proper chemotherapy treatment on the basis of age alone.[43] In fact, arbitrary dose reductions in an elderly patient may have a negative impact on survival.[46] In this section, various chemotherapy agents and their toxicities in elderly patients are discussed (Table 12-4).

Alkylating Agents

First introduced in the 1940s, these agents are still being used today. They include cyclophosphamide (Cytoxan), mechlorethamine (nitrogen mustard), busulfan, melphalan, chlorambucil (Leukeran), and ifosfamide. These agents work throughout the cell cycle by bonding to the nucleic acids and inhibiting mitosis. They are particularly useful in treating lymphoma, breast carcinoma, ovarian carcinoma, melanoma, and multiple myeloma. These agents cause a rapid destruction of tumor mass, which can then lead to an increase in purine and pyrimidine breakdown products. Uric acid nephropathy is a common toxicity.[47] Patients, particularly the elderly with preexisting kidney dysfunction, must be hydrated during therapy. Allopurinol is administered routinely, along with alkalization of their urine. The dose-limiting toxicity of these agents is severe bone marrow suppression, resulting in anemia, agranulocytosis, and thrombocytopenia. It usually occurs during therapy and resolves within a few months. This can be quite serious in the elderly, who have a limited ability to withstand this intense myelosuppression. Growth factors have been tried in these circumstances.[44] Busulfan, chlorambucil, melphalan, and cyclophosphamide have been associated with pulmonary toxicity in all age groups. The exact mechanism is unknown; however, a direct effect on pulmonary epithelial

Table 12-4 Toxicities associated with chemotherapy

Agent	Major toxicity
Cyclophosphamide (Cytoxan)	Myelosuppression, hemorrhagic cystitis, water retention, pulmonary fibrosis, plasma cholinesterase inhibition
Nitrogen mustard (mechlorethamine)	Myelosuppression, local tissue damage
Vincristine	Neurotoxicity, dilutional hyponatremia
Vinblastine	Myelosuppression
Methotrexate	Renal tubular injury
5-Fluorouracil and Ara-C	Hemorrhagic enteritis, diarrhea myelosuppression
Adriamycin	Cardiac toxicity
Bleomycin	Pulmonary toxicity
Mitomycin C	Pulmonary toxicity
Cisplatin	Renal toxicity, neurotoxicity
Nitroureas (BCNU, CCNU)	Myelosuppression, renal and pulmonary toxicity
Taxol	Hypersensitivity reaction, myelosuppression, cardiac and peripheral neuropathy
Interferon and IL-2	Immune deficiency syndrome
Growth factors	Pulmonary edema, pericardial and pleural effusions

cells resulting in alveolar fibrosis is involved. The symptoms start with a nonproductive cough, dyspnea, and cyanosis and can lead to lung fibrosis and death. Discontinuation of therapy at the first signs is essential. While this will not reverse the process, it should provide stabilization. These patients will always have compromised lung function, and this must be determined by pulmonary function studies before the delivery of an anesthetic. Cyclophosphamide, one of the most commonly used chemotherapy agents, can be given orally as well as intravenously. Nausea, vomiting, and alopecia are the typical toxicities seen with this agent. Inappropriate water retention resulting from a direct effect on renal tubules can, if severe enough, lead to hyponatremia, seizures, and coma.[48] This agent is excreted in the urine, and its metabolites are active. Hemorrhagic cystitis often results, requiring surgical coagulation.[49] When these patients present for surgery and anesthesia, an important consideration is the ability of cyclophosphamide to inhibit plasma cholinesterase.[50,51] This, of course, can lead to prolongation of the depolarizing muscle relaxant effects.

Nitrogen mustard is not commonly used today, except in isolated limb perfusion for metastatic malignant melanoma.[52] This technique involves the perfusion of the chemotherapy agent directly into the arterial circulation of the affected limb. The arterial inflow tract and the venous outflow tract are cannulated, and, via an extracorporeal pump, the perfusion is controlled for an exact period of time. The advantage of this technique is that it concentrates the chemotherapy agent in the affected limb and limits the amount that enters the general circulation. However, there is always a small leak, depending on the surgical ability to isolate the limb. It is important to stabilize pump flow before starting the chemotherapy agent or an overdose could be given. General anesthesia is generally used because of the length of the procedure, and if there is a considerable leak, systemic toxicity can be severe. Tumor necrosis factor is also being tried for this technique.

Plant Alkaloids

Vincristine sulfate (Oncovin) and vinblastine (Velban) are the two important agents in this class. They arrest mitosis by binding to microtubules in the cell. They are most useful in the treatment of testicular carcinoma, sarcoma, Hodgkin's and non-Hodgkin's lymphoma, and some leukemias. Myelosuppression is the major toxicity of vinblastine, with a few reports of neurotoxicity.[53] Vincristine, by contrast, is associated with progressive and disabling neurotoxicity. This occurs mostly in the elderly and those with preexisting neuromuscular disorders. A glove-and-stocking sensory and motor peripheral neuropathy results. Decreasing deep tendon reflexes, peripheral parathesias, ataxia, and foot drop are common. These effects can be permanent and can lead to muscle wasting and incapacitation. The amount of muscle wasting can be of concern with the administration of succinycholine and the development of hyperkalemia. Vincristine has also been associated with stimulation of antidiuretic hormone secretion and the development of dilutional hyponatremia.[54]

Antimetabolites

Methotrexate, 5 fluorouracil (5-FU), and cytarabine (cytosine arabinoside; Ara-C) are the agents most frequently used in this class. They are structural analogues of normal cellular metabolites and are therefore accepted by the cell as substrate and interfere with function. They are used in the treatment of gastrointestinal and pulmonary carcinomas, sarcomas, and some leukemias. Bone marrow suppression, severe diarrhea, nausea, and vomiting are their major toxicities. Ara-C and 5-FU can cause a wide range of pathological changes in the gastrointestinal tract, from superficial ulcerations to hemorrhagic enteritis and perforation.[55] Methotrexate is associated with renal tubular damage in 10 percent of the general population, and this number rises even higher in elderly patients with preexisting renal dysfunction. A rising blood urea nitrogen (BUN) and creatinine with a decreasing urinary volume are often encountered. Hydration and urine alkalization constitute an important treatment initiated routinely with high-dose methotrexate therapy. However, in the elderly, high-dose therapy is not recommended.[46] Methotrexate has also been implicated in causing an obstructive nephropathy because of its precipitation in the renal calyx. Hepatotoxicity has also been reported with these agents.[56] An advantage seen with these agents is that they can be used intrathecally to control CNS metastasis; however, a rise in CNS pressure may result during therapy or immediately after completion. This needs to be evaluated before anesthesia.

Antibiotics

This class of chemotherapy agents contains the most potent agents as well as the most toxic, particularly in the elderly. Included in this class are bleomycin, mitomycin C, and the anthracyclines, doxorubicin hydrochloride (Adriamycin) and daunorubicin (Cerubidin). These compounds form stable complexes with DNA and thus inhibit DNA and RNA synthesis.

The anthracyclines are used in the treatment of lymphomas and solid tumors such as breast, lung, thyroid, and ovarian tumors. Cardiac toxicity is their dose-limiting toxicity. This occurs in two phases: acute and chronic. The acute phase can occur hours to days after the initiation of treatment and is unrelated to the dose. The incidence is increased with preexisting cardiac disease, and the elderly therefore, are at a higher risk. This can be manifested as mild and transient electrocardiographic (ECG) changes or overt pump failure. Acute decreases in ejection fraction on gated pool studies within 24 to 48 h have been reported.[57,58] The ECG changes are usually benign nonspecific changes in 10 percent of patients, ranging from supraventricular tachyarrhythmias, heart block, and ventricular arrhythmias to simply decreased QRS voltage.[57] These changes usually resolve 1 to 2 months after therapy. The chronic form of anthracycline-induced cardiac toxicity is a dose-dependent chronic cardiomyopathy that leads to congestive heart failure in 2 to 10 percent of patients. Once the toxic process begins, it is irreversible in 59 percent of patients because of focal cell death and biventricular failure. Table 12-5 lists the risk factors associated with this toxicity, with age over 65 years being one of them. Endocardial biopsy is used to make the definitive diagnosis. Vacuolar degeneration, coalescence of the sarcotubular system with myofibrillar loss, and mitochondrial damage in the heart are seen on biopsy.[59] The exact mechanism is unclear; however, oxygen free radical formation seems to be involved. Heart tissue is low in an essential enzyme, catalase, that is used to break down free radicals. It has been theorized that these free radicals injure the myocardium, causing dilatation of the sarcoplasmic reticulum and a buildup of calcium in the myocytes that results in profound pump failure. Calcium chelators and free radical scavengers have been used with varying success.[60] Patients receiving anthracycline therapy are routinely followed by echocardiography and/or radionucleide cardioangiography. Serial ejection fractions are sensitive indicators of myocardial damage, while echocardiography shows early diastolic dysfunction.[58] Preoperative evaluation of these patients should include a complete cardiac workup and comparison with prechemotherapy function. Patients with damaged myocardium resulting from anthracycline therapy require full hemodynamic monitoring, as would be appropriate with other idiopathic cardiomyopathies. These patients seem to do better with an anesthetic technique that provides a low systemic vascular resistance.[61]

Bleomycin is used primarily in the treatment of testicular carcinoma, sarcomas, and carcinomas of the esophagus and lung. Its mechanism of action is to produce single- and double-stranded breaks in the DNA molecule. After bleomycin binds to DNA, the ferrous ion on the bleomycin undergoes oxidation to the ferric state and the electron that is liberated is accepted by oxygen, forming superoxide and oxygen free radicals.[62] The amount of radicals formed determines the anticancer activity as well as the drug's toxicity. The main toxicity of bleomycin is pulmonary, and it is dose-limiting. Table 12-5 lists the risk factors associated with pulmonary toxicity, and again, age over 65 is important. Pulmonary complications develop in 5 to 10 percent of bleomycin-treated patients and occur in two forms: an acute and a chronic pneumonitis. Some patients progress to pulmonary fibrosis and death. A nonproductive cough, dyspnea, and fever are the first symptoms, the onset of which can be delayed for up to 4 to 10 weeks after therapy. Pulmonary function studies, including diffusion capacity, should be done before the initiation of therapy and should be routinely followed for signs of developing interstitial damage. The decrease in diffusion capacity is the best and earliest predictor of bleomycin toxicity, which would require the discontinuation of therapy.[63] Once the process has started, the chest x-ray will show bibasilar pulmonary infiltrates that can mimic other infectious processes. An open lung biopsy is often required for definitive diagnosis. The lung is the target organ for toxicity because it is rich in the essential substrate oxygen and low in the enzyme bleomycin hydrolase, a metabolic deactivator. In a normal lung, the type 2 pneumocytes act as free radical scavengers. However, in a bleomycin lung, they are overwhelmed and cannot respond.[64,65] There is then a proliferation of alveolar macrophages that eventually cause lung fibrosis. The bleomycin must be discontinued at the first sign to prevent further damage. The use of corticosteriods has been recommended. For the anesthesiologist, the amount of lung damage that has occurred needs to be assessed preoperatively. The issue of oxygen toxicity in patients receiving bleomycin is a real concern. Numerous animal studies have shown that exposure to increasing oxygen concentrations with bleomycin or after

Table 12-5 Risk factors for antibiotic chemotherapeutic agents

Agent	Adriamycin	Bleomycin
Total cumulative dose	> 550 mg/m^2	> 200 mg
Concomitant therapy	Cyclophosphamides	Thoracic radiation
Age (years)	> 65	> 65
Positive past medical history	Cardiac disease	Lung disease
Increased oxygen concentrations	No	Possibly

bleomycin administration results in an increased incidence of pulmonary toxicity and death.[66,67] Goldiner and colleagues,[68] in a study published in 1978, suggested that the use of intraoperative oxygen concentrations greater than 28% in previously treated bleomycin patients significantly increases their risk of developing adult respiratory distress syndrome. There are numerous studies debating this issue; however, it is recommended that the perioperative oxygen concentration be limited as long as adequate tissue oxygenation can be maintained.

Mitomycin C, another chemotherapy agent in this class, was first introduced in the 1970s. It was found to be active in gastrointestinal, lung, and breast cancer. Its activation involves an enzymatic reduction process that induces lipid peroxidation and forms oxygen free radicals. The activated mitomycin inhibits DNA cellular function, causing cell death. Initially, myelosuppression was its dose-limiting toxicity. However, the pulmonary complications reported, similar to those found in bleomycin patients, are of greater concern.[69,70] Here again the lung is the toxicity target organ as well as the chemotherapy target organ. This is due to the lung's high concentration of NADPH cytochrome P450 reductase (mitomycin's activator) and the availability of oxygen as a substrate. The production of oxygen free radicals causes the pulmonary damage.[71] Unlike bleomycin, this pulmonary toxicity seems to be unrelated to the dose. The clinical presentation is a triad of fever, cough, and dyspnea. Tissue diagnosis is often needed to rule out an infectious process. Corticosteroids have been successful in these patients and should be started at the earliest signs of pulmonary compromise. Prednisone 60 mg a day for 2 to 3 weeks and then tapering over 4 weeks is recommended.[72] Again the anesthesiologist is faced with the oxygen toxicity issue. In the authors' experience, the incidence of postoperative pulmonary complications seen in mitomycin-treated patients is related to the amount of preoperative lung damage. The preoperative diffusion capacity is the best indicator of mitomycin-induced interstitial damage. Ideally, one would like to compare this with the prechemotherapy diffusion capacity to determine if there has been a decrease. In patients with a low diffusion capacity or a decrease after mitomycin, we recommend the use of low oxygen concentrations of less than 28%, if possible, while maintaining adequate oxygenation.

Miscellaneous

In this category are included cisplatin, (cisplatinum), carboplatin (carboplatinum), taxol, and the nitroureas BCNU (carmustine) and CCNU (lomustine).

Cisplatin and carboplatin are heavy metal compounds used in the treatment of testicular carcinoma, bladder carcinoma, head and neck tumors, and other solid tumors. They attack DNA and change its configuration and inhibit its synthesis. Myelosuppression and renal toxicity are their dose-limiting toxicities. Thirty percent of patients receiving cisplatin develop renal toxicity, especially if they are not properly hydrated during therapy. Hydration consists of 1 liter of intravenous fluid before cisplatin treatment and mannitol 25 to 50 g to maintain adequate urinary output.[73] Patients receiving aminoglycosides have an increased risk for the development of renal toxicity.[74] There is a coagulation necrosis of the distal renal tubules and collecting ducts, causing a reduction in renal blood flow and glomerular filtration rate with magnesium and potassium wasting.[75] The magnesium loss can lead to symptomatic tetany. Elderly patients with poor renal function before chemotherapy are particularly sensitive to these agents and must be followed closely. Preoperative BUN and creatinine are good indicators of renal damage and should be checked frequently. Intraoperative fluid management and the maintenance of an adequate urine output are vital. Mannitol is the drug of choice to maintain urine output once intravascular volume has been optimized. Cisplatin has been reported to cause nerve deafness at high doses.

BCNU and CCNU are lipid-soluble and cross the blood-brain barrier. They are used to treat lymphoma, malignant melanoma, brain neoplasm, and gastrointestinal carcinomas. Myelosuppression is their dose-limiting toxicity and can lead to nadir sepsis. The pulmonary toxicity level occurs when doses exceed 1000 mg\m^2. These agents cause direct injury to the pulmonary epithelium and lead to alveolar fibrosis. Renal toxicity is seen when the dose exceeds 1,200 mg\m^2.[76]

Taxol, a relatively new chemotherapy agent, is derived from the bark of the yew tree.[77] It is used primarily in the treatment of breast, lung, and ovarian carcinomas. However, it is under investigation in numerous other cancer treatments and in combination with other agents. Taxol promotes microtubule assembly in the absence of guanosine triphosphate (GTP) and microtubular-associated proteins (MAPs).[78] These tubules accumulate in the cell and disrupt cellular division, leading to cell death. Taxol is highly insoluble and requires a derivative of castor oil and ethylene oxide (Cremophor El) in its formulation. When it was first introduced, there was a 10 percent rate of hypersensitivity-type reactions. However, now taxol is administered over a 24-h period and the patient is premedicated with an antihistamine and corticosteriods to reduce the occurrence of these reactions. The hypersensitivity reaction usually occurs with the first or second dose and has the features of a type 1 hypersensitivity reaction (HSR).[79] Dyspnea, bronchospasm, urticaria, flushing, angioedema, erythematous rash, and hypotension are typical. Treatment with epinephrine, diphenhydramine, and fluids usually aborts further manifestations. The exact cause of this reaction is still unclear, but some feel it involves Cremophor El. As was demonstrated with propofol, which initially was solubilized in Cremophor El, a high incidence of hypersensitivity reactions will occur until the formulation is modified. This toxicity should not affect anesthetic management, since it occurs during treatment. Myelosuppression and peripheral neuropathies are the dose-limiting toxicities. The neutropenia can be severe after high-dose taxol, with counts reaching their nadir in 10 days and returning to normal by 21 days. Surgical procedures should be scheduled after recovery. The peripheral neuropathy is sensory with a glove-and-stocking distribution characterized by numbness and paresthesias. Patients with preexisting neuropathies, such as those from cisplatin, vincristine, and vinblastine, can also develop motor and autonomic dysfunction. Cardiac toxicity has been reported with this agent, characterized by conduction abnormalities such as asymptomatic bradycardia, Mobitz type I and type II, atrioventricular block, third-degree block, and atypical chest pain. This cardiac toxicity must be evaluated preoperatively, especially in an elderly patient with preexisting heart disease. In recent studies, taxol administered in the elderly for the treatment of ovarian carcinoma showed no increased incidence of toxicity and was tolerated well.[80]

Immunotherapy Agents

Interferon and interleukin-2 (IL-2) are used in the treatment of malignant melanoma, renal cell carcinoma, Kaposi's sarcoma, and various leukemias and lymphomas. Interferon is synthesized in normal cells as a response to a viral infection.[81] Theoretically, malignancies induced by a virally mediated change in nucleic acids may respond to interferon. IL-2 is used to activate naturally occurring killer T cells and tumor-infiltrating lymphocytes. Patients undergoing treatment with these agents require intensive care management because of the severe immune deficiency syndromes that develop, along with hypotension, hyperthermia, and sepsis.[82] These complications resolve after therapy and should not pose a problem to the anesthesiologist unless the patient requires emergency surgery during therapy.

Growth Factors

Although not chemotherapeutic agents in themselves, growth factors are being incorporated into most chemotherapy regimens. Severe hematopoietic toxicity is often the dose-limiting factor, especially in elderly patients with a reduced capacity for recovery. The use of G-CSF (granulocyte colony-stimulating factor) and GM-CSF (granulocyte-macrophage colony-stimulating factor) decreases the period of neutropenia, lessening the risk of infection and allowing longer use of higher doses of chemotherapeutic agents.[83] These drugs work by regulating the development of stem cells into erythrocytes, granulocytes, and megakaryocytes. The toxicity seen with these agents is a generalized leaky capillary syndrome that leads to pleural and pericardial effusions.[84]

SUMMARY

The doses, monitoring, and toxicity management of chemotherapeutic agents in the geriatric population are not well defined. Studies reveal conflicting documentation, with some showing increased toxicity while others show no difference with respect to age.[1] It is clear, however, that cancer has an increased prevalence in patients over 65 years of age. It was not until 1989 that the

National Cancer Institute allowed patients over age 70 to be enrolled in its chemotherapy protocols. In the future, anesthesiologists will see more and more elderly patients presenting for surgery who have received or are undergoing chemotherapy treatment. The preoperative evaluation is as important in this patient population as it is in any patient scheduled for surgery. Renal, pulmonary, and cardiac function need to be assessed, with particular emphasis on the type of chemotherapy agent the patient has received and the patient's physiological response to it.[85,86] The anesthetic management needs to take into account the patient's preexisting organ dysfunction as well as the chemotherapy and cancer-related problems.

REFERENCES

1. Kennedy BJ: Specific considerations for the older patient with cancer, in Calabresi P, Schein P (eds): *Medical Oncology*, 2d ed. New York: McGraw-Hill, 1993, pp 1219–1229.
2. Seidman H, Silverberg E, Bodden A: Probabilities of eventually developing and dying of cancers (risk among persons previously undiagnosed with cancer). *Cancer* 28:33, 1978.
3. Hosking MP, Warner MA, Lobdella CM, et al: Outcomes of surgery in patients 90 years of age and older. *JAMA* 261:1909, 1989.
4. Lewis AAM, Khoury GA: Resection of colorectal cancer in the very old: Are the risks too high? *Br Med J* 296:459, 1988.
5. Benton C, Favre JP, Brizon J: Surgery for carcinoma of the colon in people aged 75 years and older. *Int J Color Dis* 5:25, 1990.
6. Miller R, Marlar K, Silvay G: Anesthesia for patients aged over ninety years. *NY State J Med* Aug 1977, p 1421.
7. Daly JM, Wanebo H, DeCosse J: Principles of surgical oncology, in Calabresi P, Schein P (eds): *Medical Oncology*, 2d ed. New York: McGraw-Hill, 1993, p 239.
8. Chung F: Cancer chemotherapy and anesthesia. *Can Anaesth Soc J* 29:4, 1982.
9. Van Hoff DD, Rosencweig M, Picart M: The cardiotoxicity of anticancer agents. *Semin Oncol* 9:1, 1982.
10. Zaret B, Wachers FJ: Medical progress: Nuclear cardiology. *N Engl J Med* 329:855, 1993.
11. Schwartz RG, MacKenzie WB, Alexander J, et al: Congestive heart failure and left ventricular dysfunction complicating doxorubicin therapy: Seven year experience using serial radionuclide angiocardiography. *Am J Med* 82:1109, 1987.
12. Bogeat A, Chirolero R, Baylon P, et al: Perioperative cardiovascular collapse in patients previously treated with doxorubicin. *Anesth Analg* 67:1189, 1988.
13. Groth S, Zaric A, Srensen PB, et al: Regional lung function impairment following postoperative radiotherapy for breast cancer using direct or tangential field techniques. *Br J Radiol* 59:445, 1986.
14. Pierri MK: Heart Disease, in Groeger J (ed): *Critical Care of the Cancer Patient*, 2d ed. St. Louis: Mosby–Year Book, 1991, pp 76–77.
15. Mitchell EP, Glickman AS, Schein PS: Acute and late effects of cancer therapy and their management, in Calabresi P, Schein PS (eds): *Medical Oncology*, 2d ed. New York: McGraw-Hill, 1993, p 347.

16. Applefield MM: Long term cardiovascular evaluation of patients with Hodgkin's disease treated by thoracic mantle radiation therapy. *Cancer Treat Rep* 66:1003, 1992.
17. Fajardo LF, Stewart JR, Cohn KE: Morphology of radiation induced heart disease. *Arch Pathol Lab Med* 86:512, 1968.
18. Bajournas D: Disorders of endocrine function, in Groeger J (ed): *Critical Care of the Cancer Patient.* St. Louis: Mosby–Year Book, 1991, p 193.
19. Theriault RL: Hypercalcemia of malignancy: Pathophysiology and implications for treatment. *Oncology* 7:47, 1993.
20. Warrell RP Jr: Etiology and current management of cancer related hypercalcemia. *Oncology* 6:37, 1992.
21. Thomas CR, Dodhia N: Common emergencies in cancer medicine: Metabolic syndromes. *J Natl Med Assoc* 83:809, 1991.
22. DeDeuxchaisnes CN, Krane SM: Hypoparathyroidism, in Avioli LV, Krane SM (eds): *Metabolic Bone Disease.* New York: Academic Press, 1978, vol 2, pp 417–445.
23. Scheiner E, Isaacs M, Vanamee P: Water and electrolyte disturbances in cancer patients. *Med Clin North Am* 50:711, 1976.
24. Williams AV: Hyponatremia: Manifestations and treatment. *J SC Med Assoc* 88:285, 1992.
25. Kopec I, Groeger J: Life threatening fluid and electrolyte abnormalities associated with cancer. *Crit Care Clin* 4:81, 1988.
26. Lam KS, Kung AW, Young RT: Postirradiation hypopituitarism presenting as severe hyponatremia. *Am J Med* 2:219, 1992.
27. Flombaum CD: Electrolyte and renal abnormalities, in Groeger J (ed): *Critical Care of the Cancer Patient.* St. Louis: Mosby–Year Book, 1991, p 150.
28. Kennedy BJ: Aging and cancer, in Balducci L, Lyman G, Erschler WB (eds): *Geriatric Oncology.* Philadelphia: Lippincott, 1992, p 4.
29. Wiig JN: Blood transfusion in cancer of the colon and rectum: Friend or foe of the surgeon? A review. *Tidsskr Norske Laegeforening* 110:503, 1990.
30. Busch ORC, Hop WCJ, Hoynck van Papendrecht MAW, et al: Blood transfusions and prognosis in colorectal cancer. *N Engl J Med* 328:1372, 1993.
31. Tarlten PI: Blood transfusions and infectious complications following colorectal surgery. *Br J Surg* 75:789, 1988.
32. Kurz A, Plattner O, Sessler D, et al: The threshold for thermoregulatory vasoconstriction during nitrous oxide/isoflurane anesthesia is lower in elderly than in young patients. *Anesthesiology* 79:465, 1993.
33. Adjiman S, Zerbib M, Conquy S, et al: Morbidity of radical prostatectomy for localized cancer of the prostate. *J D Urologie* 98:73, 1992.
34. Yeager MP, Glass DD, Neff RK, et al: Epidural anesthesia and analgesia in high risk surgical patients. *Anesthesiology* 66:729, 1987.
35. Baldwin ML, Piantadosi S: Prostate cancer recurrence in radical surgery in patients receiving autologous or homologous blood. *Transfusion* 32:31, 1992.
36. Maier H, Dietz A, Gewelke U: Tobacco and alcohol and the risk of head and neck cancer. *Clin Invest* 70:320, 1992.
37. Sanders AD, Blom ED, Singer MI: Reconstructive and rehabilitative aspects of head and neck cancer in the elderly. *Otolaryngol Clin North Am* 23:1159, 1990.
38. Golden KJ: Anesthetic considerations in head and neck cancer, in Myers EN, Suen JY (eds): *Cancer of the Head and Neck*, 2d ed. New York: Churchill Livingstone, 1989, pp 145–157.
39. Kross R: Perioperative considerations, in Groeger J (ed): *Critical Care of the Cancer Patient*, 2d ed. St. Louis: Mosby–Yearbook, 1991, pp 324–328.

40. Von Doersten P, Cruz RM, Selby JV, Hilsinger RL Jr: Transfusion recurrence, and infection in head and neck cancer surgery. *Otolaryngol-Head Neck Surg* 106:60, 1992.
41. McColloch TM, Glenn MG, Riley D, et al: Blood use in head and neck tumor surgery: Potential for autologous blood. *Arch Otolaryngol Head Neck Surg* 115:1314, 1989.
42. Derby SE: Ageism in cancer care of the elderly. *Oncol Nurs Forum* 18:921, 1991.
43. Chevallier B, Monnier A, Metz R, et al: Phase II study of oral idarubicin in elderly patients with advanced breast cancer. *Am J Clin Oncol* 13:436, 1990.
44. Stone RM, Mayer RJ: The approach to the elderly patient with acute myeloid leukemia. *Hematol Oncol Clin North Am* 7:65, 1993.
45. Begg CB, Carbone PP: Clinical trials and drug toxicity in the elderly: The experience of the Eastern Cooperative Oncology Group. *Cancer* 52:1986, 1983.
46. Hutchins LF, Lipschitz DA: Cancer, clinical pharmacology, and aging. *Clin Geriatr Med* 3:483, 1987.
47. Rundles RW, Wyngaarden JB, Hitchings GH, Elion GB: Drugs and uric acid. *Ann Rev Pharmacol Toxicol* 6:345, 1969.
48. Green TP, Mirkin BL: Prevention of cyclophosphamide-induced antidiuresis by furosimide infusion. *Clin Pharmacol Ther* 29:634, 1981.
49. Cox PJ: Cyclophosphamide cystitis: Identification of acrolein as the causative agent. *Biochem Pharmacol* 28:2045, 1979.
50. Gruman GM: Prolonged apnea after succinylcholine in a case treated with cytostatics for cancer. *Anesth Analg* 51:761, 1972.
51. Zsigmond EK, Robins G: The effects of a series of anticancer drugs on plasma cholinesterase activity. *Can Anaesth Soc J* 19:75, 1972.
52. Coit DG: Hyperthermic isolation limb perfusion for malignant melanoma: A review. *Cancer Invest* 10:277, 1992.
53. Miller BR: Neurotoxicity and vincristine. *JAMA* 253:2045, 1985.
54. Robertson GL, Bhoopalam N, Zelkowitz LJ: Vincristine neurotoxicity and abnormal secretion of antidiuretic hormone. *Arch Intern Med* 132:717, 1973.
55. Selvin BL: Cancer chemotherapy: Implications for the anesthesiologist. *Anesth Analg* 60:450, 1981.
56. Desiderio DP: Anesthetic-antineoplastic drug interactions. *Semin Anesth* 12:68, 1992.
57. Jones SE, Ewy GA, Grove BM: Electrocardiographic detection of adriamycin heart disease. *Proc Am Soc Clin Oncol* 16:228, 1975.
58. Myers CE, Chabner BA: Anthracyclines, in Chabner BA, Collins JM (eds): *Cancer Chemotherapy: Principles and Practice.* Philadelphia: Lippincott, 1990, pp 356–381.
59. Bacon DR, Nuzzo RJ: Anthracycline antineoplastic chemotherapy agents: Anesthetic implications. *Semin Anesth* 12:74, 1993.
60. Kantrowitz NE, Bristow MR: Cardiotoxicity of antitumor agents. *Prog Cardiovasc Dis* 27:195, 1984.
61. Thorne AC, Orazem JP, Shah NK, et al: Isoflurane versus fentanyl: Hemodynamic effects in cancer patients treated with anthracyclines. *J Cardiothorac Vasc Anesth* 7:307, 1993.
62. Sikic BI: Biochemical and cellular determinants of bleomycin cytotoxicity. *Cancer Surv* 5:81, 1986.
63. Sorensen PG, Rossing N, Rorth M: Carbon monoxide diffusing capacity: A reliable indicator of bleomycin-induced pulmonary toxicity. *Eur J Respir Dis* 66:333, 1985.
64. Goad MEP, Tryka AF, Witschi HP: Acute respiratory failure induced by bleomycin

and hyperoxia: Pulmonary edema, cell kinetics, and morphology. *Toxicol Appl Pharmacol* 90:10, 1987.
65. Goldiner PL, Shamsi A: Bleomycin-oxygen interaction. *Semin Anesth* 12:79, 1993.
66. Toledo CH, Ross WE, Hood CI, Block ER: Potentiation of bleomycin toxicity by oxygen. *Cancer Treat Rep* 66:359, 1982.
67. Sogal RN, Gottlieb AA, Boutros AR, et al: Effects of oxygen on bleomycin-induced lung damage. *Cleve Clin J Med* 54:503, 1987.
68. Goldiner PL, Carlon GC, Cvitkovic E, et al: Factors influencing postoperative morbidity and mortality in patients treated with bleomycin. *Br Med J* 1:1664, 1978.
69. Doyle LA, Ihde DC, Carney DN, et al: Combination of chemotherapy with doxorubicin and mitomycin c in non-small cell bronchogenic carcinoma. *Am J Clin Oncol* 7:719, 1984.
70. Buzdar AU, Legha SS, Luna MA, et al: Pulmonary toxicity of mitomycin. *Cancer* 45:236, 1980.
71. Pritsos CA, Sartorelli AC: Generation of reactive oxygen radicals through bioactivation of mitomycin antibiotics. *Cancer Res* 46:3528, 1986.
72. Chang AY, Kuebler JP, Pandya KJ, et al: Pulmonary toxicity induced by mitomycin c is highly responsive to glucocorticoids. *Cancer* 57:2285, 1986.
73. Midias NE, Harrington JT: Platinum nephrotoxicity. *Am J Med* 65:307, 1978.
74. Gonzales-Vitale JC, Hayes DM, Cvitkovic E, Sternberg SS: Acute renal failure after cis-dichlorodiammineplatinum (II) and gentamycin-cephalothin therapies. *Cancer Treat Rep* 62:693, 1978.
75. Schilsky RL, Anderson T: Hypomagnesemia and renal magnesium wasting in patients receiving cisplatinum. *Ann Intern Med* 90:929, 1979.
76. Colvin M, Chabner BA: Alkylating agents, in Chabner BA, Collins JM (eds): *Cancer Chemotherapy: Principles and Practice.* Philadelphia: Lippincott, 1990, pp 276–313.
77. Slichenmyer WJ, Von Hoff DD: Taxol: A new and effective anti-cancer drug. *Anticancer Drugs* 2:519, 1991.
78. Hawkins MJ: New anticancer agents: Taxol, campotothecin analogs, and anthrapyrazoles. *Oncology* 6:17, 1992.
79. Weiss RB: Hypersensitivity reactions. *Semin Oncol* 19:458, 1992.
80. Bicher A, Sarosy GH, Kohn E, et al: Age does not influence taxol dose intensity in recurrent carcinoma of the ovary. *Cancer* 71:594, 1993.
81. Chabner BA, Myers CE: Clinical pharmacology of cancer chemotherapy, in Devita VT, Hellman S, Rosenberg SA (eds): *Cancer Principles and Practice of Oncology.* Philadelphia: Lippincott, 1989, pp 349–395.
82. Scott GM, Secher DS, Flowers D, et al: Toxicity of interferone. *Br Med J* 282:1345, 1981.
83. Krakoff IH: Cancer chemotherapeutic and biologic agents. *CA* 41:264, 1991.
84. Tobias JD, Furman WL: Anesthetic considerations in patients receiving colony-stimulating factors (G-CSF and GM-CSF). *Anesthesiology* 75:536, 1991.
85. Desiderio DP, Kross R, Bedford RF: Evaluation of the patient with oncologic disease, in Rogers MC, Tinker JH, Covino BG, Longnecker DE (eds): *Principles and Practice of Anesthesiology.* St. Louis: Mosby–Year Book, 1992, pp 377–394.
86. Desiderio DP: Cancer chemotherapy: Complications and interactions with anesthesia. *Hosp Form* 25:176, 1990.

CHAPTER 13

Cardiac Anesthesia for Geriatric Patients

Robert D. Lyons
Joseph J. Naples

INTRODUCTION

Atherosclerotic heart disease is the most prevalent cardiac disease among the aged and is responsible for more than two-thirds of all cardiac deaths in the elderly population.[1] Although significant advances have been made in the medical and surgical management of ischemic heart disease, it remains a predominant cause of mortality in the United States. It is inevitable that elderly patients will continue to form an increasing proportion of the cardiac surgical caseload (Fig. 13-1). People over age 65 constitute the fastest growing age group in the United States. The growth of the group that includes those age 85 years and older has been especially rapid, increasing almost 30 percent between 1980 and 1988.[2] Although coronary heart disease has declined in those age 65 and older since 1968, utilization of hospital services for the treatment of cardiovascular disease has increased. In 1992, people 65 years or older accounted for 63 percent of hospital discharges for heart and cerebrovascular disease.[3]

Although risk factors have remained constant, the profile of patients who require cardiac surgery is changing. In recent years, a greater percentage of patients are in the older age group and are at considerably higher risk (Fig. 13-2). Cardiac surgery in the elderly is in itself high-risk because so many patients have concomitant systemic disease and other disabilities. Because of advanced age and potentially serious concomitant organ dysfunction, the early

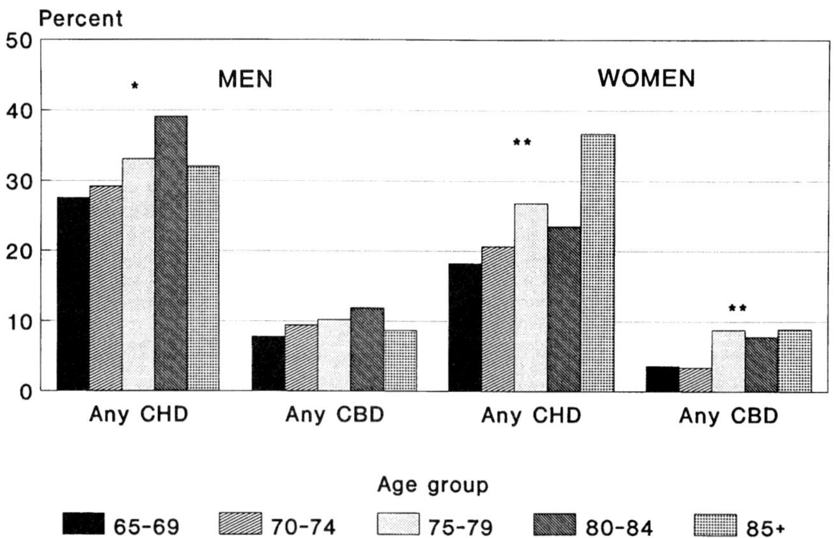

Figure 13-1 Prevalence of coronary heart disease (CAD) and cerebrovascular disease (CBD) among men and women in five age groups.
*$p<0.005$ **$p<0.0001$. CHD = coronary heart disease. CBD = cerebrovascular disease. (*Reprinted with permission from Bild DE, Fitzpatrick A, Fried IP, et al: Age-related trends in cardiovascular morbidity and physical functioning in the elderly: The cardiovascular health study. J Am Geriatr Soc 41:1054, 1993.*)

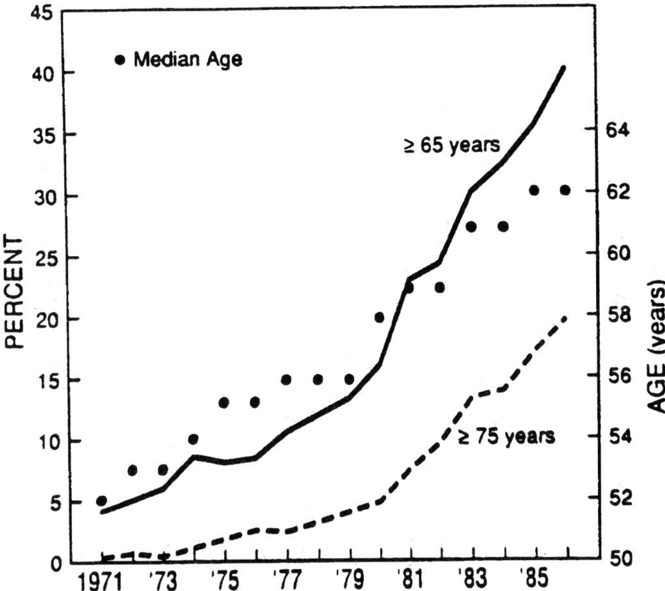

Figure 13-2 Aging of the cardiac surgery population at the Cleveland Clinic from 1971 to 1986. (*Reprinted with permission from Loop FD, Lytle BW, Cosgrove DM, et al: Coronary artery bypass graft surgery in the elderly. Cleve Clin J Med 55:23, 1988.*)

and late risk of coronary artery bypass graft (CABG) surgery and the overall efficacy of the operation in these patients have been questioned.[4] These questions are even more relevant in economic terms because of a potential funding crisis in the health care system.

The extraordinary growth of interventional cardiology has also influenced the type of patient being considered for bypass surgery. The use of percutaneous transluminal coronary angioplasty (PTCA) in the elderly is somewhat controversial because of the associated increased risk of morbidity and mortality.[5] Acute ischemic events complicating elective angioplasty in the elderly (>80 years) have been reported in up to 19 percent of patients, considerably higher than in younger age groups. However, the incidence of acute ischemic events in carefully chosen patients age 70 to 79 years is near that of younger patients. Fatal outcomes with PTCA in patients older than 65 years are much more common than they are in younger patients. As the use of PTCA continues to evolve, it is contributing to the number of high-risk patients undergoing surgical revascularization in that lower-risk patients are removed as candidates for CABG. The PTCA procedure itself results in emergency operation in about 5 percent of cases.[6]

Thrombolytic therapy in acute myocardial infarction has been shown to reduce mortality. Several large trials of thrombolytic therapy have included the elderly and have demonstrated a reduction in short-term mortality in this group.[7] Although the elderly are at an increased risk for intracerebral bleeding compared with younger patients, other disease states, such as hypertension, diabetes, and cerebrovascular disease, must be taken into account. Age should no longer be a criterion for excluding patients from thrombolytic therapy.

The decision to proceed with elective cardiac surgery or to continue medical therapy in elderly patients depends on the immediate and long-term benefits of the therapeutic options. Concern over rising operative mortality rates prompted a large risk assessment study by the Veterans Administration. The overall operative mortality rate in this study was 4.8 percent. Risk factors associated with a twofold or greater increase in operative mortality included ejection fraction less than 20 percent, emergency surgery, cardiac reoperation, forced expiratory volume less than 1.25 liters, and age over 80 years.[8] Substantial improvements in surgical technique, cardiac anesthesia, cardioplegic protection, and intensive care have made cardiac surgery a reasonable treatment modality in selected elderly patients. High-risk patients older than 65 years in the Coronary Artery Surgery Study (CASS) had a greater improvement in survival rate and greater freedom from chest pain with surgical than with medical management.[9] A recent report compared outcomes in four age groups of patients undergoing myocardial revascularization and found that patients age 60 and older had the greatest improvement in quality of life[10] (Fig. 13-3).

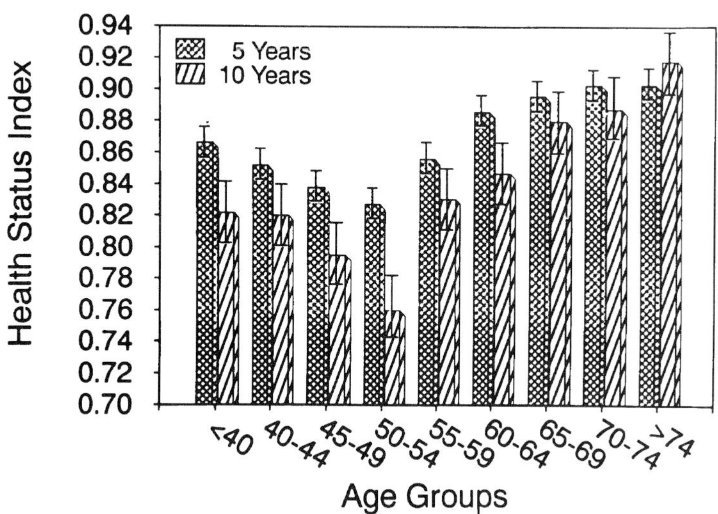

Figure 13-3 **Quality of life for age groups. Mean health status index data for years 1 to 5 and years 6 to 10 for age groups at 5-year intervals. Patients requiring associated valve replacement and those with preoperative cardiogenic shock are excluded. Data include information from surviving patients only. $p < 0.001$ by analysis of variance for data at 5 and 10 years.** (*Reprinted with permission from Carey JS, Cukingnan RA, Singer LKM: Quality of life after myocardial revascularization. J Thorac Cardiovasc Surg 103:108, 1992.*)

CARDIOVASCULAR PHYSIOLOGY

The changes in cardiac function that occur with aging may potentiate disease-related impairment of cardiac performance (Table 13-1). An increase in vascular stiffness leads to increased impedance to left ventricular ejection, prolongation of the cardiac contraction and relaxation times, decreased catecholamine responsiveness, and decreased myocardial compliance. No age-related changes occur in resting cardiac output (CO) or ejection fraction. Even with vigorous exercise, CO is not altered with age. However, there are age-related increases in end-diastolic volume and stroke volume, emphasizing the dependence of the increase in stroke volume on diastolic filling. There is an age-related decrease in exercise heart rate and exercise ejection fraction.[11] This decrease in intrinsic heart rate with aging is independent of physical activity. However, maximal oxygen uptake in elderly sedentary individuals is from 10 to 20 percent lower than that in the physically active elderly. These changes of aging, as well as the decrease in maximal oxygen uptake, decrease the functional reserve capacity of the heart and result in a diminished capacity for work and a lessened ability to tolerate a variety of stresses. The resting filling pressures of the heart are not altered with aging, but there is an accentuated pressure rise with exercise or stress as an adjustment to decreased myocardial wall distensibility. This change, combined with the increase in left ventricular mass with aging, places the elderly heart at a mechanical disadvantage. The increased filling pressure with exercise compensates for the decrease in myocardial compliance and enables the ventricles to increase their stroke volume.[12] Nevertheless, the ejection fraction may decrease with exercise in elderly subjects even in the absence of heart disease. The rate of early diastolic filling may decrease as much as 50 percent with aging, reflecting decreased ventricular compliance. The increased late diastolic filling mediated by atrial contraction helps preserve overall diastolic function. Elderly people are less able to tolerate fluid loads and are therefore predisposed to congestive heart failure (CHF).

PREOPERATIVE ASSESSMENT

The clinical assessment of an elderly patient with coronary artery disease (CAD) is often limited by the coexistence of diseases that make the interpre-

Table 13-1 Changes in cardiac parameters with increasing age

Increase	Decrease
LVEDP	Stroke volume
Pulmonary artery pressure (PAP)	Maximum heart rate
Exercise PCWP	CO
Dysrhythmia incidence	Sinus node cell number
Left ventricular wall thickness	Sinus node atropine response

tation of symptoms difficult. There may be an age-associated decline in physical activity to the point where ischemic symptoms are not present. In addition, dyspnea rather than pain may be the most prominent feature during anginal attacks. Transient features associated with acute ischemia (S_4 gallop, systolic murmur of mitral regurgitation) are often present in the elderly even in the absence of ischemia.

Drug Therapy

Elderly patients with cardiovascular disease are often on chronic therapy for myocardial disease in addition to other concomitant disease processes. Ischemic heart disease, CHF, and hypertension all may require chronic therapy. In addition, many of the elderly may require additional medications for coexisting disease states such as diabetes mellitus and chronic renal failure. Patients with one or more organ systems approaching the critical threshold are at an increased risk for adverse drug reactions. Older patients also have altered pharmacodynamic and pharmacokinetic responses to many drugs. A minimal blood level of a drug may be enough to cause an undesired side effect before the therapeutic level is reached.

Most antianginal drugs affect the balance between myocardial oxygen supply and demand (Fig. 13-4). A patient with CAD is prone to the development of myocardial ischemia, which may lead to an adverse cardiac outcome, such as myocardial infarction (MI), cardiac dysfunction, heart failure, or dysrhythmias. Coronary stenoses are dynamic conditions that are altered by hypoxia, hypotension, neural influences, and other perioperative stresses. Ischemic events may or may not be hemodynamically related. If myocardial oxygen demand outstrips limited myocardial oxygen supply, ischemia may ensue. The determinants of myocardial oxygen demand are well known and include wall tension (directly related to ventricular radius and intracavitary pressure), heart rate, and contractility. However, control of these factors may not be adequate to

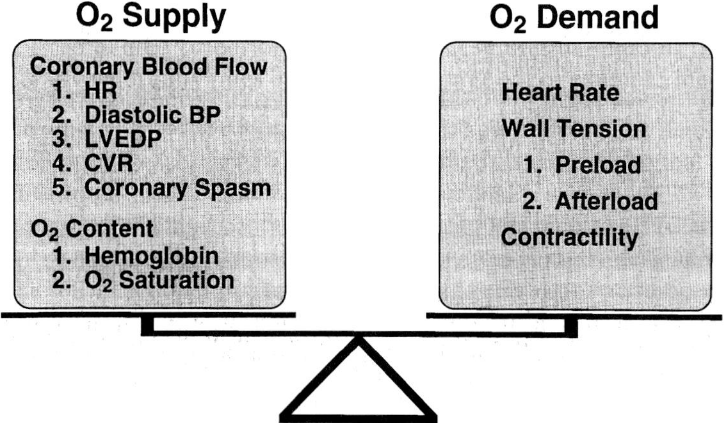

Figure 13-4 Myocardial oxygen balance.

prevent myocardial ischemia. There is an increasing body of evidence that shows that myocardial ischemia may be related to decreased coronary blood flow and oxygen supply. Critical factors governing oxygen supply to the myocardium include factors that modify coronary blood flow, including perfusion pressure, diastolic time, coronary vascular tone, and obstructions in the coronary vessels. The oxygen content of course must be maintained. Hypotension, coronary vasospasm, and acute thrombosis may all decrease coronary blood flow and therefore limit oxygen delivery to the myocardium.

In patients with cardiovascular disease presenting for cardiac surgery, the more common preoperative chronic medications include antihypertensive agents, nitrates, beta-blockers, calcium channel blockers, diuretics, and digitalis. In general, most of these agents are continued up to and including the day of surgery. Exceptions could be diuretics and digitalis preparations.

Nitroglycerin (NTG) primarily reduces wall tension and increases regional blood flow through coronary vasodilation. Venodilation reduces venous return, resulting in a reduction in wall tension. NTG also has a direct vasodilatory effect on the coronary vasculature, reducing coronary spasm. The few studies specifically addressing the issue of nitrate therapy in the elderly suggest that nitrates may play a particularly beneficial role in elderly patients with angina pectoris and congestive heart disease.[13] Evidence suggests that elderly patients are especially sensitive to vasodilators, resulting in exaggerated hemodynamic responses compared with their use in younger patients.[14]

Beta-adrenergic blockers reduce heart rate and contractility and improve myocardial oxygen balance, thus decreasing the frequency of anginal attacks. Beta-adrenergic blocking agents pose unique problems in the elderly because of the low ratio of lean body mass to fat in these patients, thus sustaining the effects of lipid-soluble agents.[15] Higher peak plasma levels may be seen as well. Hepatic and renal clearance may be diminished, and plasma protein binding may be altered. Finally, beta-adrenergic sensitivity is diminished in the elderly. Abrupt withdrawal of beta blockers has been associated with exacerbation of angina, silent ischemia, arrhythmias, and sudden blood pressure elevation.[16]

Calcium channel blockers affect myocardial oxygen supply and demand. These agents may decrease mixed venous oxygen content by peripheral arterial vasodilation and through their negative inotropic effect. Additionally, coronary blood flow may increase as a result of direct coronary vasodilation.[17] Calcium channel blockers may be potentially good choices in an elderly patient with coexisting angina pectoris and systemic hypertension. Hypotension, CHF, bradycardia, and asystole have all occurred with calcium channel blockers. These adverse effects are more likely to occur with combination therapies that include beta-blockers or digoxin.[18] Many interactions occur between calcium channel blockers and other drugs. Serum digoxin levels are increased with the use of calcium channel blockers, probably because of reduced renal clearance. For verapamil, diltiazem, and nifedipine, both the normotensive and the hypertensive elderly have reduced clearance relative to younger controls, perhaps as a result of decreased first-pass extraction.[19]

Digitalis is often prescribed for patients with CHF. Its usefulness stems from its positive inotropic effect of increasing myocardial contractility. This positive inotropy most likely results from altered excitation-contraction coupling and the resultant increased intracellular calcium concentration. Another important effect of digitalis is its ability to slow the ventricular response during atrial flutter.[18] Several pharmacokinetic parameters of digoxin, including volume of distribution, total body clearance, and drug half-life, are altered in the elderly. The effects of digoxin on cardiac contractility may occur at very low serum levels. In addition, older patients remain at higher risk for digoxin toxicity.[19]

An important potential adverse effect of digoxin therapy is dysrhythmia, which occurs as an extension of the increase in intracellular calcium responsible for increases in inotropy. Toxicity is enhanced by the presence of hypoxia, electrolyte imbalances (such as hyper- or hypokalemia), hypercalcemia, and the concurrent administration of drugs such as quinidine, verapamil, and diuretics. The digoxin serum level should be evaluated preoperatively, and if no clinical evidence of toxicity exists, the patient may take the usual dose before surgery.[18]

Angiotensin-converting enzyme (ACE) inhibitors are frequently effective in the management of hypertension in the elderly. As a result of the decrease in glomerular filtration that occurs with aging, there may be exaggerated responses to ACE inhibitors (e.g., enalapril) that are excreted by the kidneys.[20] In addition to the treatment of hypertension, this class of drugs is often prescribed for chronic CHF.

Many elderly patients receive chronic diuretic therapy to enhance renal blood flow. Diuretics include various classes of drugs with various sites of action and are beyond the scope of this chapter. Combinations of diuretics are often used to increase the probability of an effective response. Acute treatment of cardiac failure and pulmonary edema may incorporate the use of diuretics. Renal free water clearance and natriuretic capacity both decline with advancing age, predisposing older patients to hyponatremia especially during thiazide therapy.[21] A decrease in effective blood volume may also be seen early in diuretic therapy and may be evident as hypovolemia during the induction of anesthesia.

Any drug therapy is more likely to be associated with unwanted side effects in the elderly population despite strict adherence to drug regimens.[22] The standard parameters of absorption, distribution, metabolism, and excretion have all been shown to undergo changes secondary to aging. These changes tend to increase the risk of dose-related adverse reactions, which can generally be avoided by means of dosage reduction, careful titration, and monitoring of serum drug concentrations.

Diagnostic Testing

Elderly patients may be at increased risk for complications secondary to diagnostic testing. However, these evaluations may be of critical importance since the information gained from the history and physical examination may be limited because of other disease processes or drug therapy. The sequencing and selection of these tests must be individualized. Dysrhythmias and other electrocardiographic (ECG) abnormalities increase in incidence with increasing age. Any tachyarrhythmia or bradyarrhythmia may compromise cardiac function because of the resultant decrease in CO. Loss of pacemaker cells predisposes the elderly to sinus node dysfunction.[23]

The presence of left ventricular hypertrophy (LVH) on ECG, often found in cardiac patients, is frequently a result of the effects of hypertension, which is more prevalent in the elderly population. Other common ECG abnormalities in older patients include decreases in T wave amplitude and T wave inversions. First-degree heart block, left anterior hemiblock, and right bundle branch block are also seen with increased frequency.[23]

Cardiac catheterization is usually well tolerated in the elderly and is routinely performed in nearly all patients undergoing heart surgery. This procedure remains the "gold standard" of diagnostic testing in preoperative patients. Coronary angiography reveals coronary vessel anatomy, delineating stenotic or occluded areas and the extent of collateral circulation. Ventriculography is useful in assessing regional wall motion. Normal areas show concentric inward movement during systole, hypokinetic areas show reduced inward movement, and akinetic areas show no movement. Left ventricular end-diastolic pressure (LVEDP) and left ventricular ejection fraction (LVEF) also may be measured. Cardiac catheterization also allows for the measurement of other hemodynamic parameters, including CO, oxygen consumption, and saturation in the various chambers.

Noninvasive cardiac testing may be an important part of the overall preoperative assessment of cardiac patients at risk who are undergoing cardiac as well as noncardiac procedures. Exercise stress testing alone may not always be an accurate predictor of cardiac risk.[24] As a result, additional procedures may be required. These procedures vary from the simple (e.g., preoperative ambulatory ECG recording) to the highly invasive and more complex (e.g., preoperative cardiac catheterization) in patients undergoing vascular surgery. Hertzer and coworkers[25] have demonstrated that long-term morbidity may be improved by performing coronary artery bypass before vascular surgery in certain subsets of patients. However, the potential complications associated with invasive diagnostic procedures such as cardiac catheterization, as well as with cardiac surgery, are well known. Therefore, additional noninvasive testing may be used [e.g., thallium imaging (exercise or dipyridamole), echocardiography (surface or transesophageal), and radionuclide angiocardiography (multiple-unit gated acquisition scan)]. All these tests may be useful in the detection of underlying ischemic heart disease and abnormalities of ventricular function.

Echocardiography is very useful in older patients to evaluate regional wall motion, wall thickening, global ventricular function, and coronary anatomy. Also, ejection fraction (EF) can be estimated using end-systolic and end-diastolic measurements. It is important to remember that in elderly individuals the EF increases less with exercise, probably as a result of decreased beta-adrenergic responsiveness as reflected in failure to decrease end-systolic volume.[26]

Dipyridamole-thallium imaging has been found to be a useful predictor of cardiac morbidity in vascular surgery. Boucher and colleagues[27] studied 54 patients who were undergoing vascular surgery and had positive risk factors for

CAD. Among these patients, 32 had negative dipyridamole-thallium scans and went on to have their vascular procedures with no cardiac morbidity. Among the 22 who had positive dipyridamole-thallium scans, 1 refused coronary artery bypass, 1 had a lesser vascular procedure, and 4 underwent coronary bypass before an uneventful vascular procedure. Among the remaining 16, no additional workup was done after the positive dipyridamole-thallium scan, and 8 of those 16 patients (50 percent) had an adverse outcome that included cardiac morbidity. Subsequently, additional studies have shown results similar to those of Boucher.[28] As a result, many consider this the new "gold standard" of diagnostic testing for patients with cardiac risk factors who undergo vascular surgery. However, this test has limitations in regard to the preoperative screening of patients undergoing vascular surgery.[29,30] Mangano and colleagues[31] studied 60 patients preoperatively with dipyridamole imaging and found that testing had limited sensitivity for the detection of perioperative ischemia and/or an adverse cardiac outcome. Also, the negative predictive value was lower than that found in the previous studies of Boucher and Eagle.[27,28]

Raby and coworkers[32] have proposed the use of preoperative ambulatory ECG monitoring for a 48-h period for the detection of silent myocardial ischemia and as a predictor of perioperative cardiac outcome. They found it to have excellent negative predictive value in that the absence of silent myocardial ischemia was associated with an excellent cardiac outcome. In a more recent study of 115 patients undergoing vascular surgery, Raby and colleagues[33] found that monitoring of ambulatory ECGs preoperatively, intraoperatively, and up to 72 h postoperatively was very useful in detecting underlying silent myocardial ischemia and was a very good predictor of perioperative cardiac events. Overall, perioperative ischemia by ECG was positive in 14 of 16 patients who had an adverse cardiac outcome.

In an attempt to compare the two preceding testing regimens in the same cohort of patients, Abraham and coworkers[34] studied 48 patients undergoing mainly vascular surgery. These patients were thought to be at high risk in that they possessed one or more of several risk factors, including history of angina, prior MI or CHF, Q waves on ECG, diabetes, dysrhythmias being treated, and age over 70 years. Seven of the 48 patients either had a perioperative cardiac event or were subsequently found to have high-grade coronary disease. All were identified by thallium scan; however, only four of seven were identified by ambulatory monitoring. The dipyridamole-thallium scan had a much greater sensitivity for the detection of underlying coronary disease than did ambulatory ECG monitoring (100 percent versus 57 percent); however, ECG monitoring was more specific (86 percent versus 56 percent).

ANESTHESIA FOR MYOCARDIAL REVASCULARIZATION

The American Society of Anesthesiologists (ASA) physical status classification describes the overall preoperative physical condition of surgical patients and correlates well with overall morbidity and mortality in all age populations.

Defining the risk of CABG for a patient is imperative in determining which therapy (medical, PTCA, or surgery) is in that patient's best interest. Outcome data published from the CASS study showed a mortality rate of 2.3 percent.[9] Recent data on outcomes in patients older than 75 years showed a mortality of 10.8 percent.[35] This discrepancy is probably due to an older surgical population, more complex cases, and a higher percentage of emergency procedures. A study performed at the Cleveland Clinic compared operative mortality in patients over 70 years of age (1.2 to 10.5 percent) with that of patients under 70 years of age (0.6 to 3.5 percent).[36] Various preoperative scoring systems have been devised in attempts to identify the risk factors for death after cardiac surgery. Although physiological age is a better indicator of risk than is chronological age, older patients have consistently been shown to be at higher risk. Because of the higher morbidity seen in older patients, risk factors predictive of prolonged hospital stay are of increasing interest. The most important preoperative risk factors in candidates for CABG surgery are listed in Table 13-2.[37]

Preparation

Many elderly cardiac patients benefit from pharmacologic anxiolysis, but care must be taken to individualize the pretreatment plan. The preoperative level of anxiety, age, concomitant medical conditions, and ventricular function are

Table 13-2 Clinical severity scoring system

Preoperative factors	Score
Emergency case	6
Serum creatinine,	
≥141 and ≤167 μmol/L (≥1.6 and ≤1.8 mg/dL)	1
≥168 μmol/L (≥1.9 mg/dL)	4
Severe left ventricular dysfunction	3
Reoperation	3
Operative mitral valve insufficiency	3
Age ≥65 and ≤74 y	1
Age ≥75 y	2
Prior vascular surgery	2
Chronic obstructive pulmonary disease	2
Anemia (hematocrit ≤0.34)	2
Operative aortic valve stenosis	1
Weight ≤65 kg	1
Diabetes, on oral or insulin therapy	1
Cerebrovascular disease	1

SOURCE: Reprinted with permission from Higgins TL, Estafanous FG, Loop FD, et al: Stratification of morbidity and mortality outcome by preoperative risk factors in coronary artery bypass patients: A clinical severity score. *JAMA* 267:2344, 1992.

important considerations in elderly patients. Various pretreatment strategies are available. Oral lorazepam and intravenous midazolam have proved to be effective for preoperative sedation in this patient population.

Monitoring plays a key role in the management of an older patient for cardiac surgery. Standard monitors include pulse oximetry, capnography, direct arterial blood pressure, temperature probe, and urinary catheter. The need to understand cardiac function during cardiac surgery has resulted in the use of more invasive monitors in all age groups, but the elderly especially benefit because of their limited physiological reserve. Controversy concerning the use of monitors such as pulmonary artery (PA) catheters and transesophageal echocardiography (TEE) has revolved around the issue of better outcome with their use. In determining the extent of monitoring necessary, it is important to consider that the risk of complications from their use is higher. Insertion of PA catheters is more likely to produce dysrhythmias in elderly patients.[38] Radial artery cannulation may be complicated by a tortuous artery secondary to atherosclerosis. Overall, the benefits of invasive monitoring in an elderly patient with limited cardiac reserve justify its application. The usefulness and cost-effectiveness of the PA catheter during geriatric CABG surgery have been questioned.[39] Advancing age may be associated with the clinical need to use PA catheter monitoring rather than central venous pressure (CVP) monitoring during CABG surgery.

Choice of Agent

The ideal anesthetic for a cardiac patient at risk who is undergoing a major stressful surgical procedure is one that would provide the four major components of general anesthesia: hypnosis, amnesia, analgesia, and muscle relaxation. In addition, the anesthetic agent should have minimal effects on hemodynamics, should not depress myocardial function, and at the same time should provide good attenuation of the stress response to anesthesia and surgery. The latter includes suppression of autonomic, endocrine, and hemodynamic responses to noxious stimuli. The myocardial oxygen balance should not be adversely affected (no increase in heart rate, decrease in blood pressure, or ECG/TEE detection of ischemia). Also, there should be no adverse effects on vital organs. No single anesthetic agent has been developed that provides all these important characteristics without adverse side effects.

Since morphine was reintroduced into clinical anesthesia for cardiac cases nearly 25 years ago by Lowenstein and colleagues,[40] opioids have been employed widely. The newer synthetic narcotics (e.g., fentanyl) seem ideal for patients with cardiovascular disease because of the lack of cardiac depressant effects. In fact, these agents possess several traits that are attractive for cardiac patients at risk undergoing a major noncardiac procedure: (1) intense analgesia, (2) profound attenuation of the autonomic stress response, and (3) hemodynamic stability. Many of these agents have become popular as base agents on which to build a total anesthetic regimen. Opioids fall short of the ideal anesthetic in the areas of amnesia and hypnosis. There have been many reports of awareness and recall during high-dose opioid anesthesia in which few or no adjunctive agents were utilized. Controversy remains as to the future of high-dose opioid anesthesia,[41] although recent evidence has shown that anesthesia continued well into the postoperative period may be associated with decreased cardiac complications.[42]

Controversy remains concerning the advantages of one agent over another despite efforts to resolve these problems. Nine primary anesthetic techniques (agents) and more than 2000 patients were studied by two groups of investigators who looked at anesthetics, CAD, and outcome.[43,44] Although no significant advantage was observed for one anesthetic regimen over any other, it is difficult to predict the extent of cardiovascular changes effected by certain agents in individual patients.

Despite the fact that most studies have been unable to show a difference in outcome utilizing different general anesthetic techniques for patients with cardiovascular disease, there have been a few exceptions. One was a study by Benefiel and coworkers,[45] which looked at morbidity during aortic surgery utilizing sufentanil versus isoflurane for anesthesia. One hundred patients undergoing aortic reconstruction were administered either sufentanil-based anesthesia with nitrous oxide and thiopental sodium supplementation or isoflurane-based anesthesia with similar supplementation. There were significantly more complications, including renal insufficiency and CHF, in patients receiving primarily isoflurane anesthesia versus those receiving primarily sufentanil anesthesia. This did not seem to be related to hemodynamics, since there were no significant differences in hemodynamics; however, in a further analysis of the data,[46] a statistically significant correlation was found between elevations in peak plasma epinephrine concentrations and postoperative complications in those patients. Thus, it was concluded that the stress response to anesthesia and surgery, rather than any hemodynamic change, seemed to be a predictor of postoperative complications, and the inference was that the opioid-based anesthesia (sufentanil) provided better attenuation of the perioperative stress response.

Induction of anesthesia can be accomplished through the use of a single agent alone or a combination of two or three agents each possessing one or more of the ideal characteristics listed above. In the authors' experience, repeated titratable doses of sedative hypnotics as an adjunct to predominantly narcotic-based anesthesia have been the most successful. The cardiovascular effects vary but should not be confused with those produced by a simple loss of consciousness: a decline of about 10 percent in blood pressure, heart rate, and CO.

At the authors' institution, several anesthetic regimens are employed. The authors' personal preference is a total intravenous technique, combining the pharmacologic effects of an opioid (analgesia, hemodynamic stability, attenuation of stress response) and those of a benzodiazepine (amnesia, hypnosis, anxiolysis). The agents are prepared in a fixed concentration ratio and administered with the use of a syringe pump. Induction and maintenance are accomplished using a two-stage infusion technique based on the known pharmacokinetic profiles of the agents. Initially, a loading dose of sufentanil (3 μg/kg) and midazolam (60 μg/kg) is administered slowly over a 6-min period. After intubation, the infusion rate is decreased progressively to a maintenance level of approximately 1 to 2 μg/kg per hour of sufentanil and 20 to 40 μg/kg per hour of midazolam. Total doses of each agent for a 4- to 5-hour case may range from 10 to 15 μg/kg of sufentanil and 0.2 to 0.3 mg/kg of midazolam. Neuromuscular relaxation is usually provided with the use of vecuronium or doxacurium initially, followed by maintenance with doxacurium.

Surgical Technique

Surgical technique has played a major role in decreasing morbidity and mortality rates in elderly patients. Routine internal mammary artery (IMA) grafting has resulted in a better early outcome after revascularization when used for anterior wall revascularization. In an extensive study of the efficacy of IMA grafting, the reduction in operative mortality in these patients from 9.7 to 4.9 percent was significant; also, IMA grafting was one of several independent predictors of improvement in the survival of patients older than 70 years.[47] Other data suggest that long-term survival was greater and the probability of recurrent angina and reoperation was lower in elderly patients with IMA conduits.[48]

ANESTHESIA FOR VALVULAR SURGERY

Aortic Stenosis

Aortic stenosis (AS) remains the most common valvular lesion in the elderly. Among patients older than 65 years with calcific AS, the valve is tricuspid in more than 90 percent of cases. Stenosis is produced by calcium deposits that prevent the cusps from opening normally. Calcific AS appears to result from years of normal mechanical wear and tear on the valvular apparatus. Because the commissures are not fused, significant aortic regurgitation occurs infrequently.

As the aortic valve becomes stenotic, concentric hypertrophy of the left ventricle develops to compensate for the pressure load. This serves to normalize wall stress and overcome the increased afterload. Left ventricular function remains intact until late in the history of the disease, which classically evolves slowly. However, in some elderly patients with degenerative calcification, the disease may develop rapidly. This may be due in part to the cardiac alterations and decreased left ventricular compliance, which exacerbate the pathophysiological response to AS.

The clinical presentation of AS differs in inactive elderly patients, since exertionally provoked symptoms may not be noted. Left ventricle failure, not angina, is the most common presenting symptom.[49] The mortality rate is high for patients with severe symptomatic AS who are treated medically. Survival averages 1½ years in those presenting with CHF. Aortic ejection murmurs are heard in 30 percent of patients older than 65 years and to an even greater degree in elderly hypertensive patients.[49] Therefore, it is important to distinguish benign murmurs from murmurs of critical AS. In an elderly patient with AS, the decreased arterial compliance may cause a brisk carotid upstroke and systolic hypertension. The calcified valves are immobile; thus, no ejection click is heard.

Because the patient's history may be unreliable and the results of physical examination may be equivocal, noninvasive studies are the cornerstone in evaluating valvular obstruction. The ECG shows LVH in patients with significant AS, but this finding is often present in elderly hypertensive patients, possibly making this a nonspecific finding. The frequent occurrence of CAD and conduction defects also may confuse the issue.

Echocardiography is the most important noninvasive technique for assessing the severity of AS. Doppler echocardiography is the procedure of choice for routine evaluation of aortic valvular disease. Continuous-wave Doppler echocardiography permits noninvasive determination of flow velocities between two cardiac chambers, allowing for calculation of pressure gradients across the valve. Two dimensional (2-D) echo can reveal valve characteristics, such as thickening of the valve and leaflet mobility, but in elderly patients with extensive valvular calcification, valve separation during systole may not be clearly visualized.[50] Aortic valve replacement (AVR) has been undertaken using only echo-derived data, but the high percentage of CAD in the elderly mandates that cardiac catheterization be performed to determine which candidates may benefit from more extensive combined treatment (CABG-AVR).

A poor prognosis is associated with medical therapy for symptomatic AS. The initial enthusiasm for aortic balloon valvuloplasty has been tempered by the recognition of rapid stenosis in patients with degenerative AS.[51] Despite the increased risk of valvular surgery in the elderly, AVR often results in prolonged clinical improvement. The operative mortality is between 5 and 15 percent. Octogenarians who underwent AVR for AS had survival rates of 83 and 67 percent at 1 and 5 years, respectively, in a recent report.[52]

Certain patient subsets have substantially poorer outcomes. Factors associated with greater operative risk include emergency surgery, left ventricular dysfunction (EF $<$ 45 percent), CAD, malnutrition, smaller prosthetic valve, and concomitant surgical procedures.[53] Concomitant myocardial revascularization increases surgical risk in the elderly, especially in the "oldest old" group.[54] The combination of ventricular hypertrophy and stenotic lesions may compromise a patient's ability to maintain adequate cardioplegia when coronary vascularization is not undertaken. As a consequence, myocardial protection may be inadequate and left ventricular dysfunction may result. Surgical mortality is between 6.6 and 8.8 percent in patients receiving combined CABG-AVR and falls to about 5 percent in those undergoing only valve replacement. Those with concomitant mitral valve surgery have higher earlier mortality.[55]

Many patients with AS are candidates for bioprostheses or aortic root homografts because of advanced age. Both techniques allow acceptable safety from thromboembolism without the risks of anticoagulation. Limited durability is an issue with the bioprosthesis. The homograft is proposed to overcome this problem, and early studies have yielded encouraging results.[56]

Anesthetic Management

AS is a chronic left ventricular pressure overload lesion. The left ventricle is faced with a gradual increase in the impedance to ejection. Concentric hypertrophy results in a normalization of wall stress, which allows the EF to be maintained in spite of the high impedance to ejection found in critical AS. Eventually, afterload continues to increase to a point where stroke volume diminishes and the left ventricle begins to dilate in an attempt to restore stroke volume.

Left ventricular concentric hypertrophy results in diminished left ventricular compliance and the potential for compromise of early ventricular diastolic filling. Atrial systole may contribute 30 to 40 percent of left ventricular end-diastolic volume (LVEDV) instead of the usual 20 percent. Acute loss of atrial systole leads to markedly compromised left ventricular filling and severe pulmonary congestion.

The myocardial oxygen supply-demand relationship is very complex in patients with AS. Tachycardia is detrimental because the time for subendocardial perfusion is reduced. Also, the reduction in diastolic filling leads to diminished diastolic volume and low aortic diastolic pressure, further compromising coronary perfusion pressure. Bradycardia increases the valve gradient, resulting in systemic hypertension and subendocardial ischemia. More than half the elderly population with significant AS and angina also has coexistent CAD.

Afterload reduction results in very little augmentation of CO in patients with critical AS. Agents such as sodium nitroprusside (SNP) that are used to reduce afterload, also decrease aortic diastolic pressure and compromise subendocardial blood flow. Right atrial pressure greatly underestimates the pulmonary capillary wedge pressure (PCWP) and LVEDP. The PA catheter facilitates optimization of preload and afterload and maintenance of adequate stroke volume. LVEDP can best be approximated using the A wave in the wedge tracing.

The use of a narcotic technique avoids the significant myocardial depression often associated with volatile agents. A hemodynamically stable induction may be achieved with the administration of midazolam with either fentanyl or sufentanil. Opioid infusions have been shown to decrease the need for supplemental anesthesia or vasodilatory therapy by blunting reflex sympathetic responses to surgical stimulation. The choice of a neuromuscular blocking agent largely depends on the resting heart rate.

In patients with AS, the subendocardium is especially prone to ischemia, yet LVH may mask ECG signs of ischemia. Immediate treatment of hypotension is imperative to prevent a decrease in coronary perfusion pressure. Initial treatment with small doses (50 to 100 μg) of phenylephrine hydrochloride raises the blood pressure and coronary perfusion pressure and allows time for evaluation of the possible etiologies of hypotension (hypovolemia, nodal rhythm, etc.)

After valve replacement, the reduction in the valve gradient leads to a reduction of end-systolic volume and results in increased EF and increased CO. Vasodilatory therapy may be beneficial in patients with increased afterload after cardiopulmonary bypass (CPB). Patients with AS may require inotropic support to separate from bypass, as left ventricular systolic function may be compromised by inadequate myocardial protection. The use of inotropes for this purpose is discussed below.

The compliance characteristics of the left ventricle remain unchanged for up to a year after AVR; therefore, maintenance of adequate preload and sinus rhythm remains essential. After removal of the "fixed obstruction," hypertension may result, which may be effectively treated with vasodilators and/or beta-adrenergic blocking agents.

Aortic Insufficiency

In contrast to AS, isolated severe aortic regurgitation (AR) is uncommon in the elderly. Among elderly patients undergoing AVR, fewer than 20 percent have primary AR. The etiology of chronic AR in the elderly is associated with either intrinsic valvular disease or pathology of the aortic root.[57] Aortic root abnormalities may be the most common cause of valve incompetence in the aged. Degenerative dilation of the aortic root can result in regurgitation as the commissures widen and the valve cusps stretch. Acute severe AR in the elderly may result from aortic dissection or infective endocarditis.

Patients with chronic AR may remain asymptomatic for many years, during which time the left ventricle undergoes progressive eccentric enlargement. Exertional dyspnea is a common clinical presentation caused by pulmonary venous congestion. It is important to remember that coexistent coronary disease is common in the elderly and may dominate the clinical picture. Angina may occur early in the disease process and appears to result from diminished diastolic coronary perfusion pressures and impaired coronary flow reserve. Widened pulse pressure is noted on physical examination. The presentation of acute AR is much different because its rapid onset prevents left ventricular compensation and stroke volume changes. Pulmonary venous congestion and tachycardia dominate the clinical picture. The pulse pressure may not be widened.

The ECG in chronic severe AR is characterized by signs of ventricular hypertrophy. Left bundle branch block is a common finding. Chest x-ray may show left ventricular enlargement and dilation of the ascending aorta.

Echocardiography is the most reliable noninvasive method of detecting the presence of AR. It provides an objective evaluation of left ventricular size and function and allows for ongoing assessment of the changes that occur with chronic volume overload. 2-D echocardiography may assist in determining whether the pathology involves the valve or the aortic root. Serial measurements may identify impending decompensation and may be useful in the decision to consider valve replacement. Doppler echocardiography is useful in quantitatively assessing the severity of AR and determining the regurgitant fraction. Estimates of regurgitant volume are based on careful mapping of the left ventricular cavity. Color-flow imaging provides visualization of regurgitant jet area and width and correlates well with the severity of AR seen with cardiac catheterization. The latter should be performed in elderly patients with symptomatic chronic AR to assess left ventricular performance and examine the coronary anatomy.

The pathophysiology of AR includes chronic volume overloading that results in left ventricular dilation and eccentric hypertrophy. Because dilation increases compliance, end-diastolic pressure is not elevated. Stroke volume is augmented by the Starling mechanism. Compensatory hypertrophy prevents a marked increase in wall stress. As chronic AR progresses, left ventricular dysfunction occurs secondary to inadequate hypertrophy to overcome increased wall stress. As the volume overloading continues, the intrinsic contractility worsens, and any increase in venous return may increase the volume load on the heart, with subsequent transmission of volume to the pulmonary vasculature. Pulmonary venous congestion may develop earlier in the course of AR in the elderly as a result of impaired diastolic function. The slower heart rate that occurs with aging may increase the duration of diastole and the regurgitant volume.[58]

The presentation of acute AR is one of acute, severe diastolic overload to the left ventricle, resulting in an abrupt increase in LVEDP with no change in end-diastolic volume and fiber length. Wall stress rises quickly and stroke volume falls, as no compensatory hypertrophy takes place. The decrease in CO causes a reflex activation of the sympathetic nervous system that leads to an increased heart rate and systemic vascular resistance (SVR).

Surgical Concern and Outcome

The timing of AVR for chronic AR remains controversial. In some studies, preoperative left ventricular dysfunction at rest can identify patients at increased risk for death or heart failure after valve replacement. Identification of early contractile impairment using clinical and noninvasive assessment may optimize the timing of surgery. Reduction of left ventricular mass after AVR for AR is often unpredictable, even when improvement in ventricular function is seen. Therefore, the longer the duration of preoperative dysfunction, the less likely the return of normal ventricular function after valve replacement.[59] Measurements of ventricular function used to stratify risks include EF <45 percent and cardiac index <2.2 l/min per square meter. Other predictors of risk include preoperative CHF and cardiomegaly on chest x-ray. In carefully selected elderly patients, the surgical risk for AVR for chronic regurgitation is similar to that for AS, with a mortality of 5 to 15 percent and a favorable long-term clinical outcome.[59]

Anesthetic Management

Patients requiring AVR for chronic AR are managed in a manner similar to that for patients with AS. The PA catheter allows for the optimization of preload and afterload. In patients with preserved left ventricular function, a mean PCWP of 10 to 15 mmHg will assure optimal LVEDV. In patients with depressed ventricular function, PCWP will be in the range of 20 to 25 mmHg when preload is adequate. Maintaining intravascular volume is essential for hemodynamic stability. Partial compensation for the regurgitation can be achieved by maintaining preload and stroke volume. In these patients, afterload reduction helps reduce the diastolic pressure gradient and increase the CO. Since venodilators may cause a detrimental reduction in preload, primarily arteriolar vasodilators, such as sodium nitroprusside, may be preferred for afterload reduction as long as careful attention is paid to CO, arterial blood pressure, and LVEDP.

Bradycardia increases the regurgitant volume, which compromises forward stroke volume and CO because the regurgitant volume represents a large portion of the total stroke volume. Ventricular distension and increased LVEDP may result from extreme bradycardia. A moderately elevated heart rate is usually tolerated better in patients with AR. Ventricular distension from bradycardia or retrograde pump flow through an incompetent valve may occur with the onset of CPB. This may be prevented by venting the left ventricle or cross-clamping the aorta.

After AVR for AR, the regurgitant fraction is eliminated; thus, both LVEDV and LVEDP decrease and CO increases. Positive inotropic agents may be beneficial in maintaining systolic perfusion pressure, especially in patients with preoperative left ventricular dysfunction. Also, myocardial protection may be inadequate in elderly patients with hypertrophic ventricles and CAD.

Patients with AR are often operated on emergently, with the added risk of pulmonary aspiration. Rapid-sequence induction with sufentanil (1 μg/kg) followed by etomidate (0.2 mg/kg) and succinylcholine provides good intubating conditions within 60 s. The premature closure of the mitral valve will cause the PCWP to underestimate the LVEDP.[58] When ventricular dilation results in MR, PCWP will overestimate the LVEDV. Immediately after AVR for acute AR, the elimination of the regurgitant fraction allows the ventricle to maintain CO with lower LVEDV and LVEDP. Inotropic support should be available to bolster systolic function.

Mitral Stenosis

Calcification of the leaflets or the mitral anulus is frequently present in older patients. From the time of initial diagnosis, patients with symptomatic mitral stenosis (MS) have a mortality of 20 percent at 5 years.[60] With the progression of stenosis, increases in left atrial pressures are transmitted to the pulmonary vasculature, with a resultant reduction in pulmonary compliance and increased work of breathing. The effects of sustained elevated left atrial pressure may lead to left atrial dilation, which can result in atrial fibrillation. The effects of sustained high PA pressure may lead to right ventricular dilation and hypertrophy. Left ventricular dysfunction, when it occurs, has been attributed to calcification of the mitral valve and fibrosis of papillary muscles, resulting in regional areas of hypocontractility.

The clinical presentation of MS in the elderly differs little from that in younger patients except for the frequent occurrence of valvular calcification and the higher frequency of atrial fibrillation. Symptoms usually result from elevated left atrial and pulmonary venous pressures, which are transmitted to the pulmonary vasculature and the right side of the heart, generally leading to increased work of breathing and shortness of breath. Symptoms of lethargy and dyspnea on exertion occur as the valve area decreases to less than 2 cm. Elderly patients may present with evidence of a systemic embolus, and because of coexisting chronic conditions such as hypertension and atrial fibrillation, the diagnosis of MS may be missed.

The presence and severity of MS can invariably be diagnosed by ECG. Two-dimensional and Doppler echocardiography can be used to evaluate the severity of the stenosis. In elderly patients, as a result of decreased ventricular compliance affecting mitral pressure half-time, an overestimation of the valve area may occur.[61]

Cardiac catheterization should be performed in any elderly patient to confirm the severity of MS, assess the degree of pulmonary hypertension, and exclude the possibility of additional valvular lesions. Since a large percentage of elderly patients have CAD, the angiographic data are extremely valuable. Several studies have cited an increase in mortality in patients with CAD who receive mitral valve replacement (MVR).[62,63]

The merits of percutaneous mitral valvuloplasty (PMV) versus MVR continue to be debated. Elderly patients with MS more frequently undergo PMV. The advantages of PMV are shorter hospitalization, initial lower morbidity and mortality (3 and 1 percent, respectively), and avoidance of valve-related complications such as thromboembolism and endocarditis.[64] There is some concern over the long-term results of this technique, and the patient may eventually require valve replacement. However, there may remain a substantial time interval between PMV and MVR, which may be an added advantage to elderly patients. Echocardiographic evaluation of the subvalvular and valvular apparatus helps identify which patients will benefit from PMV and which would be better served by MVR. When valve replacement is required for MS, mortality is about 10 to 15 percent in those older than 70 years.[65]

Anesthetic Management

Caution should be exercised when one orders narcotics that could be associated with preoperative hypoventilation and hypoxia. Tachycardia is detrimental because of the increase in the pressure gradient across the diseased valve and the decrease in the time for ventricular filling. Maintenance of preload allows for an adequate volume gradient across the mitral valve. PA catheters are useful in assessing volume status and the effects of anesthetic agents. PCWP overestimates LVEDP because of the mitral valve gradient, especially with heart rate increases. Since prevention of pulmonary hypertension and right ventricular dysfunction is important, it is crucial to avoid precipitating causes such as hypoxia, hypercarbia, and sympathetic stimulation.

Although volatile agents may be used, the authors' preference is for a high-dose narcotic technique, as was described earlier (see "Choice of Agent"), for hemodynamic control. Treatment of hypotensive episodes may pose a dilemma. Volume loading may be beneficial, although CHF may be present. Alpha-adrenergic agonists may cause pulmonary hypertension, while beta-adrenergic agonists may cause tachycardia. Inotropic support with dopamine or dobutamine may solve the problem of hypotension without the untoward effects of vasopressors.

The mitral is probably the valve most suitable for evaluation by intraoperative TEE because it lies so close to the transducer. TEE may be beneficial in the postbypass period. After commissurotomy, some degree of mitral regurgitation will exist, and TEE helps assess the regurgitant flow. This technique also can be useful in evaluating the mechanical prosthetic device and in detecting the presence of periprosthetic leaks.

After MVR for MS, there is significant improvement in left ventricular filling via the left atrium; therefore, CO should increase. PA pressures should decrease; however, some subsets of patients continue to have elevated pulmonary vascular resistance. A phosphodiesterase inhibitor such as amrinone or milrinone may be useful for its combined vasodilating and inotropic effects. Supraventricular dysrhythmias, especially atrial fibrillation, often complicate the postoperative course after MVR.

Mitral Regurgitation

In elderly patients mitral regurgitation (MR) is a more common finding than is MS. MR can result from a variety of etiologies, including infectious endocarditis, mitral anular calcification, myxomatous degeneration of the mitral valve, and papillary muscle dysfunction. As aging progresses, pathological changes may occur that affect the functional integrity of the valve.[66] MR imposes a large volume overload on the left ventricle. Almost half the regurgitant volume may be ejected into the left atrium before the aortic valve opens.[67]

The regurgitant volume depends on the size of the mitral orifice as well as the pressure gradient across the valve. In patients with chronic MR, eccentric hypertrophy and dilatation of the LV further reduce afterload. Symptomatic patients may often have some degree of impairment of myocardial contractility, yet EF will overestimate systolic function as a result of the unique unloading conditions present (double-outlet left ventricle).

In acute MR, the ventricle does not have the enormous preload reserve, since ventricular hypertrophy does not have time to develop. A small, noncompliant left atrium exists, resulting in high left atrial pressures (LAP), and the regurgitant volume is reflected as a V wave on the PCWP or LAP wave trace.

The increased pressure is transmitted to the pulmonary circulation, and pulmonary congestion may be present (Fig. 13-5).

Elderly patients with MR typically complain of weakness, palpitations, and dyspnea on exertion. The ECG may show evidence of atrial fibrillation and left atrial hypertrophy. Two-dimensional echocardiography is more useful for determining the etiology and hemodynamic consequences of MR than for quantifying its severity.[66] Both color-flow and Doppler techniques correlate well with angiographic methods for estimating the severity of MR.[67] In addition to confirmation and quantification of valvular disease, serial noninvasive examinations can monitor the progression of valvular insufficiency objectively. Because CAD is common in the elderly and untreated CAD may adversely affect the outcome in patients undergoing mitral valve surgery, preoperative angiography is indicated in the elderly.

Anesthetic Management

Premedication is given according to the degree of ventricular dysfunction and is usually best avoided in acute MR. Direct arterial pressure monitoring helps guide vasodilatory therapy. The PA catheter allows preload and afterload to be optimized before the induction of anesthesia. The size of the V wave of the PCWP tracing corresponds to the regurgitant volume and may guide vasodilatory therapy.

In acute MR, there are very large V waves and LVEDP is elevated because of a lack of compensatory atrial and ventricular enlargement. Acute MR often occurs in the setting of acute MI and because there is often ongoing ischemia. Therapy is directed at lowering LVEDP, decreasing ventricular radius, improving aortic diastolic blood pressure, and decreasing the heart rate as much as possible without worsening the regurgitant fraction. When pharmacologic interventions fail, the use of an intraaortic balloon pump (IABP) may be indicated.

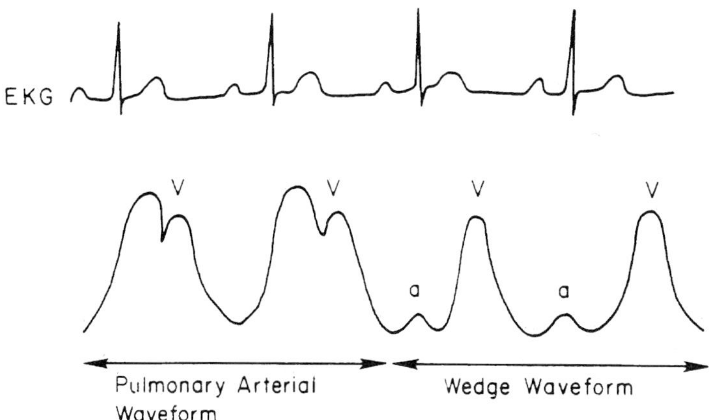

Figure 13-5 **Presence of a large V wave with mitral regurgitation.** (*Reprinted with permission from Nadeau S, Noble WH: Misinterpretation of pressure measurements from the pulmonary artery catheter. Can Anaesth Soc J 33:352, 1986.*)

A high-dose narcotic technique is often chosen because of its minimal effects on myocardial contractility and peripheral vascular resistance. Afterload can be manipulated to reduce the pressure gradient to enhance forward flow. Vasodilators may lead to profound hypotension, which may impair coronary perfusion. Vasopressors may worsen matters by leading to an increase in the regurgitant volume. Inotropic agents are a good choice for hypotension when heart rate and preload are optimal. Maintenance of heart rate at the preoperative level is usually desirable, especially if the patient functions well at this rate. Mild tachycardia may decrease the regurgitant volume.

Many patients with acute MR with infarction or ischemia are in cardiogenic shock with pulmonary congestion and may arrive in the operating room ventilated with an IABP in place. Etomidate (0.2–0.3 mg/kg) is a good choice for induction because it provides hemodynamic stability and a rapid onset of action.

Immediately after mitral valve surgery, maintenance of optimal myocardial performance is crucial because the favorable loading conditions have been eliminated. Poor systolic function may result from elevated wall stress, which accompanies elimination of the regurgitant volume. Afterload reduction and inotropic support of the systolic function are indicated therapies. The ideal pharmacologic support should include the combination of controlled vasodilation and inotropic effects without a significant increase in myocardial oxygen requirement. In patients with pulmonary hypertension, a phosphodiesterase inhibitor such as amrinone or milrinone may be effective in combining pulmonary vasodilation with an inotropic effect.

Intraoperative TEE is performed before and after CPB and allows characterization of leaflet and jet abnormalities. Determination of the origin, direction, and extent of the regurgitant jet aid in understanding the mechanism of mitral valve dysfunction. After surgical correction, the hemodynamic status is normalized, the valve function is assessed, and any residual regurgitation is quantified. One study suggests that even moderate regurgitation is associated with progressive postoperative regurgitation and more complications.[66]

Surgical Outcome

In most presentations of MR in the elderly, the etiology is degenerative changes including myxomatous valves and leaflet prolapse. Mitral valve repair is associated with a lower risk for operative mortality because left ventricular function is preserved. Operative mortality is 2 to 4 percent for repair and about 10 percent for replacement.[68] With an extremely low surgical mortality and a lack of valve-associated complications (e.g., thromboembolism), which obviates the need for anticoagulation, mitral valve repair may be the procedure of choice for MR in patients of any age.

Predictors of mortality after MVR for MR have been analyzed retrospectively.[69] Advanced patient age at the time of MVR correlated with the poorest survival, with patients older than 60 years being at greatest risk. Factors indicative of ischemic disease were the most important predictors of early mortality, possibly because these groups of patients required longer periods of CPB and aortic cross-clamping times. Patients undergoing combined procedures (e.g., MVR-CABG) had higher mortality rates than did those who received isolated valve replacement (27.8 versus 11.4 percent), possibly reflecting a greater degree of damage to both the valve and the myocardium.[68] Patients with severe CHF symptoms had higher postoperative mortality and poorer long-term survival.

In the last decade, the number of heart valve reoperations has increased steadily because of the improved results of first-time valve surgery, resulting in longer survival. Older age dramatically increases the mortality rate in reoperations to more than 50 percent in patients over 70 years of age.[70,71]

COMPLICATIONS OF CARDIAC SURGERY

Cardiac Dysfunction

Perioperative low CO states have become increasingly more common in the cardiac surgery setting because of the types of procedures being undertaken and the patients on whom surgery is being performed. At present, the patient population is older and has a greater degree of preoperative cardiac dysfunction.[72] Nearly 20 percent of coronary bypass procedures in the authors' institution are reoperations, and in some centers that figure may approach 40 percent. Many patients present for surgery after treatment for acute MI.

Acute heart failure during the perioperative period may be a result of preexisting ventricular dysfunction or acquired intraoperative dysfunction generally secondary to myocardial ischemia or infarction. Insult to the myocardium may occur at the time of operation as a result of prolonged ischemia, thermal or reperfusion injury, or the surgery itself. The total time of aortic cross-clamping and the total time of CPB are important factors in determining how the heart will perform postoperatively. Ventricular recovery may not be uniform because of inadequate myocardial protection.

Myocardial protection requires a multidisciplinary approach, and the inherent problems in using this technique have become more evident as higher-risk patients present for cardiac surgery. Protection attempted with the use of cold cardioplegia solutions results in electromechanical quiescence and provides the ischemic heart with anaerobic substrate to ensure cell survival. Several strategies have been developed to improve cardioplegia delivery during cardiac surgery. Retrograde delivery via the coronary sinus provides homogeneous distribution for cardioplegia solutions when proximal coronary artery stenoses are present. During reoperation, retrograde infusion provides distribution of the cardioplegia solution to the bed distal to the patent graft. Recent evidence suggests that using warm blood cardioplegia leads to more complete recovery of myocardial function by enhancing the metabolic recovery of the energy-depleted heart. This result is more notable in patients undergoing urgent coronary revascularization reoperations and valve procedures. A further improvement was noted in patients receiving antegrade and retrograde cardioplegia.[73] These developments have reduced the incidence of morbidity and mortality in elderly cardiac patients.

Conditions that can aggravate acute myocardial dysfunction may be present and may be relatively simple to treat. These conditions include acid-base imbalance, hypoventilation, hypoxia, anemia, and cardiac dysrhythmias. Optimization of preload and heart rate is necessary for obtaining hemodynamic stability. An elderly cardiac patient with reduced ventricular compliance and distensibility will depend on atrial systole for adequate left ventricular filling without a pathological elevation of PCWP; therefore, some mode of atrial pacing may be necessary. The placement of both atrial and ventricular epicardial pacing wires facilitates the treatment of rhythm disturbances.

The initial pharmacologic approach toward improvement in ventricular performance begins with the use of inotropic agents. The goals of inotropic therapy include (1) improved myocardial contractility, (2) reduced ventricular dimension, (3) normalized CO, (4) optimized blood pressure and tissue perfusion, and (5) relieved pulmonary congestion. An ideal inotropic agent would increase myocardial contractility without various side effects, including tachycardia, other arrhythmias, and hypertension, and increase myocardial oxygen consumption. No inotropic agent can be classified as ideal. In fact, to approach the ideal, combinations of agents are more effective than is a single inotropic agent. Inotropic agents that are useful in the cardiac surgical setting include catecholamines and several noncatecholamine inotropes, including synthetic sympathomimetics, calcium, digitalis, and phosphodiesterase inhibitors.

Vasodilators have been used for many years in the treatment of heart failure.[74] The use of these agents in this setting represents an attempt to improve myocardial contractility and reduce the workload of the heart. Reduction of the myocardial workload is an important adjunct in the care of cardiac patients. Vasodilation results in reduction of cardiac work and an increase in forward flow, which serve to reduce ventricular end-diastolic and pulmonary pressures. Vasodilators may also enhance organ perfusion.

Failure to wean from CPB leads to two additional options: (1) restoring CPB with an additional increment of perfusion time, which may result in improved myocardial performance, and (2) inserting a mechanical assist device. In the authors' experience, inserting an IABP early in the treatment of severe intractable heart failure is recommended over insertion after the myocardium has been damaged beyond the degree at which it may not recover. This is obviously a surgical decision, but experience dictates that an "early balloon" may be lifesaving. When several inotrope-vasodilator combinations have been tried and have failed, it is recommended than an IABP be instituted while the patient's heart is being rested on CPB. This may also save heart muscle that could potentially be damaged beyond recovery. If the use of an IABP is not possible because of anatomic problems or is ineffective, new alternatives have become available. Left or right heart bypass or biventricular bypass may be used for a time (several hours to several days) until the myocardium recovers. However, an overall favorable outcome remains to be proved with these extreme measures of mechanical support.[75]

Neurological Impairment

The incidence of neurological complications depends on a number of factors, including the type of operation, the age of the patient population, and the sensitivity of the testing. There is evidence that although the mortality associated with cardiac operations is decreasing, the incidence of neurological injury has increased substantially. In patients older than 75 years, the rate approaches 9 percent[76] (Fig. 13-6).

The presence of preoperative neurological abnormalities is predictive of postoperative neurological complications because the already impaired cerebral blood flow is at higher risk of further compromise during extracorporeal circulation. Cerebral embolism is strongly implicated in bypass-associated cerebral injury. Macroembolization of air from the heart or open aorta and calcium from the mitral or aortic valve leaflets are possible causes. Microemboli of gas from bubble oxygenators and fat from cardiotomy suction also have been implicated.

A number of techniques are available to assess cerebral injury, including cerebral blood flow and metabolism measurements, electroencephalography, and evoked potentials. Embolic detection with transcranial Doppler ultrasound provides a new technique for assessing potential neurological injury during bypass, but it is not yet possible to define the size and type of the embolus reliably. Pharmacologic intervention offers the most promise in the prevention of cerebral injury. Nimodipine is the most promising of the currently available agents.[77] It has beneficial effects on focal and global animal models and is currently used in the treatment of subarachnoid hemorrhage.

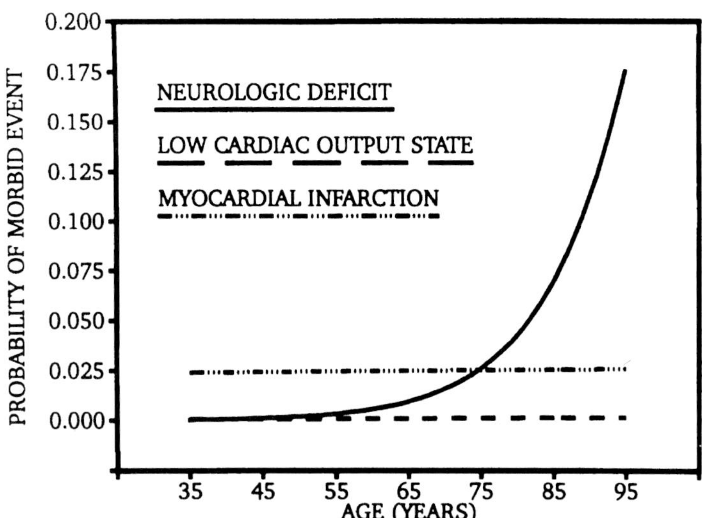

Figure 13-6 Effect of advanced age on the predicted probability of neurological and cardiac morbidity. (*Reprinted with permission from Tuman KJ, McCarthy RJ, Najafi H, et al: Differential effects of advanced age on neurologic and cardiac risks of coronary artery operations. J Thorac Cardiovasc Surg 104:1510, 1992.*)

It has been repeatedly demonstrated that during hypothermic CPB, cerebral autoregulation is preserved down to a mean arterial pressure (MAP) of 30 mmHg or a cerebral perfusion pressure (CPP) of 20 mmHg, although patients with concomitant diseases such as untreated hypertension or cerebrovascular disease usually were omitted from these investigations.[78] However, loss of autoregulation does occur in diabetic patients and elderly diabetic patients may be at increased risk for developing postoperative neurological dysfunction. Because of concern about the possibility of occult cerebrovascular disease, at the authors' institution the MAP is maintained above 50 mmHg during bypass in older individuals.

Other Noncardiac Morbidity

Other noncardiac morbidity, such as pulmonary, renal, and infectious complications, also occurs with greater frequency in the elderly. The leading noncardiac complication after cardiac surgery is infection, with the average length of hospital stay being 13 days postoperatively for a noninfected patient and approximately 30 days for an infected patient.[79] Factors that have been shown to increase the likelihood of sternal and mediastinal infections include the presence of postoperative hemorrhage, reoperation, sternal disruption resulting from cardiopulmonary resuscitation, and a low CO state. Single administration of a long-acting cephalosporin is probably as efficacious as any regimen in preventing postoperative infections.

In a patient with normal hemodynamics after cardiac surgery, failure to extubate indicates a respiratory problem if other underlying precipitating factors can be excluded. Respiratory complications occur frequently in patients with prior pulmonary disease. Early institution of bronchodilators, control of secretions, and careful monitoring of hemodynamics and fluid status are crucial factors in avoiding long-term intubation.

The etiology of renal failure after CPB remains unclear. Age, preexisting renal dysfunction as measured by elevated serum creatinine concentration and decreased 24-h urine creatinine clearance, and left ventricular dysfunction help identify patients at risk for renal failure.[80] Advancing age is associated with a progressive decline in renal blood flow and glomerular filtration rate. As a result, an elderly patient is vulnerable to fluid overload, cortical hypotension, and the cumulative effects of drugs that depend on renal clearance. Nonoliguric renal failure occurs more often after cardiac surgery and carries a mortality rate of about 15 percent. Treatment consists of maximization of CO and blood pressure to ensure adequate glomerular filtration pressures. Oliguric renal failure carries a mortality rate above 60 percent; dialysis is the universal treatment.[81]

Postbypass Surgical Bleeding

Excessive bleeding associated with CPB has always been a major concern. Defective platelets, fibrinolysis, and dilution of coagulation factors are recognized consequences of CPB. Abnormal coagulation during CPB is associated with an acquired platelet defect resulting from the exposure of blood to a large thrombogenic surface. The duration of bypass and the degree of hypothermia are related to the degree of platelet dysfunction. Hemodilution secondary to the initiation of CPB leads to mild thrombocytopenia, but the platelet count usually remains adequate and cannot explain postbypass bleeding. Defects in platelet function are the predominant cause of abnormal bleeding after CPB. Evidence for this includes formation of platelet aggregates during and after CPB and the fact that platelets lose their ability to adhere to foreign surfaces. Platelet membrane receptors (glycoproteins) are lost during exposure to CPB.[82]

Isovolemic hemodilution is commonly used in cardiac surgery to decrease transfusion requirements and facilitate hypothermia. During hypothermic CPB, temperature effects such as increased blood viscosity limit organ blood flow and tissue oxygen delivery in the absence of hemodilution. Pharmacologic reduction of bleeding associated with CPB offers the advantages of easy administration and ready availability. In addition, other measures to decrease blood loss, meticulous attention to surgical hemostasis, autologous transfusion, and stricter criteria for transfusion decrease the need for homologous blood and blood products. Avoidance of the risks and complications associated with homologous transfusions helps enhance outcomes in elderly patients undergoing cardiac surgery.

Acute plasmapheresis performed after the induction of anesthesia but before CPB may be of benefit to cardiac surgery patients. Intravascular volume is maintained by the administration of a volume of fluid equal to the volume removed, thus maintaining the hemotocrit. The platelet-rich plasma is returned to the patient after CPB, following reversal of heparinization. The basis for this technique is that compromised platelet function is the most important cause of impaired clotting after bypass. When the patient's own platelets are isolated from the CPB circuit and returned to the patient after bypass, platelet function may be preserved. Improved hemostasis by augmenting clotting factors appears to be the reason for less pronounced bleeding. Withdrawal of autologous platelet-rich plasma also may make it possible to avoid the administration of homologous blood products.

Many elderly patients take platelet-inhibiting drugs, and plateletpheresis may not be advantageous. Patients undergoing repeat cardiac procedures experience greater blood loss and are much more likely to require allogeneic blood product transfusions. If plateletpheresis is likely to improve hemostasis after cardiac surgery, it is more likely to benefit patients undergoing reoperations.

It is difficult to know by what criteria the success or failure of administration of autologous platelet-rich plasma should be judged. There is little doubt that patients receiving platelet-rich plasma have higher platelet counts and better platelet aggregation, yet platelet counts correlate poorly with postoperative bleeding during cardiac surgery. Several studies have found a decrease in perioperative blood loss and transfusion requirements,[83,84] although other studies dispute these findings.[85] While not indicated in all cardiac surgical procedures, the use of platelet-rich autologous blood may benefit patients in whom the withdrawal of autologous whole blood cannot be performed and those expected to have long CPB procedures. Further definition of the role of acute plasmapheresis during cardiac surgery is being sought.

Both antiplasmin effects and antikallikrein properties have been proposed as the mechanism of action of aprotinin. Both mechanisms postulate that an acquired platelet defect is responsible for increased bleeding after CPB. The antiplasmin mechanism is based on the demonstration that plasmin lowers the number of platelet receptors (GP1b), reducing platelet adhesion after CPB. Aprotinin preserves GP1b platelet receptors and preserves the adhesive capacity of platelets in the postoperative period. The antikallikrein effects of aprotinin inhibit the contact phase of coagulation, leading to diminished generation of thrombin. Thrombin is a platelet aggregator, and platelet aggregation during CPB is thought to lead to postoperative platelet dysfunction. Because aprotinin is a kallikrein inhibitor, it has the potential to prolong clotting tests that depend on contact activation, such as whole blood activated clotting time (ACT). This is independent of prolongation of ACT by heparin, which works via factor VIII activation. A current recommendation is maintenance of heparin anticoagulation by increasing the ACT minimum to 750 s.[86]

Some controversy has surrounded early saphenous vein graft patency and the use of aprotinin. Specifically, the concern over increased perioperative MI in some patients receiving this drug has led to much investigation, which at this time seems to point to the safety of aprotinin. In one recent study, no deleterious effects on graft patency or renal function were demonstrated.[87] Aprotinin is effective in reducing bleeding and blood product transfusion rates. Because of its high cost and potential for adverse effects, identification of the patient population at highest risk of bleeding is crucial. Patients who require repeat combined procedures (revascularization and valve procedures) and repeat valve surgery are the most likely to be exposed to foreign blood products.[88]

ε-Aminocaproic acid (EACA) has antifibrinolytic activity that interferes with clot breakdown by inhibiting the fibrin-dissolving properties of plasmin. Treatment with fibrinolytic inhibitors is associated with a theoretical risk of an increased thrombotic tendency. However, controlled trials of the administration of prophylactic EACA to cardiac surgical patients have not demonstrated an increased incidence of venous, coronary, or cerebrovascular thrombosis.[89] Prophylactic administration has been shown to decrease chest tube blood loss 24 h postoperatively and the need for blood transfusions. EACA may exert its beneficial effect by inhibiting fibrinolysis, especially in the period from sternotomy to the end of CPB, but it also may help preserve platelets during and after CPB by reducing the effects of plasmin GP1b platelet receptors.

Desmopressin, an analogue of vasopressin that lacks vasoconstrictor properties, alters coagulation through its effects on circulatory endothelial cells and platelets. Factor VIII is released from storage sites, yielding a highly variable (2 to 20 times) increase in factor VIII coagulant activity. Desmopressin may be beneficial in a patient with a history of aspirin use and in a patient undergoing a reoperation or complicated combined procedures.[90]

Postoperative hemorrhage after CPB has multiple etiologies, making diagnosis and treatment difficult. Postbypass bleeding can be due to many interrelated factors, including the quality of surgical hemostasis, the nature of the coagulation defect, patient temperature, neuroendocrine responses, and drug therapy. The diagnosis of coagulation defects is often based on clinical evaluation and the results of laboratory screening tests. The selection of treatment usually is based on the hemostatic abnormalities that commonly occur in cardiac patients. Empirical therapy, however, may put patients at risk from unnecessary transfusion of blood products.

Clotting is a dynamic process that is difficult to measure using static endpoints that provide no information about the quality of the clot or the dynamics of its formation. Conventional coagulation screens (prothrombin time, partial thromboplastin time, platelet count, and fibrinogen concentration) are frequently inadequate for monitoring coagulation when there may be many potential hemostatic defects and continued blood loss may make the interpretation of sample results difficult. Thromboelastography (TEG), a test of viscoelastic clot strength, is helpful in assessing some specific abnormalities of hemostasis. Theoretically, TEG measures the entire process of clotting from the time of initial fibrin formation to eventual clot lysis. TEG allows a global assessment of hemostatic function to be made from a single blood sample, documenting the interaction of platelets with the protein coagulation cascade from the time of the initial platelet-fibrin interaction through clot strengthening and clot lysis. The generated tracing is characteristic of clotting factor activity, platelet function, and any significant fibrinolytic process within 20 to 30 min.

It has been suggested that TEG provides a unique means of assessing platelet activity and fibrinolysis, two common causes of postoperative bleeding in surgical cardiac patients. There is controversy surrounding the predictive accuracy of TEG versus routine coagulation testing.[91] The successful use of TEG as a tool for monitoring coagulation requires care and experience in performing the test and interpreting the results. Despite its limitations, it helps improve the assessment of coagulation after CPB.[92] Heparin-modified TEG assays are helpful in obtaining whole blood clotting information in the face of systemic heparinization and in the differentiation of causes of prolonged ACT values. Prospective longitudinal studies are needed to assess the specificity of TEG prediction of operative bleeding and to determine whether TEG-guided blood product administration can reduce transfusion requirements.

SUMMARY

Prediction of outcome measures such as length of stay and operative mortality is becoming an essential tool used by physicians in planning surgery. The decision to undergo elective cardiac surgery or to continue medical therapy in the elderly depends on the immediate and long-term benefits of the therapeutic options. Since the number of elderly cardiac patients is likely to continue to increase, it is necessary to gain a better understanding of the relative risks of morbidity after cardiac surgery in the aged.

Elective cardiac surgery can be performed in the elderly without prohibitive perioperative mortality and morbidity and with the anticipation of significantly improved symptomatic status and probably increased longevity. Delay of indicated operative intervention may result in the need for urgent operation with its greatly increased perioperative mortality rate. In many cases, surgical treatment has a positive impact on health care by decreasing the need for repeated acute-care hospital admissions. Awareness of facts concerning mortality, morbidity, length of hospital stay, and quality of life should guide the selection of candidates for cardiac surgery.

REFERENCES

1. National Center for Health Statistics: *Advance Data from Vital and Health Statistics.* Dept of Health and Human Services Publication (PHS) 89-1232. Washington, D.C.: U.S. Government Printing Office, 1989.
2. US Bureau of the Census: *Statistical Abstract of the United States: 1990,* 110th ed. Washington, D.C.: U.S. Government Printing Office, 1990.
3. Graves EJ: National Hospital Discharge Survey: Annual summary, 1988. National Center for Health Statistics. *Vital Health Stat* 13(106):1, 1991.
4. Weintraub WS, Craver JM, Cohen CL, et al: Influence of age on results of coronary artery surgery. *Circulation* 84(Suppl III):226, 1991.
5. Simpfendorfer C, Raymond R, Schraider J, et al: Early and long-term results of percutaneous transluminal coronary angioplasty in patients 70 years of age and older with angina pectoris. *Am J Cardiol* 62:959, 1988.
6. Kern MJ, Deligonul U, Galan K, et al: Percutaneous transluminal coronary angioplasty in octogenarians. *Am J Cardiol* 61:457, 1988.
7. GUSTO AFCR: The Global Utilization of Streptokinase and Tissue Plasminogen Activator for Occluded Coronary Arteries (GUSTO) Trial. *N Engl J Med* 329:723, 1993.
8. Grover FL, Hammermeister KE, Burchfiel C: Initial report of the Veterans Administration preoperative risk assessment study for cardiac surgery. *Ann Thorac Surg* 50:12, 1990.
9. Gersch BJ, Kronmal RA, Schaff HV, et al: Comparison of coronary artery bypass surgery and medical therapy in patients 65 years of age or older: A nonrandomized study from the Coronary Artery Surgery Study (CASS) registry. *N Engl J Med* 313:217, 1985.
10. Carey JS, Cukingnan RA, Singer LK: Quality of life after myocardial revascularization. *J Thorac Cardiovasc Surg* 103:108, 1992.
11. Bonow RO, Vitale DF, Bacharach SL, et al: Effects of aging on asynchronous left ventricular regional function and global ventricular filling in normal human subjects. *J Am Coll Cardiol* 11:50, 1988.
12. Rodeheffer RJ, Gerstenblith G, Becker LC, et al: Exercise cardiac output is maintained with advancing age in healthy human subjects: Cardiac dilatation and increased stroke volume compensate for a diminished heart rate. *Circulation* 69:203, 1984.

13. Alpert JS: Nitrate therapy in the elderly. *Am J Cardiol* 65:23J, 1990.
14. Flaherty JT, Reid PR, Kelly DT, et al: Intravenous nitroglycerin in acute myocardial infarction. *Circulation* 51:132, 1975.
15. Beck JC: Common diseases, disorders and health concerns—cardiovascular disease, in Beck JC (ed): *Geriatric Review Syllabus: A Core Curriculum in Geriatric Medicine.* New York: American Geriatrics Society, 1991, pp 265–286.
16. Egstrup K: Transient myocardial ischemia after abrupt withdrawal of antianginal therapy in chronic stable angina. *Am J Cardiol* 61:1219, 1988.
17. Durand PG, Lehot JJ, Foex P: Calcium-channel blockers and anaesthesia. *Can J Anaesth* 38:75, 1991.
18. Smith TW: Digitalis: Mechanism of action and clinical use. *N Engl J Med* 318:358, 1988.
19. Abernethy DR: Altered pharmacodynamics of cardiovascular drugs and their relation to altered pharmacokinetics in elderly patients. *Clin Geriatr Med* 6:285, 1990.
20. Williams GH: Converting enzyme inhibitors in the treatment of hypertension. *N Engl J Med* 319:1518, 1988.
21. Gundersen T, Abrahamsen, AM, Kjekshus J, et al: Timolol-related reduction in mortality and reinfarction in patients ages 65–75 years surviving acute myocardial infarction. *Circulation* 66:1179, 1982.
22. Lamy PP: Adverse drug effects. *Clin Geriatr Med* 6:293, 1990.
23. Fleg JL, Kennedy HL: Cardiac arrhythmias in a healthy elderly population: Detection by 24 hour ambulatory electrocardiography. *Chest* 81:302, 1982.
24. Carliner NH, Fisher ML, Plotnick GD, et al: Routine preoperative exercise testing in patients undergoing major noncardiac surgery. *Am J Cardiol* 56:51, 1985.
25. Hertzer NR, Young JR, Beven EG, et al: Late results of coronary bypass in patients with peripheral vascular disease: II. Five-year survival according to sex, hypertension, and diabetes. *Cleve Clin Q* 54:15, 1987.
26. Lakatta EG: Cardiovascular regulatory mechanism in advanced age. *Physiol Rev* 73:413, 1993.
27. Boucher CA, Brewster DC, Darling RC, et al: Determination of cardiac risk by dipyridamole-thallium imaging before peripheral vascular surgery. *N Engl J Med* 312:389, 1985.
28. Eagle KA, Coley CM, Newell JB, et al: Combining clinical and thallium data optimizes preoperative assessment of cardiac risk before major vascular surgery. *Ann Intern Med* 110:859, 1989.
29. Marwick TH, Underwood DA: Dipyridamole thallium imaging may not be a reliable screening test for coronary artery disease in patients undergoing vascular surgery. *Clin Cardiol* 13:14, 1990.
30. Fleisher LA, Nelson AH, Rosenbaum SH: Failure of negative dipyridamole thallium scans to predict perioperative myocardial ischaemia and infarction. *Can J Anaesth* 39:179, 1992.
31. Mangano DT, London MJ, Tubau JF, et al: Dipyridamole thallium-scintigraphy as a preoperative screening test: A reexamination of its predictive potential. *Circulation* 84:493, 1991.
32. Raby KE, Goldman L, Creager MA, et al: Correlation between preoperative ischemia and major cardiac events after peripheral vascular surgery. *N Engl J Med* 321:1296, 1989.
33. Raby KE, Barry J, Creager MA, et al: Detection and significance of intraoperative and postoperative myocardial ischemia in peripheral vascular surgery. *JAMA* 268:222, 1992.

34. Abraham SA, Coles NA, Coley CM, et al: Comparison of dipyridamole-thallium scintigraphy and ambulatory ECG monitoring in the pre-operative assessment of cardiac risk for vascular surgery (abstract). *J Am Coll Cardiol* 17:204A, 1991.
35. Horvath KA, DiSesa VJ, Peigh PS, et al: Favorable results of coronary artery bypass grafting in patients older than 75 years. *J Thorac Cardiovasc Surg* 99:92, 1990.
36. Loop FD, Lytle BW, Cosgrove DM, et al: Coronary artery bypass graft surgery in the elderly: Indications and outcome. *Cleve Clin J Med* 55:23, 1988.
37. Higgins TL, Estafanous FG, Loop FD, et al: Stratification of morbidity and mortality outcome by preoperative risk factors in coronary artery bypass patients: A clinical severity score. *JAMA* 267:2344, 1992.
38. Shah KB, Rao TLK, Laughlin S: A review of pulmonary artery catheterization in 6245 patients. *Anesthesiology* 61:271, 1984.
39. Tuman KJ, McCarthy RJ, Speiss BD, et al: Effect of pulmonary artery catheterization on outcome in patients undergoing coronary artery surgery. *Anesthesiology* 70:199, 1989.
40. Lowenstein E, Hollowell P, Levine F, et al: Cardiovascular response to large doses of intravenous morphine in man. *N Engl J Med* 281:1389, 1969.
41. Philbin DM, Rosow CE, Schneider RC, et al: Fentanyl and sufentanil anesthesia revisited: How much is enough? *Anesthesiology* 73:5, 1990.
42. Mangano DT, Siliciano D, Hollenberg M, et al: Postoperative myocardial ischemia: Therapeutic trials using intensive analgesia following surgery. *Anesthesiology* 76:342, 1992.
43. Tuman KJ, McCarthy RJ, Spiess BD, et al: Does choice of anesthetic agent significantly affect outcome after coronary artery surgery? *Anesthesiology* 70:189, 1989.
44. Slogoff S, Keats AS: Randomized trial of primary anesthetic agents on outcome of coronary bypass operations. *Anesthesiology* 70:179, 1989.
45. Benefiel DJ, Roizen, MF, Lamp GH, et al: Morbidity after aortic surgery with sufentanil versus isoflurane anesthesia. *Anesthesiology* 65:A516, 1986.
46. Roizen MF, Lampe GH, Benefiel DJ, et al: Is increased operative stress associated with worse outcome? *Anesthesiology* 67:A1, 1987.
47. Loop FD, Lytle BW, Cosgrove DM, et al: Influence of the internal-mammary-artery graft on 10-year survival and other cardiac events. *N Engl J Med* 314:1, 1986.
48. Barner HB, Swartz MT, Mudd JG, et al: Late patency of the internal mammary artery as a coronary bypass conduit. *Ann Thorac Surg* 34:408, 1982.
49. Roberts WC, Perloff JK, Costantino T: Severe valvular aortic stenosis in patients over 65 years of age: A clinicopathologic study. *Am J Cardiol* 27:497, 1971.
50. Roger VL, Tajik AJ, Bailey KR, et al: Progression of aortic stenosis in adults: New appraisal using Doppler echocardiography. *Am Heart J* 119:331, 1990.
51. Safian RD, Berman AD, Diver DJ, et al: Balloon aortic valvuloplasty in 170 consecutive patients. *N Engl J Med* 319:125, 1988.
52. Elayda MA, Hall RJ, Reul RM, et al: Aortic valve replacement in patients 80 years and older: Operative risks and long-term results. *Circulation* 88(II):11, 1993.
53. Lund O: Preoperative risk evaluation and stratification of long-term survival after valve replacement for aortic stenosis: Reasons for earlier operative intervention. *Circulation* 82:124, 1990.
54. Culliford AT, Galloway AC, Colvin SB, et al: Cardiac surgery in octogenarians: Do the risks exceed the benefit? *Am J Geriatr Cardiol* 1:15, 1992.
55. Christakis GT, Weisel RD, David TE, et al: Predictors of operative survival after valve replacement. *Circulation* 78(Suppl 1):25, 1988.

56. Matsuki O, Robles A, Gibbs S, et al: Long-term performance of 555 aortic homografts in the aortic position. *Ann Thorac Surg* 46:187, 1988.
57. Olson LJ, Subramanian R, Edwards WD: Surgical pathology of pure aortic insufficiency: A case study of 225 cases. *Mayo Clin Proc* 59:835, 1984.
58. Borow KM, Marcus RH: Aortic regurgitation: The need for an integrated physiologic approach. *J Am Coll Cardiol* 17:898, 1991.
59. Blakeman BM, Pifarre R, Sullivan HJ, et al: Aortic valve replacement in patients 75 years old and older. *Ann Thorac Surg* 44:637, 1987.
60. Limas CT: Mitral stenosis in the elderly. *Geriatrics* 26:75, 1971.
61. Thomas JD, Weyman AE: Doppler mitral pressure half-time: A clinical tool in search of theoretical justification. *J Am Coll Cardiol* 10:923, 1987.
62. Kay PH, Nunley DL, Grunkemeier GL, et al: Late results of combined mitral valve replacement and coronary bypass surgery. *J Am Coll Cardiol* 5:29, 1985.
63. Czer, LSC, Gray RJ, DeRobertis MA, et al: Mitral valve replacement: Impact of coronary artery disease and determinants of prognosis after revascularization. *Circulation* 70(Suppl I):1, 1984.
64. Deloche A, Jebara VA, Relland JYM, et al: Valve repair with Carpentier techniques, a second decade. *J Thorac Cardiovasc Surg* 99:1002, 1990.
65. Scott WC, Miller DC, Haverich A, et al: Operative risk of mitral valve replacement: Discriminant analysis of 1329 procedures. *Circulation* 72(Suppl II):108, 1985.
66. Sheikh KH, DeBruijn N, Rankin JS, et al: Utility of transesophageal echocardiography in patients undergoing cardiac valve surgery. *J Am Coll Cardiol* 13:123A, 1989.
67. Ross J: Afterload mismatch in aortic and mitral valve disease: Implications for surgical therapy. *J Am Coll Cardiol* 5:811, 1985.
68. Cosgrove DM, Stewart WJ: Mitral valvuloplasty. *Curr Probl Cardiol* 14:355, 1989.
69. Zile MR, Gaasch WH, Carroll JD, et al: Chronic mitral regurgitation: Predictive value of preoperative echocardiographic indexes of left ventricular function and wall stress. *J Am Coll Cardiol* 3:235, 1984.
70. Davis EA, Gardner TJ, Gillinov AM, et al: Valvular disease in the elderly: Influence on surgical results. *Ann Thorac Surg* 55:333, 1993.
71. Lytle BW, Cosgrove DM, Taylor PC, et al: Reoperations for valve surgery: Perioperative mortality and determinants of risk for 1,000 patients from 1958. *Ann Thorac Surg* 42:632, 1986.
72. Cosgrove DM: Evaluation of perioperative risk factors. *J Cardiac Surg* 5(Suppl 3):227, 1990.
73. Salerno TA, Houck JP, Barrozzo CAM, et al: Retrograde continuous warm blood cardioplegia: A new concept in myocardial protection. *Am J Thorac Surg* 51:245, 1991.
74. Mikulic E, Cohn JN, Franciosa JA: Comparative hemodynamic effects of inotropic and vasodilator drugs in severe heart failure. *Circulation* 56:528, 1977.
75. Cohn LH: The role of mechanical devices. *J Cardiac Surg* 5(Suppl):278, 1990.
76. Tuman KJ, McCarthy RJ, Najafi H, et al: Differential effects of advanced age on neurologic and cardiac risks of coronary artery operations. *J Thorac Cardiovasc Surg* 104:1510, 1992.
77. Petruk KC, West M, Mohr G, et al: Nimodipine treatment in poor-grade aneurysm patients: Results of a multi-center double-blind placebo-controlled trial. *J Neurosurg* 68:505, 1988.
78. Brusino FG, Reves JG, Smith LR, et al: The effect of age on cerebral blood flow during hypothermic cardiopulmonary bypass. *J Thorac Cardiovasc Surg* 97:541, 1989.

79. Loop FD, Lytle BW, Cosgrove DM, et al: Sternal wound complications after isolated coronary artery bypass grafting: Early and late mortality, morbidity and cost of care. *Ann Thorac Surg* 49:179, 1990.
80. Gailiunas P, Chawla R, Lazarus J, et al: Acute renal failure following cardiac operations. *J Thorac Cardiovasc Surg* 79:241, 1980.
81. Corwin HL, Sprague SM, DeLaria GA, et al: Acute renal failure associated with cardiac operations. *J Thorac Cardiovasc Surg* 98:1107, 1989.
82. Mammen EF, Koets MH, Washington BC: Hemostasis changes during cardiopulmonary bypass surgery. *Semin Thromb Hemost* 11:281, 1985.
83. Czer LSC: Mediastinal bleeding after cardiac surgery: Etiologies, diagnostic considerations, and blood conservation methods. *J Cardiovasc Anesth* 3:760, 1989.
84. Boldt J, von Bormann B, Kling D, et al: Preoperative plasmapheresis in patients undergoing cardiac surgery procedures. *Anesthesiology* 72:282, 1990.
85. Wong CA, Franklin ML, Wade LD: Coagulation tests, blood loss, and transfusion requirements in platelet-rich plasmapheresed versus nonpheresed cardiac surgery patients. *Anesth Analg* 78:29, 1994.
86. Hunt BJ, Segal H, Yacoub M: Aprotinin and heparin monitoring during cardiopulmonary bypass. *Circulation* 86(Suppl II):410, 1992.
87. Lemmer JH, Stanford W, Bonney SL, et al: Aprotinin for coronary bypass operations: Efficacy, safety, and influence on early saphenous vein graft patency. *J Thorac Cardiovasc Surg* 107:543, 1994.
88. Hardy JF, Perrault J, Tremblay N, et al: The stratification of cardiac surgical procedures according to use of blood products: A retrospective analysis of 1,480 cases. *Can J Anaesth* 38:511, 1991.
89. DelRossi AJ, Cernaianu AC, Botros S: Prophylactic treatment of postperfusion bleeding using EACA. *Chest* 96:27, 1989.
90. Scott WJ, Kessler R, Wernly JA: Blood conservation in cardiac surgery. *Ann Thorac Surg* 50:843, 1990.
91. Wang JS, Lin CY, Hung WT, et al: Thromboelastogram fails to predict postoperative hemorrhage in cardiac patients. *Ann Thorac Surg* 53:435, 1992.
92. Tuman KJ, Speiss BD, McCarthy RJ, et al: Comparison of viscoelastic measures of coagulation after cardiopulmonary bypass. *Anesth Analg* 69:69, 1989.

CHAPTER 14

Anesthesia for Thoracic Surgery in Geriatric Patients

Dale E. Solomon

INTRODUCTION

Thoracic surgery today predominantly consists of geriatric surgery because lung cancer, esophageal disorders, and pleural disease mostly afflict the elderly population. Since with few exceptions only the aged undergo thoracic operations, most of what is known about anesthesia for thoracic surgery has come from clinical studies involving elderly patients. Therefore, the safe conduct of thoracic anesthesia requires (1) specific knowledge of the effect of aging and disease on the physiology of the major organ systems, (2) suspicion of and a search for occult major organ disease in asymptomatic patients, (3) appreciation of the effect of aging on the pharmacokinetic and pharmacodynamic properties of anesthetic drugs, (4) recognition of the limited homeostatic responses of elderly patients to physiological perturbations caused by surgical trauma, changes in blood volume, and pain, and (5) knowledge of the unique aspects of thoracic surgery, such as positioning, the surgical incision, one-lung ventilation, and pain control.

This chapter discusses the preoperative evaluation of elderly thoracic surgery patients, reviews general considerations of patient care during thoracic surgery, discusses anesthesia for common thoracic operations, considers the complications associated with those procedures, and reviews postoperative pain management and pain control. Because the effect of aging on organ system function and drug pharmacology has been presented in Chaps. 1 through 6, these changes will be discussed only as they relate to the perioperative care of thoracic surgery patients.

PREOPERATIVE EVALUATION

Elderly patients presenting for thoracic surgery have wide variations in baseline physiological status and response to stress. Disease occurs focally in the elderly population and with widely variable degrees of severity. Many of the disease processes are occult. Thoracic surgical procedures challenge patients with a large degree of perioperative stress, resulting in some of the highest perioperative mortality rates of any elective surgery. For example, the mortality associated with pneumonectomy is about 6 to 7 percent.[1] Thus, exhaustive preoperative assessment and optimization of organ function are critically important in defining risk and optimizing outcome in thoracic surgery.

Cardiovascular Status

Most noncardiac thoracic operations today are lung resections for cancer. The patients are most often elderly and have a history of cigarette smoking. These patients have a high prevalence of coronary artery disease (CAD), most of which is clinically silent. The manifestations of CAD include angina, congestive heart failure, conduction disturbances, arrhythmias, and valvular disorders. A careful history and physical examination should be directed toward the signs and symptoms of these disorders. In addition, evidence of CAD should be investigated by noninvasive and invasive methods when necessary. Nearly all patients will have a preoperative 12-lead electrocardiogram (ECG); a normal resting ECG does not preclude the presence of CAD, but an abnormal ECG is correlated with an adverse cardiac outcome.[2] Many patients, including those with documented CAD or risk factors for CAD, require further cardiac testing. Fleisher and Barash[3] have proposed a preoperative cardiac evaluation algorithm for patients undergoing surgical procedures that place them at a high risk for perioperative ischemia, including intrathoracic procedures. Their scheme proposes further evaluation (dipyridamole thallium, thallium exercise, or coronary angiography) for patients with documented CAD and patients with poor exercise tolerance who have risk factors for CAD (age, hypertension, diabetes mellitus, male sex, lipid profile).

Pulmonary Status

Thoracic surgeons are primarily responsible for determining the resectability of lung cancers. Bronchoscopy, mediastinoscopy, and limited thoracotomy are performed to evaluate the local spread of tumor, while radiological procedures and bone marrow biopsy rule out metastatic disease. If the lesion is limited to the lung, the feasibility of a lung resection is evaluated by pulmonary testing. The goal of testing is to predict morbidity and mortality after lung resection so that futile operations are not performed and patients can make informed decisions about their care.

Male sex, older age, greater extent of surgical resection, and a compromised forced expiratory volume (FEV_1) on spirometric testing have been associated with increased morbidity and mortality after lung resection.[4] Among these factors, FEV_1 is the most controversial, with nearly half the relevant investigations failing to show a correlation of FEV_1 with the postoperative outcome. Still, most experts agree that preoperative pulmonary function tests are useful in identifying high-risk patients. The risk is higher in patients with FEV_1 below 2 liters undergoing pneumonectomy, below 1 liter for those undergoing lobectomy, and below 0.6 liter for those undergoing wedge resection.[1] These groups of patients should receive quantitative ventilation-perfusion lung scanning to determine the amount of functional lung tissue after resection. On the basis of historical data, patients are considered candidates for lung resection when the calculated FEV_1 of the remaining lung after resection is greater than 800 to 1000 ml or above 40 percent of the normal value.[5] When the calculated FEV_1 is borderline, exercise testing to assess the maximum rate of oxygen utilization ($VO_{2\,max}$) may predict mortality: A $VO_{2\,max} > 20$ ml/kg per minute is associated with low morbidity and mortality.

Several other patient variables may preoperatively identify risk factors for a poor outcome after thoracotomy. These include arterial blood gases ($Pa_{CO_2} > 45$ mmHg, $Pa_{O_2} < 50$ mmHg), dyspnea at rest, low carbon monoxide diffusing capacity (DLCO), current smoking, and pulmonary hypertension or cor pulmonale.[4–6] Most clinicians favor offering surgical treatment even to lung cancer patients at high risk for morbidity and mortality because of the dismal outcome of nonoperative therapies.

During spirometry, the response of dynamic lung volumes to bronchodilators is assessed. Patients with a beneficial response to bronchodilator therapy should receive inhaled $beta_2$ agonists beginning 1 to 2 days before the procedure and through the perioperative period. Patients with chronic bronchitis should be treated with antibiotics if there is evidence of acute infection or if the sputum has recently changed in quality or quantity. Finally, the value of preoperative teaching of incentive spirometry, inhalation of bronchodilators, and coughing techniques cannot be overemphasized.

Other Major Organ Systems

As with any elective surgical procedure, preoperative evaluation requires a search for existing diseases and medical optimization of those disease states. Of particular importance in elderly thoracic surgery patients are the evaluation of renal function and the detection of both neurological disease (including cerebrovascular disease, CNS tumors, myasthenic syndromes, Parkinson's disease, and dementia) and metabolic disorders (poor nutritional status, electrolyte imbalance, and endocrine disease). Many elderly patients have a hiatal hernia and/or gastroesophageal reflux in addition to disorders of esophageal motility. These abnormalities place them at risk for aspiration of gastric contents during the induction of anesthesia and the placement of a double-lumen endotracheal tube.

INTRAOPERATIVE CARE OF ELDERLY PATIENTS DURING THORACIC SURGERY

Monitoring

Because of the greater potential for cardiovascular stress and respiratory dysfunction imposed by thoracic operations, the level of intraoperative monitoring is usually increased, especially in older patients with more organ system disease. All patients undergoing thoracic surgery receive blood pressure, pulse oximeter, temperature, and end-tidal gas monitoring. In addition, a two-lead ECG system can detect supraventricular arrhythmias and most episodes of myocardial ischemia. However, because the ECG electrode positions must be altered during left-sided chest operations and because most patients will be in the lateral position, ST segment analysis is more difficult during thoracic surgery. Intraarterial catheters are invaluable for blood gas sampling both during surgery and postoperatively and provide instantaneous evaluation of the effects of anesthetic agents, surgical incursions, cardiac dysrhythmias, and blood loss on changes in blood pressure. Many patients undergoing thoracotomy require central venous pressure (CVP) monitoring. The CVP displays a trend that may be used as an adjunct in assessing the adequacy of intravascular volume replacement, especially when the response of the CVP to fluid challenges is analyzed. In cases where extensive pulmonary resection has caused increases in pulmonary vascular resistance and right ventricular strain, acute elevations of the CVP may be the first indicator of right-sided heart dysfunction. In addition, the CVP provides reliable and speedy access to the central circulation in a group of patients who are at increased risk for cardiac dysrhythmias. While the CVP has been presumed to give some indication of left-sided heart filling in elderly patients with cardiac and pulmonary disease, this assumption is often not reliable.[7] In this group of patients, especially when extensive pulmonary resection is planned or when the potential for blood loss is great, pulmonary artery catheter monitoring is recommended to judge the adequacy of cardiac preload and function. It should be noted that the pulmonary artery occlusion pressure (PAOP) may give falsely low readings after a pneumonectomy, probably as a result of balloon occlusion causing a decrease in left-sided heart filling when the pulmonary vascular cross-sectional area is diminished.[8] Also, care must be taken to redirect the pulmonary artery catheter into the nonoperative lung before clamping of the pulmonary artery during pneumonectomy.

Choice of Anesthetic Agents

The choice of anesthetic agents is influenced by multiple factors, including the patient's preanesthetic physiological condition, the type and duration of the proposed operation, and the anesthesiologist's skill and experience with specific anesthetic techniques and drugs. Various combinations of volatile anesthetics, opioids, and muscle relaxants can provide safe anesthesia for thoracic surgery in the elderly. Patients with significant bronchospastic disease and airway resistance may benefit from a volatile anesthetic-based regimen that avoids the use of histamine-releasing drugs such as morphine and curare. Even during one-lung ventilation, the effect of volatile anesthetics in reducing hypoxic pulmonary vasoconstriction and causing arterial hypoxemia is clinically unimportant. For patients in whom extubation of the trachea is planned at the end of surgery, careful dosing of opioids to allow spontaneous ventilation while providing adequate analgesia at the end of surgery can be a challenge because of the great variability of the pharmacokinetics and pharmacodynamics of opioids in the elderly. Elderly patients metabolize opioid analgesics nearly as quickly as does the younger population, but the pharmacodynamic effect at the same serum concentration may be exaggerated, leading to more pronounced sedation and respiratory depression. Many patients with known CAD require an opioid-based anesthetic because of the beneficial effects on hemodynamic variables. A study comparing high-dose fentanyl with halothane for thoracic surgery found greater suppression of the cardiovascular and hormonal response to surgical stress with fentanyl but also more postoperative respiratory depression.[9]

Elderly patients may benefit from combined epidural analgesia–general anesthesia for thoracic operations, but prospective randomized outcome studies showing a beneficial effect of this technique are lacking.[10] The potential advantages of combining epidural analgesia with general anesthesia include (1) the effect of preemptive analgesia in attenuating postoperative pain, (2) lower dose requirements for volatile anesthetics and opioids, resulting in lessened postoperative CNS and respiratory depression, (3) favorable hemodynamic changes, including venous and arterial dilation, resulting in decreased cardiac preload and afterload, (4) cardiac sympatholysis, and (5) chest wall relaxation without the use of muscle relaxants. However, epidural anesthesia may result in significant hypotension, requiring fluid administration and preventing the use of the higher doses of the volatile anesthetics that may be needed to treat bronchospasm.

Positioning

Many thoracic operations (mediastinoscopy, lung biopsy, thymectomy) can be performed in the supine or tilted position, but most lung surgery is performed in the lateral decubitus position to allow a posterolateral thoracotomy incision. This position is associated with many potential nerve injury syndromes, including brachial plexus injury, ulnar nerve injury, peroneal nerve injury, and Horner's syndrome. In addition, ligamentous injury to the neck can occur, as well as ocular damage (retinal artery thrombosis) caused by excessive pressure on the eyeball.[11] Patients with glaucoma appear to be at greater risk for the latter complication. The elderly may be more prone to position-related injuries caused by vascular and nutritional disease, loss of musculoskeletal elasticity, and loss of subcutaneous tissue protecting peripheral nerves. However, no study has indicated that the elderly have an increased incidence of nerve injury during positioning for thoracic surgery.

Careful attention during positioning to prevent compression of the axilla, pad superficial nerves, relieve pressure on the eye, and maintain the normal anatomic relations of the head, arms, and legs will prevent most injuries associated with the lateral decubitus position. This position has important effects on pulmonary physiology that are discussed under "Pulmonary Resection," below.

The Incision

Advances in technology now allow many thoracic procedures to be performed endoscopically, including pulmonary and mediastinal lymph node biopsies, airway and esophageal laser surgery, and esophageal dilatation. A number of intrathoracic procedures are now performed with a thoracoscope, including pulmonary wedge resection, lobectomy, and pericardial procedures. Except for thoracoscopic surgery, endoscopic procedures cause minimal physiological stress and can be tolerated even by very elderly patients in poor medical condition.

By far the most common incision in thoracic surgery is the thoracotomy, an incision that provides excellent exposure for a pulmonary resection. After thoracotomy, there is an immediate decrease in vital capacity that continues to worsen until the third postoperative day.[12] The FEV_1 and functional residual capacity (FRC) decrease by at least 50 percent. The closing volume (lung volume at which small airways begin to collapse) increases with aging and eventually surpasses the FRC, resulting in alveolar collapse during tidal breathing. Further decreases in FRC associated with a chest incision exaggerate this phenomenon and result in arterial hypoxemia. Rib spreading must be performed carefully in the elderly because of the tendency of ribs to break rather than bend, and rib resection has been advocated when this difficulty is encountered. Anterolateral thoracotomy incisions seem to cause less pain and to be better tolerated than are posterolateral thoracotomy incisions. Muscle-sparing thoracotomy incisions have been found to improve postoperative pulmonary function compared with standard thoracotomy incisions (Fig. 14-1).[13] The median sternotomy incision has a less adverse effect on postoperative pulmonary function than does the thoracotomy incision but provides suboptimal surgical access for some pulmonary resections.

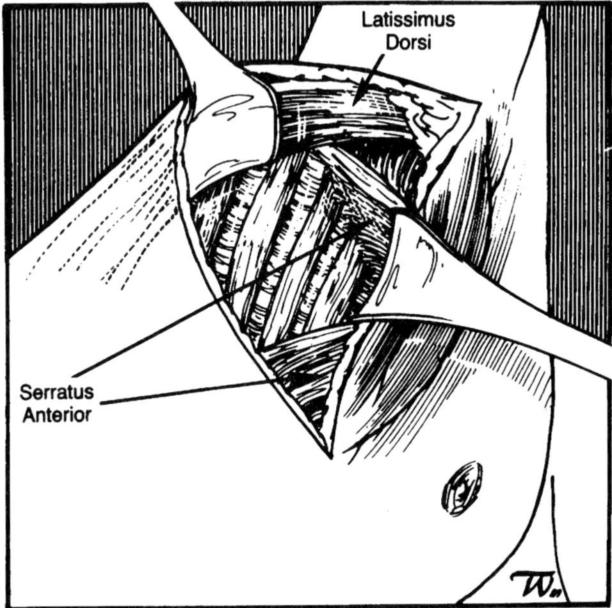

Figure 14-1 Retraction of latissimus dorsi and serratus anterior muscles during limited muscle-sparing thoracotomy incision. (*Reprinted with permission from Lemmer JH, Gomez MN, Symreng T, et al: Limited lateral thoracotomy: Improved postoperative pulmonary function. Arch Surg 125:873, 1990. Copyright 1990 American Medical Association.*)

Fluid Management

Elderly patients have a depressed homeostatic response to changes in intravascular blood volume. With blood loss, more severe hypotension occurs in the elderly compared with the young. In addition, vascular disease and altered autoregulation make episodes of hypotension much more damaging. Elevations in intravascular volume can lead to excessive preload, especially in a heart with diastolic dysfunction, which in turn leads to elevations in left atrial and pulmonary artery pressures and pulmonary edema. Excessive fluid administration during chest surgery has been associated with atrial dysrhythmias and postpneumonectomy pulmonary edema. There is no clear substantiation in the literature for preference of either crystalloid or colloid for fluid replacement. While many studies seem to indicate that cancer patients who receive allogeneic blood have an increased relapse rate,[14] not all investigators have found this to be true.[15]

Temperature Regulation

The elderly are more prone to intraoperative hypothermia.[16] During chest surgery, they may become hypothermic because of depressed thermoregulatory responses to the hypothermic operating room environment, a lowered basal metabolic rate, or exposure of the highly vascular contents of the thoracic cage to the cold, arid ambient atmosphere. Precautions should be taken to prevent hypothermia during thoracic anesthesia because of the negative consequences of postoperative hypothermia and shivering on cardiac and respiratory demand in patients who are already compromised by preexisting disease, lung resection, and postthoracotomy pain. To this end, anesthetic gases should be heated and humidified, exposure of skin to the cold operating room environment should be kept to a minimum, and intravenous fluids and blood should be warmed. In addition, the operating room should be kept relatively warm while a patient is undergoing surgical preparation.

NONCARDIAC THORACIC OPERATIONS

Mediastinoscopy

Mediastinoscopy is performed in patients before thoracotomy to make a tissue diagnosis of cancer or to verify the absence of metastatic disease before thoracotomy and lung resection. The mediastinoscope is inserted through a cervical incision just cephalad to the sternal notch and is advanced under the sternum to visualize and biopsy the mediastinal lymph nodes that drain the lungs. The position of the mediastinoscope is anterior to the trachea and posterior to the great vessels. The anterior mediastinum cannot be accessed during mediastinoscopy; for this, an anterior mediastinotomy (Chamberlain's incision) is performed. Mediastinoscopy is well tolerated even by the most frail patients, since there is usually very little postoperative pain and surgical stress response. Probably the most stressful part of the operation is the induction of anesthesia and tracheal intubation. The only absolute contraindication to mediastinoscopy is previous mediastinal surgery, since scar tissue eliminates the plane of dissection.

Most patients for mediastinoscopy receive general endotracheal anesthesia, although the procedure can be performed with local anesthesia only. Anesthesia can be induced with a variety of short-acting anesthetics and muscle relaxants in anticipation of a short surgical procedure and tracheal extubation at the end of surgery. A relatively large, armored endotracheal tube is preferred to allow flexible bronchoscopy, if needed, and prevent tracheal compression by the mediastinoscope.

Mediastinoscopy can be associated with serious complications. Accidental injury to the aorta or pulmonary vasculature can result in an exsanguinating hemorrhage. For this reason, large-bore venous access should be obtained and blood should be made available before surgical intervention; intraarterial pressure monitoring is also recommended. If the superior vena cava is lacerated, venous access in the lower extremities must be obtained. The mediastinoscope can compress the right innominate artery, compromising blood flow to both the right arm and the right carotid and vertebral arteries. Thus, right radial arterial cannulation is usually performed to detect innominate artery compression. An alternative option is left radial arterial cannulation with a right-hand pulse oximeter or Doppler to monitor innominate artery flow.

Air entrainment through the mediastinoscope can occur, especially in a patient who is allowed to breathe spontaneously. Phrenic nerve damage may result in diaphragmatic dysfunction. Pneumothorax can occur, as can injury to the recurrent laryngeal nerve, especially on the left. Finally, because many of these patients have lung cancer, they have a higher prevalence of myasthenic syndrome (Eaton-Lambert syndrome) and may exhibit exaggerated responses to nondepolarizing muscle relaxants.

Pulmonary Resection

Patients undergoing pulmonary resection are for the most part aged, and those who are most elderly are at increased risk for the perioperative complications associated with thoracotomy.[4] Resection of pulmonary tissue is performed for benign or malignant neoplasms, infectious processes, lung biopsy, or pulmonary vascular lesions. The amount of lung removed ranges from a small wedge to a complete pneumonectomy, but the anesthetic considerations are similar in that most of the procedures require a thoracotomy incision and one-lung ventilation (OLV). Pulmonary resection performed through a thoracoscope is discussed under a separate heading below.

Small pulmonary resections (e.g., lung biopsy and wedge resection) can be performed without the use of OLV. However, most lung surgeries are facilitated by OLV when the patient is in the lateral decubitus position, allowing the operative lung to deflate in the chest cavity while the dependent lung is ventilated. The only absolute indications for OLV are to separate the two lungs to prevent spillover of infection, blood, or fluid from the diseased lung to the healthy lung and to minimize the complications associated with positive-pressure ventilation in patients with a bronchopleural fistula, giant bullae, or severe unilateral disease. Otherwise, OLV improves the surgeon's operative field and makes the dissection quicker and easier. OLV is highly desirable for some operations but less so for others (Table 14-1).

Most OLV today is performed with polyvinyl chloride double-lumen tubes (DLTs) designed for the left or right mainstem bronchus. They are available in French sizes 35, 37, 39, and 41, with the smaller sizes being utilized for women and small men and the larger sizes for large men. The use of right-sided DLTs is diminishing because of the difficulty in placing the endobronchial portion of the tube without occluding the right upper lobe bronchus. Nearly all operations, including left pneumonectomy, can be performed with a left-sided DLT by pulling the bronchial portion of the tube back before clamping the mainstem bronchus.

Proper placement of the DLT is of paramount importance to assure adequate oxygenation and ventilation during OLV. Today, most clinicians verify optimal positioning of the DLT with a fiber-optic bronchoscope (FOB). When the FOB is inserted into the tracheal lumen of the DLT, passage of the bronchial portion of the DLT into the appropriate mainstem bronchus can be ascertained. The inflated bronchial balloon (blue-colored for easy recognition) should be seen just below the carina but not herniating over the top. With a pediatric FOB, the takeoff of the left or right upper lobe bronchus should be visualized past the tip of the left endobronchial tube or through a special side slot in the right endobronchial tube. After the patient has been placed in the lateral decubitus position, placement should be verified again.

Recently the Univent tube, which is basically a single-lumen endotracheal tube with an integrated bronchial blocker, has become available for OLV (Fig. 14-2). The Univent tube may cause less trauma during insertion, can be used for rapid sequence induction of anesthesia, can selectively block lung segments, and eliminates the need for changing the tube at the end of anesthesia.[17] These properties may make the Univent tube advantageous for elderly patients.

The physiology of OLV predicts that a significant pulmonary shunt will occur because of atelectasis of the nondependent (deflated) lung with maintained

Table 14-1 Procedures facilitated by one-lung ventilation

High priority
Thoracic aortic aneurysm
Pneumonectomy
Upper lobectomy
Thoracoscopy
Low priority
Middle and lower lobectomies and wedge resections
Esophageal surgery
Thoracic spine operations

SOURCE: Adapted from Benumof JL: *Anesthesia for Thoracic Surgery*. Philadelphia: Saunders, 1987, p 224.

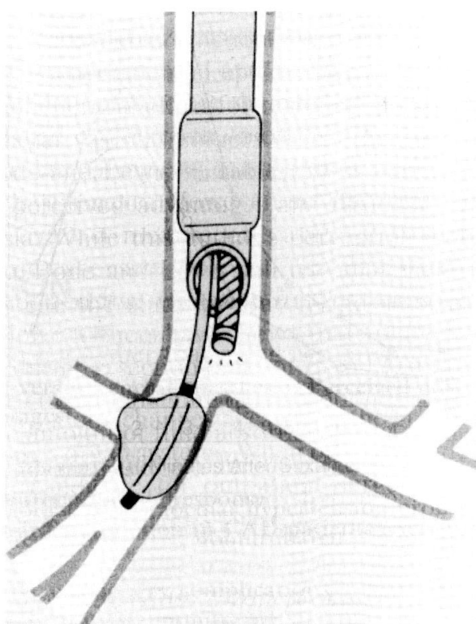

Figure 14-2 The Univent tube. Bronchoscopic verification of proper blocker placement in the right mainstem bronchus. (*Reprinted with permission from Fuji Systems Corporation, Tokyo, Japan.*)

perfusion. The lateral decubitus position and the effect of hypoxic pulmonary vasoconstriction (HPV), which tends to limit pulmonary blood flow to hypoxic areas of lung, diminish blood flow to the nonventilated nondependent lung. Elderly patients may have conditions that inhibit the effectiveness of HPV in preventing hypoxemia. For example, elevations in left atrial pressure and pulmonary arterial pressure allow blood to flow past the limitation imposed at the level of the precapillary pulmonary arterioles, allowing greater perfusion of poorly ventilated alveoli. In addition, as pulmonary function worsens with age, baseline V/Q mismatching and pulmonary shunt are additive to the detrimental effects of OLV, allowing hypoxemia during OLV. Volatile anesthetics, pulmonary vasodilators, and alkalosis all tend to inhibit the effect of HPV. As was mentioned earlier, the clinical effect of volatile anesthetics on arterial oxygen pressure (Pa_{O_2}) during OLV appears to be minimal.

However, in a study examining patient variables that are associated with arterial hypoxemia during OLV, age was not an independent variable. The Pa_{O_2} during OLV was found to be predicted by (1) which lung was operated on, (2) the preoperative FEV_1 percent, and (3) the intraoperative Pa_{O_2} during two-lung ventilation.[18]

Problems with hypoxemia during OLV are treated by increasing the F_iO_2, assuring proper DLT placement, supplying continuous positive airway pressure (CPAP) to the nondependent lung and/or supplying positive end-expiratory pressure (PEEP) to the dependent lung. Normocarbia should be maintained to optimize HPV, and in elderly patients this may require a lower minute ventilation compared with the young, since carbon dioxide production (V_{CO_2}) declines with age.

Two complications frequently associated with pneumonectomy deserve mention: atrial fibrillation (AF) and postpneumonectomy pulmonary edema. There is a high prevalence of AF in the elderly population, probably because of atrial enlargement, CAD, conduction system disease, and elevated circulating catecholamines. Elderly patients are more susceptible to the detrimental effects of AF because they are more dependent on synchronized atrial contraction to maintain cardiac output and are less able to tolerate transient episodes of hypotension associated with AF. About 15 percent of elderly patients develop AF after thoracotomy, and patients who develop atrial dysrhythmias have a higher mortality. Older patients have been reported to be at increased risk for the onset of AF after thoracotomy, although this finding is not constant. Atrial fibrillation appears to occur more frequently after pneumonectomy compared with lobectomy, and intrapericardial dissection is a predisposing factor.[19]

Digoxin has been administered prophylactically to patients undergoing lung resection, with some studies showing a decreased incidence of cardiac dysrhythmias. More recent prospective randomized trials have failed to show a benefit of digoxin after thoracotomy,[20,21] and the use of digoxin to prevent or treat AF in other clinical situations is being reevaluated.[22] Intravenous diltiazem has become available for the treatment of AF with rapid ventricular response.[23] Prevention of AF depends on limiting increases in atrial size and circulating catecholamine levels. To this end, judicious fluid administration, prevention of anemia, and pain control may be beneficial.

Postpneumonectomy pulmonary edema occurs in about 5 percent of patients up to 6 days after pneumonectomy.[24] Its occurrence appears to be increased after right pneumonectomy and when the perioperative fluid balance is distinctly positive. The pulmonary artery occlusion pressure is usually low, in a range where the diagnosis of noncardiogenic pulmonary edema is made. Autopsy findings in patients who die with postpneumonectomy pulmonary edema most often reveal histological evidence of ARDS. Etiologic factors may include endothelial cell injury and capillary leak, decreased lymphatic drainage, and decreased plasma oncotic pressure.[25] Elderly patients may be at increased risk for postpneumonectomy pulmonary edema because of an elevated pulmonary arterial pressure, elevated pulmonary artery occlusion pressure, decreased serum protein concentrations, and decreased surface area of the pulmonary capillary bed resulting from the emphysematous changes associated with aging. Treatment of the pulmonary edema is much the same as with other causes of pulmonary edema: oxygen, positive-pressure airway therapy, diuresis, and fluid restriction.

Esophageal Surgery

Esophageal diseases that afflict primarily the elderly often require surgical intervention: esophageal diverticulum, achalasia, and cancer. Most surgical procedures performed on the esophagus require left thoracotomy and OLV.

These patients often come to surgery in a debilitated, nutritionally compromised condition and are at risk for pulmonary aspiration of esophageal and gastric contents during the induction of anesthesia. Esophagectomy is performed by many surgeons now as a transhiatal operation carried out with abdominal and cervical incisions. The stomach is pulled up to the neck through the bed of the esophagus, and a cervical esophagogastrostomy is performed. Manipulation of the mediastinum during freeing of the esophagus results in a high incidence of cardiac arrhythmias, including premature ventricular contractions (PVCs) and AF. Blood loss can be excessive, and large-bore intravenous access is recommended. Elderly patients appear to have a higher rate of postoperative pulmonary complications and a higher mortality.[26]

Thymectomy

Thymoma is more frequently associated with myasthenia gravis in the elderly,[27] and it has been recommended that all elderly patients with myasthenia gravis undergo thymectomy. The procedure can be undertaken through either a cervical incision or a sternotomy. The procedure is tolerated well in most elderly patients. While the perioperative management of myasthenia gravis is beyond the scope of this chapter, it should be emphasized that plasmapheresis has been found to be of benefit in improving neuromuscular function postoperatively.[28]

Thoracoscopic Surgery

Chest surgery performed through a thoracoscope [video-assisted thoracic surgery (VATS)] has become widespread since 1992. Procedures that can be performed with VATS include wedge resection, lung biopsy, lobectomy, pleural biopsy, pleurectomy, and several other procedures involving intrathoracic structures, including pericardial drainage and biopsy. The technique requires OLV and the lateral decubitus position. Three small incisions less than 3 cm each are necessary for insertion of the video telescope and surgical instruments (Fig. 14-3).[29] Before the insertion of the instruments, the lung is deflated and collapse is verified by digital examination. A relatively large proportion of patients (up to 20 percent) require conversion to full thoracotomy because of inability to locate the lung mass or because a difficult resection is encountered. The respiratory compromise imposed by OLV occurs with VATS, but the surgical stress is much less and postoperative pain and pulmonary dysfunction are probably greatly diminished. For instance, patients undergoing lung resection via muscle-sparing thoracotomy have greater postoperative morphine requirements, greater pain perception scores, worsened FEV_1 on postoperative day 3, and a greater number of postoperative pulmonary complications compared with patients undergoing VATS.[30] Compared with younger patients undergoing VATS, older patients (> age 75 years) have a longer hospital stay and a greater incidence of pulmonary air leaks and cardiac dysrhythmias.[31]

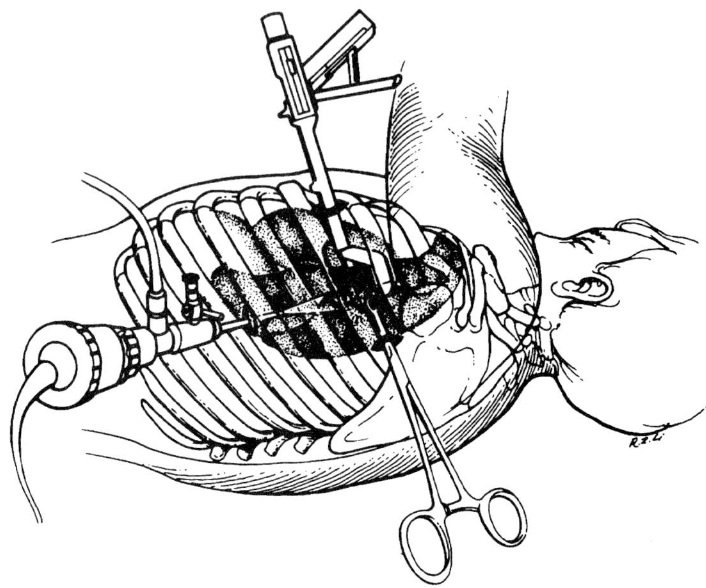

Figure 14-3 Incisions for thoracoscope and instruments during VATS. (*Reprinted with permission from Lewis RJ, Caccavale RJ, Sisler GE, Mackenzie JW: One hundred consecutive patients undergoing video-assisted thoracic operations. Ann Thorac Surg 54:421, 1992.*)

POSTOPERATIVE MANAGEMENT

Most elderly patients require intensive hemodynamic and respiratory support after thoracic surgery because the physiological insults caused by surgical stress, pain, loss of pulmonary tissue, and changes in intravascular volume are poorly compensated for by the limited cardiopulmonary reserve of the aged. The leading cause of postoperative morbidity after thoracotomy is pulmonary dysfunction, which is related at least in part to the fact that these patients have significant preexisting pulmonary disease. In addition, the effects of the thoracotomy are such that diaphragmatic function is depressed.[32] Pain control improves respiratory function and allows adequate coughing and deep breathing to assist in clearance of secretions and in preventing atelectasis. Many patients require a period of postoperative mechanical ventilatory support while respiratory therapy maneuvers and hemodynamic manipulations are performed to optimize cardiopulmonary function.

There are many indications for postoperative mechanical ventilation (Table 14-2). Patients with borderline major organ system function, many of whom are elderly, benefit from a period of postoperative mechanical ventilation, allowing full evaluation and optimization of respiratory and cardiac function, pain relief, surgical hemostasis, and adjustment of intravascular volume status. The use of PEEP and tidal volumes adjusted to the steep portion of the compliance curve

Table 14-2 Indications for postoperative mechanical ventilation

Slow emergence, obtunded mental status
Ventilatory insufficiency
High V_{CO_2}
Large dead space ventilation
Central respiratory depression
Poor alveolar ventilation
Increased work of breathing
Muscle weakness or fatigue
Hypoxemia:
High FiO_2 requirement
Large Q_s/Q_t
Large amount of blood or secretions in airways
Radiographic abnormalities
Pulmonary edema
Pneumothorax
Pulmonary contusion
Large pleural effusion
Large pulmonary air leak
Poor pulmonary compliance
Hemodynamic instability
Other major organ dysfunction that may cause respiratory insufficiency

of the remaining lung, bronchodilators, tracheal suctioning, and chest physiotherapy are therapeutic maneuvers that improve respiratory function in most patients.

When the patient's clinical condition is optimized, traditional weaning parameters can be used to determine the suitability of ventilator weaning. These parameters include vital capacity (VC), dead space ventilation, negative inspiratory force (NIF), and oxygen index (Pa_{O_2}/FiO_2). When one is evaluating the weaning parameters in elderly postthoracotomy patients, it must be remembered that the elderly have a depressed baseline VC and that the loss of functional lung tissue further decreases measured lung volumes. A multitude of physiological and psychological variables cause failure to wean and may have to be optimized before successful weaning. Concurrent minitracheostomy with thoracotomy has been found to decrease the incidence of atelectasis and radiographic evidence of pulmonary infiltrates, because secretions can be easily suctioned from the airway.[33] A variety of techniques can be used to wean elderly patients from the ventilator. Most weaning techniques gradually or intermittently withdraw ventilator support and allow the patient to assume a greater proportion of the work of breathing. Most practitioners employ intermittent mandatory ventilation (IMV) weaning, in which the number of mechanically supported breaths is gradually diminished until the patient provides nearly all the work of breathing.

Once the trachea has been extubated, the patient is started on an intense regimen of pulmonary toilet, including incentive spirometry, bronchodilators, and chest physiotherapy. CPAP by mask is an effective method of improving lung volumes and reversing hypoxemia in patients who have adequate ventilatory function.

POSTOPERATIVE COMPLICATIONS

In a series involving 369 patients undergoing lobectomy, patients over 60 years of age had a 50 percent incidence of major complications, compared with 36 percent in patients below age 60.[34] A variety of postoperative complications that are mostly unique to thoracic surgery probably have a higher incidence in elderly patients.[19] These complications include cardiac herniation through a pericardial defect, lobar torsion and gangrene, bronchopleural fistula, and postpneumonectomy pulmonary edema. In addition, an elderly thoracic patient is more susceptible to many postoperative complications that also occur after other major surgeries, such as major cardiac events, pulmonary atelectasis, pneumonia, pulmonary embolism, and respiratory failure.

POSTOPERATIVE PAIN CONTROL

Surgeons, anesthesiologists, and patients agree that adequate pain control is one of the most important aspects of perioperative care in thoracic surgery. The thoracotomy incision is a very painful incision that inhibits coughing and deep breathing, causing atelectasis and retention of secretions. In addition, inhibitory reflexes mediated at the spinal cord level depress the contractility of the diaphragm.[32] The goal of pain relief is to provide patient comfort and improve patient outcome. A number of techniques have been used to attain this goal.

Epidural and Subarachnoid Analgesia

When local anesthetics and opioids enter the cerebrospinal fluid (CSF), they migrate into the spinal cord and inhibit the cephalad migration of pain impulses, preventing the central perception of pain. The epidural space and the subarachnoid space can be used as reservoirs of local anesthetics and opioids; drugs are deposited by bolus injection through a needle or by continuous infusion through a catheter.

Many thoracic surgeons consider epidural opioid analgesia the standard of care for thoracotomy pain.[30] Epidural analgesia is usually administered in a continuous fashion through a catheter inserted at the lumbar or thoracic spinal level. The elderly are more susceptible to the respiratory depressant effects of the epidural opioids and have lower dose requirements for effective analgesia. Thus, lower doses and/or concentrations of opioids should be administered to the elderly.[35]

Low concentrations of local anesthetic mixed with the opioid infusion allow lower doses of opioid to be used; local anesthetic requirements are probably also decreased in the elderly.[36] Thoracic epidural fentanyl has been reported to provide superior analgesia compared with lumbar epidural fentanyl, but other investigators have been unable to confirm a superiority of the thoracic over the lumbar route of administration.[37,38] Currently, lumbar epidural fentanyl alone is not recommended for thoracotomy pain.[39] Several clinical studies indicate that epidurally administered fentanyl provides its analgesic effect primarily through systemic absorption that reaches analgesic serum concentrations of fentanyl even when the catheter insertion site is close to the dermatomal level of painful stimulation.[38,40] Thus, when fentanyl is used for epidural analgesia, the catheter probably should be inserted at the thoracic level and the opioid should be mixed with low concentrations of local anesthetic. It should be noted that the depth of the epidural space from the skin increases with age.[41] Morphine, being less lipophilic than fentanyl, can be injected into the lumbar epidural space and can provide adequate thoracic analgesia for a prolonged period. The usual dose is 2 to 5 mg.

Preservative-free morphine placed in the subarachnoid space at the lumbar level can also provide good pain relief for thoracic incisions.[42] The dose should be diminished for elderly patients because cephalad spread may cause greater degrees of respiratory depression than occur in younger patients. Urinary retention may also be a problem in elderly men, but most thoracic surgery patients will have a Foley catheter for several days postoperatively. Most patients will have an adequate analgesic effect using 0.25 to 0.5 mg of subarachnoid preservative-free morphine.

Other Pain Treatment Modalities

Several other modalities have been shown to provide adequate analgesia for thoracotomy pain. Intercostal nerve block by continuous infusion of local anesthetic has been shown to provide pain relief equivalent to that of epidural opioids without the side effects of spinal opioids.[43] Patient-controlled analgesia (PCA), which involves the injection of systemic opioids, can provide adequate analgesia and is well liked because the patient controls his or her own pain management, but pain relief is probably less than with properly administered epidural opioids.[44] Thoracic paravertebral block and interpleural block are other modalities useful in the treatment of acute chest pain.

SUMMARY

Most patients presenting for thoracic surgery are elderly and have multiple organ system diseases. A thorough presurgical evaluation is necessary to identify and optimize the treatment of preexisting medical conditions. Once prepared for surgery, the patient will be subjected to many unique stresses, including one-lung ventilation, the thoracotomy incision, the lateral decubitus position, and loss of lung tissue. Optimal patient outcome requires specific knowledge of the unique complications that occur as a result of thoracic surgery.

REFERENCES

1. Lee-Chiong TL Jr, Matthay RA: Lung cancer in the elderly patient. *Clin Chest Med* 14:453, 1993.
2. Ross AF, Tinker JH: Cardiovascular disease, in Brown DL (ed): *Risk and Outcome in Anesthesia*. Philadelphia: Lippincott, 1992, pp 39–76.
3. Fleisher LA, Barash PG: Preoperative cardiac evaluation for noncardiac surgery: A functional approach. *Anesth Analg* 74:586, 1992.
4. Dales RE, Dionne G, Leech JA, et al: Preoperative prediction of pulmonary complications following thoracic surgery. *Chest* 104:155, 1993.
5. Reilly JJ: Preoperative assessment of patients undergoing pulmonary resection. *Chest* 103:342S, 1993.
6. Shields TW: Surgical therapy for carcinoma of the lung. *Clin Chest Med* 14:121, 1993.
7. Ansley DM, Ransay JG, Whalley DG, et al: The relationship between central venous pressure and pulmonary capillary wedge pressure during aortic surgery. *Can J Anaesth* 34:594, 1987.
8. Wittnich C, Trudel J, Zidulka A, Chiu RC: Misleading "pulmonary wedge pressure" after pneumonectomy: Its importance in postoperative fluid therapy. *Ann Thorac Surg* 42:192, 1986.
9. Sofianos E, Alevizou F, Zissis N, et al: Hormonal response in thoracic surgery: Effects of high-dose fentanyl anesthesia, compared to halothane anesthesia. *Acta Anaesthiol Belg* 36:89, 1985.
10. Temeck BK, Schafer PW, Park WY, Harmon JW: Epidural anesthesia in patients undergoing thoracic surgery. *Arch Surg* 124:415, 1989.
11. Lawson NW: The lateral decubitus position, in Martin JT (ed): *Positioning in Anesthesia and Surgery*. Philadelphia: Saunders, 1987, pp 155–179.
12. Slinger PD: Anaesthesia for lung resection. *Can J Anaesth* 37:Sxv, 1990.
13. Lemmer JH, Gomez MN, Symreng T, et al: Limited lateral thoracotomy: Improved postoperative pulmonary function. *Arch Surg* 125:873, 1990.
14. Blumberg N, Heal JM: Transfusion-induced immunomodulation and its possible role in cancer recurrence and perioperative bacterial infection. *Yale J Biol Med* 63:429, 1990.
15. Pena CM, Rice TW, Ahmad M, Medendorp SV: Significance of perioperative blood transfusions in patients undergoing resection of stage I and II non-small-cell lung cancers. *Chest* 102:84, 1992.
16. Frank SM, Beattie C, Christopherson R, et al: Epidural versus general anesthesia, ambient operating room temperature, and patient age as predictors of inadvertent hypothermia. *Anesthesiology* 77:252, 1992.
17. Gayes JM: Pro: One-lung ventilation is best accomplished with the Univent endotracheal tube. *J Cardiothorac Vasc Anesth* 7:103, 1993.
18. Slinger P, Suissa S, Triolet W: Predicting arterial oxygenation during one-lung anaesthesia. *Can J Anaesth* 39:1030, 1992.
19. Piccione W, Faber LP: Management of complications related to pulmonary resec-

tion, in Waldhausen JA, Orringer MB (eds): *Complications in Cardiothoracic Surgery*. St. Louis: Mosby–Year Book, 1991, pp 336–353.
20. Ritchie AJ, Tolan M, Whiteside M, et al: Prophylactic digitalization fails to control dysrhythmia in thoracic esophageal operations. *Ann Thorac Surg* 55:86, 1993.
21. Ritchie AJ, Bowe P, Gibbons JR: Prophylactic digitalization for thoracotomy: A reassessment. *Ann Thorac Surg* 50:86, 1990.
22. Falk RH, Leavitt JI: Digoxin for atrial fibrillation: A drug whose time has gone? *Ann Intern Med* 114:573, 1991.
23. Bolognesi R: The pharmacologic treatment of atrial fibrillation. *Cardiovasc Drugs Ther* 5:617, 1991.
24. Shapira OM, Shahian DM: Postpneumonectomy pulmonary edema. *Ann Thorac Surg* 56:190, 1993.
25. Turnage WS, Lunn JJ: Postpneumonectomy pulmonary edema: A retrospective analysis of associated variables. *Chest* 103:1646, 1993.
26. Katlic MR: Thoracic surgery in the elderly, in Katlic MR (ed): *Geriatric Surgery*. Baltimore: Urban & Schwarzenberg, 1990, pp 419–443.
27. Peters RM: Pulmonary disease and mediastinal surgery for the elderly, in Adkins RB Jr, Scott HW Jr (eds): *Surgical Care for the Elderly*. Baltimore: Williams & Wilkins, 1988, pp 221–236.
28. D'Empaire G, Hoaglin D, Perlo V, et al: Effect of prethymectomy plasma exchange on post-operative respiratory function in myasthenia gravis. *J Thorac Cardiovasc Surg* 89:592, 1985.
29. Lewis RJ, Caccavale RJ, Sisler GE, Mackenzie JW: One hundred consecutive patients undergoing video-assisted thoracic operations. *Ann Thorac Surg* 54:421, 1992.
30. Landreneau RJ, Hazelrigg SR, Mack MJ, et al: Postoperative pain-related morbidity: Video-assisted thoracic surgery versus thoracotomy. *Ann Thorac Surg* 56:1285, 1993.
31. Hazelrigg SR, Nunchuck SK, LoCicero J III: Video assisted thoracic surgery study group data. *Ann Thorac Surg* 56:1039, 1993.
32. Fratacci MD, Kimball WR, Wain JC, et al: Diaphragmatic shortening after thoracic surgery in humans: Effects of mechanical ventilation and thoracic epidural anesthesia. *Anesthesiology* 79:654, 1993.
33. Randell TT, Tierla EK, Lepantalo MJ, Lindgren L: Prophylactic mini-tracheostomy after thoracotomy: A prospective random control, clinical trial. *Eur J Surg* 157:501, 1991.
34. Keagy BA, Lores ME, Starek PJ, et al: Elective pulmonary lobectomy: Factors associated with morbidity and operative mortality. *Ann Thorac Surg* 40:349, 1985.
35. Moore AK, Vilderman S, Lubenskyi W, et al: Differences in epidural morphine requirements between elderly and young patients after abdominal surgery. *Anesth Analg* 70:316, 1990.
36. Nydahl PA, Philipson L, Axelsson K, Johansson JE: Epidural anesthesia with 0.5% bupivacaine: Influence of age on sensory and motor blockade. *Anesth Analg* 73:780, 1991.
37. Coe A, Sarginson R, Smith MW, et al: Pain following thoracotomy: A randomised, double-blind comparison of lumbar versus thoracic epidural fentanyl. *Anaesthesia* 46:919, 1991.
38. Guinard JP, Mavrocordatos P, Chiolero R, Carpenter RL: A randomized comparison of intravenous versus lumbar and thoracic epidural fentanyl for analgesia after thoracotomy. *Anesthesiology* 77:1108, 1992.

39. Ferrante FM, VandeBoncouer TR: Epidural and subarachnoid analgesia for thoracic surgery, in Gravlee GP, Ranch RL (eds): *Pain Management in Cardiothoracic Surgery*. Philadelphia: Lippincott, 1993, pp 1–24.
40. Sandler AN, Stringer D, Panos L, et al: A randomized, double-blind comparison of lumbar epidural and intravenous fentanyl infusions for postthoracotomy pain relief: Analgesic, pharmacokinetic, and respiratory effects. *Anesthesiology* 77:626, 1992.
41. Matsumoto J, Mitsuhata H, Matsumoto S, et al: Skin-epidural distance in human lumbar region. *Masui* 40:250, 1991.
42. Neustein SM, Cohen E: Intrathecal morphine during thoracotomy: II. Effect on postoperative meperidine requirements and pulmonary function tests. *J Cardiothorac Vasc Anesth* 7:157, 1993.
43. Richardson J, Sabanathan S, Eng J, et al: Continuous intercostal nerve block versus epidural morphine for postthoracotomy analgesia. *Ann Thorac Surg* 55:377, 1993.
44. Benzon HT, Wong HY, Belavic AM Jr, et al: A randomized double-blind comparison of epidural fentanyl infusion versus patient-controlled analgesia with morphine for postthoracotomy pain. *Anesth Analg* 76:316, 1993.

CHAPTER 15

Anesthesia for Major Vascular Surgery in Geriatric Patients

Christopher A. Bracken

INTRODUCTION

There continues to be debate over the significance of age as a predictor of morbidity and/or mortality for anesthetic exposures. The Goldman classification scheme still assigns a point for age over 70 years but gives much greater significance to a prior history of congestive heart failure (CHF), previous myocardial infarction (MI), and current peripheral edema. The American Society of Anesthesiologists' (ASA) physical status classification scale does not include an age criterion, although most centers still separately classify age extremes (<1 year old and >70 years old). A large prospective study in France[1] looked at the results of almost 200,000 anesthetics. It clearly indicated that the associated disease state was much more significant in affecting the complication rate than was age alone but also demonstrated that elderly people are more likely to have associated disease states that negatively affect their ability to withstand the insult of anesthesia and surgery. Furthermore, at each equivalent level of disease state, the elderly had a higher complication rate. The greater the number of disease states present preoperatively, the greater the distinction between a younger adult and an elderly patient. Older patients with advanced disease are significantly more likely to have a complication associated with an anesthetic than are either younger patients with equivalent advanced disease or equally old patients with significantly less disease, even at a fairly minimal disease level (Fig. 15-1).

Vascular surgery by definition is predominantly geriatric surgery. Most of these patients are chronologically elderly or have degrees of concurrent sys-

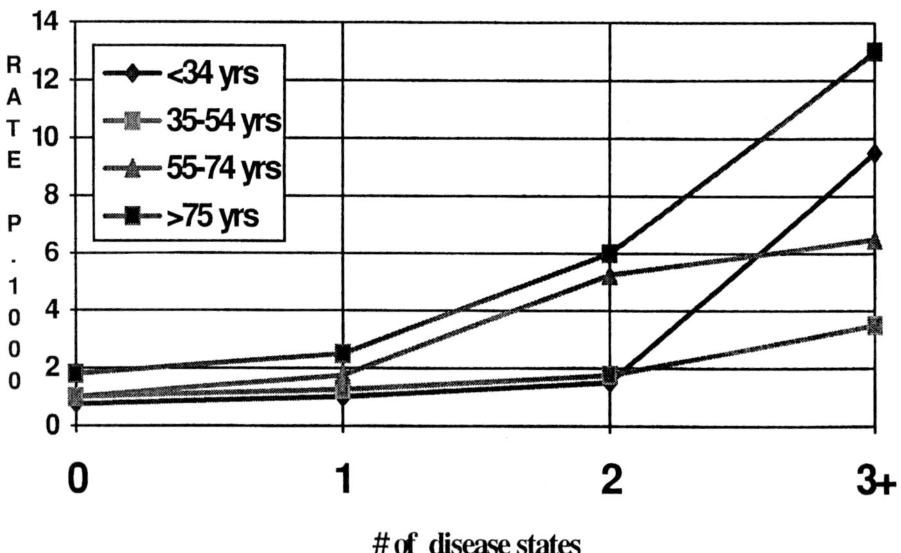

Figure 15-1 Complication rate per 1000 anesthetics, as a function of age and concurrent disease states.

temic diseases that have caused them to "age beyond their time." Concurrent diabetes mellitus, hypertension, chronic obstructive pulmonary disease (COPD), and elevated serum lipids combine to destroy organs and the vascular tree at an accelerated rate. These patients quite often have a significant smoking history that has contributed to their general deterioration. Patients scheduled for major vascular surgery often function with minimal reserve capacity. All of them must be considered to have at least small vessel coronary artery disease despite a lack of overt symptomatology. The assaults of vascular surgery in this population historically carry an extremely high complication rate. In the mid-1960s, major aortic reconstruction was associated with a 25 percent 6-day mortality rate.[2] Today that rate has fallen to 1 to 2 percent, primarily because of a better understanding of the pathology involved and more meticulous attention to detail.

Most of the mortality associated with vascular surgery is cardiac in origin. Patients requiring vascular surgery have been demonstrated to have a high incidence of hemodynamically significant coronary occlusion, with a resultant significant perioperative cardiac morbidity and mortality.[3] Tables 15-1 and 15-2 clearly show that most of the mortality for carotid endarterectomy and aortic reconstruction, respectively, is associated with cardiac causes. Figure 15-2 graphically shows the pathophysiology of acute coronary syndromes in the perioperative period.[4]

Major vascular surgery is an enormous stressor to the system and most often provokes a stress response, demanding increased cardiac output. The major mechanism by which older people enhance cardiac output is through an increased reliance on the Frank-Starling mechanism rather than an increasing heart rate. Advancing age attenuates the chronotropic ability of the heart secondary to metabolic demand. The increase in stroke volume results in an increased end-diastolic volume. Over time, the heart either hypertrophies or

Table 15-1 Mortality after carotid endarterectomy

			% patients with serious morbidity or mortality from	
Senior author	Year of publication	No. patients studied	Cardiac causes	CNS causes
Sundt	1981	1145	50	31
Hertzer	1981	355	60	17
Ennix	1979	1546	60	30
Callow	1982	1141	67	33
Gewertz	1986	105	100	0
Smith	1988	60	0	100

SOURCE: Reprinted with permission from Roizen MF: Anesthesia for vascular surgery, in Barash PG, Cullen BF, Stoelting RK (eds): *Clinical Anesthesia*. New York: Lippincott, 1989, chap 36, p 1016.

Table 15-2 Percentages of perioperative mortality related to cardiac events

Aortic reconstruction series	Deaths/total no. patients	Mortality caused by cardiac dysfunction, %
Szilagyi et al (1966)	59/401	48
Young et al (1977)	7/144	100
Hicks et al (1975)	19/225	53
Thompson et al (1975)	6/108	83
Mulcare et al (1978)	14/140	79
Whittemore et al (1980)	1/110	100
Crawford et al (1981)	41/860	54
Hertzer (1983)	22/523	64
Yeager et al (1986)	4/97	100
Benefiel et al (1986)	3/96	67

SOURCE: Reprinted with permission from Roizen MF: Anesthesia for vascular surgery, in Barash PG, Cullen BF, Stoelting RK (eds): *Clinical Anesthesia*. New York: Lippincott, 1989, chap 36, p 1017.

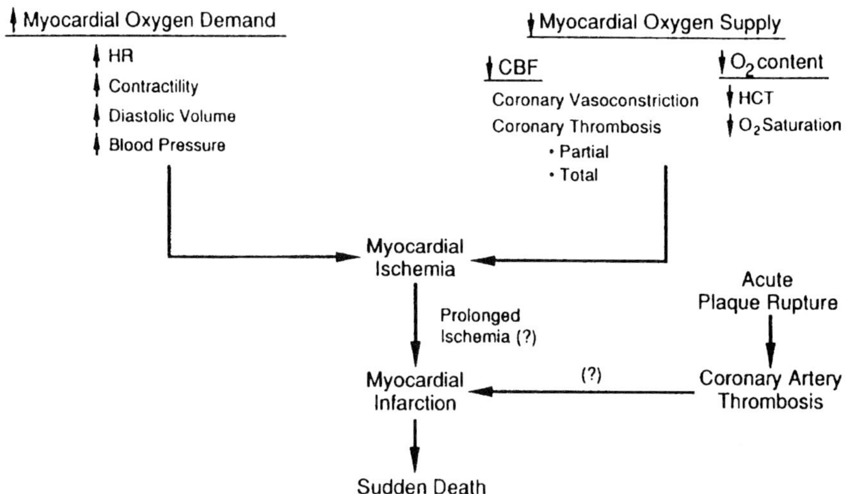

Figure 15-2 Pathophysiology of acute coronary syndromes during the perioperative period. In the setting of a coronary stenosis, the normal ability of vasculature to adjust flow and meet an increase in myocardial oxygen demand is limited. Even if demand is steady, acute decreases in oxygen supply can occur. Both conditions may lead to myocardial ischemia. Prolonged ischemia in turn may lead to infarction, although an alternative hypothesis implicates plaque rupture and thrombus formation at a noncritical stenosis. HR = heart rate; CBF = coronary blood flow; HCT = hematocrit. (*Reproduced with permission from Beattie C, Fleisher LA: Perioperative myocardial ischemia and infarction. Int Anesthesiol Clin 30(1):xx, 1992.*)

dilates. Dilation leads to frank CHF. Hypertrophy entails elevated filling pressures for any given level of end-diastolic volume, resulting in a steeper pressure-volume curve. After dilation or hypertrophy, elderly people are much more volume-sensitive, tolerating neither volume depletion nor fluid loading.

Anesthesiologists need to remember that elderly patients not only have a lessened ability to tolerate tachycardia but also display less of a heart rate response to a given level of stress or exogenously administered catecholamines. Thus, it is more difficult to maintain a proper anesthetic level.

PREOPERATIVE EVALUATION

Initial examination of an elderly patient may not reveal much about the deterioration of the cardiovascular reserve that has occurred. If elderly patients have a sedentary lifestyle, they are more likely to have both accelerated deterioration of cardiovascular reserve and little symptomatology to warn the physician about how little reserve function they maintain. Despite this lack of symptomatology, most elderly patients have a significant degree of coronary artery disease and must be treated as such. A variety of evaluation practices have been proposed over the years in an effort to determine the optimal workup modality.[5–7] A detailed study was conducted to survey the type of evaluation performed by cardiovascular anesthesiologists before major vascular surgery.[8] Interestingly, the spectrum of clinical practice at private and university hospitals was not significantly different. More than 60 percent of the approximately 400,000 patients in the United States who undergo major vascular procedures annually also undergo an expensive and potentially risky preoperative evaluation. The survey implied that preoperative testing resulted in modification of perioperative monitoring in 85 percent of cases. The authors did not state whether the modification resulted in greater or lesser degrees of monitoring, but the implication is that more monitoring was used as a result of the preoperative evaluation. Table 15-3 shows that for aortic surgery, more than 97 percent of the patients received at least a central venous pressure (CVP) line, with 85 to 95 percent receiving a pulmonary artery (PA) catheter.[8] In this case, preoperative testing is used to determine who does not need a PA catheter. Some might argue it is cheaper and safer to use only a PA catheter in all cases. For peripheral vascular surgery, both the testing and the invasive monitoring tend to be less. The question of which type of preoperative testing is most effective continues to be debated, especially in this age of increasingly cost-conscious third-party payer examination. In an attempt to quantitate cost-benefit ratios, researchers are comparing the sensitivity and specificity of various tests in detecting coronary artery disease and then attempting to do population prevalence studies to predict which patients can benefit from a particular testing modality. Cost is then factored into the equation in ways that have not yet been fully established. Table 15-4 compares the sensitivities, specificities, and estimated cost of eight different testing modali-

Table 15-3 Percentage of patients with invasive monitoring by surgical procedure

	University practice	Private practice
Aorta		
CVP	13 ± 18	5 ± 9
PA*	84 ± 21	94 ± 10
Carotid		
CVP*	23 ± 34	6 ± 17
PA	12 ± 21	6 ± 11
Lower extremity		
CVP†	27 ± 26	14 ± 20
PA	24 ± 28	21 ± 25

*$p < 0.05$.

†$p = 0.05$.

SOURCE: Reprinted with permission from Fleischer LA, Beattie C: Current practice in the preoperative evaluation of patients undergoing major vascular surgery: A survey of cardiovascular anesthesiologists. *J Cardiothorac Vasc Anesth* 7:650, 1993.

ties that might be considered in evaluating a patient before major noncardiac surgery. In most cases, the surgeon or cardiologist initiates the preoperative testing, but the anesthesiologist is always the final hurdle. Norris and Fleischer[10] concluded that the decision to test should be based on the preoperative cardiac morbidity and mortality rates for the planned surgical procedure at the institution in question.

Table 15-4 Sensitivity and specificity of various diagnostic tests for detecting coronary artery disease

Test	Sensitivity, %	Specificity, %	Cost, $
Ambulatory electrocardiography	70	85	280
	81	66	450
Exercise electrocardiography			
Exercise thallium imaging			
Qualitative planar	84	87	1200
Quantitative planar	89	89	1200
SPECT	94	82	1200
	85	90	1200
Dipyridamole thallium imaging			
	80–90	80–90	600
Stress echocardiography			
	70–80	70–80	900
Stress radionuclide angiography			

SOURCE: Reprinted with permission from Fleischer LA, Hulyalker A: Cardiovascular testing for the 1990s. *Adv Anesth* 11:27, 1993.

The anesthesiologist needs to concentrate on factors that prevent myocardial damage perioperatively in patients undergoing vascular surgery. After more than 25 years of investigation, exactly what serves as adequate evaluation and what is prognostic have not been elucidated entirely. Some general conclusions have been postulated. In 1977, Goldman and colleagues[11] reported that postoperative risk can be related to heart failure, recent infarction, preoperative rhythm disturbance, type of surgical procedure, age over 70 years, presence of significant valvular stenosis, and "poor general condition." In 1985, another group, looking particularly at geriatric noncardiac surgery, implicated only the patient's history, exercise tolerance for stairs, and inability to perform supine bicycle exercise for 2 min to raise the heart rate to 99 beats per minute (bpm) as predictors of cardiac complications after vascular surgery.[12] In 1992, Mangano's group from UCSF published a series of articles[13–16] discussing myocardial risk factors and perioperative methodologies for at-risk populations.

Five major predictors of postoperative myocardial ischemia were identified by the UCSF study group: left ventricular hypertrophy (LVH) by electrocardiography (ECG), history of hypertension, diabetes mellitus, definite coronary artery disease, and use of digoxin.[13] The risk of ischemia was cumulative, rising with the increasing number of risk factors, from 22 percent in those with no risk factors to 31 percent, 46 percent, 70 percent, and 77 percent in those with one, two, three, or four risk factors, respectively. When analyzed for mortality risk factors, the same patients revealed slightly different prognostic clues. Hypertension, severely limited activity level, and creatinine clearance less than 0.83 ml/s were all independently associated with an increased risk of short-term postoperative mortality. Patients with two or more of these risk factors had a 20 percent hospital mortality. Deaths occurred from 2 to 69 days postoperatively (5 percent overall), 23 percent (6 of 26) from septic causes and 23 percent (6 of 26) from cardiac causes. A 2-year follow-up had another 18 percent mortality rate (5 + 18 = 23 percent overall); cancer, renal dysfunction, CHF, and COPD were independently associated with long-term mortality.[16] In a further evaluation of long-term cardiac prognosis, patients with acute perioperative ischemic events were determined to be at significantly increased risk for long-term cardiac death and probably warranted more aggressive long-term follow-up. They in essence failed "an intraoperative stress test."[17] Figure 15-3 shows how patients with an in-hospital cardiac event had approximately a 75 percent 2-year mortality rate.

The UCSF study was able to show that 111 of 285 patients at high risk for coronary artery disease who received noncardiac surgery had ischemic events, and all negative perioperative events (ischemic outcomes, CHF, and ventricular tachycardia) were associated with intraoperative ischemia detection. Of interest, they concluded that compared with routine two-lead ECG monitoring, aggressive monitoring for ischemia using transesophageal echocardiography (TEE) and/or 12-lead ECG had "little incremental clinical value in identifying patients at high risk for perioperative ischemic outcomes."[14]

In another phase of the UCSF study designed to determine if ventricular arrhythmias can be used as a predictor of risk, the authors concluded that while

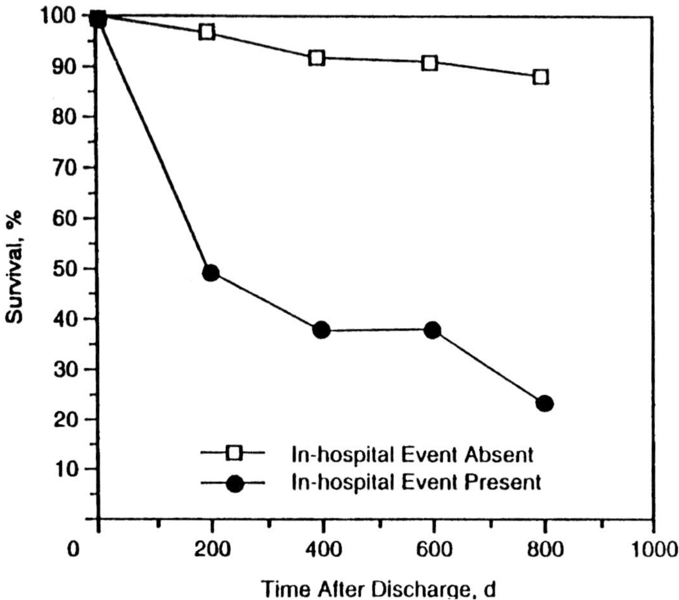

Figure 15-3 Freedom from cardiac complications occurring after hospital discharge in patients with and without in-hospital event (postoperative myocardial infarction or unstable angina). (*Reproduced with permission from Mangano DT, Browner WS, Hollenberg M, et al: Long-term cardiac prognosis following noncardiac surgery. JAMA 268:233, 1992. Copyright 1992, American Medical Association.*)

almost half the high-risk patients had frequent ventricular dysrhythmias [premature ventricular contractions (PVCs) >30/min or nonsustained ventricular tachycardia], these arrhythmias were not prognostic of further deterioration if no other signs or symptoms were associated. They concluded that isolated dysrhythmias do not require aggressive monitoring or treatment during the perioperative period.[15]

The same issue of *JAMA* also had an article from Boston dealing with the same subject.[18] No intraoperative deaths were reported. The consensus supported the statement that perioperative (1 day before to 3 days after an operation) cardiac stability is the most critical element in reducing morbidity and mortality, especially in the geriatric population. As was intuitively suspected, the detection and treatment of preoperative ischemia are both prognostic and therapeutic. Raby and colleagues[18] found that preoperative ischemia was closely correlated with intraoperative (18 percent) and postoperative (30 percent) ischemia in patients undergoing peripheral vascular surgery. Furthermore, ischemia preceded cardiac events in 14 of 16 patients (87 percent). They concluded that in high-risk patients with preoperative ischemia, perioperative monitoring detects the silent ischemia that commonly precedes clinical events and may afford options for early treatment. An accompanying editorial[19] commented that the difficult clinical challenge posed by peripheral vascular patients is the high incidence of coronary artery disease masked by inactivity. The surgery is risky, but it is the only therapy available to reduce suffering and improve the quality of life. Therefore, the ability to reduce postoperative mortality by instituting improved patient selection is not a feasible option. Roizen[20] pointed out that no one really knows which preoperative testing modalities can provide the best information for reducing perioperative risk. Mangano concluded that four areas of future research are rational: (1) control of hemodynamics, (2) investigation of the present and new anti-ischemic therapies (nitrates, beta-blockers, calcium channel blockers, adenosine-regulating agents), (3) antithrombotics, and (4) stress modulation (alpha$_2$ agonists).[21] After subset identification, patients will be maintained on a combination of these therapies, depending on the chronic disease state and the anticipated stresses that will be induced perioperatively. Until these modalities are further defined, the consensus is that a fragile geriatric patient should be handled gently and the anesthetic should be achieved in as simple a fashion as possible.

REGIONAL OR GENERAL?

A classic debate in anesthesiology concerns the relative effectiveness and benefits of regional versus general anesthesia, particularly for peripheral vascular surgery in the elderly population. A 1992 private practice retrospective study discussed carotid endarterectomy under local anesthesia.[22] This article alluded to the generalized increased risk of operating on the elderly and discussed the perceived benefits of conducting the operation under local anesthesia. The authors felt that the major benefit was the ability to avoid shunt placement in 80 percent of the operations as well as the lesser hemodynamic manipulation achieved with local anesthesia in this elderly, myocardially unstable population. A group in the Netherlands looked at endocrine responses to abdominal aortic aneurysm (AAA) reconstruction under either epidural or general anesthesia and demonstrated higher cortisol and catecholamine levels in the general anesthesia group, suggesting an attenuation of the stress response with epidural anesthesia.[23] Subsequently, a similar study carried out by Gold and coworkers confirmed these results.[24] Another group demonstrated that patients with combined epidural and general anesthesia for aortic reconstruction were able to be extubated earlier and required significantly less postoperative opioid.[25] They postulated that this would be an advantage in a patient with marginal pulmonary function, which is often a consideration in an elderly patient. A well-constructed study conducted at Johns Hopkins was unable to demonstrate any significant differences in outcome between groups randomized to epidural or to general anesthesia who had elective lower extremity vascular reconstruction.[26] However, a significant difference in the rate of reoperation for regrafting or embolectomy was noted. In the general anesthesia group, 11 of 50 (22 percent) required a second operation, while only 2 of 50 (4 percent) in the epidural group required a second operation. The investigators concluded that while no long-term outcome differences could be documented, the lower rate of reoperation could justify the choice of epidural anesthesia for revascularization of the lower extremities.

A pair of studies examined the issue of temperature regulation in the elderly population under regional versus general anesthesia.[27,28] They concluded that core temperature profiles are not affected by the choice of anesthetic technique. Epidural anesthesia was associated with less intraoperative upper body thermoregulatory impairment but greater and more persistent postoperative lower extremity thermoregulatory impairment. Younger patients appeared to be better able to maintain thermoregulatory activity under epidural anesthesia than were older patients, while the age-related differences were minimal in the general anesthesia group (Fig. 15-4). Another study concluded that epidural anesthesia reduced the vasoconstriction threshold during general anesthesia, markedly increasing the rate of core cooling when epidural was combined with general anesthesia.[29] Finally, some anesthesiologists prefer regional because it seems to calm the patient in the postoperative period beyond mere pain relief. Hannallah and Mundt[30] demonstrated that after a 3-h latency period, an analgesic dose of epidural morphine decreased the requirement for intraoperative midazolam during long peripheral vascular operations. Thus, the systemic absorption provides some sedation. The issue of regional anesthesia benefits will be discussed in greater detail below in the sections covering each major type of operation.

CAROTID ARTERY SURGERY

Carotid artery surgery has been the subject of much controversy over the last decade both in the United States and overseas.[31–33] For a while it was reported (along with abdominal hysterectomy) as one of the surgeries most frequently performed for the least appropriate indications. However, several large multicenter randomized studies published in the last 2 years clearly have indicated that carotid artery surgery is indicated in most cases of symptomatic carotid artery stenosis and in a specific subset of asymptomatic stenosis. This surgery still carries a significant morbidity and mortality, depending most on the preoperative neurological and cardiac status of the patient. However, several investigators have implicated age as a significant contributor to morbidity. Glaser[34] documented a strong correlation between age and both cardiac and CNS morbidity.

Patients scheduled for carotid surgery present for two reasons. They have either recurrent transient ischemic attacks (TIAs) suggestive of embolic disease or neurological deficits caused by critical narrowing of the carotid artery, resulting in hemodynamic insufficiency (occlusive disease). Occlusive disease patients rely on collateral circulation, which has little autoregulatory capacity. Therefore, they may not tolerate decreases in blood pressure and may require aggressive treatment of hypotensive episodes. These patients frequently have significant coronary disease (50 to 70 percent) and hypertension. The literature

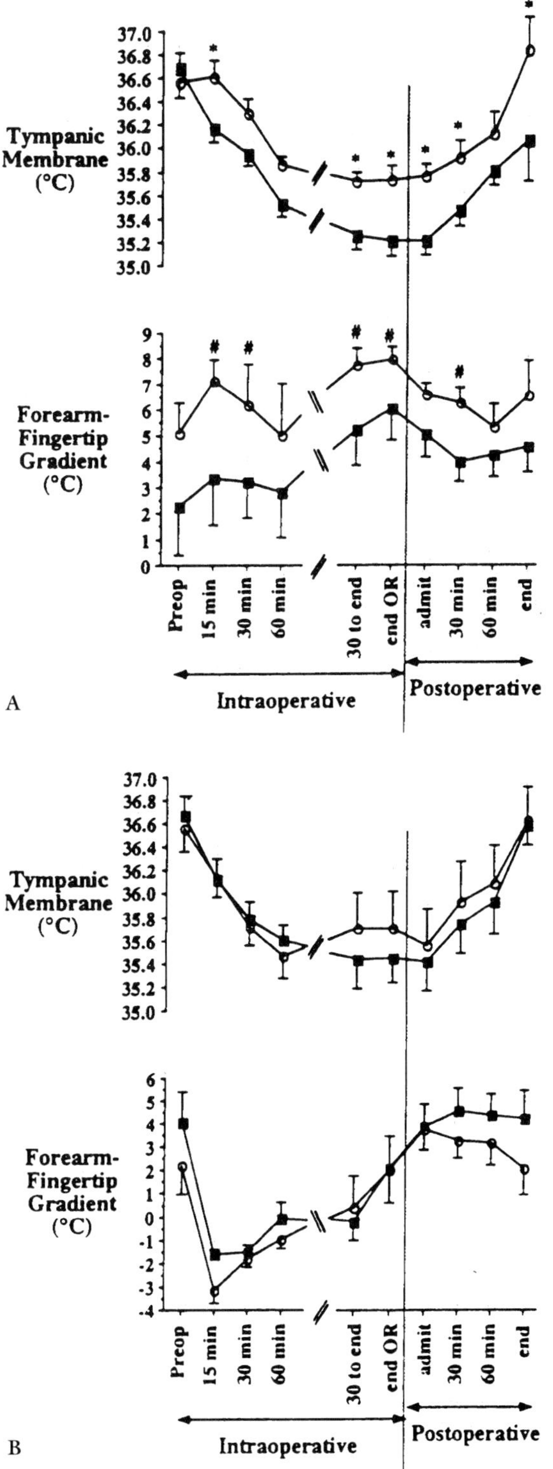

Figure 15-4 Comparison of core temperatures and forearm-fingertip skin-surface temperature gradients in younger and older patient subgroups during the perioperative period. A. Epidural anesthesia: ○, younger patients; ■, older patients. B. General anesthesia: ○, younger patients; ■, older patients. (*Reprodued with permission from Frank SM, Shir Y, Raja SN, et al: Core hypothermia and skin-surface temperature gradients: Epidural versus general anesthesia and the effects of age. Anesthesiology 80:502, 1994.*)

confirms a greater risk of perioperative myocardial infarction than of perioperative stroke.[35]

In the early 1980s, several clinical trials were initiated to determine the efficacy of carotid endarterectomy in various circumstances. In 1991, interim reports were published for the North American Symptomatic Carotid Endarterectomy Trial (NASCET)[36] and the European Carotid Surgery Trial (ECST).[37] Both reported efficacy of surgery in patients with symptomatic carotid artery stenosis greater than 70 percent. In addition, functional status was judged to be better in the surgery subgroup than in the medically managed subgroup. They did identify age as an important risk factor but found surgery to be more beneficial than medical management. NASCET and ECST continued for symptomatic patients with stenoses between 30 and 69 percent. Patients randomized to medical management who had ulcerated plaques had a 24-month risk of ipsilateral stroke that increased from 26.3 to 73.2 percent as stenosis increased from 50 to 95 percent.[38] Patients with no ulcer had a 21.3 percent risk of stroke regardless of the degree of stenosis. Overall, carotid endarterectomy reduced the risk of ipsilateral stroke at 24 months by at least 50 percent. The study concluded that carotid endarterectomy is beneficial in reducing the risk of stroke regardless of plaque ulceration and the degree of stenosis severity. A retrospective study from the Massachusetts General Hospital separated out patients with unstable and compelling neurological conditions.[39] The authors concluded that carotid endarterectomy performed for compelling or unstable neurological conditions carries a low morbidity and mortality rate and that early aggressive surgical therapy is warranted. The implication that surgery is protective in symptomatic carotid ulceration is quite clear.

While the justification for operating on patients with neurologic symptoms is rapidly becoming accepted, the rationale for operating on asymptomatic patients with bruits is much more controversial. Several trials involving asymptomatic patients were begun in an attempt to settle this debate. A nonrandomized retrospective review from UCLA examined the results of 141 carotid endarterectomies in 123 patients with stenosis over 75 percent but with no other symptoms.[40] Natural history for nonoperative outcome was used as a control equivalent. Study patients were followed from 3 to 10 years. No perioperative deaths were reported, but there were two contralateral perioperative strokes in the follow-up period. Recurrent stenosis occurred in 2.8 percent of the patients. This was in contrast to the reported natural history of a 1-year neurological event rate of 18 percent and a 1-year stroke rate of 5 percent. A comparative European study examined the "natural history" of 188 asymptomatic patients for up to 8 years without surgery.[41] At a mean of 4 years, there were six deaths and seven cerebrovascular accidents (CVAs), with the higher-grade stenosis patients having more frequent events (Table 15-5). They concluded from these data that a conservative approach to asymptomatic carotid stenosis should be followed.

To better address these conflicting data, three large trials in asymptomatic patients were conducted: (1) the Mayo Asymptomatic Trial,[42] (2) the Carotid Artery Stenosis with Asymptomatic Narrowing: Operation versus Aspirin trial,

Table 15-5 Asymptomatic carotid stenosis: Natural history

No. patients	Stenosis, %	TIA	CVA	Deaths
96	<50		2 (2%)	3 (3%)
33	50–79	(2%)	1 (4%)	2 (6%)
59	>80	4 (7%)	4 (7%)	1 (2%)

SOURCE: Adapted from Shanik GD, Moore DJ, Leahy A, et al: Asymptomatic carotid stenosis: A benign lesion? *Eur J Vasc Surg* 6:10, 1992.

and, (3) the Veterans Administration Asymptomatic Trial (Cooperative Studies Protocol 167 of the VA).[43–45] Although no statistically significant benefit from surgery in regard to the prevention of stroke or death was shown, none of the studies was sufficiently large to exclude such a benefit. The large Asymptomatic Carotid Atherosclerosis Study (ACAS) is still in progress. The Mayo Clinic Study was terminated early because of a significantly higher number of MIs and TIAs in the surgical group.[42] Most of these events were not temporally related to the surgical procedure, but there was evidence that they could have been related to the absence of aspirin therapy in the surgical group. The VA 167 study identified eight prospective indicators of accelerated mortality: coronary artery disease, angina, CHF, abnormal ECG at entry, peripheral vascular disease, claudication, diabetes, and a history of hypertension.[43,44] Patients with two or three risk factors had annual mortality rates of 11.3 and 13 percent, respectively. This study concluded that adult male patients with high-grade asymptomatic carotid artery stenosis have a 37 percent mortality rate at 4 years. Although age per se was not identified as a risk factor, the elderly population has a higher incidence of the factors that were identified: hypertension, diabetes, coronary artery disease, and peripheral vascular disease. Thompson and Talkington in 1993[46] and Easton and Wilterdink in 1994[33] reviewed all these studies.

A study specifically designed to examine the appropriateness of carotid endarterectomy in the elderly was published in 1992.[47] One hundred forty-six patients age 80 or over underwent 183 carotid endarterectomies from 1964 through 1990. Only three patients (1.6 percent of operations) had a perioperative stroke resulting in a residual deficit, and three patients died (1.6 percent), all from MIs. The authors concluded that carotid endarterectomy is a viable option for elderly patients because of the low incidence of complications. A similar study in France looked at 69 patients over age 75 who underwent 81 carotid endarterectomies.[48] Nine patients required a combined procedure (six cardiac, three vascular). The perioperative mortality rate was 3.7 percent, compared with a perioperative mortality rate of 1.2 percent for patients under 75 years of age. The early stroke rate of 6.1 percent was in contrast to 5.3 percent for younger patients. Actuarial 10-year survival was 58 percent, and freedom from stroke at 10 years was 86 percent. The authors concluded that surgery did not significantly prolong life expectancy in this elderly population, as mortality depended mainly on cardiac events, but that it did improve quality of life, significantly reducing the risk of stroke.

Determining quantitative cardiac risk during evaluation before carotid endarterectomy remains controversial. A common "baseline" assumption is that all carotid endarterectomy patients are cardiac risk patients. An Italian study attempted to justify that assumption.[49] The authors looked at 106 patients with high-grade stenosis without any history of symptoms of coronary artery disease (CAD). While 25 percent were found to have reversible ischemia on thallium-exercise tolerance testing (TETT), none had any intraoperative cardiac events, although five (18.5 percent) died of MI within 5 years. After 7 years, the Kaplan-Meier estimated survival free from coronary events was 51 percent in the positive TETT group and 98 percent in the CAD-free group. Risk factors identified as being prognostic for CAD were male sex, carotid lesions > 90 percent, and bilateral carotid lesions. The conclusion was that even when there is no history or symptoms of CAD, 25 percent of carotid patients have significant ischemia, particularly those in the risk groups mentioned. A response[50] criticized the conclusions drawn, pointing out that the sensitivity of exercise ECG detection of CAD is low, probably less than 70 percent.[51] The authors also pointed out that thallium scintigraphy has been shown to have a sensitivity for detection of significant CAD of only 84 percent and, when limited to patients without a history of an infarction, is only 79 percent sensitive.[52] This means that the Italian study significantly underestimated the incidence of significant CAD. The commentary also points out that the patients in the Italian study who had documented CAD were treated differently from those without it. Thus, the statement that there was no intraoperative difference was not valid, as the two groups were not treated equally. The commentary concluded that patients without clinical, ECG, or echocardiographic evidence of CAD undergoing elective carotid endarterectomy for asymptomatic disease are at low risk for perioperative cardiovascular morbidity and mortality provided that those with abnormal exercise ECG and thallium scintigraphy receive anti-ischemic prophylaxis during the perioperative period. A population-based study from the Mayo Clinic confirmed the high prevalence of MI in patients with CAD and elective carotid endarterectomy and suggested that these patients may represent a population with rapidly progressive atherosclerosis who should be monitored closely and treated more aggressively.[53] The issue of when and how aggressively to screen for asymptomatic disease, especially if the treatment is either marginal or is routinely instituted in any case, remains controversial.

The question of when carotid disease has an impact on other cardiac or vascular surgery has also been debated and investigated. A study designed to determine the role of preoperative carotid screening before cardiac surgery included 1087 patients older than 65 years.[54] Carotid duplex ultrasonography revealed a 17 percent incidence of stenosis greater than 50 percent and a 5.9 percent incidence of stenosis greater than 80 percent. Five predictors of stenosis greater than 80 percent were identified: female sex, peripheral vascular disease, history of TIA or CVA, left main coronary disease, and history of smoking. The authors concluded that screening all patients with one of these risk factors would identify 95 percent of patients with 80 percent stenosis. Among the 1087 patients studied, 46 received combined cardiac-carotid surgery. The overall stroke rate was 2 percent (22 patients), and the 30-day mortality was 5.2 percent (56 patients). An Australian study also examined the stroke risk in patients with carotid artery stenosis discovered before coronary artery or major vascular surgery.[55] The authors concluded that prophylactic endarterectomy was not justified in asymptomatic patients, as the stroke incidence in their study was only 1 of 309 (0.3 percent).[55] Again, this presents conflicting data.

Frequently, after a patient is fully evaluated and both lesions are determined to be appropriate surgical pathology, the question is which lesion to operate on first. The relative priorities among an AAA, severe carotid stenosis, and major CAD are not easy to assign and must be evaluated individually. The question of whether it is better to have staged procedures or a combined procedure is still debated, as well as the order of operation, whether it is staged or combined. A Swiss study looked at the results of combining coronary artery bypass graft (CABG) and carotid endarterectomy in 52 patients.[56] Overall hospital mortality was 3.8 percent. Early mortality was much higher in urgent and emergency cases. An 8-year follow-up revealed an actuarial survival of 86 percent. A control group of 45 patients had a staged procedure (carotid endarterectomy followed by CABG several weeks later), and 42 more patients had CABG in the presence of carotid bruits (<75 percent occlusion). Early cardiac complication in the first group and early neurological complication in the second group were much more common than they were in the combined procedures. The authors concluded that combined procedure is the optimum choice. A similar study conducted in the United States reached similar conclusions.[57] A variation of the combined technique was reported in which the carotid endarterectomy was performed during the aortic cross-clamp period in the belief that superior cerebral protection would be provided.[58] The patients were cooled to 20°C on the cardiac bypass machine before aortic cross-clamping, and then carotid endarterectomy and CABG were accomplished during the cross-clamp time. In this population, 83 percent were over 65 years old. Sixty-one percent had other associated vascular pathological conditions, including peripheral vascular occlusive disease, renal artery stenosis, and AAA. The results in this elderly population were very good. A review of the literature published in 1991[59] concluded that patients with symptomatic coronary and carotid disease should undergo a combined operation in the presence of unstable angina or left main coronary disease but should have a staged procedure (carotid endarterectomy followed by CABG) in the presence of stable angina. Patients with symptomatic coronary disease and asymptomatic severe (>80 percent) carotid disease should also have a staged procedure not to prevent perioperative stroke but rather to prevent late stroke. They emphasized that carotid surgeons must have a good track record with a combined morbidity and mortality below 5 percent in symptomatic patients and below 3 percent in asymptomatic patients.

The question of monitoring CNS function during carotid surgery continues to generate discussion. This is a surgery that conceivably can be performed under deep and superficial cervical plexus block. The advantage is that the patient is awake; mental status serves as the neurological monitor. This is the thrust of the paper by Donato and Hill that was mentioned earlier.[22] Bergeron and coworkers used a similar approach but combined it with preoperative transcranial Doppler screening to identify high-risk patients for shunting.[60] Figure 15-5[61] shows how a transcranial Doppler can be used to monitor cerebral blood flow. The negative aspects of this awake technique are an uncontrolled airway immediately adjacent to the surgical field, an inability to sedate the patient to a significant degree, and the necessity for the patient to remain motionless and under claustrophobia-inducing drapes. In an elderly patient, these concerns are often magnified. Stump pressure monitoring during carotid endarterectomy is controversial. Stump pressures are generally no longer thought to be informative; however, a recent article indicates that a stump pressure less than 35 mmHg, when combined with local anesthesia (LA) and a documented contralateral carotid stenosis greater than 80 percent, is a reliable predictor of "high risk" for CVA.[62] Nationally, few anesthesiologists choose the awake patient. Most anesthesiologists opt to proceed with a general anesthetic and make a decision about appropriate neurological monitoring on that basis. A stronger case for monitoring could be made for elderly patients, as they have even less reserve and less of an ability to handle insults. Table 15-6 compares some of the available monitoring techniques. A review was published recently.[63]

After operative repair of the stenosis, a significant percentage of patients restenose. An elegant French study examined the postoperative course of 278 patients for an average of 30 months. In that time there were 10 deaths, 4 from MI. There were 11 infarctions (6 percent) at 36 months.[64] Twenty-five patients had ischemic episodes, four required a CABG, and seven received percutane-

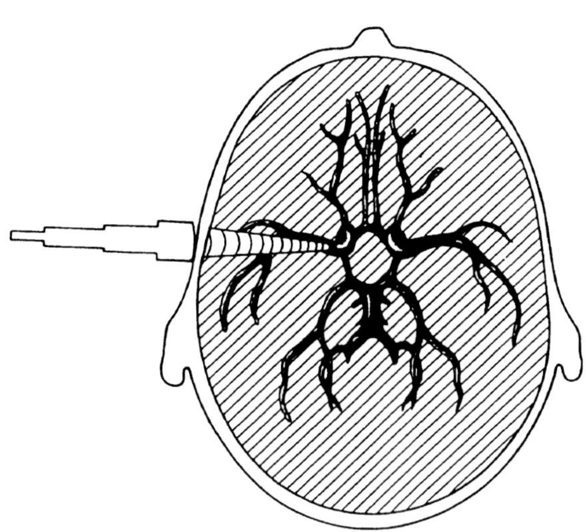

Figure 15-5 **Schematic of transcranial Doppler ultrasound. Blood flow velocity is measured by determining the Doppler shift of sound waves reflected from blood cells moving in the basal arteries of the brain.** (***Reprinted with permission from Mahla ME: Carotid artery surgery: Anesthesia and monitoring update. Semin Anesth 13:75, 1994.***)

Table 15-6 Monitors of the CNS during carotid surgery

Monitor	Ease of application	Continuous	Parameter measured	Ease of interpretation
Awake patient	1	Yes	Neurological exam	1
EEG	2,3,4	Yes	Spontaneous cortical electrical activity	2,3,4
Somatosensory evoked potential	3	Yes	Evoked cortical electrical activity	2
Transcranial Doppler	2	Yes	Cerebral artery blood flow velocity	1
Cerebral blood flow	3	No	Cerebral blood flow	1
Internal carotid stump pressure	1	No	Collateral transmitted pressure	1

KEY TO TABLE: 1—Easy, requires no special training; 2—Requires some training, can be done without technical assistance; 3—Requires training, is better accomplished with technical assistance; 4—Requires extensive training, must have technical assistance.

SOURCE: Reprinted with permission from Mahla M: Carotid artery surgery: Anesthesia and monitoring. Lecture 142. ASA 43d Annual Refresher Course Lectures, 1992.

ous transluminal angioplasty. The combined neurological mortality and morbidity was 1.7 percent, with actuarial rates of survival and freedom from CVAs of 94 and 95.8 percent, respectively. There were no deaths from CVA. Three patients had asymptomatic carotid restenosis greater than 80 percent and underwent reoperation. Thirty-two had contralateral stenosis greater than 80 percent (24 asymptomatic), and 28 underwent surgery. As their results indicate, even 3 years after carotid endarterectomy, despite a significant degree of stenosis (ipsilateral or contralateral), the mortality remains predominantly cardiac in origin.

AORTIC RECONSTRUCTION

As with carotid disease, surgery for aortic disease is associated with significant morbidity and mortality, again primarily cardiac in origin (Table 15-2). However, various components of the disease are also prognostic and should be considered. Aneurysmal surgery has twice the mortality and morbidity of occlusive aortic disease. Occlusive disease limited to the aortic and iliac vessels is less significant than disease involving the entire lower extremity, partly because the latter is almost always associated with coronary insufficiency. Aneurysms should be operated on if they are twice the size of the uninvolved aorta or over 5 to 6 cm in diameter. The 5-year survival of patients with an unoperated thoracic aneurysm is less than 20 percent, with half of them dying from rupture of the aneurysm. More than a third of these deaths occurred in the first year after the diagnosis.[65] Successful surgical repair leads to 70 percent

5-year survival, but rupture of the aneurysm remains the major cause of late mortality.[66]

Combined epidural and general anesthesia is very popular for aortic reconstructive surgery not only because it minimizes the required systemic anesthesia, allowing earlier extubation, but also because of the excellent postoperative pain control it affords. Much effort has been expended to show that epidural anesthesia minimizes endocrine responses to surgery. Gold and associates[24] were able to demonstrate that epidural anesthesia to a T4 level prevents norepinephrine and epinephrine increases in response to abdominal aortic surgery. Catecholamine levels were not reflected in systemic vascular resistance (SVR) changes. Another theoretical advantage that continues to be investigated is the theory of "preemptive analgesia," which seems to be most consistently achieved with a central neuraxial block. The theory states that complete blockade of all pain stimuli at the spinal cord level (profound neuraxial blockade) preemptively diminishes the incidence of early and late postoperative pain.[67] By contrast, some anesthesiologists feel uncomfortable with epidurals in aortic patients for several reasons. First, they are leery of placing a catheter in a patient who may at some point have a coagulopathy either because of iatrogenic anticoagulation or because of bleeding during the operation. Several case reports of epidural hematomas have been associated with anticoagulated patients.[68–70] A second reason for concern is the loss of all reactive vasomotor constriction, removing all homeostatic safeguards. Several investigations into the hemodynamic consequences of adding an epidural to the anesthetic plan have been reported. Saada and coworkers[71] attempted to examine the effects on myocardial function of adding thoracic epidural anesthesia (TEA) to general endotracheal anesthesia (GETA) in vascular surgery patients. Theoretically, TEA should minimize myocardial ischemia. TEA was found to induce a decrease in systemic arterial blood pressure, heart rate, and cardiac index. A slight improvement in wall motion parameters was observed in the TEA group. The authors concluded that TEA does not negatively affect and may positively influence cardiac performance during vascular surgery. A similar study looked at 173 patients randomized to either "balanced" general anesthesia or TEA with "light" GETA.[72] The investigators were unable to ascertain any significant difference in morbidity or mortality between the two groups. Another study looked at intraoperative hemodynamic stability and length of postoperative stay in the intensive care unit (ICU). They concluded that the epidural-general group was more stable intraoperatively and had a significantly shorter ICU stay.[73] Still another group looked at intestinal hemodynamics as a function of TEA, specifically superior mesenteric artery blood flow (SMABF) during aortic reconstruction.[74] The authors concluded that TEA causes a reduction in SMABF, resulting in intestinal reductive metabolism. This reduction in blood flow can be ameliorated by adding a dopamine infusion.

Attempts to manipulate epidural solutions to provide more hemodynamic stability constitute a popular area of investigation. Various combinations of local anesthetic, potent opioids, and drugs such as $alpha_2$ blockers have been investigated. A study comparing bupivacaine with sufentanil found little difference in the hemodynamic profiles of patients undergoing aortoiliac surgery, except for a slight reduction in heart rate and cardiac index during induction with sufentanil. They concluded that both techniques provide adequate analgesia and stable hemodynamics.[75]

Aortic reconstructive surgery is associated with a significant incidence of ischemic spinal cord damage. The location of origin for the radicular artery of Adamkiewicz is highly variable. In 75 percent of the population, the artery arises between T9 and T12, but it has also been found from T3 to as low as L5.[76] The higher the aortic cross-clamp, the more likely it is that interruption of perfusion to the spinal cord will occur. However, despite aggressive monitoring and interventional modalities [somatosensory evoked potential (SSEP) monitoring and lumbar cerebrospinal fluid (CSF) drainage], even operations limited to the distal descending thoracic aorta are associated with spinal cord ischemia in anywhere from 1 to 11 percent of cases.[77] Other reports claim incidences of paraplegia as low as 0.4 percent after elective repair of coarctations[78] to as high as 24 to 40 percent for traumatic rupture of the thoracoabdominal aorta and acute dissections of the aorta.[79] Factors thought to influence the incidence of paraplegia include the nature of the disease, etiology of the aneurysm, extent of the aneurysm, aortic clamp time, availability of collateral circulation, and anatomy of the blood supply to the spinal cord. The final common denominator is an ischemic insult of sufficient magnitude and duration to produce irreversible motor neuron damage. Methods of preventing paraplegia are summarized in Table 15-7.[80] SSEPs have been investigated as a monitoring tool over the past decade.[81] However, SSEP monitoring has several limitations. First, it directly measures the activity of the anterior sensory tracts, not the dorsal motor tracts, which seem to sustain the most damage. Second, attenuation of the signal may indicate peripheral nerve ischemia, not spinal cord dysfunction.[82] Because of these limitations, studies continue to investigate the most appropriate ways to monitor the spinal cord. A group from Brooke Army Medical Center published a study of spinal evoked potentials (SpEPs) as a monitoring tool during aortic occlusion in pigs.[83] The study was an attempt to improve on the acknowledged limitations of SSEP in detecting damage in the motor columns of the spinal cord. Previous reports were inconclusive about the reliability of this modality in predicting motor neuron damage.[84,85] It appears that to be a reliable predictor of damage, the evoked potentials must monitor the low lumbar (L4) area of the spinal cord. Mongan's group[83] claimed 92.8 percent sensitivity and 90.9 percent specificity for the prediction of early postoperative motor dysfunction after the loss of the L4 SpEP. The time of loss of the SpEP was not necessarily related to the ischemic time of the cord, but continued ischemia after loss of the SpEP was consistently followed by motor dysfunction. As was mentioned above, temperature is another variable that is thought to contribute to spinal cord preservation during ischemia. A group of investigators looked at the correlation between core temperature and intrathecal temperature during aortic surgery.[86] Earlier work had suggested that a modest reduction in temperature can delay the onset of neuronal damage, but

Table 15-7 Methods of preventing paraplegia

Left heart bypass
Heparin-coated shunts
Partial cardiopulmonary bypass
Left-sided heart bypass with a pump (centrifugal pump)
Hypothermia
Monitoring of spinal cord ischemia by
Somatosensory evoked potentials
Motor evoked potentials
Reattachment of intercostal and lumbar arteries
Identification of blood supply of spinal cord
Radiographic
Hydrogen-induced current
Enhancement of perfusion pressure of spinal cord
Use of papaverine
CSF drainage
Pharmacologic agents
Steroids
Thiopental sodium
Oxygen radical scavenger
Artificial blood (Fluosol DA)
Naloxone
Calcium channel blockers

SOURCE: Reprinted with permission from Shenaq SA, Svensson LG: Con: Cerebrospinal fluid drainage does not afford spinal cord protection during resection of thoracic aneurysms. *J Cardiothorac Vasc Anesth* 6:369, 1992.

the question remained of how to verify the appropriate level of spinal cord cooling. This study documented excellent correlations between pulmonary artery temperatures and intrathecal temperatures during all phases of aortic surgery. Work in spinal cord monitoring continues to refine the techniques used to minimize spinal cord damage.

A controversial topic is whether cerebrospinal fluid drainage (CSFD) early in the operation has a protective effect on the spinal cord during aortic cross-clamping, in the belief that drainage may improve spinal cord perfusion pressure. A retrospective analysis of the Mayo Clinic study found no untoward events associated with the CSFD but was also unable to document any beneficial effect.[87] A pro-con debate was published in 1992. Nugent argued in favor of CSFD, feeling that it was a useful adjunct to other modalities, such as mild hypothermia and avoidance of glucose solutions.[88] Shenaq and Svensson[80] argued against drainage and cited the anatomic differences between dogs and humans as part of the reasoning: Dogs lack the artery of Adamkiewicz, making them more prone to spinal cord ischemia than humans in model system studies. The authors also discussed a prospective randomized study of 98 high-risk patients that failed to demonstrate any advantage to CSFD in humans.[89] They concluded that reimplantation of critical intercostal arteries, use of antioxidants, and spinal cord cooling are the most promising strategies for increasing spinal cord preservation. Another study of 110 patients combined the use of naloxone with CSFD and concluded that this combination was effective, as they found that only 1 of 61 patients treated with the combination of naloxone and CSFD suffered a neurological deficit, while 11 of 49 patients who were not treated with the combination suffered a deficit.[90] The primary predictive risk factors these investigators identified were acute status, Crawford type II aneurysm, and extent of the aorta replaced.

The use of sodium nitroprusside (SNP) during aortic cross-clamping is also controversial. Obviously, SVR is markedly increased with the application of the aortic cross-clamp, and SNP is frequently recommended to decrease the workload on the left ventricle during this period. The controversy involves the fact that SNP not only may decrease SVR but also may decrease cerebral vascular resistance, resulting in an increase in cerebral blood flow, cerebral blood volume, and CSF pressure. At the same time, SNP reduces the aortic pressure below the aortic cross-clamp, possibly decreasing the perfusion gradient from the distal aorta to the spinal cord.[91,92] Some investigators recommend that SNP be avoided as long as the surgeon feels that the proximal aorta can withstand the higher pressures and acute left ventricular failure or myocardial ischemia does not occur.

Another area of concern is the preservation of renal function during vascular surgery. Many manipulations are done to preserve renal function. Investigations into the impact of various anesthetic regimens continue. For example, Colson and associates[93] compared the effects of isoflurane, halothane, droperidol, or flunitrazepam as the primary anesthetic drug on renal function during and after infrarenal aortic reconstruction. They found that halothane and flunitrazepam reduced glomerular filtration rate (GFR) and effective renal plasma flow (ERPF) before aortic clamping but not during the clamp period. After clamping, the GFR and ERPF rebounded strongly in patients who received these anesthetics. They contrasted these agents to droperidol, which significantly reduced these parameters during the cross-clamp period, and to isoflurane, which preserved renal function during all phases of the operation. There were no comments about long-term function. The search for the ideal anesthetic continues. To further examine the mechanisms of renal impairment, the same group examined the effects of enalapril (an angiotensin-converting enzyme inhibitor) and nicardipine (a calcium channel antagonist) on renal blood flow (RBF) during aortic cross-clamping.[94] GFR and RBF decreased in the control and enalapril patients despite a maintenance of cardiac output and SVR in the enalapril group. In contrast, the nicardipine group experienced decreased cardiac output and increased SVR, similar to the control group, but maintained better GFR and RBF. The authors concluded that the renin-angiotensin system is not an important determinant of renal vasoconstriction associated with aortic cross-clamping. They further suggested that nicardipine probably acts at the level of the preglomerular resistance vessels to maintain RBF despite a reduction in cardiac output.

Side issues are also important to consider in these patients. For example, blood transfusion is now very much on the minds of the public. Major vascular surgery is one of the operations most likely to require blood transfusion, and these are often the patients least able to tolerate a low hematocrit. Ways to avoid blood transfusion are being evaluated. Preoperative normovolemic hemodilution (PNH) has been investigated in order to evaluate patient tolerance and reduction in transfusion requirements.[95] The authors looked particularly at left ventricular segmental wall motion (SWM) by TEE to evaluate hemodynamic instability in this population prone to cardiac dysfunction. The authors concluded that PNH actually provides a better tolerance of aortic clamping.

A review of the anesthetic implications of abdominal aortic surgery was published in 1991.[96]

PERIPHERAL VASCULAR SURGERY

Operations for peripheral vascular disease are numerous and vary widely in complexity. Generally, the patient has symptoms of claudication or ischemic ulcers on the lower extremity that necessitate revascularization of the affected limb. Perioperative MI is reported to occur in up to 15 percent of patients having peripheral revascularization operations, accounting for more than 50 percent of their perioperative mortality.[97] The value of preoperative optimization of these patients cannot be overemphasized.[98] A review of controversies in the surgical management of asymptomatic peripheral vascular disease has been published.[99]

These operations are very frequently carried out under regional anesthesia, although the literature on the "proof" of benefit is still controversial. The article by Christopherson and colleagues,[26] summarizing the Perioperative Ischemia Randomized Anesthesia Trial (PIRAT) is the latest in an attempt to prove benefits for regional anesthesia, which is limited to minimizing the requirement for reoperation.[100] Several observers have commented that the rate of early graft failure in this study was very high (13 percent versus 2 to 5 percent in other studies) and thus places the other observations in doubt.[101,102] A debate about the benefits of regional anesthesia was published in 1994. Tuman and colleagues argued in favor of regional anesthesia.[103] One thrust of their argument seems to be that morbidity and mortality for vascular surgery occur mostly in the hours and days *after* the actual operation and that a regional technique allows the anesthesiologist to both smooth the transition from the operating room to recovery and provide better postoperative analgesia, thus minimizing the trauma of "postsurgery." They cite studies that document attenuation of the norepinephrine response after major vascular surgery obtained by the employment of epidural morphine for postoperative analgesia.[24,104] A randomized trial of epidural combined with "light" GETA versus GETA "cardiac style" found that the only predictors of morbidity were CHF and lack of an epidural.[105] Other investigators documented improved global and regional left ventricular function during stress-induced myocardial ischemia in CAD patients when an epidural was used.[106] All these reports are cited to suggest a beneficial effect for regional and particularly epidural anesthesia for peripheral vascular surgery. The other side of the argument was presented by Bode and Lewis.[107] Table 15-8 is adapted from this article and summarizes the perceived advantages and disadvantages of regional versus general anesthesia. While this author's perception would seem to favor regional anesthesia, Bode and Lewis still feel that there is no true advantage. Bode and Lewis cite the study by Baron and associates,[72] which found no

Table 15-8 Regional versus general anesthesia: Perceived advantages and disadvantages

Regional anesthesia: advantages

1. Attenuation of neuroendocrine response
2. Improvement in cardiac function in CAD patients (reduction of both before and after load)
3. Fewer postoperative pulmonary complications
4. Perhaps less need for invasive monitoring
5. Additional epidural benefits
   a. Slow titration of level
   b. Avoidance of rapid changes in heart rate or blood pressure
   c. Ability to continue the analgesia into postoperative period
   d. Potentially favorable effects on coagulation

Regional anesthesia: disadvantages

1. Sympathetic blockade producing vasodilation of both resistance and capacitance vessels
2. Potential hypotension, severity not necessarily related to level of sympathectomy
3. Myocardial regional wall motion abnormalities
4. Early graft thrombosis
5. Technical failures resulting in operating room delays and increased patient morbidity

General anesthesia: advantages

1. Quick onset
2. Reliability in producing surgical anesthesia
3. Securement of airway
4. Avoidance of oversedation or restlessness in "awake" patient undergoing long procedure
5. Ability to tailor anesthesia to patient's physiological needs by judicious monitoring and employment of vasoactive drugs

General anesthesia: disadvantages

1. Minimal suppression of neuroendocrine "stress response"
2. Adverse hemodynamic changes associated with induction of and emergence from general anesthesia

SOURCE: Derived from Bode RH, Lewis KP: Con: Regional anesthesia is not better than general anesthesia for lower extremity revascularization. *J Cardiothorac Vasc Anesth* 8:118, 1994.

difference in outcome in abdominal aortic surgery when specific intraoperative and postoperative guidelines for monitoring, hemodynamic maintenance, and pain control were maintained to minimize the differences between the two groups. Another study suggested that postoperative epidural analgesia does not significantly reduce the incidence of postoperative pulmonary complications.[108] The incidence of early graft closure has led other groups to investigate whether systemic heparinization can minimize graft closure. Gold had demonstrated an activated coagulation time (ACT) reduction of 8 to 10 percent after the induction of regional anesthesia.[109] The study of Martin and associates employed ACT, thromboelastography (TEG), and heparin titration monitoring in an effort to idealize the anticoagulation results.[110] Those authors concluded that variability of patient response to heparin necessitates aggressive monitoring to maintain appropriate anticoagulation during revascularization operations. A literature metaanalysis of all randomized controlled clinical trials since 1966 comparing regional and general anesthesia has been published.[111] More than 5000 patients were involved in the reviewed studies, most for surgery below the umbilicus. No statistically significant differences in overall mortality, cardiac morbidity, postoperative pulmonary complications, or pulmonary emboli were documented after the metaanalysis. Bode's own group has presented a large (706 patients) study examining anesthesia techniques (spinal versus epidural versus general) in patients scheduled for lower extremity revascularization.[112] Four hundred twenty-three patients were prospectively randomized, while 283 patients were followed up in a nonrandomized group. No significant differences were found in regard to cardiac morbidity, mortality, and length of hospital stay among the three anesthetic techniques. The overall incidences of perioperative MI and death were 4.5 and 2.6 percent, respectively, in the randomized population. The proof of regional benefit remains elusive.

It appears that the predominance of regional techniques employed for these operations or the belief that more limited hemodynamic alterations are encountered causes the incidence of invasive monitoring to be significantly lower than it is in other types of vascular surgery. Perhaps the "truest" statement is that the anesthesia technique should be tailored to both the patient and the experience level of the anesthesiologist. Appropriate monitoring combined with vigilant control of hemodynamic variables during the perioperative period is probably more important than the choice of anesthesia technique in determining the outcome. Reviews of factors affecting outcomes in peripheral vascular surgery were published in *Anesthesiology* in 1993 and 1994.[113,114]

DIALYSIS ACCESS SURGERY

Dialysis access patients are frequently among the most fragile patients an anesthesiologist encounters. They are by definition end-stage renal failure (ESRF) patients, with the associated problems of electrolyte imbalances, fluid imbalance (dry or wet), probable diabetes, CHF, hypertension, poor vascular access, frequent severe anemia with numerous cross-reactivities to blood typing (often with hepatitis or HIV infections), frequent CAD, and a low tolerance of further invasive medical care. The surgeon is frequently not happy to be asked to "once again" establish a dialysis shunt, a difficult and time-consuming procedure with little reward. The surgeon does not consider these patients as his or her patients but feels that he or she is "merely operating on them for someone else" (the dialysis physician). Therefore, the surgeon is usually not interested in "tuning them up" for surgery. These patients are generally given minimal to no anesthesia, yet the anesthesiologist is responsible for their hemodynamic stability and must attempt to keep them calm, pain-free, and motionless during the procedure. Axillary blocks are controversial. Some surgeons routinely request their placement because they provide an excellent surgical field and help vasodilate the vessels in the arm. Other surgeons dislike axillary blocks, feeling that they too frequently fail to provide a good surgical field and that violation of the axillary artery by a transvascular approach compromises the long-term patency of the graft because of clot formation and embolization. These surgeons may even complain about the sympathetic vasodilation, claiming that it misleads them into grafting into vessels inherently too small to maintain patency after the block resolves. These surgeons frequently rely on nearly toxic doses of local anesthetic in an effort to gain control of a local field. It is imperative that the anesthesiologist establish good communication with the surgeon to map out an acceptable plan.

SUMMARY

Vascular surgery is predominantly geriatric surgery. Most of these patients have multiple organ system involvement. Cardiac morbidity and mortality remains the major complication despite attempts to assess risk factors and determine optimum evaluation and monitoring protocols. Indications for these surgeries are becoming clearer as multicenter prospective studies are reported. This is particularly true for carotid surgery. Beyond eliminating smoking and attempting to stabilize concurrent metabolic diseases, little can be done to prevent the progression of these diseases. This surgical specialty will become more prevalent as the elderly population increases in number. Continued research into more efficient management of the cardiac evaluation and into the risks and benefits of regional versus general anesthesia will make anesthesia for this surgery more rational.

REFERENCES

1. Tiret L, Desmonts JM, Hatton F, et al: Complications associated with anesthesia—a prospective survey in France. *Can Anaesth Soc J* 33:336, 1986.
2. Roizen MF: Anesthesia for vascular surgery, in Barash PG, Cullen BF, Stoelting RK (eds): *Clinical Anesthesia*. New York: Lippincott, 1989, chap 36, p 1015.

3. Hertzer NR, Bevan EG, Young JR, et al: Coronary artery disease in peripheral vascular patients: A classification of 1000 coronary angiograms and results of surgical management. *Ann Surg* 199:223, 1984.
4. Beattie C, Fleisher LA: Perioperative myocardial ischemia and infarction. *Int Anesthesiol Clin* 30(1):xx, 1992.
5. Boucher CA, Brewster DC, Darling RC, et al: Determination of cardiac risk by dipyridamole-thallium imaging before peripheral vascular surgery. *N Engl J Med* 312:389, 1985.
6. Blunt T: The role of a defined protocol for cardiac risk assessment in decreasing perioperative myocardial infarction in vascular surgery. *J Vasc Surg* 15:626, 1992.
7. Fleisher LA, Barash PG: Preoperative cardiac evaluation for noncardiac surgery: A functional approach. *Anesth Analg* 74:586, 1992.
8. Fleischer LA, Beattie C: Current practice in the preoperative evaluation of patients undergoing major vascular surgery: A survey of cardiovascular anesthesiologists. *J Cardiothorac Vasc Anesth* 7:650, 1993.
9. Fleischer LA, Hulyalker A: Cardiovascular testing for the 1990s. *Adv Anesth* 11:27, 1993.
10. Norris EJ, Fleischer LA: Preoperative cardiac risk assessment in patients presenting for major vascular surgery. *Semin Anesth* 13:2, 1994.
11. Goldman L, Caldera DL, Nussbaum SR, et al: Multifactorial index of cardiac risk in noncardiac surgical patients. *N Engl J Med* 297:845, 1977.
12. Gerson MC, Hurst JM, Hertzberg VS, et al: Cardiac prognosis in noncardiac geriatric surgery. *Ann Intern Med* 103:832, 1985.
13. Hollenberg M, Mangano DT, Browner WS, et al: Predictors of postoperative myocardial ischemia in patients undergoing noncardiac surgery. *JAMA* 268:205, 1992.
14. Eisenberg MJ, London MJ, Leung JM, et al: Monitoring the myocardial ischemia during noncardiac surgery: A technology assessment of transesophageal echocardiography and 12-lead electrocardiography. *JAMA* 268:210, 1992.
15. O'Kelly B, Browner WS, Massie B, et al: Ventricular arrhythmias in patients undergoing noncardiac surgery. *JAMA* 268:217, 1992.
16. Browner WS, Li J, Mangano DT, et al: In-hospital and long-term mortality in male veterans following noncardiac surgery. *JAMA* 268:228, 1992.
17. Mangano DT, Browner WS, Hollenberg M, et al: Long-term cardiac prognosis following noncardiac surgery. *JAMA* 268:233, 1992.
18. Raby KE, Barry J, Dreager MA, et al: Detection and significance of intraoperative and postoperative myocardial ischemia in peripheral vascular surgery. *JAMA* 268:222, 1992.
19. Killip T: Anesthesia and major noncardiac surgery (editorial). *JAMA* 268:252, 1992.
20. Roizen MF: Preoperative evaluation of vascular access patients: Are the benefits worth the cost? *J Cardiothorac Vasc Anesth* 7:645, 1993.
21. Mangano DT: Perioperative myocardial infarction, stroke and CNS dysfunction. Orlando, FL: IARS Review Course Lectures, 1994, pp 58–60.
22. Donato AT, Hill SL: Carotid arterial surgery using local anesthesia: A private practice retrospective study. *Am Surg* 58:466, 1992.
23. Smeets HJ, Kievit J, Dulfer FT, van Kleef JW: Endocrine-metabolic response to abdominal aortic surgery: A randomized trial of general anesthesia versus general plus epidural anesthesia. *World J Surg* 17:601, 1993.
24. Gold MS, DeCrosta D, Rizzuto C, et al: The effect of lumbar epidural and general anesthesia on plasma catecholamines and hemodynamics during abdominal aortic aneurysm repair. *Anesth Analg* 78:225, 1994.

25. Mason RA, Newton GB, Cassel W, et al: Combined epidural and general anesthesia in aortic surgery. *J Cardiovasc Surg* 31:442, 1990.
26. Christopherson R, Beattie C, Frank SM, et al: Perioperative morbidity in patients randomized to epidural or general anesthesia for lower extremity vascular surgery. *Anesthesiology* 79:422, 1993.
27. Frank SM, Beattie C, Christopherson R, et al: Epidural versus general anesthesia, ambient operation room temperature, and patient age as predictors of inadvertent hypothermia. *Anesthesiology* 77:252, 1992.
28. Frank SM, Shir Y, Raja SN, et al: Core hypothermia and skin-surface temperature gradients: Epidural versus general anesthesia and the effects of age. *Anesthesiology* 80:502, 1994.
29. Joris J, Ozaki M, Sessler DI, et al: Epidural anesthesia impairs both central and peripheral thermoregulatory control during general anesthesia. *Anesthesiology* 80:268, 1994.
30. Hannallah MS, Mundt DJ: Effect of epidural morphine on sedation requirements during regional anesthesia. *J Clin Anesth* 6:10, 1994.
31. Dyken ML: Carotid endarterectomy: A continuing cause for concern (editorial). *Stroke* 23:1047, 1992.
32. Bridgewater BJ, Naylor AR, Ratliff DA, Bell PR: Benefits of carotid endarterectomy: The message is not getting through. *Br J Surg* 80:722, 1993.
33. Easton JD, Wilterdink JL: Carotid endarterectomy: Trials and tribulations (review). *Ann Neurol* 35:5, 1994.
34. Glaser RB: Morbidity and mortality resulting from vascular surgery, in Roizen MF (ed): *Anesthesia for Vascular Surgery*. New York: Churchill Livingstone, 1989.
35. Mahla ME: Carotid artery surgery: Anesthesia and monitoring. 43rd Annual Refresher Course Lectures, ASA, New Orleans, October 1992, lecture 142.
36. Barnett HJ: Status report on the North American Symptomatic Carotid Surgery Trial (review). *J Mal Vasc* 18:202, 1993.
37. Warlow CP: Symptomatic patients: The European Carotid Surgery Trial (ECST). *J Mal Vasc* 18:198, 1993.
38. Eliasziw M, Streifler JY, Fox AJ, et al: Significance of plaque ulceration in symptomatic patients with high-grade carotid stenosis: North American Symptomatic Carotid Endarterectomy Trial. *Stroke* 25:304, 1994.
39. Gertler JP, Blankensteijn JD, Brewster DC, et al: Carotid endarterectomy for unstable and compelling neurologic conditions: Do results justify an aggressive approach? (review). *J Vasc Surg* 19:32, 1994.
40. Freischlag JA, Hanna D, Moore WS: Improved prognosis for asymptomatic carotid stenosis with prophylactic carotid endarterectomy. *Stroke* 23:479, 1992.
41. Shanik GD, Moore DJ, Leahy A, et al: Asymptomatic carotid stenosis: A benign lesion? *Eur J Vasc Surg* 6:10, 1992.
42. Results of a randomized controlled trial of carotid endarterectomy for asymptomatic carotid stenosis: Mayo Asymptomatic Carotid Endarterectomy Study Group. *Mayo Clin Proc* 67:597, 1992.
43. Cohen SN, Hobson RW II, Weiss DG, Chimowitz M: Death associated with asymptomatic carotid artery stenosis: Long-term clinical evaluation: VA Cooperative Study 167 Group (review). *J Vasc Surg* 18:1002, 1993.
44. Hobson RW II, Weiss DG, Fields WS, et al: Efficacy of carotid endarterectomy for asymptomatic carotid stenosis: The Veterans Affairs Cooperative Study Group. *N Engl J Med* 328:221, 1993.

45. Barnett HJ, Haines SJ: Carotid endarterectomy for asymptomatic carotid stenosis (editorial). *N Engl J Med* 328:276, 1993.
46. Thompson JE, Talkington CM: Carotid endarterectomy (review). *Adv Surg* 26:99, 1993.
47. Treiman RL, Wagner WH, Foran RF, et al: Carotid endarterectomy in the elderly. *Ann Vasc Surg* 6:321, 1992.
48. Roques XF, Baudet EM, Clerc F: Results of carotid endarterectomy in patients 75 years of age and older. *J Cardiovasc Surg* 32:726, 1991.
49. Urbinati S, Di Pasquale G, Andreoli A, et al: Frequency and prognostic significance of silent coronary artery disease in patients with cerebral ischemia undergoing carotid endarterectomy. *Am J Cardiol* 69:1166, 1992.
50. Chaffee RB: Silent coronary artery disease in patients to undergo carotid endarterectomy. *Am J Cardiol* 71:498, 1993.
51. Gianrossi R, Detrano R, Mulvihill D, et al: Exercise-induced ST depression in the diagnosis of coronary artery disease: A meta-analysis. *Circulation* 80:87, 1989.
52. Kotler TS, Diamond GA: Exercise thallium-201 scintigraphy in the diagnosis and prognosis of coronary artery disease. *Ann Intern Med* 113:684, 1990.
53. Rihal CS, Gersh BJ, Whisnant JP, et al: Influence of coronary heart disease on morbidity and mortality after carotid endarterectomy: A population-based study in Olmsted County, Minnesota (1970–1988). *J Am Coll Cardiol* 19:1254, 1992.
54. Berens ES, Kouchoukos NT, Murphy SF, Wareing TH: Preoperative carotid artery screening in elderly patients undergoing cardiac surgery. *J Vasc Surg* 15:313, 1992.
55. Gerraty RP, Gates PC, Doyle JC: Carotid stenosis and perioperative stroke risk in symptomatic and asymptomatic patients undergoing vascular or coronary surgery. *Stroke* 24:1115, 1993.
56. Carrel T, Stillhard G, Turina M: Combined carotid and coronary artery surgery: Early and late results. *Cardiology* 80:118, 1992.
57. Bernstein EF: Staged versus simultaneous carotid endarterectomy in patients undergoing cardiac surgery. *J Vasc Surg* 15:870, 1992.
58. Weiss SJ, Sutter FP, Shannon TO, Goldman SM: Combined cardiac operation and carotid endartectomy during aortic cross-clamping. *Ann Thorac Surg* 55:813, 1992.
59. Gugulakis A, Kalodiki E, Nicolaides AN: Combined carotid endarterectomy and coronary artery bypass grafting: A literature review. *Int Angiol* 10:167, 1991.
60. Bergeron P, Benichou H, Rudondy P, et al: Stroke prevention during carotid surgery in high risk patients (value of the transcranial Doppler and local anesthesia). *J Cardiovasc Surg* 32:713, 1991.
61. Mahla ME: Carotid artery surgery: Anesthesia and monitoring update. *Semin Anesth* 13:75, 1994.
62. Burke PE, Prendiville E, Tadros E, et al: Contralateral stenosis and stump pressures: Parameters to identify the high risk patient undergoing carotid endarterectomy under local anesthesia. *Eur J Vasc Surg* 7:317, 1993.
63. Naylor AR, Bell PR, Ruckley CV: Monitoring and cerebral protection during carotid endarterectomy (review). *Br J Surg* 79:735, 1992.
64. Ricco JB, Gauthier JB, Richer JP, et al: The evolution of carotid and coronary artery disease after operation for carotid stenosis. *Ann Vasc Surg* 6:408, 1992.
65. Nacht A: Anesthesia for surgery on the thoracic aorta. *Semin Anesth* 13:63, 1994.
66. Griepp RB, Ergin MA, Lansman SL, et al: The natural history of thoracic aortic aneurysms. *Semin Thorac Cardiovasc Surg* 3:258, 1991.

67. Katz J, Kavanagh MB, Sandler AN, et al: Preemptive analgesia: Clinical evidence of neuroplasticity contributing to postoperative pain. *Anesthesiology* 77:439, 1992.
68. Dickman CA, Shedd SA, Spetzler RF, et al: Spinal epidural hematoma associated with epidural anesthesia: Complications of systemic heparinization in patients receiving peripheral vascular thrombolytic therapy. *Anesthesiology* 72:947, 1990.
69. DeAngelis J: Hazards of subdural and epidural anesthesia during anticoagulant therapy: A case report and review. *Anesth Analg* 51:676, 1972.
70. Wille-Jorgensen P, Jorgensen LN, Rasmussen LS: Lumbar regional anaesthesia and prophylactic anticoagulation therapy: Is the combination safe? *Anaesthesia* 46:623, 1991.
71. Saada M, Catoire P, Bonnet F, et al: Effect of thoracic epidural anesthesia combined with general anesthesia on segmental wall motion assessed by transesophageal echocardiography. *Anesth Analg* 75:329, 1992.
72. Baron JF, Bertrand M, Barre E, et al: Combined epidural and general anesthesia versus general anesthesia for abdominal aortic surgery. *Anesthesiology* 75:611, 1991.
73. Her C, Kizelshteyn G, Walker V, et al: Combined epidural and general anesthesia for abdominal aortic surgery. *J Cardiothorac Anesth* 4:552, 1990.
74. Lundberg J, Lundberg D, Norgren L, et al: Intestinal hemodynamics during laparotomy: Effects of thoracic epidural anesthesia and dopamine in humans. *Anesth Analg* 71:9, 1990.
75. Houweling PL, Ionescu TI: Epidural bupivacaine versus epidural sufentanil anesthesia: Hemodynamic differences during induction of anesthesia and abdominal dissection in aortic surgery. *Acta Anaesthesiol Belg* 43:227, 1992.
76. Wadouh F, Lindemann EM, Arndt CF, et al: The arteria radicularis magna anterior as a decisive factor influencing spinal cord damage during aortic occlusion. *J Thorac Cardiovasc Surg* 88:1, 1984.
77. Crawford ES, Walker HSJ, Saleh SA, et al: Graft replacement of aneurysm in descending thoracic aorta: Results without bypass or shunting. *Surgery* 89:73, 1981.
78. Brewer LA III, Fosburg RG, Mulder GA, et al: Spinal cord complications following surgery for coarctation of the aorta. *J Thorac Cardiovasc Surg* 64:368, 1972.
79. Crawford ES, Crawford JL, Safi HJ, et al: Thoracoabdominal aortic aneurysms: Preoperative and intraoperative factors determining immediate and long-term results of operations in 605 patients. *J Vasc Surg* 3:389, 1986.
80. Shenaq SA, Svensson LG: Con: Cerebrospinal fluid drainage does not afford spinal cord protection during resection of thoracic aneurysms. *J Cardiothorac Vasc Anesth* 6:369, 1992.
81. Crawford ES, Mizrahi EM, Hess KR, et al: The impact of distal aortic perfusion and somatosensory evoked potential monitoring on prevention of paraplegia after aortic aneurysm operation. *J Thorac Cardiovasc Surg* 95:357, 1988.
82. North RB, Drenger B, Beattie C, et al: Monitoring of spinal cord stimulation evoked potentials during thoracoabdominal aneurysm surgery. *Neurosurgery* 28:325, 1991.
83. Mongan PD, Peterson RE, Williams D: Spinal evoked potentials are predictive of neurologic function in a porcine model of aortic occlusion. *Anesth Analg* 78:257, 1994.
84. Owen JH, Jenny AB, Naito M, et al: Effects of spinal cord lesioning on somatosensory and neurogenic-motor evoked potentials. *Spine* 15:618, 1989.
85. Elmore JR, Gloviczki P, Harper CM, et al: Failure of motor evoked potentials to predict neurologic outcome in experimental thoracic aortic occlusion. *J Vasc Surg* 14:131, 1991.

86. Kumar M, Murray MJ, Werner E, Lanier WL: Monitoring intrathecal temperature: Does core temperature reflect intrathecal temperature during aortic surgery? *J Cardiothorac Vasc Anesth* 8:35, 1994.
87. Murray MJ, Bower TC, Oliver WC, et al: Effects of cerebrospinal fluid drainage in patients undergoing thoracic and thoracoabdominal aortic surgery. *J Cardiothorac Vasc Anesth* 7:266, 1993.
88. Nugent M: Pro: Cerebral spinal fluid drainage prevents paraplegia. *J Cardiothorac Vasc Anesth* 6:366, 1992.
89. Crawford ES, Svensson LG, Hess KR, et al: A prospective randomized study of cerebrospinal fluid drainage to prevent paraplegia after high-risk surgery on the thoracoabdominal aorta. *J Vasc Surg* 13:36, 1990.
90. Acher CW, Wynn MM, Hoch JR, et al: Combined use of cerebral spinal fluid drainage and naloxone reduces the risk of paraplegia in thoracoabdominal aneurysm repair. *J Vasc Surg* 19:236, 1994.
91. Shine T, Nugent M: Sodium nitroprusside decreases spinal cord perfusion pressure during descending thoracic aortic cross-clamping in the dog. *J Cardiothorac Anesth* 4:185, 1990.
92. Marini CP, Grubbs PE, Toporoff B, et al: Effect of sodium nitroprusside on spinal cord perfusion and paraplegia during aortic cross-clamping. *Ann Thorac Surg* 47:379, 1989.
93. Colson P, Capdevilla X, Cuchet D, et al: Does the choice of anesthetic influence renal function during infrarenal aortic surgery? *Anesth Analg* 74:481, 1992.
94. Colson P, Ribstein J, Sequin JR, et al: Mechanisms of renal hemodynamic impairment during infrarenal aortic cross-clamping. *Anesth Analg* 75:18, 1992.
95. Catoire P, Saada M, Liu N, et al: Effect of preoperative normovolemic hemodilution on left ventricular segmental wall motion during abdominal aortic surgery. *Anesth Analg* 75:654, 1992.
96. Cunningham AJ: Abdominal aortic surgery: Anesthetic implications. *Yale J Biol Med* 64:309, 1991.
97. Mangano DT: Perioperative cardiac morbidity. *Anesthesiology* 72:153, 1990.
98. Berlauk JF, Abrams JH, Gilmour IJ, et al: Preoperative optimization of cardiovascular hemodynamics improves outcome in peripheral vascular surgery. *Ann Surg* 214:289, 1991.
99. Flynn TC: Controversies in surgical management of asymptomatic peripheral vascular disease (review). *Surg Annu* 24(2):191, 1992.
100. Rosenfeld BA, Beattie C, Christopherson R, et al: The Perioperative Ischemia Randomized Anesthesia Trial Study Group: The effects of different anesthetic regimens on fibrinolysis and the development of postoperative arterial thrombosis. *Anesthesiology* 79:435, 1993.
101. Kupeli IA: Factors affecting outcome in patients undergoing peripheral vascular surgery: I. *Anesthesiology* 80:483, 1994.
102. Badner N: Factors affecting outcome in patients undergoing peripheral vascular surgery: II. *Anesthesiology* 80:485, 1994.
103. Tuman KJ, McCarthy RJ, March RJ, et al: Effects of epidural anesthesia and analgesia on coagulation and outcome after major vascular surgery. *Anesth Analg* 73:696, 1991.
104. Kajata J: Thoracolumbar epidural anesthesia and isoflurane to prevent hypertension and tachycardia in patients undergoing abdominal aortic surgery. *Eur J Anaesthesiol* 8:427, 1991.
105. Tuman KJ, Ivankovich AD: Pro: Regional anesthesia is better than general anes-

thesia for lower extremity revascularization. *J Cardiothorac Vasc Anesth* 8:114, 1994.

106. Kock M, Blomberg S, Emanuelsson H, et al: Thoracic epidural anesthesia improves global and regional left ventricular function during stress-induced myocardial ischemia in patients with coronary artery disease. *Anesth Analg* 71:625, 1990.
107. Bode RH, Lewis KP: Con: Regional anesthesia is not better than general anesthesia for lower extremity revascularization. *J Cardiothorac Vasc Anesth* 8:118, 1994.
108. Jayr C, Thomas H, Rey A, et al: Postoperative pulmonary complications: Epidural anesthesia using bupivacaine and opioids versus parenteral opioids. *Anesthesiology* 78:666, 1993.
109. Gold MS: The effect of epidural/general and cervical plexus block anesthesia on activated clotting time in patients undergoing vascular surgery. *Anesth Analg* 76:701, 1993.
110. Martin P, Greenstein D, Gupta NK, et al: Systemic heparinization during peripheral vascular surgery: Thromboelastographic activated coagulation time, and heparin titration monitoring. *J Cardiothorac Vasc Anesth* 8:150, 1994.
111. Sorensen RM, Pace NL: Mortality and morbidity of regional vs general anesthesia: A meta-analysis. *Anesthesiology* 75:A1053, 1991.
112. Bode RH, Lewis KP, Sarich SW, et al: Anesthesia does not alter cardiac outcome of peripheral vascular surgery. 15th Annual Meeting of the Society of Cardiovascular Anesthesiologists, Montreal, April 1993, p 244.
113. Gelman S: General versus regional anesthesia for peripheral vascular surgery: Is the problem solved? *Anesthesiology* 79:415, 1993.
114. Waskell L: Factors affecting outcome in patients undergoing peripheral vascular surgery. *Anesthesiology* 80:486, 1994.

CHAPTER 16

Anesthesia for Orthopedic Surgery in Elderly Patients

Harald Breivik

INTRODUCTION

The growing elderly population consists of a heterogeneous group of people with widely varying physiological and organic changes resulting from disease and degeneration; this pertains to the musculoskeletal and joint systems in particular. Orthopedic surgery is one of the most common areas that present both elective and urgent cases for major surgery in the elderly. Urgent as well as elective orthopedic operations are good examples of the increasingly acknowledged fact that investment in optimum treatment of chronologically old patients often yields rich dividends through the avoidance of expensive long-term dependency.

URGENT ORTHOPEDIC SURGERY FOR TRAUMA

Age- and disuse-related weakening of skeletal muscles, degeneration, and structural weakening of the skeleton; age- and disease-related reduction in vital organ functions, vision, proprioceptive senses, and mobility; and acute medical problems all predispose octogenarians to falls and trauma. Patients admitted for surgery for fractures near the hip occupy a large proportion of orthopedic hospital beds. There appears to be an overall increase in the incidence of femoral neck fractures, and the rapidly growing number of elderly people in the population will cause the presentation of this age-specific condition to increase dramatically in the near future.[1] Possible mechanisms for the rise in the incidence of hip fractures in the last two decades include the effects of reduction in physical activity on bone mass and an increase in smoking among women. An increasing use of sedative and hypnotic drugs may have an influence on home accidents and the tendency to fall.

There is considerable mortality in excess of that of healthy age-matched controls after femoral neck fractures, making this one of the most common causes of demise among the elderly female population. The 6-month postoperative mortality varies widely in recently published series, ranging from 14 to 29 percent, mirroring in part the volume and specialization of the individual hospital.[2–5]

Two broad groups of patients sustain hip fractures. The first group consists of individuals who are physically and mentally healthy and active. They usually fracture their hips outdoors when engaging in strenuous activity such as running for the bus, shopping, and ballroom dancing.[6] However, the second group sustaining hip fractures includes those who have coexistent medical disease, have impaired mobility, and usually sustain a fracture indoors. In many of these cases, the hip fracture may be the presenting sign of a medical condition. Mortality is positively correlated to medical problems such as cardiac impairment, CNS disease, dementia, delirium, and low body weight (malnutrition) and to higher age, living in an institution, poor mobility, and falling indoors. All of the latter causes are usually associated with medical illness.[7] It is therefore not reasonable to attribute to surgical or anesthetic mishaps the "excess" deaths that occur weeks or months after anesthesia and surgery for hip fracture.

Trochanteric and femoral neck fractures are the most common urgent orthopedic injuries that require surgery in the elderly. There is a long list of other fractures, many of which are best dealt with by internal fixation to get the elderly person up and mobile and home to his or her familiar environment as soon as possible. Table 16-1 summarizes the common fractures of elderly patients and describes how they are handled surgically.[1]

An impending or established pathological fracture is an indication for immediate internal fixation, followed by radiotherapy. Amputation above or below the knee to relieve the sequelae of occlusive arterial disease is another urgent orthopedic operation that can improve the quality of life for these patients.

Emergency orthopedic operations in elderly patients include surgery for acute paraplegia from a secondary deposit pressing on the spinal cord. Speed is essential in securing a cure and avoiding a miserable terminal phase with paraplegia and double incontinence. If a spinal decompression can be done within 8 h of the onset of paraplegia, functional recovery can be good.[1]

ELECTIVE SURGERY FOR DEGENERATIVE AND RHEUMATOID ARTHRITIS

When the quality of life is reduced by pain and immobility from osteoarthritis or rheumatoid arthritis to the degree that the patient is a social cripple, is mentally depressed, and is deprived of the ability to live at home, surgery such as total hip replacement, total knee replacement, or reconstructive surgery of other joints is strongly indicated. Such surgery has been shown to be highly cost-effective, with physical, psychological, and social benefits for the patients and their relatives. The overall economic balance for society is also highly positive with such procedures, a fact that has caused Norwegian health authorities to offer hospitals an extra "premium" for each total hip replacement. In the United Kingdom, total hip replacement is now the most common major surgical procedure performed.[1]

Elective surgery for degenerative and inflammatory joint disease is done in patients who are often 10 to 20 years younger than those who present with urgent orthopedic conditions such as hip fractures. Still, these patients present many of the same challenges to the anesthesia care team as does a patient with a traumatic orthopedic condition.

An increasing number of patients now come for revision hip arthroplasty. These patients are older, the operation takes at least twice as long, and blood loss during surgery and through drains in the postoperative period is much larger. Thermal balance problems during surgery are therefore more of a problem. Postoperative thromboembolism, myocardial infarction, and prosthetic infection are all more common than is seen after primary hip replacement.

Table 16-1 Fractures in elderly patients[1]

Fracture site	Comments
Spine	Osteoporotic women who slip from the chair, sit down heavily. A painful injury, usually stable, treated conservatively, with "aggressive" mobilization and appropriate analgesics.
Pelvis	Fractures of the pubis are usually stable compression fractures and are treated conservatively with immobilization and analgesics. Unstable fractures of the pelvis can be treated with external fixation, which provides relief from pain and allows early mobilization.
Clavicle	Not common in the elderly. Treated with slings.
Neck of humerus	Internal fixation of this often extremely painful fracture relieves pain and allows the patient to get home quickly.
Elbow	A "shattered elbow" is usually treated conservatively with early movement.
Olecranon	Internal fixation followed by early movements.
Colles' fracture	A very common fracture in the elderly that calls for immediate reduction and plaster fixation and active movement of fingers, elbow, and shoulder.
Femur	Trochanteric and femoral neck fractures are treated with internal fixation to allow early mobilization. Femoral shaft fractures are more common in the very elderly and in frail osteoporotic patients. Intramedullary nailing is still a major surgical and anesthetic challenge. Fractures of the femoral condyles should be internally fixed to allow early walking.
Patella	Stellate fractures require plaster for pain relief and support.
Tibia	Internal fixation and plaster to allow the patient to ambulate.
Fibula	Usually treated with simple support and encouragement to walk.
Lateral malleolus	Internal fixation and a light walking cast to allow the patient to ambulate immediately.
Tarsal bones	Firm, supportive bandage and encouragement to walk.

PREANESTHETIC ASSESSMENT AND PREPARATION

Elderly patients presenting for elective major orthopedic surgery should have a preanesthetic assessment according to the general guidelines given in Chaps. 10 and 20. The optimal treatment of hypertension, ischemic and congestive heart disease, obstructive lung disease, and diabetes should be ascertained. The nutritional status of patients who have suffered from arthritic pain and immobility for a long time must also be evaluated and corrected as much as possible before major elective orthopedic surgery.

Urgent surgery in patients with a complex medical history, those with reduced vital organ functional reserves, those on multiple medications, and those who may be difficult to communicate with effectively poses particular challenges to the anesthetist doing the preoperative evaluation and planning the anesthetic procedure. Eighty percent of patients with fractured hips have concomitant medical problems, especially cardiovascular, respiratory, and CNS diseases.[8]

Perioperative morbidity and mortality increase markedly if correctable medical problems are not taken care of before urgent orthopedic surgery. Fast supraventricular dysrhythmias, untreated congestive heart failure, and untreated diabetes can be dealt with rapidly. There is no excuse for deferring surgery for days for such reasons. Prolonged immobility leads to thromboembolic complications, bedsores, pneumonia, hypoxemia, unnecessary suffering, and increased mortality.[9–12]

Surgery for hip fracture in a very sick geriatric patient should be performed during the "window of opportunity," lasting at most a few days, during which the clinical status of the patient may be improved. Even a very frail patient without an obviously correctable medical problem should have the benefit of internal fixation of a near hip fracture, provided that the patient is not in a state of obvious "impending death."[1]

Premedication

Provided that a patient has appropriate analgesic treatment for the fracture and a supportive preanesthetic visit and discussion with the anesthesiologist, premedication usually is unnecessary until the patient arrives in the operating room. At that point, an intravenously titrated dose of a rapidly acting opioid should make the induction of general or regional anesthesia pain-free for the patient. If an anticholinergic effect is needed, glycopyrrolate should be given intravenously rather than atropine, which causes central anticholinergic sedation and prolonged confusion in the elderly.[13,14]

GENERAL OR REGIONAL ANESTHESIA

The aim of orthopedic surgery is to correct the pathology and make the patient mobile and capable of returning to the home environment with intact or improved functions for daily activity. After a fracture of the hip, any delay in surgery beyond approximately 24 h increases postoperative morbidity and mortality.[9] For this early surgery to be possible, the anesthetic management has to provide perioperative cardiovascular stability, intact pulmonary gas exchange, intact skeletal muscle strength, intact gastrointestinal function, intact mental functions, and avoidance of postoperative hypoxemia, immobility, and reduced nutritional status. This requires not only expert handling of operative anesthesia but also provision for optimal perioperative analgesia. Provided that the patient is appropriately assessed and pretreated, both general and regional anesthesia, administered with due respect for the pharmacodynamic and pharmacokinetic changes that occur in the elderly (Chaps. 6–9), can be administered safely and with excellent results for both the surgeon and the patient.

The orthopedic-anesthetic tradition in different parts of the western world varies tremendously. In the United Kingdom, most orthopedic surgery is apparently done under general anesthesia, which is preferred by both anesthesiologists and patients.[1,15] In Scandinavia, general anesthesia is used less often for geriatric orthopedic surgery, with the preferred techniques being spinal, epidural, or combined epidural and spinal anesthesia. Spinal anesthesia is often deepened and prolonged with minidose morphine or fentanyl, as is epidural anesthesia.[16] Epidural anesthesia is continued as postoperative epidural analgesia with low-dose bupivacaine and a low-dose opioid.

Potential Benefits from Optimal Regional Anesthesia for Orthopedic Surgery

This general topic is reviewed in Chap. 6. However, since much of the discussion and controversy surrounding general versus regional anesthesia has centered on anesthesia for elderly orthopedic patients, a summary of the topic is appropriate in this chapter.

Physicians who have been enthusiastically providing optimal regional anesthesia for elderly patients undergoing major orthopedic surgery have never claimed that regional anesthesia is a cure-all that prevents all postoperative problems. However, there is no doubt that patients and ward nurses in Scandinavia are in favor of post-hip-replacement patients receiving epidural anesthesia-analgesia. This allows the patient to be pain-free and alert, able to read the evening newspaper, and enjoy a cup of tea during the afternoon of the day of surgery. These patients are mobile with intact muscle strength, able to stand and walk with support the next morning, able to void, and without emesis or orthostatic blood pressure problems. This ideal immediate postoperative situation cannot quite be mimicked even by the most expertly administered general anesthetic.

The spinal/epidural anesthesia-analgesia technique, however, can also be grossly mismanaged to the degree where the patient not only is pain-free but also has motor blockade of both lower extremities, is unable to void, has repeated vomiting from spinal morphine, is orthostatically unstable, and even develops pressure sores on the heels because of immobility and hypotension. One of the worst ways to manage a frail old lady for urgent amputation of the leg is to use a single-shot spinal anesthetic with lidocaine. When this anesthetic wears off and no other pain relief has been provided, the patient suddenly finds herself in agonizing pain. The ward nurses are usually unable to catch up with the pain because of the fear of side effects from parenteral opioid analgesics. This is a glaring example of the fact that so-called preemptive analgesia is not obtainable with local anesthesia alone for surgery.

It is also appropriate to comment on the technical difficulties and possible severe complications from spinal/epidural blockade. There are patients in whom anatomic obstructions to correct needle and catheter placement exist, making it foolish to continue attempting to establish a central blockade. Patients with a clinically increased bleeding tendency, patients on full anticoagulant doses of warfarin (Coumadin) or heparin, and patients who had fibrinolytic therapy less than 48 h previously all should be given general anesthesia for orthopedic surgery. However, in Scandinavia, thromboprophylactic therapy with dextran or low-dose heparin/low-molecular-weight heparin and nonsteroidal anti-inflammatory drugs (NSAIDs) therapy are not considered contraindications for spinal or epidural analgesia.[17–19] However, there remain about 5 to 10 percent of these patients who because of such contraindications or for technical reasons cannot benefit from central regional anesthesia techniques.

Table 16-2 lists some of the potential benefits of optimally managed perioperative regional anesthesia-analgesia techniques for orthopedic surgery in elderly patients. Each of these areas is discussed below.

Reduced Blood Loss

In comparative studies, under epidural or spinal anesthesia for total hip replacement, blood loss has consistently been up to 50 percent less than under general anesthesia.[20,21] Under general anesthesia, blood loss correlates with mean arterial pressure and can be reduced by means of deliberate hypotension. This correlation between arterial pressure and blood loss does not exist for epidural or spinal anesthesia, probably because venous bleeding is reduced by the effect on venous pressure. Although modern surgical techniques reduce

Table 16-2 Possible benefits from optimally managed spinal/epidural anesthesia and postoperative regional analgesia for orthopedic surgery in elderly patients

Reduced blood loss
Reduced thromboembolism
Reduced immediate postoperative morbidity
Less impairment of immediate postoperative mental functions
Improved immediate postoperative pain relief
Maintenance of postoperative pulmonary function and gas exchange
Perioperative cardiovascular stability
Less impairment of immune functions
Suppression of the traumatic stress response

operative blood loss[22] and the differences between general and regional anesthesia are not marked during internal fixation of a femoral neck fracture, even a moderate reduction in operative blood loss may be of significance in many frail elderly patients.

Reduced Deep Vein Thrombosis and Postoperative Thromboembolism

The majority of randomized prospective studies comparing the incidence of postoperative deep vein thrombosis after major orthopedic surgery have documented an approximate 50 percent reduction in the incidence when comparing patients who received general anesthesia (average, 55 percent) with those who received an epidural or spinal anesthetic (average, 27 percent).[23–26]

This effect is brought about by effects on all three components of Virchow's triad in that local anesthetic drugs appear to protect blood vessel walls by preventing leukocyte adhesion, reducing the surgery-induced postoperative hypercoagulable state[23] in part by reducing the traumatic stress response, and maintaining a higher blood flow in leg veins.[27] In patients receiving effective prophylaxis against postoperative deep vein thrombosis with low-molecular-weight heparin, the difference between epidural/spinal anesthesia and general anesthesia is less evident.[21]

Pulmonary embolism is still the major cause of death in old patients after major orthopedic surgery.[1] Since medical prophylaxis against postoperative thromboembolism is never 100 percent effective in these high-risk patients, the potential beneficial effects of regional anesthesia and analgesia should be included in the management of elderly patients undergoing major orthopedic surgery whenever feasible.

Improved Immediate Postoperative Mental Functions

Although it has not been possible to show any difference in the long-term effect on cognitive functions after major orthopedic surgery when general has been compared with regional anesthesia,[28,29] mental impairment and confusion are more common immediately after general anesthesia. Confusion in the first postoperative week occurs more frequently in patients with a history of mental depression, when anticholinergic drugs have been used, and in patients with hypoxemia after general anesthesia.[30] In as many as 25 percent of patients, signs of mental disturbance may persist for several weeks.[1] Confused patients have a longer hospitalization time because of more postoperative complications.[30]

Improved Cardiovascular Stability

Spinal and epidural anesthesia may result in improved cardiovascular stability during cement insertion for total hip arthroplasty.[31] Aggravation of cardiovascular changes by air embolism during general anesthesia with nitrous oxide is possible.[15] The cardiotoxic effects of free methacrylic acid (methyl methacrylate) monomer are no longer thought to be important in the sudden cardiovascular collapse that may occur during femoral reaming and cement insertion. These cardiotoxic effects are seen more often during replacement arthroplasty for transcervical fracture than in elective hip arthroplasty.[21] Release of marrow contents into the circulation and embolization to the lungs can cause pulmonary hypertension, impaired right-sided heart function, and hypoxemia.[32] Subsequent release of vasoactive substances from the lungs may cause vasodilatation and systemic arterial hypotension.[32]

Marked hemodynamic changes during urgent as well as elective procedures appear more likely to be related to the preexisting medical condition of the patient, especially hypertension, ischemic heart disease, renal insufficiency, and diabetes, than to the specific anesthetic technique.[15]

Improved Postoperative Pulmonary Function and Gas Exchange

There is a fall in arterial oxygen tension during insertion of the prosthesis material for total hip or knee replacement. This is caused by increased ventilation-perfusion mismatching and increased dead space from the bronchial and pulmonary vascular effects of embolic material resulting from the surgeon's interference with the bone marrow.[33,34] Postoperative hypoxemia is less pronounced after epidural or spinal anesthesia than it is after general anesthesia.[35] Although most studies have shown only transient enhancement of oxygenation after regional anesthesia compared with general anesthesia for hip surgery, these effects come at a critical period in which the postoperative hypoxemia often is added to the preoperative hypoxemia of patients with fractured hips.[8,36] As was noted above, hypoxemia after general anesthesia is associated with postoperative confusion and increased postoperative complications and prolonged hospitalization.[30]

Less Impairment of Immune Functions after Major Orthopedic Surgery

Pre- and postoperative impairment of immune functions appears to be related to humoral factors released from the site of injury and to the neuroendocrine response to surgery. Part of this inhibition of the immune system is ameliorated by spinal or epidural anesthesia. Postoperative lymphopenia is prevented and lymphocyte and monocyte/macrophage functions are unchanged or improved under spinal epidural anesthesia and epidural plus general anesthesia but impaired under sole general anesthesia for total hip arthroplasty.[37,38] The clinical importance of these findings is not known.

Suppression of the Traumatic Stress Response after Orthopedic Surgery

The neuroendocrine stress response to major orthopedic surgery, illustrated by the rise in blood cortisol and glucose concentrations, can be suppressed completely or partially by spinal or epidural anesthesia.[20,39–41] This suppression of the traumatic neuroendocrine stress response may, at least in part, mediate the beneficial effects of regional anesthesia on hemostasis, immune functions, and carbohydrate and nitrogen metabolism after orthopedic surgery. Intuitively, these effects would appear to be of benefit to a frail elderly patient undergoing major surgery with a demanding postoperative rehabilitation phase. However, the real clinical value of these effects of regional anesthesia-analgesia has not been evaluated. Most likely, these effects by themselves may not be of great importance. However, if they are exploited in a comprehensive perioperative rehabilitation regimen with stress-free anesthesia, optimal postoperative analgesia, early postoperative nutrition, and an active mobilization and rehabilitation program, a significant improvement in speed and quality of recovery may be seen.[42]

Reduced Immediate Postoperative Morbidity after Urgent Orthopedic Surgery

There has been a decade-long debate on whether regional anesthesia has effects on mortality after surgery for fractured hips in elderly patients. This debate was initiated by the study of McLaren and colleagues[43] in 1978, which showed a marked difference in hospital mortality between patients operated on under spinal anesthesia and those who received general anesthesia. This has finally been resolved, as several prospective studies conclusively show that there is no major difference in immediate or late mortality after fractured hip surgery under spinal versus general anesthesia.[11,12] The average 1-month mortality of 6 to 8 percent and 1-year mortality of 20 percent were not markedly influenced by anesthetic technique but were determined by the medical condition of the patient and by the adequacy of assessment and preoperative treatment of an elderly patient with preexisting medical problems.[11,12]

However, postoperative morbidity and hospital stay are increased by hypoxemia after general anesthesia.[30] More dramatic effects on the postoperative course have been obtained by prolonging epidural anesthesia to balanced postoperative epidural analgesia and exploiting this for a radically more active rehabilitation regimen.[44]

Improved Immediate Postoperative Pain Relief

In the recent debate on the value of preemptive analgesia, proponents maintain that afferent blockade and opioid analgesics suppress the obligatory central sensitization of the nociceptive system and therefore diminish subsequent pain perception.[45,46] The preemptive analgesia effect is real but transient. Analgesic treatment must be continued as long as pain stimuli are generated from the surgical wound.[46] Well-conducted balanced spinal and/or epidural anesthesia with local anesthetics and opioids, continued into the postoperative period as long as needed, should give the patient maximal comfort. The possibility also exists that prolonged perioperative epidural analgesia reduces the incidence of incapacitating postamputation phantom limb pain.[47]

PAIN RELIEF AFTER ORTHOPEDIC SURGERY

Patients who have been plagued by chronic, often nocturnal, pain from osteoarthritis and patients who have had excruciating pain on movement after a fractured hip are so obviously helped by their operations that they often do not complain of pain after surgery. Still, perioperative pain relief should be managed systematically and optimally in all patients to allow early mobilization and rehabilitation.[44] Postorthopedic surgery pain often responds well to nonopioid analgesics such as acetaminophen (paracetamol, Tylenol) and NSAIDs. These drugs should always be used as the basic analgesic therapy, before opioid analgesics are added. Paracetamol does not have the ulcerogenic, hemostatic, and renal side effects that may occasionally be of significance when NSAID analgesics are used in elderly patients.

For surgery on femoral neck fractures, the addition of morphine 0.1 to 0.2 mg to spinal bupivacaine not only will deepen and prolong operative spinal anesthesia but also will render most patients pain-free for the first 24 to 40 h after surgery, so that they will need only paracetamol or NSAID analgesics for the remaining postoperative period. A similar effect can be obtained with the addition of morphine 2 mg to an epidural anesthetic dose of bupivacaine.[48] However, there is a narrow dosing range: Adding a little more to a total of 0.3 mg morphine in the subarachnoid space will cause 11 percent of patients to develop respiratory depression that can come on at any time during the subsequent 28 h.[16]

Local anesthetic drugs, opioid analgesics, and adrenergic agonists all have antinociceptive effects in the spinal cord. Local anesthetics inhibit excitation, while opioids and adrenergic agonists enhance inhibition of pain impulse transmission between the primary afferent nociceptive neuron and the secondary nociceptive neuron in the dorsal horn of the spinal cord.[49] These three different types of spinal analgesic agents have different side effect profiles but show analgesic synergy.[49] Provided that an epidural catheter is placed correctly near the segmental part of the spinal cord receiving pain impulses from the surgical wound, a mixture of low concentrations of bupivacaine (0.6–1 mg/ml), fentanyl (2 μg/ml), and adrenaline (2 μg/ml) will provide excellent analgesia.[50] The side effects of prolonged epidural anesthesia with local anesthetics alone (muscle paralysis, hypotension, urinary retention) or epidural opioids alone (respiratory depression, urinary retention, nausea, pruritus), which have discredited epidural analgesia after orthopedic surgery,[15] are virtually absent.[51] However, if the catheter is placed in the lumbar area, below the spinal cord, the local anesthetic effect on the spinal nerve roots causes motor blockade and lower extremity paresis and urinary retention in more than 15 percent of cases.

In the recent report from Kehlet's group,[44,52] bupivacaine 2.5 mg/h and morphine 0.2 mg/h in continuous epidural infusion were used for 4 days after hip replacement in combination with an NSAID and an "aggressive" mobilization and rehabilitation regimen. By exploiting optimal epidural analgesia in this way, the authors were able to reduce the hospital stay from 10 to 13 days to 6 to 8 days.

Patient-controlled analgesia (PCA) with intravenous morphine can be used with advantage after orthopedic operations, but a few elderly patients are unable to benefit from PCA because they are confused after surgery.[53]

Continuous peripheral nerve blockade with local anesthetic drug infusion is possible for lower extremity postoperative pain. Continuous infusion of a low-concentration bupivacaine solution for the femoral nerve or a "3-in-1" nerve blockade can be very effective after knee replacement.[54]

SUMMARY

Age- and disuse-related weakening of skeletal muscles, degeneration, and structural weakening of the skeleton; age- and disease-related reduction in vital organ functions, vision, and proprioceptive senses and mobility; and acute medical problems all predispose octogenarians to falls and trauma. Patients admitted for surgery for fractures near the hip occupy a large and increasing number of orthopedic hospital beds. In Scandinavia, emergency as well as elective orthopedic surgery is performed mostly under regional anesthesia with postoperative regional analgesia with local anesthetic drugs, opioids, and nonopioid analgesic drugs such as paracetamol (NSAIDs). Optimally managed regional anesthesia-analgesia has a number of potential benefits, such as reduced blood loss, thromboprophylactic effects, intact mental abilities, improved cardiovascular stability and postoperative pulmonary functions, less impairment of immune functions, suppression of the traumatic stress response, improved immediate postoperative pain relief, and reduced immediate postoperative morbidity after urgent orthopedic surgery. In about 10 percent of patients, technical difficulties or contraindications to regional anesthesia such as an increased bleeding tendency make general anesthesia preferable.

REFERENCES

1. Devas M, Plumpton FA, Seymour DG: Orthopaedics, in Crosby DL, Rees GAD, Seymour DG (eds): *The Aging Surgical Patient: Anaesthetic, Operative, and Medical Management.* New York: Wiley, 1992, chap 11, pp 329–351.
2. Jensen JS: Determining factors for the mortality following hip fractures. *Injury* 15:411, 1984.
3. Elmerson S, Zetterburg C, Andersson BJ: Ten-year survival after fractures of the proximal end of the femur. *Gerontology* 34:186, 1988.
4. Gilchrist WJ, Newman RJ, Hamblen DL, Williams BO: Prospective randomised study of an orthopaedic geriatric inpatient service. *Br Med J* 297:1116, 1988.
5. Hughes RC, Garnick DW, Luft HS, et al: Hospital volume and patient outcomes: The case of hip fracture patients. *Med Care* 26:1057, 1988.
6. Evans JG: Falls and fractures. *Age Ageing* 17:361, 1988.
7. Evans JG, Prudham D, Wandless I: A prospective study of fractured proximal femur: Factors predisposing to survival. *Age Ageing* 8:246, 1979.

8. Haljamä H, Stefansson T, Wickström I: Preanaesthetic evaluation of the female geriatric patient with hip fracture. *Acta Anaesthesiol Scand* 26:393, 1982.
9. Royal College of Physicians: Fractured neck of femur: Prevention and management. *J R Coll Physicians Lond* 23:8, 1989.
10. Wyant GM, Cocking EC: A study in geriatric anaesthesia—fractured neck of the femur. *Can Anaesth Soc J* 10:567, 1963.
11. Valentin N, Lomholt B, Jensen JS, et al: Spinal or general anaesthesia for surgery of the fractured hip? A prospective study of mortality in 578 patients. *Br J Anaesth* 58:284, 1986.
12. Davis FM, Woolner DF, Frampton C, et al: Prospective, multi-center trial of mortality following general or spinal anaesthesia for hip fracture surgery in the elderly. *Br J Anaesth* 59:1080, 1987.
13. Breivik H: The central anticholinergic syndrome and its treatment with physostigmine. *Tidss Nor Lægeforen* 95:1771, 1975.
14. Ruprecht J, Dworacek B: The central anticholinergic syndrome in the postoperative period, in Nunn JF, Utting JE, Brown BR Jr (eds): *General Anaesthesia*, 5th ed. London: Butterworth, 1989, chap 91, pp 1141–1148.
15. Davis FM: Anaesthesia for major orthopaedic surgery in the elderly. *Curr Anaesth Crit Care* 3:193, 1992.
16. Johnson A, Bengtsson M, Merits H, Löfström JB: Anesthesia for major hip surgery: A clinical study of spinal and general anesthesia in 244 patients. *Reg Anesth* 11:83, 1986.
17. Bergqvist D, Lindblad B, Mätzsch T: Low molecular weight heparin for thromboprophylaxis and epidural/spinal anaesthesia—is there a risk? *Acta Anaesthesiol Scand* 36:605, 1992.
18. Modig J: Spinal or epidural anaesthesia with low molecular weight heparin for thromboprophylaxis requires careful postoperative neurological observation. *Acta Anaesthesiol Scand* 36:603, 1992.
19. Stenseth R, Breivik H, Grimstad J: Consensus report of Norwegian Association of Anaesthesiologists on regional anaesthesia/analgesia for patients with obvious or potential bleeding problems. Norwegian Association of Anaesthesiologists, Annual Meeting, Oslo, Oct. 28, 1993.
20. Hole A, Terjesen T, Breivik H: Epidural versus general anaesthesia for total hip arthroplasty in elderly patients. *Acta Anaesthesiol Scand* 24:279, 1980.
21. Davis FM: Anaesthesia for hip surgery: Comparative studies of spinal anaesthesia and general anaesthesia for elective total hip replacement and internal fixation of fractures of the femoral neck in the elderly (MD thesis). Dunedin, New Zealand: University of Otago, 1988.
22. Planes A, Vochelle N, Fagola M, et al: Prevention of deep vein thrombosis after total hip replacement: The effect of low-molecular weight heparin with spinal and general anaesthesia. *J Bone Joint Surg [Br]* 73-B:418, 1991.
23. Modig J: The role of lumbar epidural anaesthesia as antithrombotic prophylaxis in total hip replacement. *Acta Chir Scand* 151:589, 1985.
24. McKenzie PJ, Wishart HY, Gray I, Smith G: Effects of anaesthetic technique on deep vein thrombosis: A comparison of subarachnoid and general anaesthesia. *Br J Anaesth* 57:853, 1985.
25. Davis FM, Laurenson VG, Gillespie WJ, et al: Deep vein thrombosis after total hip replacement: A comparison between spinal and general anaesthesia. *J Bone Joint Surg [Br]* 71-B:181, 1989.
26. Jørgensen LN, Rasmussen LS, Nielsen PT, et al: Antithrombotic efficacy of continuous extradural analgesia after knee replacement. *Br J Anaesth* 66:8, 1991.

27. Davis FM, Laurenson VG, Gillespie WJ, et al: Leg blood flow during total hip replacement under spinal or general anaesthesia. *Anaesth Intensive Care* 17:136, 1989.
28. Jones MJT, Piggott SE, Vaughan RS, et al: Cognitive and functional competence after anaesthesia in patients aged over 60: Controlled trial of general and regional anaesthesia for elective hip or knee replacement. *Br Med J* 300:1683, 1990.
29. Nielson WR, Gelb AW, Casey JE, et al: Long-term cognitive and social sequelae of general versus regional anesthesia during arthroplasty in the elderly. *Anesthesiology* 73:1103, 1990.
30. Berggren D, Gustafsson Y, Eriksson B, et al: Postoperative confusion after anesthesia in elderly patients with femoral neck fractures. *Anesth Analg* 66:497, 1987.
31. James ML: Anaesthetic and metabolic complications, in Ling RSM (ed): *Complications of Total Hip Replacement: Current Problems in Orthopaedics.* Edinburgh: Churchill Livingstone, 1984, pp 1–17.
32. Modig J, Busch C, Olerud S, et al: Arterial hypotension and hypoxaemia during total hip replacement: The importance of thromboplastic products, fat embolism and acrylic monomers. *Acta Anaesthesiol Scand* 19:28, 1975.
33. Hedenstierna G, Mebius C, Bygdeman S: Ventilation-perfusion relationship during hip arthroplasty. *Acta Anaesthesiol Scand* 27:56, 1983.
34. Mebius C, Hedenstierna G: Airway closure and gas distribution during hip arthroplasty. *Acta Anaesthesiol Scand* 26:72, 1982.
35. Hedenstierna G, Löfström J: Effect of anaesthesia on respiratory function after major lower extremity surgery: A comparison between bupivacaine spinal analgesia with low-dose morphine and general anaesthesia. *Acta Anaesthesiol Scand* 29:55, 1985.
36. McKenzie PJ, Wishart HY, Dewar KMS, et al: Comparison of the effects of spinal anaesthesia and general anaesthesia on postoperative oxygenation and perioperative mortality. *Br J Anaesth* 52:49, 1980.
37. Hole A, Unsgaard G, Breivik H: Monocyte functions are depressed during and after surgery under general anaesthesia but not under epidural anaesthesia. *Acta Anaesthesiol Scand* 26:301, 1982.
38. Salo M, Nissila M: Cell-mediated and humoral immune responses to total hip replacement under spinal or general anaesthesia. *Acta Anaesthesiol Scand* 34:241, 1990.
39. Stefansson T, Wickström I, Haljamae H: Effects of neurolept and epidural analgesia on cardiovascular function and tissue metabolism in the geriatric patient. *Acta Anaesthesiol Scand* 26:386, 1982.
40. Davis FM, Laurenson VG, Lewis J, et al: Metabolic response to total hip arthroplasty under hypobaric subarachnoid or general anaesthesia. *Br J Anaesth* 59:725, 1987.
41. Davis FM, McDermott E, Hicton C, et al: Influence of spinal and general anaesthesia on haemostasis during total hip arthroplasty. *Br J Anaesth* 59:561, 1987.
42. Kehlet H: The importance of postoperative pain relief. *Acta Anaesthesiol Scand* 37(Supp 100):122, 1993.
43. McLaren AD, Stockwell MC, Reid VT: Anaesthetic techniques for surgical correction of fractured neck of femur: A comparative study of spinal and general anaesthesia in the elderly. *Anaesthesia* 33:10, 1978.
44. Møiniche S, Hansen BL, Christensen S-E, et al: Activity of patients and duration of hospitalisation following hip-replacement with balanced treatment of pain and early mobilization. *Ugeskr Laeger* 154:1495, 1992.

45. Wall PD: The prevention of postoperative pain. *Pain* 33:289, 1988.
46. Woolf CJ, Chong M-S: Preemptive analgesia—treating postoperative pain by preventing the establishment of central sensitization. *Anesth Analg* 77:362, 1993.
47. Bach S, Nordberg MF, Tjelden NU: Phantom limb pain in amputees during the first 12 months following limb amputation, after preoperative lumbar epidural blockade. *Pain* 33:297, 1988.
48. Stenseth R, Sellevold O, Breivik H: Epidural morphine for postoperative pain: Experience with 1085 patients. *Acta Anaesthesiol Scand* 29:148, 1985.
49. Maves TJ, Gebhart GF: Antinociceptive synergy between intrathecal morphine and lidocaine during visceral and somatic nociception in the rat. *Anesthesiology* 76:91, 1992.
50. Breivik H: Epidural opioids: current use. *Curr Opin Anaesth* 5:661, 1992.
51. Högström H, Breivik H, Stalder B, et al: Balanced epidural analgesia for postoperative pain on surgical wards in a large university hospital. *Int Monit Reg Anaesth* 5(*Eur Soc Reg Anaesth*, Dublin, Sept. 8–10, 1993, Abstracts):46, 1993.
52. Møiniche S, Dahl JB, Hansen BL, Kehlet H: The effect of balanced analgesia and reinforced rehabilitation on convalescence after major orthopaedic and abdominal surgery. *Reg Anesth* 18(Supp 2):84, 1993.
53. Stalder B, Breivik H, Högström H, et al: Intravenous PCA on surgical wards in a large university hospital. *Int Monit Reg Anaesth* 5(*Eur Soc Reg Anaesth*, Dublin, Sept. 8–10, 1993, Abstracts):59, 1993.
54. Edwards ND, Wright EM: Continuous low-dose 3-in-1 nerve blockade for postoperative pain relief after total knee replacement. *Anesth Analg* 75:265, 1992.

CHAPTER 17

Anesthesia for Ophthalmic Surgery in Geriatric Patients

R. Brian Smith

INTRODUCTION

Other than infrequent trauma or congenital malformation, ophthalmic surgery is predominately focused on the geriatric population. Frequently these patients have multisystem involvement and are on multiple medications. In addition, ophthalmic surgery is almost entirely performed as an outpatient procedure, meaning the anesthesiologist has a very limited period of contact available to evaluate the patient and make any desired interventions. Most of these patients are very anxious to have their surgery, as their activities of daily living are highly dependent on their visual accuity. It is anticipated that the surgery will require very limited anesthesia (local or conscious sedation), so frequently little is done to maximize the patients' medical management prior to the procedure. This misconception can place a patient at increased risk if an allergic or vagal reaction occurs necessitating the need for general anesthesia. This chapter will help to explain what is happening to the eye to necessitate surgery, how various ophthalmic drugs interact with systemic drugs, including anesthetic drugs, and then discuss the anesthetic options.

PHYSIOLOGY OF THE EYE

It is necessary to review the physiology of the eye before discussing the effects of anesthetic agents on the eye.

It is important to maintain intraocular pressure (IOP) in the normal physiological range of 10 to 22 mmHg. IOP is usually considered pathological when it is above 25 mmHg, and there is a normal diurnal variation of 2 to 3 mmHg. IOP is higher than the pressure in any other tissue or organ, excluding the cardiovascular system. This high pressure is needed to maintain the optical properties of the refracting surface of the eye. During anesthesia or postoperatively, a rise in IOP can lead to permanent loss of vision. If the eye is suddenly opened when IOP is high, hemorrhage may occur as a result of ruptured blood vessels. The IOP becomes atmospheric once the cornea has been incised. Any increase in pressure can result in loss of vitreous and prolapse of the lens and iris. There is central control of IOP from areas in the diencephalon that, when stimulated, can cause alterations in IOP through nerve impulses, hormonal effects, or both.

Aqueous humor helps maintain IOP and is a source of nutrition for the lens and the posterior part of the cornea, as these structures have no blood vessels. The circulation of aqueous humor is shown in Fig. 17-1. It is formed mainly in the posterior chamber by the epithelial cells of the ciliary process and circulates to the anterior chamber of the eye through the pupil to be drained at the angle of the eye. It then passes through small channels called spaces of Fontana to drain through Schlemm's canal. It is carried to aqueous veins and ends in the ophthalmic veins. These veins have anastomosis outside the skull with the superior ophthalmic vein and the facial vein. The ophthalmic vein drains into

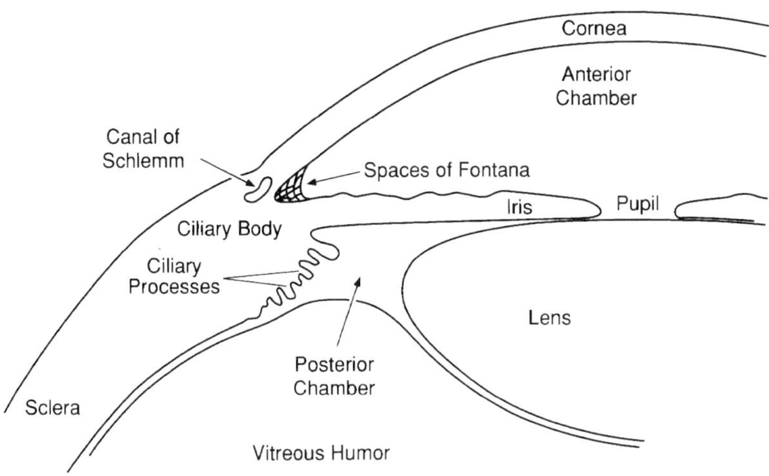

Figure 17-1 **Circulation of the aqueous humor.** *(Reprinted with permission from Aboul-Eish: Physiology of the eye pertinent to anesthesia, in Smith RB (ed): Anesthesia in Ophthalmology. International Ophthalmology Clinics, 1973. Boston: Little, Brown, 1973, vol 13, no 2, p 1.)*

the cavernous sinus (Fig. 17-2). As this venous system is without valves, any rise in central venous pressure immediately affects the IOP (i.e., vomiting, coughing, or straining from any other cause).

Changes in arterial blood pressure do not significantly affect IOP. The rise in IOP is only about 10 percent of the rise in blood pressure. This is due to changes in blood volume in the eye, not overproduction of aqueous humor.

CHANGES IN THE EYE CAUSED BY THE AGING PROCESS

Glaucoma

Glaucoma is a disease process associated with an elevation in IOP. Eventually this rise in IOP impairs blood flow to the optic nerve.

The incidence of glaucoma is approximately 2 percent in the adult population, and this disease is seen more frequently with advancing age. If IOP exceeds 30 mmHg, this disease eventually will progress to optic nerve changes with visual field loss. The initial pressure rise is usually caused by obstruction to the outflow of the aqueous humor in the trabecular network. The classification of the causes of glaucoma is of little relevance to the anesthesiologist except to indicate that there are acute and chronic forms of the disease. The pharmacology and drug interactions that may occur during treatment are of considerable importance. The drugs used include parasympathomimetics (pilocarpine, carbachol), anticholinesterases (echothiophate iodide), sympathomimetics (phenylephrine hydrochloride), adrenergics (epinephrine), beta blockers (timolol, betaxolol),

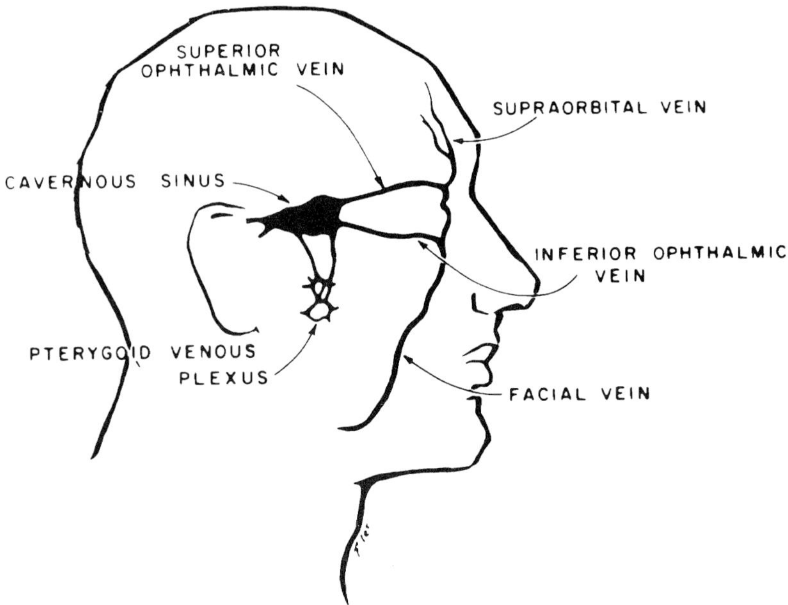

Figure 17-2 Aqueous and venous drainage of the eye. [*Reprinted with permission from Aboul-Eish: Physiology of the eye pertinent to anesthesia, in Smith RB (ed): Anesthesia in Ophthalmology. International Ophthalmology Clinics, 1973. Boston: Little, Brown, 1973, vol 13, no 2, p 7.*]

and carbonic anhydrase inhibitors (acetazolamide). Details about the drugs will be dealt with below under "Ocular Drugs." Failure of medical treatment to contain the disorder may result in a need for surgical filtration procedures to improve outflow and reduce pressure. These procedures include trabeculectomy, trephines, sclerotomy, and many others.

Because of their mydriatic effect, atropine and scopolamine can have a deleterious effect in patients with narrow-angle glaucoma. However, the doses of atropine used for premedication are probably safe. Because scopolamine produces more mydriasis than does atropine and has a propensity to cause disorientation, its use should be avoided.

Vitreous and Retinal Disease

Diabetes mellitus is a common cause of retinopathy resulting from ischemic changes. Probably less than 10 percent of the total diabetic population becomes blind. One of the early treatments of diabetic retinopathy is photocoagulation. Argon laser retinal photocoagulation has been shown to be 60 percent effective in preventing loss of vision secondary to vascular proliferation. Photocoagulation does not usually require the skills of an anesthesiologist. It should be noted, however, that retrobulbar block may be employed frequently to ensure immobility of the eye. In advanced disease, vitrectomy may be performed to remove opaque material filling the globe. Because of the duration of the procedure, anesthesiologists are usually involved. Local and regional anesthesia with monitored anesthesia care or general anesthesia may be used.

The aging human eye undergoes considerable changes, including anatomic changes in vitreo-retinal relations. Vitreous in the young is a semisolid gel. In an older patient, the vitreous frequently undergoes segregation of the collagenous elements from the water and acid molecule, resulting in some liquefaction. Separation of the vitreous becomes fairly common in the elderly. In adults over 70 years of age, separation of the vitreous from the posterior retina occurs 50 percent of the time.

The annual incidence of retinal detachment in the general population is about 1 in 15,000. It occurs in about 2 percent of patients after cataract surgery. A large proportion of retinal detachments occur in patients over age 60 years. Cryosurgical techniques have greatly reduced the need for extensive surgery such as scleral buckling. In addition to vitrectomy, air or inert intraocular gas can be used (such as sulfur hexafluoride) to maintain retinal integrity.

Cataract

It has been estimated that more than 500,000 persons undergo cataract surgery in the United States annually, and the majority of these patients are elderly. The degenerative cataract begins with a gradual loss of transparency. Senile degeneration is the most common cause. Other causes include x-rays, heat from infrared rays, trauma, systemic disease (diabetes), and systemic medication (steroids).

INTRAOCULAR PRESSURE

Intravenous Agents

The commonly used intravenous barbiturate induction agents (thiopental sodium, thiamylal, and methohexital sodium) are all considered to lower IOP. In a study by deRoetth and Schwartz,[1] IOP dropped 19 mmHg after the administration of thiopental. The more recently introduced intravenous induction agent propofol has also been shown to reduce IOP. Mirakhur and colleagues[2] compared the effects of thiopental and propofol in 30 patients. Both agents caused a lowering of IOP that was slightly more marked with propofol. Unfortunately, there was also more hypotension with propofol, and this may be undesirable in the elderly.[2] The fall in IOP is probably secondary to depression of the diencephalon and in part facilitates aqueous humor outflow. Relaxation of the extraocular muscles also may play a role.

There is some controversy about the use of ketamine. An early study by Corssen and Hoy[3] reported a slight but statistically significant rise in IOP. However, in a subsequent study by Peuler and associates,[4] 2 mg/kg of ketamine was given intravenously to adults and did not cause a significant rise in IOP.

Ketamine is of questionable value as an anesthetic agent in an elderly patient undergoing ophthalmic surgery. It causes a systemic rise in blood pressure and is associated with postoperative hallucinations. In addition, it frequently causes nystagmus and blepharospasm, which are troublesome in ophthalmic surgery.

Inhalational Agents

The inhalational agents enflurane and isoflurane have been shown to lower IOP. Studies on halothane have not demonstrated a consistent reduction in IOP. However, a comparison of the effects of halothane and isoflurane on IOP in patients when Pa_{CO_2} and posture were controlled demonstrated a similar fall in IOP with both agents.[5] This fall did not appear to be dose-related. The mechanism of the fall is probably similar to that of the barbiturates, supplemented by the relaxant effects of these agents on the extraocular muscles.

All the CNS depressants used in anesthesia, such as opioids, tranquilizers, neuroleptics, and hypnotics, appear to lower IOP.

Muscle Relaxants

The nondepolarizing muscle relaxants *d*-tubocurarine, pancuronium, vecuronium, atracurium, and mivacurium are all associated with a fall in IOP. There is a consensus that this fall is caused by relaxation of the extraocular muscles. The widely used nondepolarizing muscle relaxant succinylcholine (SCC) is well known for causing an increase in IOP. This rise is hypothesized to be caused primarily by contraction of the extraocular muscles, which in turn squeeze the globe. Studies on the effects of SCC are somewhat complicated because of the well-known rise in IOP caused by tracheal intubation. In 1970, Pandey and colleagues[6] studied the effects of SCC on IOP in patients with and without tracheal intubation (Fig. 17-3). The rise in IOP was higher when SCC was followed by tracheal intubation. Subsequently, many studies have attempted to prevent the rise in IOP caused by SCC and tracheal intubation. Pretreatment with a nondepolarizing muscle relaxant has been shown to attenuate but not prevent the rise in IOP (Fig. 17-4). One study compared a group of patients pretreated with *d*-tubocurarine with intubation after SCC with a group intubated after pancuronium.[7] The use of intravenous lidocaine as a pretreatment has also been shown in a number of experiments to attenuate but not prevent the rise in IOP. Pretreatment with propanolol has been shown to prevent the rise in IOP during a thiopental-succinylcholine intubation sequence.[8] The narcotics alfentanil and sufentanil given intravenously before SCC and tracheal intubation will blunt any rise in IOP.

SCC can be used to facilitate intubation in selected patients with open eye injuries. For example, it can be used in patients in whom rapid onset of paralysis is required before intubation, such as those with a full stomach or extreme obesity. However, in these cases, SCC must be pretreated with a nondepolarizing muscle relaxant. In general, SCC can be used to facilitate intubation in patients undergoing elective ophthalmic surgery before incision of the cornea.

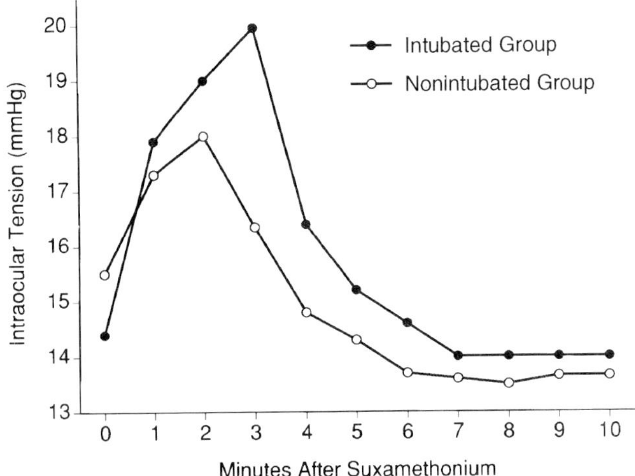

Figure 17-3 Time course of intraocular hypertension produced by succinylcholine. -●-, Intubated group; -○-, nonintubated group. *(Reprinted from Pandey K, Badola RP, Kumar S: Time course of intraocular hypertension produced by suxamethonium. Br J Anaesth 191:44, 1972. With permission.)*

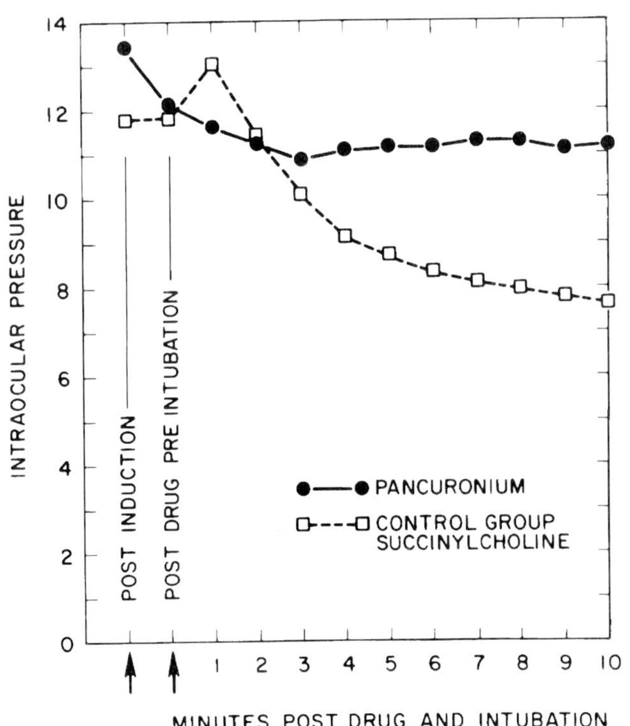

Figure 17-4 Intraocular pressure after pancuronium. ● — ●, Pancuronium; □----□, control group succinylcholine. *(Reprinted from Smith RB, Leano N: Intraocular pressure following pancuronium. Can Anaesth Soc J 744:20, 1973. With permission.)*

Any rise in IOP caused by the SCC will be dissipated within the 15 to 20 min it takes to prepare the patient. It should be noted that SCC, by causing prolonged tonic contraction of the extraocular muscles, can impair the forced duction test, which is used frequently in patients with strabismus.

Nitrous Oxide

Caution must be exercised when nitrous oxide is administered to patients who have air or sulfahexafluoride (SF6) in the vitreous cavity. Smith and colleagues[9] reported a significant rise in IOP during nitrous oxide administration in eyes of rhesus monkeys containing intravitreal air (Fig. 17-5). This is explained on the basis that nitrous oxide is a highly soluble gas compared with nitrogen and SF6. During administration, nitrous oxide diffuses rapidly into the air or SF6 and the inert gas diffuses very slowly out of the eye, increasing the risk for raised IOP. It is recommended that the use of nitrous oxide be avoided in these cases.

Adjuvant Drugs

Intravenous hypertonic solutions decrease aqueous humor formation and lower IOP by elevating plasma oncotic pressure. This rise in plasma oncotic pressure causes fluid to flow out of the eye and into the plasma. Dextran and mannitol are probably the most commonly used hypertonic solutions.

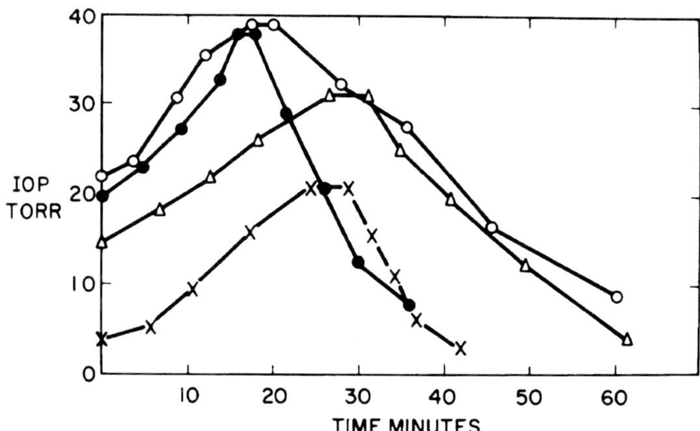

Figure 17-5 Effect of nitrous oxide on air in vitreous. *(Reprinted from Smith RB, Carl B, Linn J, Nemoto E: Effect of nitrous oxide on air in vitreous. Am J Ophthalmol 78:314, 1974. Published with permission from The American Journal of Ophthalmology. Copyright by The Ophthalmic Publishing Company.)*

Ventilation

Alterations in Pa_{CO_2} have a significant effect on IOP. An anesthesiologist can manipulate this factor during general anesthesia by controlling the ventilation. Hyperventilation reduces IOP to a small degree and contributes to a "soft eye." Conversely, hypoventilation significantly increases IOP. These effects have been shown to closely follow intracranial pressure and are probably vascular in origin.

Positive End-Expiratory Pressure

Because positive end-expiratory pressure (PEEP) raises central venous pressure, it would be expected to cause a rise in IOP. As PEEP is frequently used with mechanical ventilation, it is important to be aware of its effects on the eye. Figure 17-6 shows the effect of PEEP on IOP in cats. In this study, the Pa_{CO_2} was kept constant.[10]

OCULOCARDIAC REFLEX

The oculocardiac reflex was first described independently by Bernard Aschner[11] and Giuseppe Dagnini in 1908.[12] Traction on the extraocular muscles and pressure on the eyeball can evoke this reflex, which is manifested by bradycardia and cardiac dysrhythmias. The afferent pathway consists of fibers that run through the short ciliary nerves to the ciliary ganglion and then pass with

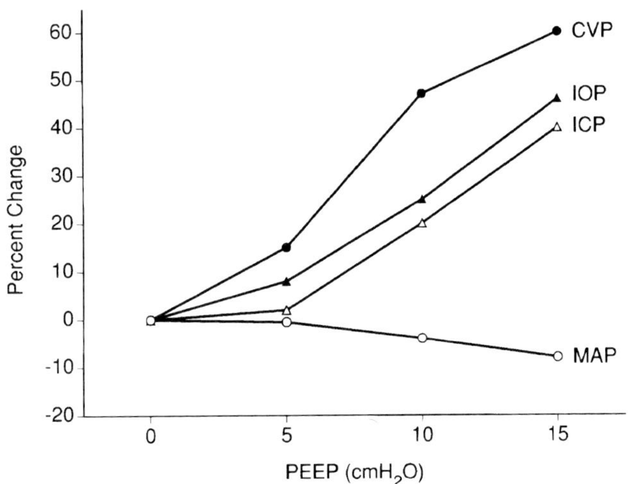

Figure 17-6 **Effect of PEEP on IOP.** ***(Reprinted from Niminogadda U, Joseph NJ, Salem MR, et al: Positive end-expiratory pressure and the intraocular pressure. Anesthesiology 67:A132, 1987. With permission.)***

the ophthalmic division of the trigeminal nerve to the trigeminal ganglion. Afferent fibers also pass in the long ciliary nerve and then again in the ophthalmic division of the trigeminal nerve to the trigeminal ganglion. From this ganglion, both groups of afferent fibers terminate in the main central nucleus of the trigeminal nerve in the fourth ventricle. The efferent limb is the vagus nerve; thus, the reflex is trigeminal and vagal (Fig. 17-7).

A number of cardiac arrests have been associated with this reflex. Kirsch and colleagues[13] reported a rate of 1 arrest in every 3500 patients presenting for anesthesia and operation on the eye. Knoblock and Lorenz[14] found that among 300,000 patients, 60 died while undergoing operations for strabismus.

Numerous methods of blocking the afferent or efferent pathways have been tried with varying degrees of success. It appears that the preoperative use of intramuscular or subcutaneous atropine is of little or no value in prevention of the reflex; however, when given intravenously in the operating room before anesthesia, atropine is of considerable value. The dose of atropine required to block the vagus completely in an adult is 2 to 3 mg. This dose cannot be used safely in elderly patients because of the risk of tachydysrhythmias, but smaller doses up to 0.6 mg may be given. The disadvantages seen with atropine, such as tachydysrhythmias and disorientation in the elderly, can be largely avoided by using glycopyrrolate. Glycopyrrolate has the advantage over atropine that it does not cross the blood-brain barrier and has less of a tendency to produce

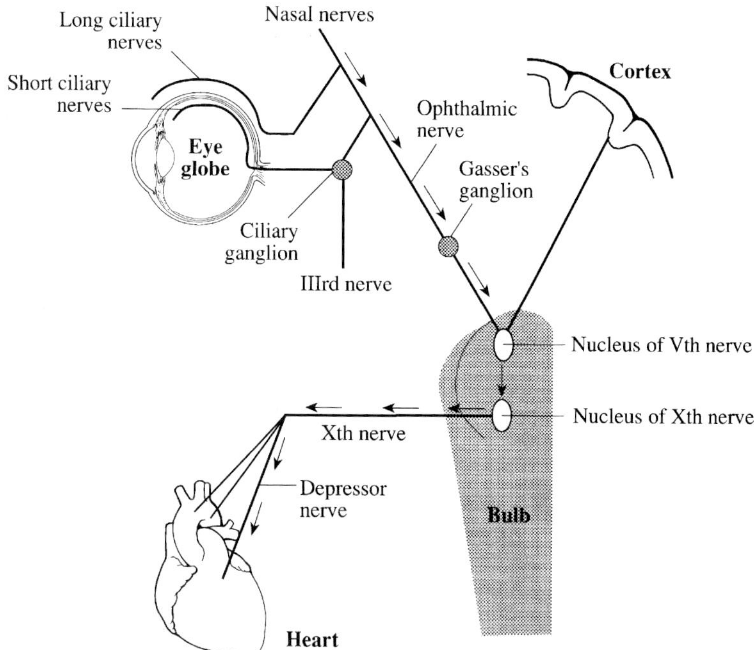

Figure 17-7 The oculocardiac reflex.

tachycardia. There is good evidence that glycopyrrolate also blocks the oculocardiac reflex.

It is well known that a retrobulbar block can block the oculocardiac reflex. It is important to remember that the block itself can elicit the reflex. In one study, a retrobulbar block elicited the reflex in 44 percent of patients. Smith and coworkers[15] reported two cases of sinoatrial arrest in patients who had a retrobulbar block (Fig. 17-8) while undergoing local anesthesia under monitored anesthetic care.

Anesthetic agents also can influence the degree of vagal tone, thus affecting the severity of the reflex. For example, halothane has a strong vagotonic effect and is likely to exaggerate the reflex, whereas the muscle relaxant pancuronium has a vagolytic effect and should offer some protection against the reflex.

OCULAR DRUGS

Anticholinesterases

The anticholinesterases isoflurophate and echothiophate iodide are widely used in the treatment of patients with glaucoma. Prolonged apnea from SCC has been reported in patients taking an anticholinesterase. SCC, a depolarizing muscle relaxant, is hydrolyzed by pseudocholinesterase in the plasma.

Systemic effects may be seen after the use of an anticholinesterase. Because bronchospasm may occur, anticholinesterase agents are contraindicated in asthmatic patients. Abdominal colic and diarrhea are not uncommon and may lead to a mistaken diagnosis. A case of apparent cardiac arrest was reported in a patient taking echothiophate therapy. The arrest was hypothesized to be due to excessive vagal tone.

Ellis and Esterdahl[16] studied blood cholinesterase levels in patients treated with one drop of 0.06% echothiophate iodide daily for 8 to 12 weeks. The blood cholinesterase levels fell in all patients. This decline began within the first 2 weeks after treatment was started, and the maximal drop occurred

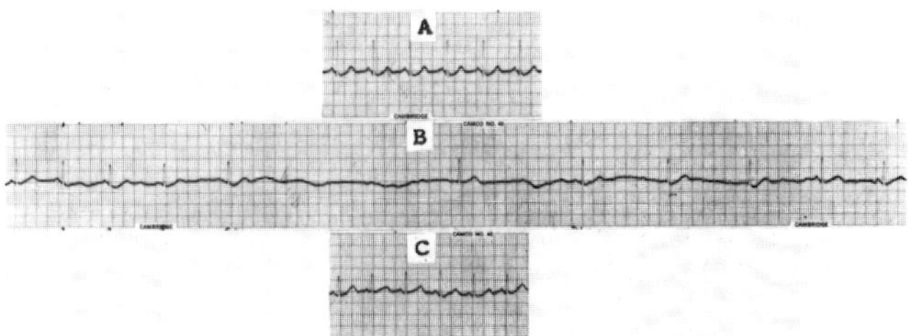

Figure 17-8 **The oculocardiac reflex and sinoatrial arrest. ECG findings. (A) Before retrobulbar block. Normal sinus rhythm. (B) During retrobulbar block: sinoatrial block. (C) After atropine. Sinus tachycardia.** ***(Reprinted from Smith RB, Douglas MN, Petruscak J: The oculocardiac reflex and sinoatrial arrest. Can Anaesth Soc J 18:132, 1972. With permission.)***

within 5 to 7 weeks. After treatment was discontinued, it was several weeks before the cholinesterase values reached their pretreatment levels. The authors recommended the avoidance of SCC in patients who have been treated with echothiophate iodide within 6 weeks immediately preceding surgery.

It should be emphasized that patients taking anticholinesterase therapy should be given an adequate dose of atropine (0.4–1.0 mg) or glycopyrrolate (0.01–0.02 mg/kg) intravenously before starting anesthesia. (These doses of atropine and glycopyrrolate do not raise IOP in patients with glaucoma.) Atropine blocks the undesirable muscarinic effects of acetylcholine, such as salivation and bronchospasm. It also may be effective in reducing the high incidence of dysrhythmias caused by SCC. SCC can also cause severe bradycardia, particularly if it is injected repeatedly. This may be due to a breakdown product, choline, or to the SCC molecule itself, which is similar to acetylcholine.

Acetylcholine

Acetylcholine is used to produce miosis during cataract extraction. The effects of this drug when it is administered systemically are well known; they include bronchospasm and increases in bronchial secretions, salivation, and bradycardia. Until recently, systemic effects from topical use in the eye were not reported. Rongey and Weisman[17] described a patient who developed hypotension and bradycardia after receiving acetylcholine eyedrops subsequent to cataract extraction under local anesthesia. The effects were rapidly reversed with intravenous atropine.

The effects of acetylcholine might be expected to be increased in patients under halothane anesthesia, which has a vagotonic effect. A possible systemic reaction to acetylcholine injected into the anterior chamber of the eye was reported by Babinski and coworkers[18] in a 65-year-old patient who had a cataract extraction while under general anesthesia. After cataract extraction, 20 mg of acetylcholine chloride was injected into the anterior chamber of the eye, and hypotension and bradycardia immediately occurred.

A case of bronchospasm has been reported after acetylcholine injection into the anterior chamber of the eye of a patient taking metoprolol for hypertension.[19] This suggests an interaction between acetylcholine and a beta-adrenergic blocking drug.

Phenylephrine

Ten percent phenylephrine ophthalmic solution is widely used in ophthalmic surgery for both capillary decongestion and dilatation. Although the cardiovascular effects of parenteral phenylephrine are recognized, the systemic effects of the drug when applied topically have received little documentation. Because this drug is often used preoperatively and at the conclusion of ophthalmologic procedures, anesthesiologists may be confronted with these systemic effects.

Reports describing adverse systemic reactions to the topical application of phenylephrine ophthalmic solutions are rare. Lansche[20] reported a patient who developed severe hypotension and an occipital headache after the instillation of one drop of 10% phenylephrine. This patient had previously manifested a similar reaction to ophthalmic epinephrine. McReynolds and coworkers[21] reported a case of extreme hypertension and occipital headache that progressed to subarachnoid hemorrhage after cotton wicks soaked in phenylephrine were applied to the lower conjunctival cul-de-sac. Both patients recovered without sequelae. When McReynolds and coworkers[21] instilled 10% phenylephrine into 100 hypertensive patients, only 6 developed elevations in blood pressure and all elevations were less than 10 mmHg. The same authors also reported finding no significant elevations of blood pressure in 20 patients who received topical phenylephrine after an operation on the arm muscles. However, none of these three studies was controlled, nor were the precise doses of phenylephrine documented.

Even in view of these studies, it seems likely that severe hypertension can occur after the topical application of 10% phenylephrine ophthalmic solutions. Such hypertension is especially dangerous in elderly patients, who are more likely to suffer vascular accidents or pulmonary edema. In addition, marked hypertension postoperatively may promote intraocular hemorrhage in situations where the eye has been opened during the operation. Systemic absorption may be enhanced by a diseased or postsurgical eye. Certain individuals may be more susceptible to the effect of a systemically absorbed drug. Finally, it is possible that the hypertensive effects of phenylephrine may be caused by a combination of phenylephrine with other drugs, such as cyclopentolate. Also, it is not clear whether the main site of absorption is the conjunctival or the nasal mucosa after drainage by the tear ducts.

Ten percent phenylephrine solution probably should not be used because of its potentially hazardous cardiovascular side effects. It seems likely that these side effects could be avoided by using a solution of lower concentrations, as less drug would be available for absorption. A possible objection is that solutions below 10% may not produce sufficient mydriasis to be clinically useful. However, Haddad and colleagues[22] prepared a dose-response curve using solutions ranging from 0.1 to 10% and showed that there was very little increase in mydriatic effect with solutions above 5%. The issue is somewhat clouded, however, in that they used freshly prepared aqueous solutions. The 10% commercial preparation, which they also tested, produced only as much mydriasis as did the 2.25% fresh solution. They suggested differences in pH, addition of preservatives to the commercial solution, and instability of the drug during storage as possible explanations for the disparity. Smith and coworkers[23] studied the mydriatic effect of phenylephrine in patients undergoing elective cataract surgery under local anesthesia. They compared the commercially available 10% solution with a 2.5% solution of phenylephrine and found no significant difference in regard to the mydriatic effects.

Cyclopentolate

Cyclopentolate is used to cause pupillary dilation and is administered topically to the eye. CNS toxicity may develop after ocular instillation of cyclopentolate, with symptoms including dysarthria and disorientation. The symptoms occur within 30 to 45 min and persist for several hours. Binkhorst and associates,[24] in a pilot study on the effect of 2% cyclopentolate in 40 patients, found that 5 patients had psychotic reactions. In a double-blind study, 7 of 10 patients had a psychotic reaction with 2% cyclopentolate and 1 of 13 had a psychotic reaction with 1% solution of this drug. When confusion occurs in an elderly patient, it must be remembered that it can be caused by cyclopentolate. It may theoretically be possible to reverse the effects with physostigmine; however, the authors know of no work to support this possibility. Convulsions have also been reported after the use of cyclopentolate in children, but it appears that this is a dose-related phenomenon.

Topical Beta Blockers

Increased IOP in glaucoma can be treated with beta-adrenergic blocking agents administered topically. Recent evidence indicates that these drugs may have systemic effects because of their high lipid solubility and ease of tissue penetration. Bradycardia was reported in a 73-year-old patient applying 0.25% timolol one drop in each eye twice daily for 3 months.[25] Caution must be exercised in administering beta-adrenergic blocking drugs to patients with bronchospastic disease, as this may be worsened. The newer beta blocker, butaxolol, is considered to have fewer systemic effects than does timolol. However, the use of topical beta blockers is contraindicated in patients with sinus bradycardia, congestive heart failure, heart block, and myocardial failure.

The concomitant use of beta-adrenergic blocking drugs (topically or systemically) and phenylephrine eyedrops is potentially dangerous. In a patient already taking propanolol, this drug may prevent the vasodilation mediated by beta-adrenergic receptors that would have reduced the pressure response to phenylephrine.[26]

Epinephrine

Halogenated hydrocarbon anesthetics may sensitize the heart to epinephrine and lead to serious dysrhythmias. Epinephrine may be administered under certain controlled circumstances during halothane anesthesia, but there is a much lower risk of dysrhythmias with enflurane or isoflurane.

For infiltration of local anesthesia for nerve blocks, the following guidelines for the safe use of epinephrine with halothane have been recommended: Ventilation should be assured, epinephrine should be used in a solution of 1:100,000 to 1:200,000, and the dose in adults should not exceed 10 ml of 1:100,000 solution (100 μg) in any 10-min period (30 ml/h).

Topical application of epinephrine to the eye has been associated with a systemic effect. Ballin and coworkers[27] studied the incidence of dysrhythmias in patients undergoing tonography. The incidence of premature ventricular contractions was found to be high in patients receiving topical epinephrine. Although topical application of epinephrine in concentrations of 0.5 to 2.0% is used in the treatment of open-angle glaucoma, it is probably inadvisable to use it in the eyes of patients anesthetized with halothane.

Enflurane and isoflurane appear to be safer to use with epinephrine because they contain an ether linkage in the molecule that confers greater conduction stability to the heart. The author, however, recommends employing the above guidelines for halothane when these two agents are used with epinephrine.

Serious drug interactions may occur when exogenous epinephrine or another catecholamine is administered. The following drugs make the patient more sensitive: tricyclic antidepressants, cocaine, guanethidine, reserpine, monamine oxidase inhibitors, and levodopa. This list is by no means complete but provides a representative sample.

Smith and associates[28] reported on the administration of epinephrine into the anterior chamber of the eye in patients undergoing cataract surgery by phacoemulsification and aspiration. They concluded that it appears to be safe to administer epinephrine in doses as high as 68 μg/kg into the anterior chamber of the eyes of patients with cataract aspiration by phacoemulsification with halothane anesthesia. They postulated that because the iris is richly supplied with adrenergic receptors, it may be able to capture the epinephrine injected into the eye very rapidly, before it is systemically distributed.

GENERAL VERSUS LOCAL ANESTHETICS

Anesthesiologists and ophthalmologists generally agree that local anesthesia is preferable to general anesthesia when feasible, particularly in the elderly. It was easy to see how this philosophy developed in the early days of general anesthesia, when the agents ether and cyclopropane were primarily used. However, more recent techniques for general anesthesia have provided considerable safety and comfort for the patient and excellent working conditions for the ophthalmologist.

A prospective randomized study of local versus general anesthesia for cataract surgery was reported recently.[29] One hundred sixty-nine patients aged 65 to 98 years were randomized to receive either local or general anesthesia for cataract surgery. Cognitive function was assessed using numerous psychometric tests for up to 3 months postoperatively. Blood pressure, heart rate, and oxygen saturation were monitored and recorded. Sixty-one percent of the patients in the general anesthesia group experienced falls in blood pressure greater than 30 percent of the preinduction value. Blood pressures in the local anesthesia group were relatively stable. Also in the general anesthesia group,

19 percent of the patients experienced at least one episode of oxygen desaturation during the procedure, while none of the patients in the local anesthesia group experienced desaturation. Importantly, no evidence of long-term postoperative cognitive dysfunction was detected in either group. Other significant differences between the two groups were 6 cases of urinary retention and 33 cases of sore throat in the general anesthesia group compared with no retention and 1 sore throat in the local anesthesia group.

The mortality associated with ophthalmologic surgery from 1962 to 1971 at the Eye and Ear Hospital in Pittsburgh was reviewed by Petruscak and associates[30] to evaluate the death rate, causes of death, and results from improvement of management of the patients.

In the first 5-year period, the patients treated with local anesthesia were premedicated by the surgeons. They were not monitored intraoperatively. Patients selected for operation under general anesthesia were managed in the same manner in both 5-year periods. In the second period, patients operated on under local anesthesia were premedicated by the anesthesiologist. Many had intraoperative sedation consisting of diazepam (2.5–5.0 mg) and fentanyl (0.05–0.1 mg), and all were monitored intraoperatively.

In the first 5-year period, the mortality for all ocular surgery was 0.71 per 1000. A total of 14,167 procedures were performed with 10 deaths, 2 of which occurred intraoperatively with the patients under local anesthesia.

In the second 5-year period, there were nine deaths among 17,155 procedures, none of which occurred intraoperatively. The death rates related to general anesthesia and local anesthesia were 0.69 per 1000 and 0.35 per 1000, respectively. All deaths occurred in patients aged 70 to 90 years and occurred from 1 to 18 days postoperatively. The intraoperative death rate fell from 2 per 14,167 or 0.14 per 1000 in the first period to 0 per 17,155 in the second period.

From this study, it was concluded that the most important factor contributing to the death of a patient undergoing ocular surgery is the preexisting medical condition. There appeared to be little difference between the results of general anesthesia and those of local anesthesia. The reduction in intraoperative mortality from the first to the second 5-year period was believed to be secondary to preoperative evaluation by an anesthesiologist and intraoperative monitoring of all patients. The residual death rate associated with cataract surgery was believed to reflect the normal mortality for patients in the age range of 70 to 90 years. The results of five studies investigating deaths and the use of local and general anesthesia in ophthalmic surgery are shown in Table 17-1.[31]

When one is using local anesthesia in an elderly patient, there are considerable advantages to providing monitored anesthesia care. A patient receiving such care has important aspects of his or her physiological status assessed repeatedly. This includes level of consciousness, respirations, electrocardiogram, blood pressure, hemoglobin saturation, and heart rate. In this way, sedative drugs can be administered safely and undesirable drug effects or surgically induced effects can be corrected.

Table 17-1 Deaths by type of anesthesia

Author	General anesthesia			Local anesthesia			Time interval
	No. cases	No. deaths	Deaths/1000	No. cases	No. deaths	Deaths/1000	
Bejat	2,162	2	0.30	14,874	10	0.68	1942–1958
Kristensen	3,327	1	0.92	5,517	34	6.16	1931–1964
Strub	2,510	—	—	10,472	19	1.81	1953–1966
Duncalf et al.	70,744	46	0.65	129,909	79	0.62	1967
Petruscak et al.	8,452	3	0.35	8,703	6	0.69	1967–1971

SOURCE: From Smith RB: Mortality related to ophthalmological surgery. *Arch Ophthalmol* 90:343, 1973.

Table 17-2 Suggested maximum doses of local anesthetics

Local anesthetic	Dose, mg/kg
Mepivacaine (Carbocaine)	7.0*
Lidocaine	2.9
Lidocaine + epinephrine	7.0
Bupivacaine (Marcaine)	2.0

*These are suggested maximum doses and are not necessarily safe doses. Severe reactions may occur at lower doses.

LOCAL ANESTHETICS

The most widely used local anesthetic agents in ophthalmology today are lidocaine, mepivacaine, and bupivacaine. Suggested maximum doses are shown in Table 17-2. The addition of bupivacaine in 1974[32] to the ophthalmologist's armamentarium was especially valuable because of its prolonged anesthetic effect. It is 3 to 4 times as potent as lidocaine and considerably longer in duration of action.

Since 1981, a significant number of occurrences of accidental brainstem anesthesia from retrobulbar block have been reported. It has been postulated that the local anesthetic gains access to the subarachnoid space. This could occur by means of perforation of the meningeal sheath that surrounds the optic nerve. The onset of unconsciousness and apnea occurs over a period of about 7 min.[33] Convulsions may also be seen. This potential though rare complication can easily be fatal if it is not recognized and managed effectively. The possibility of brainstem anesthesia and oculocardiac reflex makes a good case for monitored anesthesia care becoming the accepted standard.

SUMMARY

Providing anesthesia for opthalmic surgery in a geriatric patient can be a challenge. One must be familiar not only with the physiological changes of aging but also with the potential for drug interactions. It stands to reason that the fewer the drugs given, the less the chance for interactions. Monitored anesthesia care provides this advantage.

REFERENCES

1. DeRoetth A Jr, Schwartz H: Aqueous humor dynamics in glaucoma: Effect of ganglionic blocking agents and thiopental sodium (Pentothal) anesthesia on aqueous humor dynamics. *AMA Arch Ophthalmol* 55:755, 1956.

2. Mirakhur RK, Shepherd WFI, Darrau WC: Propofol or thiopentone: Effects on intraocular pressure associated with induction of anaesthesia and tracheal intubation (facilitated with suxamethonium). *Br J Anaesth* 59:431, 1987.
3. Corssen G, Hoy JE: A new parenteral anesthetic—C1-581: Its effect on intraocular pressure. *J Pediatr Ophthalmol* 4:20, 1967.
4. Peuler M, Glass DD, Arens JF: Ketamine and intraocular pressure. *Anesthesiology* 43:575, 1975.
5. Mirakhur RK, Elliot P, Shepherd WFI, McGalliard J: Comparison of the effects of isoflurane and halothane on intraocular pressure. *Acta Anaesthesiol Scand* 34:282, 1990.
6. Pandey K, Badola RP, Kumar S: Time course of intraocular hypertension produced by suxamethonium. *Br J Anaesth* 44:191, 1972.
7. Smith RB, Leano N: Intraocular pressure following pancuronium. *Can Anaesth Soc J* 20:742, 1973.
8. Cook JH, Feneck RO, Smith MB: Effect of pretreatment with propanolol on intraocular pressure changes during induction of anesthesia. *Eur J Anaesth* 3:449, 1986.
9. Smith RB, Carl B, Linn J, Nemoto E: Effect of nitrous oxide on air in vitreous. *Am J Ophthalmol* 78:314, 1974.
10. Niminogadda U, Joseph NJ, Salem MR, et al: Positive end-expiratory pressure and the intraocular pressure. *Anesthesiology* 67:A132, 1987.
11. Aschner B: Uber einen bisher noch nicht beschriebenen reflex von auge auf kreislauf und atmung: Verschwinden des rapialpulses bei druck auf das auge. *Wien Klin Wochenschr* 21:1529, 1908.
12. Dagnini G: Intorno ad un riflesso provocato in alcuni emiplegici collo stimolo della cornea e colla pressione sul bulbo oculare. *Bull Sci Med* 8:380, 1908.
13. Kirsch RE, Samet P, Kugel V, Axelrod S: Electrocardiographic changes during ocular surgery and their prevention by retrobulbar injection. *AMA Arch Ophthalmol* 58:348, 1957.
14. Knoblock R, Lorenz A: Uber ernste komplikationen nach schieloperationen. *Klin Monatsbl Augenheilkd* 141:348, 1962.
15. Smith RB, Douglas HN, Petruscak J: The oculocardiac reflex and sinoatrial arrest. *Can Anaesth Soc J* 18:132, 1972.
16. Ellis PP, Esterdahl M: Echothiophate iodide therapy in children: Effect upon blood cholinesterase levels. *Arch Ophthalmol* 77:598, 1967.
17. Rongey KA, Weisman H: Hypotension following intraocular acetylcholine (correspondence). *Anesthesiology* 36:412, 1972.
18. Babinski M, Smith RB, Wickerham P: Hypotension and bradycardia following intraocular acetylcholine injection. *Arch Ophthalmol* 94:675, 1976.
19. Rasch D, Holt J, Wilson NM, Smith RB: Bronchospasm following intraocular injection of acetylcholine in a patient taking metoprolol. *Anesthesiology* 59:91, 1983.
20. Lansche RK: Systemic reactions to topical epinephrine and phenylephrine. *Am J Ophthalmol* 61:95, 1966.
21. McReynolds WU, Havener WH, Henderson JW: Hazards of the use of sympathomimetic drugs in ophthalmology. *AMA Arch Ophthalmol* 56:176, 1956.
22. Haddad NJ, Moyer NJ, Riley FC: Mydriatic effect of phenylephrine hydrochloride. *Am J Ophthalmol* 70:729, 1970.
23. Smith RB, Read S: Oczypok mydriatic effect of phenylephrine. *Eye Ear Throat Monthly* 55:133, 1976.

24. Binkhorst RD, Weinstein GW, Baretz RM, Clahane AC: Psychotic reaction induced by cyclopentolate (Cyclogyl): Results of a pilot study and a double-blind study. *Am J Ophthalmol* 55:1243, 1963.
25. Sannusch SL, Maye M: Beta receptor blockade following the use of eye drops. *Anesthesiology* 52:369, 1980.
26. Cass E, Kadar D, Stein HA: Hazards of phenylephrine topical medication in pressure taking propronolol. *Can Med Assoc J* 120:1261, 1979.
27. Ballin N, Becker B, Goldman ML: Systemic effects of epinephrine applied topically to the eye. *Invest Ophthalmol* 5:125, 1966.
28. Smith RB, Douglas HN, Petruscak J, et al: Safety of intraocular adrenaline with halothane anaesthesia. *Br J Anaesth* 44:1314, 1972.
29. Campbell DNC, Lim M, Muir MK, et al: A prospective randomized study of local versus general anaesthetics for cataract surgery. *Anaesthesia* 48:422, 1993.
30. Petruscak J, Smith RB, Breslin P: Mortality related to ophthalmological surgery. *Arch Ophthalmol* 89:106, 1973.
31. Smith RB: Mortality related to ophthalmological surgery. *Arch Ophthalmol* 90:343, 1973.
32. Smith RB, Linn JG: Retrobulbar block for anesthesia and akinesia. *Invest Ophthalmol* 13:157, 1974.
33. Chang JK, Gonzales AE, Larson CE: Brainstem anesthesia following retrobulbar block. *Anesthesiology* 61:789, 1984.

CHAPTER 18

Anesthesia for Urologic Surgery in Geriatric Patients

Michael S. Brown
Noel W. Lawson

INTRODUCTION

The greatest incidence of urologic disease occurs in the elderly. The number of people now living into the seventh, eighth, and ninth decades will be reflected in an increased need for urologic surgery. Technological advances in equipment and improved techniques have led to less invasive urologic procedures that are particularly suitable for use in an older patient. Providing anesthesia for an elderly urologic patient requires an understanding of aging, common coexisting disease states, patient profiles, and urologic surgical techniques.

IMPLICATIONS OF AGING RELEVANT TO ANESTHESIA FOR UROLOGIC PROCEDURES

Physiological changes associated with aging are discussed in detail in Chaps. 5 and 11. However, there are three areas in which the physiological changes associated with aging have particular importance for a geriatric patient undergoing urologic surgery: (1) renal function, (2) fluid balance, and (3) temperature regulation.

Renal Function

Renal function associated with aging results from the anatomic and physiological changes that occur in the kidney. Renal mass decreases 20 to 30 percent from the third to the eighth decade of life.[1,2] The number of glomeruli is reduced by 30 to 50 percent by the eighth decade, with up to 30 percent of the remaining glomeruli having glomerular sclerosis.[3–5] Age-related changes also occur in the renal tubules, with a reduction in the size as well as the number of tubules.[1,2,6] Renal blood flow has been shown to decrease rapidly beyond age 40 at an average rate of 10 percent per decade.[7]

Glomerular filtration rate (GFR) also decreases, beginning in the third decade and accelerating after the sixth decade. There is also a decreased ability of the kidney to conserve water by concentrating the urine. Up to 40 percent of clearance is lost by age 90.[8,9] Creatinine clearance remains the most accurate clinical method for calculating GFR in the aged. Plasma creatinine levels represent the production and renal elimination of creatinine. Creatinine production is directly related or proportional to muscle mass: Muscle mass in an aging patient decreases proportionally with creatinine clearance. Therefore, creatinine levels are not useful as a guide to renal function in geriatric patients.[10]

Fluid Balance

The ability of the body to maintain a homeostatic fluid balance is dependent primarily on sodium and water metabolism. Aging has little effect on the normal range of electrolytes and osmolality. However, the ability of the body to maintain a proper fluid balance is impaired with aging.[11] Sodium homeostasis and conservation are impaired in aged patients even with sodium deprivation. Older people also take longer to achieve sodium balance.[12] Therefore, a decreased ability to conserve and/or excrete sodium in the elderly can lead to hypernatremia or hyponatremia.

Hypernatremia increases the risk of congestive heart failure in patients with minimal cardiac reserve because of the attendant increase in total body water. Correction of hypernatremia is more difficult in elderly persons because of their slower homeostatic response to a sodium load. The risk of hypernatremia also may be increased in the elderly secondary to dehydration from diuretics, heat, diarrhea, anorexia, and vomiting as well as a documented decreased perception of thirst.[13,14] Decreased response to thirst occurs even with an increase in the antidiuretic hormone response to osmolar changes.[13] Hypernatremia is usually a result of a lack of free water.

Geriatric hyponatremia can have multiple causes and cannot be regarded simply as evidence of water excess or salt depletion. Hyponatremia is commonly associated with the use of diuretics and low-sodium diets. It is also associated with chronic congestive heart failure, cirrhosis, ascites, and excess release of antidiuretic hormone.[15] The use of hypotonic irrigating solutions in urologic surgery, in conjunction with impaired sodium and water-handling ability and hypotonic intravenous solutions, predisposes elderly patients to dilutional hyponatremia and the transurethral prostatic resection (TURP) syndrome (see "TURP Syndrome") associated with prostate surgery.

The elderly often exhibit decreased autonomic responses, decreased cardiovascular reserve, and a decreased ability to manage fluid shifts. Often, anticipated changes in supine blood pressure and heart rate are impaired and do not become evident until up to 20 percent of the circulating volume has been lost. Because of this factor, many authors feel that invasive monitoring beyond the standard clinical monitors is appropriate. In some centers, this includes central venous pressure and pulmonary artery occlusion pressure in addition to urine output and temperature monitoring. Volume replacement should be limited to sodium-containing solutions. Dextrose solutions should be avoided except to replace insensible loss.[11] Dextrose metabolism in the CNS leaves only free water, which may accentuate the CNS effects of dilutional hyponatremia.

Temperature Regulation

Multiple factors influence thermoregulation in the elderly, including a decreased ability to sense and respond to changes in environmental temperature. Temperature regulation is controlled by an area in the brain that is anatomically located in, but not limited to, the anterior and posterior hypothalamus. The control area interprets incoming data from two groups of sensors. Peripheral sensors are located in the skin and respond to absolute temperature, warm and cold. They are largely located in the hands, face, neck, and chest. Central thermosensors are found in the anterior hypothalamus. The central area compares the incoming data with an internal thermostat called a *set point*. The set point itself is dynamic and can be affected by circadian rhythms, disease, medication, and aging. The response to central sensors is more rapid and potent than is the response to skin sensors. A change in temperature from the set point as little as -0.7 to $+0.5$°C is sufficient to initiate compensatory responses in the young.[18] Some elderly patients maintain normal thermoregulatory control, while others exhibit impairment of the thermoregulatory system. Catecholamine release occurs in conjunction with autonomic activity when the body temperature moves to either side of the set point. Autonomic responses vigorously defend this set point temperature even at the expense of blood volume–blood pressure imbalance.

Insulation of the body core from ambient temperature is provided by vasoactivity in the skin. Excess body heat is lost through vasodilatation and sweating. Vasodilatation occurs with hyperthermia even in the presence of hypovolemia. Similarly, vasoconstriction occurs with hypothermia and hypervolemia. Heat production is increased by lipolysis and utilization of free fatty acids, and thermogenesis is increased by shivering. The mechanism for shivering thermogenesis has also been shown to be impaired in the elderly.[19] The response in the elderly to temperature changes often is further impaired by decreased metabolic rate, decreased receptor response to circulating catecholamines, and decreased muscle mass that limits the productivity of shivering thermogenesis. The response of the afferent temperature system is limited by normal sympathetic decline with aging and peripheral vascular disease.

The changes in thermoregulation that occur with age are important considerations in a patient undergoing urologic surgery. Temperature gain is rarely a problem. However, elderly patients are exposed to multiple factors that can result in hypothermia.[20] Significant heat loss can occur before such patients reach the operating room. This heat loss may be a result of premedication and transport to the operating room. Body temperatures between 35.2 and 35.8°C have been recorded in patients on arrival in the operating room.[21]

Advanced age has also been shown to lead to a greater intraoperative decrease in body temperature.[22] The operating room temperature is an extremely important factor in temperature regulation. Temperatures of 21°C or lower produce significant hypothermia in nearly all patients. Only 30 percent of patients become hypothermic with ambient operating room temperatures between 21 and 24°C. An ambient temperature between 24 and 26°C appears to maintain normothermia.[23]

The greater the length of the operative procedure, the greater the drop in core temperature. Much of this decline may be due to an elderly patient's inability to increase heat production. Additionally, cool operative suites with high airflows increase both convective and evaporative heat losses. Conductive heat losses are increased when the patient lies on a cool operating table. In addition, an elderly urologic patient is exposed to the relatively large volumes of fluids used for bladder irrigation. This is in effect an internal conductive heat loss.

Correlation between ambient operating room temperature and types of anesthesia has also been demonstrated. A greater intraoperative decrease in temperature occurred with general anesthesia compared with epidural anesthesia in a cold operating room. Comparative temperature decreases between general anesthesia and epidural anesthesia were similar when the operating room was warm. Patient age is a determinant of postoperative rewarming, with elderly patients taking longer to rewarm postoperatively.[22]

Hypothermia can have multiple adverse physiological effects, including cardiac dysrhythmias, coagulation disturbances, altered levels of consciousness, decreased drug metabolism, impaired renal function, and a leftward shift in the hemoglobin oxygen saturation curve.[24] Oxygen delivery may be adequate, but the unloading of oxygen from hemoglobin may be impaired. Postoperative shivering can increase total body oxygen consumption by as much as 300 to 800 percent during a time of impaired delivery and utilization.[25–27] The need to increase oxygen delivery in the presence of peripheral vasoconstriction (afterload increase) may result in an increase in morbidity in patients with cardiopulmonary disease. There is an increase in myocardial work. The increased catecholamine output also increases the heart rate and predisposes the patient to cardiac dysrhythmias. Vasoconstriction can cause increasing tissue hypoxia and acidosis. Subsequent venous stagnation can increase the risk of developing deep venous thrombosis.

An aging pulmonary system with secondary disease may be unable to meet increased oxygen demands from shivering. Closing volumes increase in the elderly, producing greater ventilation-perfusion mismatches, an increased oxygen diffusion gradient, and the potential for increased postoperative atelectasis. The patient may be unable to respond by increasing hemoglobin saturation.

Additionally, the hemoglobin concentration may be reduced secondary to the dilutional effects and surgical loss in a urologic patient.

PROFILE OF PATIENTS PRESENTING FOR UROLOGIC PROCEDURES

Historically, patients were often refused surgery on the basis of age alone. When surgery was performed, the patient was admitted to the hospital, often days before surgery, so that extensive preoperative evaluations could be performed. Current trends are for increased outpatient procedures and increased admissions on the day of surgery. Age alone no longer excludes a patient from undergoing elective or emergency surgery.[28] A geriatric patient is often seen by the anesthesiologist on the day of surgery regardless of the patient's physical status or coexisting disease state. This procedural change was not a medical mandate but a matter of economics mandated by third-party payers. However, it imposed an additional medical-legal burden on the anesthesiologist to ensure patient safety. Ideally, these patients should be evaluated by the anesthesiologist as outpatients before surgery in a preanesthesia or presurgical clinic. This concept is gaining momentum, as national experience will document. Early evaluation will ensure thorough screening, including x-ray and laboratory testing when needed, and ensure that the patient's coexisting diseases are medically optimized. Surgical delays and cancellations are minimized. For a urologic patient, the preoperative diagnosis and planned procedure in conjunction with a drug history and an evaluation of the patient's cardiovascular, pulmonary, and renal systems will allow the anesthesiologist and surgeon to determine the course of anesthesia and surgery best suited for the individual patient.

COMMON DISEASE STATES REQUIRING UROLOGIC INTERVENTION

Prostatism

Prostatism is a term used to describe the symptoms of bladder outflow obstruction. Symptoms include urgency, frequency, hesitancy, decreased urine flow, and micturition dribbling. Urodynamic studies that include the urine flow rate are conducted in the urology laboratory preoperatively. Additional information regarding the prostate gland is found by means of rectal examination, transrectal ultrasound, and prostate biopsy. If the prostate biopsy reveals carcinoma, a metastatic workup is conducted.

Hematuria

Hematuria is divided into painful and painless hematuria. Painless hematuria usually results from a bladder tumor. Painful hematuria is associated with the symptoms of urgency, frequency, and burning, which usually signal the presence of bacterial cystitis.

Painless Hematuria

Bladder carcinoma affects both sexes, with a fourfold greater prevalence in males. Patients presenting with painless hematuria should undergo an intravenous pyelogram (IVP), which may not only reveal a renal cell carcinoma but also delineate the irregular filling defects present in the bladder that are characteristic of bladder tumors. Urine cytology may also reveal malignant cells. Cystopanendoscopy is another tool used to diagnose bladder tumors. Once a diagnosis is made, treatment modalities are determined on the basis of the degree of bladder invasion by the tumor. Approximately 75 percent of bladder tumors can be resected by transurethral endoscopic resection with diathermy. The decision for more radical surgery should be based on the patient's ability to withstand major surgery, not by the patient's chronological age.

Painful Hematuria

Hematuria resulting from bacterial cystitis is best treated with appropriate antibiotic therapy. However, patients with bladder tumors often present with the signs and symptoms of cystitis. Therefore, patients with bacterial infections often require an IVP and cystoscopy.

Incontinence

Elderly male patients frequently present with symptoms of nocturnal incontinence. These symptoms are secondary to chronic urinary retention and result in urine overflow. Incontinence associated with urgency also may result from infection, bladder tumors, prostatic tumors that affect the base of the bladder, and bladder calculi or may represent the sequelae of a cerebral vascular accident.

An elderly female patient can present with a similar spectrum of symptoms and etiologies, except for those of prostatic origin. Additionally, estrogen deficiencies can cause symptoms of urinary tract irritation in the absence of infection. Stress urinary incontinence is often associated with weakness of the pelvic floor. Urodynamic assessment is often necessary to further delineate the source of incontinence in women patients. When atrophic changes are determined to be the source of incontinence, they frequently respond well to systemic or local hormonal therapy. Detrussor muscle instability responds well to anticholinergic medications. Numerous procedures are available for surgical correction of incontinence secondary to pelvic floor weakness.

COMMON COEXISTING DISEASE STATES

Cardiovascular

Patients frequently present with a history of cardiovascular disease. This includes problems with coronary artery disease, dysrhythmias, peripheral vascular disease, and, most commonly, hypertension. The degree of control of hypertension should be estimated. Patients with diastolic blood pressures up to 110 mmHg, in the absence of compensatory symptoms or the physical sequelae of hypertension, have been shown to have the same surgical risk as patients of the same age without hypertension. However, patients with a diastolic pressure of 110 mmHg or greater with sequelae should have surgery delayed for better control. Patients with diastolic pressures of 120 mmHg, even without physical findings, should have surgery delayed until the pressure is controlled and stable. The benefits of long-term control of hypertension are without question, but these conditions may not be achievable within the time constraints of an obstructive or invasive urinary tract pathological condition. An estimation of the stability of cardiovascular symptoms such as angina, dyspnea, and the symptoms associated with congestive heart failure should be delineated. The highest morbidity and mortality related to surgery and anesthesia occur in patients in whom this combination exists. Plans will also have to be made to accommodate a patient with a pacemaker, in whom electrical current may interfere with pacemaker function.

Pulmonary (Chap. 2)

Patients presenting for urologic surgery often have accompanying pulmonary disease states such as chronic obstructive pulmonary disease (COPD). An evaluation of the patient's pulmonary status, including blood gases and pulmonary function tests, may be necessary.

Renal (Chap. 5)

Many elderly patients suffer from some form of acute or chronic renal insufficiency. Often patients with urinary tract obstruction show signs of acute renal insufficiency.

PREANESTHESIA EVALUATION

The history and physical should be conducted with special attention directed toward the organ systems already mentioned, because this will determine if further evaluation is necessary. Routine evaluation, although patient-specific, may include a complete blood count, electrocardiogram, and chest x-ray. Most other pertinent laboratory data related to the surgical procedure, such as urinalysis, renal function, and electrolyes, will be ordered by the surgeon. All laboratory data should be examined before anesthesia. This is one of the benefits of a preoperative clinic in that medical consultation can be obtained to determine if further workup is necessary. Cancellations or delays in a busy operating room schedule are avoided, and the patient benefits.

OUTPATIENT SURGICAL/DIAGNOSTIC PROCEDURES

Common Procedures

Cystoscopy with panendoscopic examination of the urethra and bladder is the most common outpatient urologic procedure performed. It forms the basis through which most urologic endoscopic procedures are performed (e.g., TURP). Cystpanendoscopy (CPE) is commonly used to diagnose prostatic hypertrophy. It is also used to diagnose, remove, or follow up bladder tumors; to treat urethral strictures; and for placement of retrograde urethral catheters for uroradiological diagnostic studies.[29] These procedures are performed with anesthesia ranging from urethral topical anesthesia with lidocaine jelly to light general anesthesia. Between these two extremes, the procedure is performed with or without urethral topical anesthesia and includes monitored anesthesia care, low spinal block, and epidural anesthesia.

Potential Procedures

Technological advances in urology in the last 15 years have seen urologic surgery become less invasive and more applicable to the outpatient routine. Flexible cystoscopy has been shown to be effective in fulgurating small recurrent bladder tumors (less than 1 cm), using local urethral anesthesia.[30] Endoscopic urethrotomy for urethral strictures also has been shown to be effectively performed with local urethral anesthesia in the outpatient setting.[31] Others have used various local anesthetic blocks, with sedation, to perform procedures ranging from circumcision to penile prosthesis placement on an outpatient basis.[32] Orandi,[33] using highly selected patients, employed a resectoscope equipped with an injection needle to perform bladder tumor resection, extensive bladder biopsy, meatotomy, incision and fulguration of bladder diverticuli, bladder neck contracture incision, and TURP.[33]

TURP is a major part of a urologist's work (see "Inpatient Procedures" for details). TURP, with its accompanying morbidity, mortality, and complications, is beginning to be used in the outpatient setting, and thus it is appropriate for anesthesia for TURP to be discussed as an outpatient procedure.

Improved technology, cost control, and the risk inherent in exposing an elderly patient to surgery and anesthesia initiated the performance of transurethral procedures in the outpatient setting. Several surgeons have reported success in this area.[34–38] Patient selection for each study was critical, with the criteria for rejection including age greater than 75, prostate glands thought to be greater than 50 g, and those who are thought to be unable to tolerate sedation for any reason. Anesthesia ranged from general anesthesia, to subarachnoid block, to local anesthetic block with sedation. *Sedoanalgesia* is a term that was coined to describe the combination of local anesthetic block and sedation. Procedures performed with a local block and sedation were also followed with monitored anesthesia care, including all standard ASA monitors (electrocardiogram, blood pressure monitoring, and pulse oximetry). Most studies exhibited a learning curve such that as the study progressed, patient selection was widened and anesthetic techniques were changed to reflect more use of the local anesthetic block with sedation. TURP using local anesthesia alone has also been successfully demonstrated.[34,35,39]

Sedoanalgesia

Birch and colleagues published two studies in which TURP was performed using sedoanalgesia.[40,41] Alternatives to TURP were also discussed, including balloon dilatation, closed commissurotomy, microwave hypothermia, endoprostatic stents, alpha-adrenergic blockade, penile injection, cytotoxic agents, cryotherapy, and endocrine manipulation. Each technique holds an advantage in avoiding the risk of anesthesia in a high-risk patient. However, each also was more costly in the long term than was conventional TURP. Therefore, Birch explored the use of sedoanalgesia for conventional TURP in high-risk patients (initial patients ASA classes III and IV).[40] All patients, irrespective of ASA classification, initially had prostate glands less than 40 g in weight. Each patient was given diazepam intramuscularly 30 min before surgery. After 15 min, 2% lidocaine gel was applied topically to the urethra and was retained using penile clamps. Additional midazolam and topical lidocaine gel were administered as needed in the operating room. The patient was placed in the lithotomy position, and a cystoscope equipped with an endoneedle was used for additional local anesthetic infiltration. Lidocaine (1%) was injected beneath the trigone of the bladder as well as just lateral and medial to the ureteric orifices. Additionally, a 1% lidocaine solution with 1:200,000 epinephrine was injected into the bladder neck and prostate. Prostatic injections were always done outward toward the capsule. Birch's following study used the technique of sedoanalgesia to include multiple endoscopic and open procedures.[41] This study included patients ranging in age from 16 to 98 years with more than one-third being over 70 years of age, and 16 percent were classified as ASA class III or IV. Each of the patients in this classification had been denied general anesthesia in a day surgery setting. Eighty percent of the patients were treated on a day surgery basis.

Midazolam was chosen for sedation because of its superior quality compared with diazepam and its shorter half-life. Flumazenil was used whenever needed to reverse oversedation. This study pointed out that midazolam has no analgesic properties and that adequate local anesthesia must be achieved for the procedure to be successful.

Birch and associates concluded that in their practice, "There is no doubt that sedoanalgesia had radically changed the practice of urology. Safety, efficiency and cost effectiveness, coupled with patient preference combine to make sedoanalgesia a preferable alternative to general anesthesia for many urologic procedures, both endoscopic and open."[40]

All patients underwent some form of monitoring by the surgical or anesthesia staff. Only elderly and/or ASA class III or IV patients received supplemental oxygen. Continuous electrocardiogram and automatic blood pressure monitoring were also available but were inconsistently applied. For this technique to gain widespread acceptance, it would seem imperative that all patients, irrespective of age or ASA classification, be fully monitored using an electrocardiogram, noninvasive blood pressure machine, and pulse oximeter and be given supplemental oxygen according to current standards of anesthesia practice and JCAH guidelines. Sedoanalgesia cannot supplant the need for trained personnel in the operating room.

The importance of supplemental oxygen was demonstrated when a study to determine the effects of sedation with midazolam on oxygen saturation, using pulse oximetry as a measure, was undertaken in patients undergoing surgery with regional conduction block.[42] The original study was designed to include 100 patients with ages ranging from 20 to 85 years who fit ASA classes I through III. Patients were to be randomly allocated into one of two groups: Group 1 received oxygen at 2 liters/min via a nasal cannula, and group 2 received no additional oxygen unless the saturation decreased to less than 90 percent. All patients underwent surgery with regional conduction blockade in combination with sedation, using incremental doses of midazolam 1 to 2.5 mg intravenously as needed. The study was abandoned after only 10 patients. Six of these patients had been given supplemental oxygen with no untoward events. Three of the four patients randomized into the group that would receive no supplemental oxygen desaturated to levels below 90 percent. These three patients' ages ranged from 59 to 70 years, and all were classified as ASA class I. Surgical procedures using local anesthetic block and sedation can be carried out safely and effectively if adequate monitoring of the patient's vital signs and supplemental oxygenation are provided. The axiom remains, "There are no minor anesthetics."

The trend toward an increase in the numbers and types of surgeries performed in the outpatient setting will require close observation of the types of problems encountered postoperatively that require hospitalization. In Biswas and Leery's review of 18,321 procedures performed by different specialties in a hospital-based day surgery unit, 225 patients (1.2 percent) required hospital admission.[43] The highest admission rate was found in gynecologic surgery, with the majority of these admissions occurring after laparoscopic procedures. Urologic surgery resulted in 35 admissions and was felt to represent the patient's age group and preexisting medical condition, with 13 of the admissions being for social reasons related to age. Most of the admissions by all specialties were related to multiple procedures or surgery more extensive than had originally been planned.

INPATIENT PROCEDURES

Transurethral Resection of the Prostate

TURP is the second most commonly performed operation in adult men.[44–46] It is the most commonly performed operation in urology, with 250,000 TURPs performed annually in the United States. Disease conditions resulting in prostatectomy include benign prostatic hyperplasia (BPH), bladder neck contracture, and carcinoma. BPH represents 70 percent of the total, with the remaining percentage equally shared between the other two conditions.[44,47]

Few operations subject the patient to a larger number of physiological insults than TURP.[48] Mortality is above the average associated with anesthesia, ranging from 0.4 to 5.6 percent.[44,48–50] Major morbidity occurs in between 2.5 and 20 percent of patients undergoing TURP.[49,50] The high rate of morbidity and mortality is due largely to the advanced age of these patients, their associated medical problems, and the number of profound and acute physiological changes presented to the patient. Specific factors associated with increased morbidity and mortality during TURP are age above 80, resection time greater than 150 min, weight of tissue resected greater than 80 g, experience of surgeon, blood loss, presence of azotemia, preexisting diseases, and hypothermia.[11,42]

Anatomy and Surgical Technique

The prostate is a pear-shaped gland that completely surrounds the urethra. It is the largest accessory gland in the male reproductive system. There are five anatomic lobes (one anterior, two lateral, one median, and one posterior), but only the single median lobe and the two lateral lobes become enlarged and are surgically excised during TURP. The prostate gland is enclosed by a dense fascial sheath of tissue (Fig. 18-1). An extensive venous plexus lies between the capsule of the prostate and this fascial sheath.

The prostate gland begins to enlarge in all men after age 40. After age 50, testicular hormones cause submucosal glands and smooth muscle of the prostatic urethra to undergo hyperplasia and leiomyomatous changes. The enlarging adenomatous tissue forces normal prostatic tissue to compress the fibrous capsule. This forms the so-called surgical capsule, which consists of the compressed normal gland and veins, which are often infiltrated by adenomatous growth. Transurethral prostatectomy entails resection of the prostatic tissue surrounding the neck of the bladder as far as the capsule of the gland. A modified cystoscope, or resectoscope, is inserted via the urethra. A cauterizing wire loop is used under direct vision to remove tissue and coagulate bleeding vessels. The procedure is best performed under a continuous irrigation of the

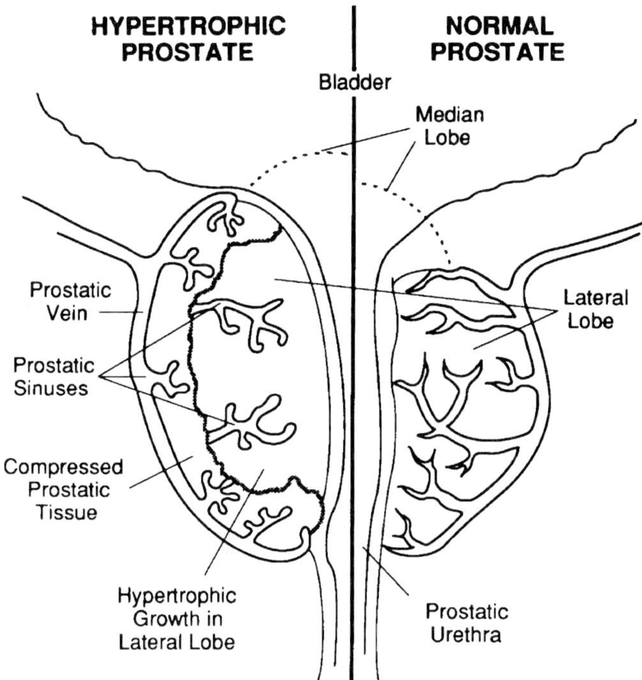

Figure 18-1 Anatomy of prostate, comparing normal lobe to hypertrophic lobe. Hypertrophic growth consisting of glandular and leiomyomatous hyperplasia of submucosal glands and smooth muscle of the prostatic urethra. A surgical capsule composed of normal prostate gland is created when the prostate is compressed by hypertrophic growth.

bladder and prostatic urethra to ensure visibility, distend the operative field, and remove dissected tissue and blood.[51]

Complications

Complications associated with TURP include pulmonary edema, water intoxication, hyponatremia, glycine and ammonia toxicity, hypovolemia, visual disturbances, hemolysis, coagulopathies, sepsis and toxemia, bladder perforation, and air embolism.[52] The most common causes of death found in one series were myocardial infarction, pulmonary edema, and renal insufficiency.[44] This is not surprising, since myocardial infarction, congestive heart failure, renal failure, and diabetes, particularly in combination, bear close association to geriatric surgical morbidity and mortality for other procedures as well.

TURP SYNDROME *TURP syndrome* is a generalized term used to describe the complications associated with TURP. The development of TURP syndrome occurs early during surgery and up to several hours postoperatively. The primary etiology is excessive absorption of irrigation solution. Specific complications, their signs and symptoms, and factors that enhance fluid absorption are discussed in later sections. The comparison of preoperative sodium levels with postoperative sodium levels allows the determination of the volume of irrigation fluid absorbed, as described by the following formula:

$$\text{Volume absorbed} = \left(\frac{\text{preoperative Serum } [Na^+]}{\text{postoperative Serum } [Na^+]} \times \text{ECF}\right) - \text{ECF}$$

Extracellular fluid (ECF) is estimated as 20 to 30 percent of the body weight in kilograms.

The treatment of TURP syndrome includes the termination of surgery, an assessment of arterial blood gas and sodium levels, fluid restriction, diuretics, and hypertonic saline as directed by the specific case.

The best treatment of TURP syndrome is avoidance of its occurrence. Surgical maneuvers include preservation of the prostatic capsule, avoidance of overdistension of the bladder, controlling the height of the irrigation solution to decrease hydrostatic pressure, and controlling resection time whenever possible. An elderly patient's physiological status should be optimized, with close attention paid to fluid and electrolyte balance. Patients susceptible to circulatory overloading secondary to poor cardiac reserve may best be managed by conservative surgery, including "channel TURP" or a staged resection. Intravenous fluid administration should be restricted. Hypotension secondary to the administration of regional anesthesia may best be treated with vasoconstrictors rather than fluid boluses. Some physicians recommend prophylactic administration of furosemide because it has been shown to maintain serum colloid-osmotic pressure gradients. A low colloid-osmotic pressure has been associated with pulmonary edema.

BLOOD LOSS Blood loss ranges from 2.6 to 4.6 ml/min of resection time and/or from 7 to 20 ml/g of tissue resected.[52–54] The blood loss ranges from 200 to 2,000 ml and averages 500 ml, with one unit or less lost in 80 percent of patients undergoing TURP.[53,55,56] The amount of blood loss during TURP is related to resection time and weight of tissue resected. An accompanying infection, associated with an indwelling catheter, can increase blood loss secondary to the presence of hyperemia and tissue congestion.[52,53] Quantification of blood loss is difficult because of dilution with irrigating fluids and the masking of signs such as hypotension and tachycardia by the increased circulatory volume secondary to the absorption of irrigation fluids through the venous sinuses.

The physiological effects of blood loss and decreased oxygen-carrying capacity may be poorly tolerated by a geriatric patient. The accompanying increased circulatory volume by itself may be insufficient to compensate for blood loss. Multiple attempts to study the effects of the type of anesthesia on blood loss have been conflicting and inconclusive (see "Anesthesia for TURP"). Other factors that may influence blood loss include increased peripheral venous pressure, shivering, coughing, straining, vascular overload, and the experience of the surgeon.[57]

Various methods have been used to quantify blood loss during TURP, including radioactive labeling of red blood cells and albumin and alterations in the electrical conductivity of an irrigant when blood or electrolytes are present. Colorimetric techniques, based on a calculation of the patient's preoperative total hemoglobin content and the subsequent measurement of hemoglobin content in hemolyzed irrigation solution, allow an estimation of blood loss during the procedure.[52,58,59] None of these techniques appears to have gained widespread use.

COAGULOPATHIES Persistent perioperative bleeding may represent a coagulation defect. Some physicians have historically believed that this results from the release of urokinase (a plasminogen activator) from prostatic tissue, ultimately resulting in fibrinolysis and causing the dissolution of freshly formed clots in the surgical field.[61] Plasminogen-activating factor inhibitors such as ϵ-aminocaproic acid (Amicar or EACA) had been used to decrease blood loss during TURP. However, the failure of EACA to control bleeding with TURP and evidence of decreased plasminogen activators after TURP have challenged this theory.[62] Current opinion now supports diffuse intravascular coagulopathy (DIC) as the cause of TURP coagulopathy.[63] This hypothesis suggests that resected prostate tissue releases thromboplastins that can trigger DIC. This observation is supported by decreased platelets and fibrinogen levels with associated increases in fibrin degradation products in patients who develop TURP coagulopathy. The treatment is the same as for any DIC, including restoration of clotting factors.

HEAT LOSS Irrigation fluid at room temperature has been shown to cause significant hypothermia in TURP patients. Warmed irrigating solution was found to prevent the hypothermia.[64] No association between warmed irrigating solutions and increased blood loss has been shown.[65]

PERFORATION OF BLADDER AND PROSTATE CAPSULE Perforation of the prostatic capsule or bladder is a surgical complication of TURP or transurethral resection of bladder tumor (TURBT). Perforation can be urethral, intraperitoneal, extraperitoneal, or capsular with periprostatic extravasation. The causes of perforation can be surgical instrumentation, overdistension of the bladder, and rarely ignition of trace hydrogen gas in the bladder.[66]

Characteristic signs and symptoms of bladder perforation depend on the site of perforation (Table 18-1). Intraperitoneal perforation produces a characteristic shoulder tip pain followed shortly by nausea and abdominal distension in

Table 18-1 Signs and symptoms of bladder perforation

Intraperitoneal	Shoulder tip pain followed rapidly by nausea and abdominal distension
Extraperitoneal	Nausea followed by abdominal distension; slow to develop; no shoulder tip pain
Extravasation into periprostatic tissue	Low suprapubic discomfort; suprapubic space can be visibly distended and firm; blood pressure increases; bradycardia; nausea and vomiting

rapid sequence. Extraperitoneal perforation produces similar signs, but without shoulder pain. It is often of slower onset. Extravasation into periprostatic tissue produces suprapubic discomfort, and the suprapubic space may be visibly distended and firm. An experienced surgeon will become aware of an irregular irrigating pattern and/or a loss of irrigant fluid. Patients may complain of abdominal pain, which may be generalized or localized, as was previously mentioned. Conscious patients may complain of periumbilical, suprapubic, or inguinal pain. Patients under spinal anesthesia with levels greater than T_{10} may be unable to report these symptoms. However, other suspicious clinical signs include pallor, diaphoresis, abdominal rigidity, nausea and vomiting, hypertension or hypotension, shortness of breath, and bradycardia.[67] Hiccups may also accompany subdiaphragmatic irritation. A shocklike state can develop. In patients who are under general anesthesia, making the diagnosis of perforation is difficult.

The treatment of perforations depends on the site and extent. Localized extraperitoneal, periprostatic, and urethral tears can be treated with an indwelling catheter and appropriate antibiotics. Major perivesical extravasations and intraperitoneal involvement may necessitate surgical exploration. Perforation repair and drainage of the perivesical space may be needed. Often, both suprapubic and urethral catheters are kept in place.

Radioisotope studies have shown that only about 30 percent of absorbed glycine directly enters the circulation, with the remainder entering the extravascular spaces for later absorption. Intraperitoneal fluid is eventually excreted by the kidneys without difficulty.[68]

ADDUCTOR SPASM Adductor contraction secondary to obturator nerve stimulation occasionally occurs during TURP. The incidence is increased to about one in five patients with large intraurethral adenomas and tumors of the lateral vesicle walls.[69] Adductor contraction may cause bladder perforation and dissemination of tumor cells and delay or postpone the surgical procedure. Stimulation occurs distal to the regional block and requires either generalized muscle relaxation (impractical in an awake patient) or local obturator nerve block. Local obturator nerve block has been effective in preventing adductor spasm, but a blind approach to obturator nerve block is difficult and has a low success rate. Others have advocated the use of a nerve stimulator to locate the obturator nerve accurately (Figs. 18-2 and 18-3). This method has proved to be safe and highly accurate. No complications were reported from performing the block with the use of a nerve stimulator.[70] Plasma levels of local anesthetics remain at nontoxic levels with the use of spinal anesthesia and obturator nerve block. Fujita and coworkers concluded that the two procedures can be performed simultaneously without exposing the patient to dangerous levels of local anesthetic.[71]

BACTEREMIA, SEPTICEMIA, TOXICITY During TURP, bacteria can enter the circulation from the prostate by way of the prostatic venous sinus. The prostate gland often contains bacteria, especially in the presence of urinary obstruction. Approximately 30 percent of all patients undergoing TURP have infected urine at the time of surgery.[72] Increased hydrostatic pressure of the irrigation

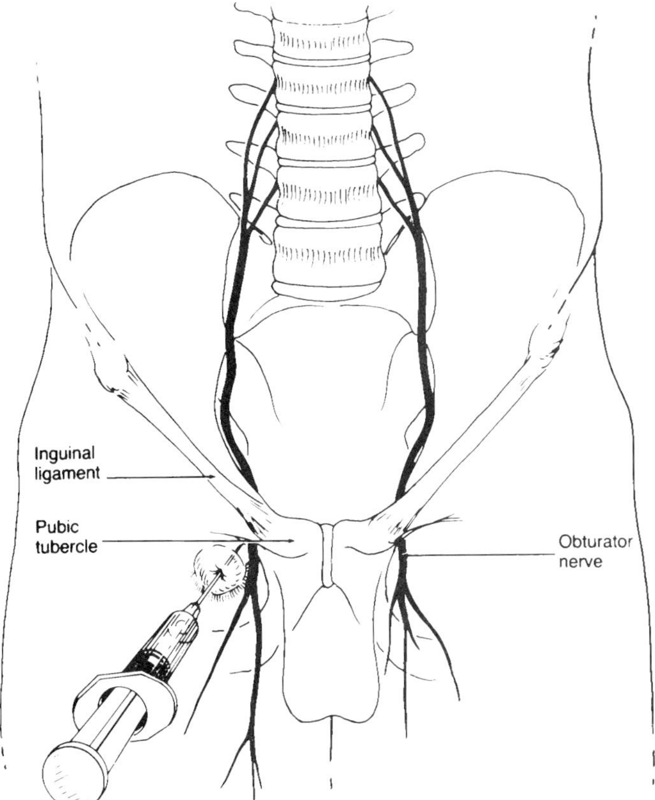

Figure 18-2 Block needle inserted 1 to 2 cm lateral and inferior to pubic tubercle.

solution in conjunction with surgical entry of venous plexuses facilitates bacteremia, which is usually transient and asymptomatic. When symptomatic, bacteremia includes rigor, fever, and hypotension. Approximately 6 percent of patients with bacteremia are complicated by septicemia,[51] which is a common cause of postoperative morbidity and mortality after TURP. Clinically significant septicemia usually develops in the recovery room. Common signs include fever, chills, hypotension, and tachycardia and/or bradycardia. Bradycardia and new-onset dysrhythmias are also characteristic of gram-negative septicemia. Mortality rates range from 25 to 75 percent, increasing with patient age. Blood cultures should be drawn when a diagnosis of sepsis is made or suspected. Broad-spectrum antibiotic therapy should be initiated. Additional supportive therapy as indicated by the vital signs is warranted. Organisms commonly associated with bacterial sepsis during TURP include *Escherichia coli*, *Pseudomonas*, *Proteus*, *Aerobacter*, *Klebsiella*, and *Staphylococcus*.[52]

A short-term toxic state occasionally develops postoperatively, characterized by hypotension, severe chills, fever, and capillary dilatation. It differs from the more serious form because patients are usually symptomatic only for

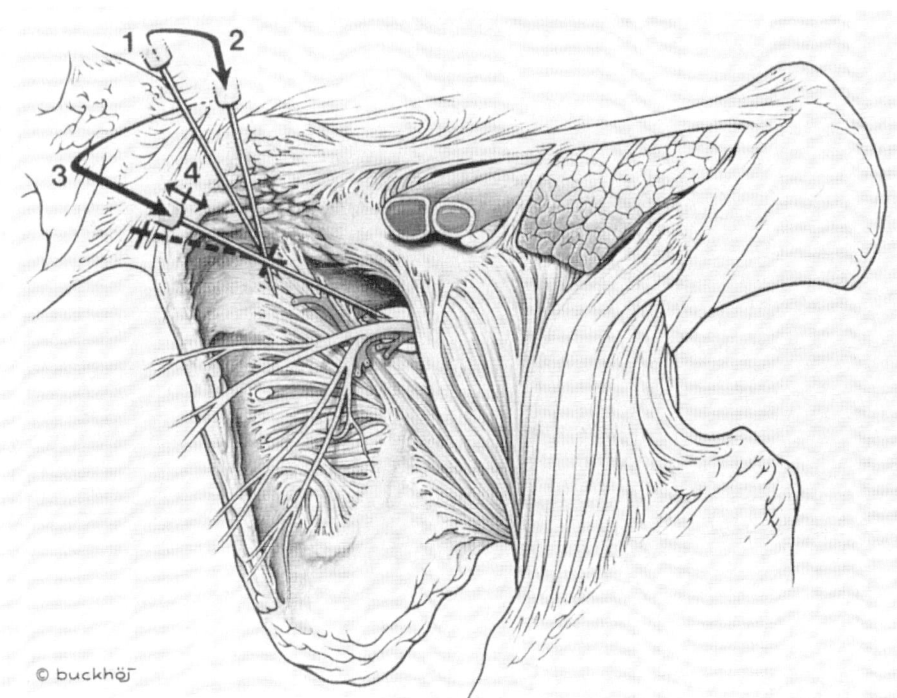

Figure 18-3 **After insertion, the needle is directed upward, backward, and laterally (1 and 2) to contact the pubic tubercle. It is then directed inferior (3 and 4) to the pubic ramus into the obturator foramen. Use of a nerve stimulator needle will elicit adductor muscle twitch.** *(Reprinted with permission from Butterworth JF IV: Lower extremity nerve blocks, in Atlas of Procedures in Anesthesia and Critical Care. Philadelphia: Saunders, 1992, p 171.)*

a few hours and complete recovery is observed. The etiology is thought to be absorption of a bacterial endotoxin or toxic by-products of cauterized prostatic tissue.[51]

ERECTION Penile erection is an infrequent occurrence during transurethral instrumentation. It makes the procedure difficult for the surgeon and can be distressing to the patient. Treatment of penile erection by the anesthesiologist is often difficult. The physiology of erection is complex but is thought to be a predominantly parasympathetic response. Spinal anesthesia does not prevent erection. The use of ketamine has been suggested but has shown a greater efficacy in children than in adults. The use of beta blockers such as propanolol has been suggested and shown to be effective.

ABSORPTION OF IRRIGATION SOLUTION Irrigation solutions allow adequate visualization of the operative field and facilitate the washing away of blood and resected prostate parts. An ideal irrigating solution would be isotonic, electrically inert, nontoxic, transparent, rapidly excreted, inexpensive, and easily sterilized. Water, which has many of these properties, causes hemolysis upon absorption. This has led to renal insufficiency. Lactated Ringer's and normal saline would solve problems of isotonicity but are not electrically neutral. Several solutions have been used and are available for endoscopic irrigation (Table 18-2). Cytol and glycine are the most frequently used. Glycine concentrations of 1.2% and 1.5% are the most frequently used worldwide because they are inexpensive. Glycine is not isotonic, as a 2.1% solution would be required to reach isotonicity. However, its other properties fulfill the criteria for an irrigant. Cytol, a mixture of sorbitol 2.7% and mannitol 0.54%, is isosmotic but more expensive.

It has been reported that irrigation fluid is absorbed at a rate of 10 to 30 ml/min of resection.[73] Others have shown that volumes as great as 6 to 8 liters can be absorbed during resection times of 75 to 120 min.[74] The choice of irrigating fluid has little effect on the rate of absorption.[75] Beal and colleagues concur that reducing the amount of fluid absorbed is best managed by decreasing the pressure of the irrigating fluid and limiting the operative time to 60 min.[76]

Glycine is a nonessential fatty acid that also functions as an inhibitory neurotransmitter. Normal serum levels range between 13 and 17 μg/liter. Glycine is metabolized by several different pathways to ammonia, glyoxalic acid, and oxalic acid. Large amounts have toxic effects on the heart and retina in dogs.[51] The addition of arginine blunts or blocks the toxic effects of glycine.[77] Glycine has the greatest incidence of neurological sequlae; this may be the result of direct neurotoxic effects.[76]

The signs and symptoms of glycine toxicity include vomiting, bradypnea, apnea, cyanosis, seizures, hypotension, oliguria, and anuria. Death may occur. Visual disturbances and transient blindness can be associated with TURP. This may occur during the surgery or in the postanesthesia care unit, with patients complaining of blurred or "foggy" vision and objects surrounded by a "halo." These visual disturbances are usually isolated but can occur with other signs of TURP syndrome. Intraocular pressure and optic disks are normal, but the pupils are dilated and unresponsive. Most symptoms usually resolve within 48 h.[78] Evidence suggests a retinal etiology rather than cortical blindness, which would be associated with cerebral cortex edema. Glycine, a neuroinhibitor with known toxic retinal effects, is thought to be the cause of this transient blindness.[78] An inverse relation between glycine and visual acuity has been demonstrated.[78]

Table 18-2 **The osmolality of various irrigation solutions used for transurethral prostatectomy**

Solution	Concentration, %	Osmolality, mOsmol
Glycine	1.2	175
Glycine	1.5	220
Cytol		178
Glucose	2.5	139
Urea	1.0	167
Water		0

Ammonia is a by-product of glycine metabolism. Hyperammonemia is a rare but potential complication of glycine absorption.[51] Normal blood levels of ammonia are 11 to 35 μmol per liter, with symptoms of ammonia toxicity developing at 150 μmol per liter. The signs of ammonia toxicity usually develop within 1 h after surgery, characterized by nausea and vomiting followed by coma. The coma can last up to 10 to 12 h, and the patient awakens when blood levels fall below 150 μmol/liter. Patients with liver dysfunction or arginine deficiency are thought to be at greater risk for hyperammonemia. However, no evidence supports liver dysfunction as a cause.[68,79] The metabolism of ammonia to urea in the liver relies on the presence of arginine. Patients deficient in arginine accumulate excess ammonia. Arginine has been shown to increase the uptake of ammonia in animals.[80]

Oxalic acid is another product of glycine metabolism. Hyperoxaluria secondary to increased oxalate secretion can last up to 2 weeks. If the patient is not well hydrated, formation of oxalate crystals in the kidney can occur.

WATER INTOXICATION The incidence of water intoxication during TURP has been reported to be as high as 10 percent of cases.[81] Fourteen of 2,000 patients in another series developed coma. All were older, had larger prostate glands, and had longer resection times. All these patients exhibited lower serum sodium levels at the end of resection. Water intoxication is a consequence of the absorption of nonelectrolyte irrigation solutions. The result is a hypervolemic and hyponatremic state. Water intoxication is heralded by the triad bradycardia, hypertension with increased pulse pressure and cerebral agitation, and/or depression.[82] Progressive increases in arterial, central venous, or pulmonary capillary wedge pressure can be an early sign of excessive fluid absorption.[83] CNS symptoms, secondary to cerebral swelling and increased intracranial pressure, consist of somnolence and/or confusion that progresses to agitation. Seizures and a progression to coma can occur. Papilledema with dilated and slow pupillary response may be found. Comatose patients may assume a decerebrate posture with clonus and Babinski's sign. Bilateral low-voltage electroencephalographic (EEG) signals occur. The increased intracerebral pressure correlates with the increased body weight and blood pressure associated with hypervolemia.[82] Water intoxication usually develops at the end of surgery but can occur early during resection. The length of the coma is variable, lasting from several hours to several days. In one series,[75] the onset of coma occurred between the completion of and up to 10 h after surgery.

HYPONATREMIA Sodium is necessary for the proper functioning of excitable cells, especially in the heart and brain. Hyponatremia during TURP results from the absorption of nonelectrolytic irrigation solution. Sodium levels of 120 mEq/liter or lower produce abnormal myocardial and CNS dysfunction. The signs and symptoms associated with hyponatremia and its effect on the cardiac system and CNS are well known (Table 18-3). The average decline in serum sodium during TURP is between 3.65 and 10 mEq/liter.[51] Several factors contribute to the etiology of hyponatremia, including excessive absorption of the irrigation solution, sodium loss into irrigation fluid as it passes through the

Table 18-3 Symptoms and acute changes in serum Na^+

Serum Na^+	Electrocardiogram	Central nervous system
120 mmol/liter^{-1}	Possibly widening QRS*	Restlessness, confusion
115 mmol/liter^{-1}	Widened QRS, elevated ST segment	Nausea, semicoma
100 mmol/liter^{-1}	Ventricular tachycardia or fibrillation	Seizures, coma

*QRS = principal deflection in an electrocardiogram.

SOURCE: Jensen V: The TURP syndrome. *Can J Anaesth* 38:92, 1991.

resection site, and diffusion loss into pockets of irrigation solution in the periprostatic and retroperitoneal spaces. Investigations into the correlation between the degree of hyponatremia and the amount of irrigation fluid absorbed have not been consistent. Some propose a direct correlation, while others find no correlation. The decline in serum sodium may be related to the rate of absorption rather than to the total volume of irrigation solution absorbed.[50,84] The occurrence of coma and seizures appears to depend on the acuteness and severity of the hyponatremia. However, a correlation between the incidence of neurological symptoms and serum sodium levels is less clear. In some patients a moderate decrease in serum sodium results in CNS symptomatology, while in others with serum sodium levels well below 100 mmol/liter, no CNS symptomatology appears.[75] There does, however, appear to be a correlation between the rate of decrease in serum sodium and an increased incidence of neurological symptoms.[85] Others have demonstrated a correlation between decreases in serum osmolality and the occurrence of CNS symptoms. Desmond found that a decrease in both serum sodium and serum osmolality was necessary for the development of CNS symptoms.[48]

The cardiac symptoms associated with hyponatremia appear to have a direct correlation with the degree of hyponatremia. The lower the serum sodium falls, the graver are the cardiac signs and symptoms that occur.[51]

Correction of hyponatremia is oftentimes unnecessary and may prove fatal to the patient. Levels above 120 mEq/liter need not be corrected. Spontaneous or induced diuresis can correct hyponatremia associated with TURP in several hours.

Attempts to correct hyponatremia with 3% or 5% hypertonic saline should be undertaken with caution. These patients already exhibit signs of circulatory overload, and the infusion of hypertonic saline may induce cardiovascular collapse. A diuretic should always be given before saline administration. Rapid correction of hyponatremia with hypertonic saline is associated with central pontine myelinolysis, which is a fatal neurological complication of unknown cause. It has been recommended that serum sodium levels be corrected at a rate no faster than 0.5 mEq/liter per hour and that fluid infusion rates be kept at 100 ml/h or less.[86]

Anesthesia for TURP

Anesthesiologists should allow the patient's preference, not the patient's condition, to determine the anesthetic technique for surgery. While many physicians feel that regional anesthesia is safer in elderly patients and therefore is the method of choice, there is not much evidence to support this theory. Relatively recent research has studied several aspects of this controversy, including morbidity and mortality, cognitive function, postoperative pain relief, surgical stress, blood loss, and heat loss. When one compares regional and general anesthesia, a clearly superior technique does not surface from these data, with each having some advantages and disadvantages.

Several authors feel that regional anesthesia is the technique of choice for TURP.[51,52] Regional anesthesia allows the detection of changes in mentation and other signs and symptoms that would allow for earlier recognition of TURP syndrome. Additionally, the use of a regional anesthetic provides postoperative analgesia. Also, there is some evidence that the peripheral pooling of blood may reduce circulatory overloading and that low spinal anesthesia helps maintain a stable cardiovascular system. Evidence clearly supports the theory that regional anesthesia to a level of T_{12} to T_{10} allows adequate surgical anesthesia and maintains cardiovascular stability while allowing most signs and symptoms of TURP syndrome to be determined.

If regional anesthesia is contraindicated and general anesthesia is chosen, there appears to be no advantage in using one general anesthetic rather than another. However, the use of a relaxant technique may decrease straining that could lead to increased absorption of the irrigant fluid.

Transurethral Resection of Bladder Tumor

While many bladder tumors are resected in the outpatient setting, some are too large or involve extensive areas of the bladder and are therefore resected in an inpatient setting. In general, these patients are not exposed to the altered circulatory volumes, electrolyte changes, and osmolality changes seen with prostatic resection.

OPEN PROSTATECTOMY

Only 10 percent of patients undergoing prostatectomy for urinary obstruction have open prostatectomies. Open prostatectomy for cancer of the prostate is the treatment of choice where appropriate. The choice of open prostatectomy rather than transurethral resection is based predominantly on the size of the prostate gland to be removed. In general, prostates greater than 80 g are more conveniently removed by open prostatectomy. Open prostatectomy can be achieved by suprapubic (transvesicle), retropubic, or perineal prostatectomy. In general, retropubic and perineal prostatectomies are performed more commonly.

Open prostatectomy can be performed under general anesthesia, regional anesthesia, or combined regional and light general anesthesia.

Perineal prostatectomy utilizes an exaggerated lithotomy position with a head-down tilt. This provides superior exposure, including a very dry field for the surgeon, but impairs the cardiovascular and respiratory systems of the patient. The effects of lithotomy and Trendelenburg's position may have a greater impact on an elderly patient.[89]

CYSTECTOMY

Radical cystectomy with urinary diversion is a long procedure associated with considerable blood loss, large third space fluid losses, prolonged abdominal exposure, and pelvic instrumentation. These patients require invasive monitoring, including arterial, central venous, or pulmonary artery wedge pressure. Core and peripheral temperature measurement is essential, and precautions to prevent excessive heat loss should be taken.

RADIOLOGICAL PROCEDURES

Advances in technology have led to an increase in less invasive or totally noninvasive radiological techniques that primarily facilitate stone management. The two most common techniques are described below.

Extracorporeal Shock Wave Lithotripsy

Extracorporeal shock wave lithotripsy (ESWL) was introduced in 1980. By 1985, it was estimated that 85 percent of renal calculi were treated by this technique. First-generation models directed approximately 20 KV from a capacitor through an underwater electrode to produce an instantaneous spark. This spark was immediately vaporized within the electro gap, producing shock waves that were focused onto the calculus by the ellipsoid-shaped reflector. The energy of these shock waves was released when there was a change in the medium through which the shock waves were passing. The greatest energy was released at the soft tissue–stone interface, since the interface between water and soft tissue is negligible. Earlier machines required the patient to be immersed in a bath of water.

Immersion in a warm water bath, usually 36°C, results in heat loss that averages 0.5°C. Additionally, immersion in the bath has a compression effect similar to that seen with mast trousers. This leads to a rise in right atrial and pulmonary capillary wedge pressures up from 3 to 16.5 mmHg and 6.5 to 17.5

mmHg, respectively.[90] The degree of rise is proportional to the degree of immersion in the water bath. This increase in preload can lead to circulatory collapse in patients with cardiovascular failure.

The original machines used asynchronous triggering of shock waves, which resulted in an approximately 80 percent incidence of cardiac dysrhythmias. Newer machines utilize an R wave from an electrocardiogram (ECG) to trigger discharges. Heart rate is also important, because a length of time is necessary to recharge the capacitor, and if a rapid heart rate is present, insufficient time to recharge the capacitor may lead to low-voltage discharges. Bradycardia, while not lowering voltage discharges, also can extend the time of treatment.

The two most common anesthetic techniques employed are epidural anesthesia and general anesthesia with controlled ventilation. Both have advantages and disadvantages, but neither is superior to the other. However, as a result of immersion in water, head-elevated positioning, and the known occurrence of postural hypotension requiring fluid preload and vasopressors, epidural anesthesia may be contraindicated in some patients with decreased cardiac reserve.[91]

Second-generation machines no longer require immersion in a water bath, and the shock waves are less powerful, resulting in a lessened requirement for anesthesia.

Percutaneous Nephrolithotomy

This procedure has been performed more frequently over the last few years and is now recommended by some workers instead of ESWL.[92] It involves Seldinger-type wires to be placed into the renal pelvis with radiological assistance. The radiological technique employed requires identification of the renal pelvis, using contrast dye placed via a ureteral catheter inserted after the induction of anesthesia. The patient is then turned prone, and a radiologically guided needle is placed into the renal pelvis. The position of the needle in the renal pelvis is confirmed by aspiration of contrast. The guide wire is then introduced, and increasingly large dilators are passed over the wire until a nephroscope can be passed into the renal pelvis. The stone can then be removed or broken up into fragments with ultrasound probes and removed in pieces.

Potential problems from this procedure are related primarily to anatomy and the need to have the patient prone. Pneumothorax is a possibility, as forced inspiration with an expiratory pause is often necessary to place the kidney in an accessible position. Damage to renal vessels can occur. Additionally, damage to or perforation of the renal pelvis may occur during dilation or manipulation, with resultant absorption of irrigation fluid.

The anesthetic management of these patients requires anesthesia from a level of T_{10} downward and a large-bore IV in case unexpected blood loss occurs. There is no anesthetic technique of choice for this type of procedure.

Postoperatively, occult bleeding and hypothermia, as well as pain, are the biggest complications. Hypothermia can occur in these patients if the procedure is prolonged.

SUMMARY

The challenges presented to the anesthesiology team by an aging patient who presents for urologic surgery are best met by a thorough understanding of aging, coexisting diseases, the physiological impact of the surgical technique, and the potential complications. For example, TURP syndrome is best treated by avoiding its occurrence. An understanding of its etiology, precipitation factors, and the ability to make an early diagnosis and effect proper treatment are necessary in treating an elderly patient.

REFERENCES

1. Lindeman RD, Goldman R: Anatomic and physiologic age changes in the kidney. *Exp Gerontol* 21:379, 1986.
2. Lindeman RD: Kidney and body fluids, in Masro EJ (ed): *CRC Handbook of Physiology and Aging*. Boca Raton, CRC Press, 1981, p 175.
3. Atul Roy T, et al: Renal failure in older people: UCLA grand rounds. *J Am Geriatr Soc* 38:239, 1990.
4. Frocht A, Phillit H: Renal disease in the geriatric patient. *J Am Geriatr Soc* 32:28, 1984.
5. McLachlan MSF, Guthrie JC, Anderson CK, et al: Vascular and glomerular changes in the aging kidney. *J Pathol* 121:65, 1977.
6. Darmady EM, Offur J, Woodhouse MA: The parameters of the aging kidney. *J Pathol* 109:195, 1973.
7. Wesson LG: Renal hemodynamics in physiologic states. *Physiology of the Human Kidney*. New York: Grune & Stratton, 1969, pp 96–108.
8. Rowe JW, Andres R, Tobikn S, et al: The effects of age on creatinine clearance in man: A cross sectional longitudinal study. *J Gerontol* 31:155, 1976.
9. Kapmann J, Siesbaek M, Nielson K, et al: Rapid evaluation of creatine clearance. *Acta Med Scand* 196:517, 1974.
10. Lindeman RD: Assessment of renal function in the old: Special considerations. *Clin Lab Med* 13:269, 1993.
11. Gingell JC, Dodds C: Urology in the aging surgical patient, in Crosby, Rees, and Seymour (eds): *Anesthetic, Operative, and Medical Management*. Wiley, 1992.
12. Epstein M, Hollenberg NK: Age as determinant of renal sodium conservation in normal man. *J Lab Clin Med* 87:411, 1972.
13. Helderman JH, Vestal RE, Rowe JW, et al: The response of arginine vasopressin to intravenous ethanol and hypertonic saline: The impact of aging. *J Gerontol* 33:39, 1978.
14. Gold I, Roxe DM: Severe hypernatremia caused by age, isolation, and obstructive uropathy. *South Med J* 72:1198, 1979.

15. Roxe DM: Renal function, aging and drug therapy. *Compr Ther* 15:13, 1989.
16. Dontas AS, Marketos S, Papaayiouton P: Mechanisms of renal tubular defect in old age. *Postgrad Med* 48:295, 1972.
17. Lindeman RD, Lee TD Jr, Yiengst MJ, et al: Influence of age, renal disease, hypertension, diuretics and calcium on the antidiuretic responses to suboptimal infusions of vasopressin. *J Lab Clin Med* 68:206, 1968.
18. Benzinger TH, Pratt AW, Kitzinger CH: The thermostatic control of human metabolic heat production. *Proc Natl Acad Sci USA* 47:730, 1961.
19. Collins KJ, Eston JC, Exton-Smith AM: Shivering thermogenesis and vasomotor responses with convective cooling in the elderly. *J Physiol* 320:76, 1981.
20. Collins KJ, Exton-Smith AM, Dore C: Urban hypothermia: Preferred temperature and thermal perception in old age. *Br Med J* 282:175, 1981.
21. Carli F, Itiaba K: Effective heat conservation during and after major abdominal surgery on muscle protein breakdown. *Br J Anaesth* 58:502, 1986.
22. Frank SM, Battie C, Kristopherson R, et al: Epidural versus general anesthesia, ambient operating room temperature and patient age as predictors of inadvertent hypothermia. *Anesthesiology* 77:252, 1992.
23. Morris RH: Operating room temperature in the anesthetized paralyzed patient. *Arch Surg* 102:95, 1971.
24. Conim SW: Accidental hypothermia. *Anaesthesia* 34:250, 1979.
25. Bay J, Nunn JF, Prys-Roberts C: Factors influencing arterial PO_2 during recovery from anaesthesia. *Br J Anaesth* 40:398, 1968.
26. Horvath SM, Spurr GB, Hutt BK, et al: Metabolic cost of shivering. *J Appl Physiol* 8:145, 1956.
27. Benzinger TH: Heat regulation: Homeostasis of central temperature in man. *Physiol Rev* 49:671, 1969.
28. Catlic MR: Surgery in centenarians. *JAMA* 253:3139, 1985.
29. Deutsch S: Anesthesia for urologic surgery, in *ASA Refresher Courses.* Park Ridge, IL: American Society of Anesthesiologists, 1991, vol 20, pp 1–14.
30. German K, Hasan ST, Derry C: Cystodiathermy under local anesthesia using flexible cystoscope. *Br J Neurol* 69:518, 1992.
31. Greenland JE, Lynch TH, Wallis DMA: Optical urethrotomy under local urethral anaesthesia. *Br J Neurol* 67:385, 1991.
32. Kaye KW: Surgery using local anesthesia in the elderly: Urologic care in the elderly. *Clin Geriatr Med* 6:85–119, 1990.
33. Orandi A: Urologic endoscopic surgery under local anesthesia: A cost reducing idea. *J Urol* 132:1146, 1984.
34. Sinha B, Haikel G, Lange PH, et al: Transurethral resection of the prostate with local anesthesia in 100 patients. *J Urol* 135:719, 1986.
35. Moffet NA: Transurethral prostatic resections under local anesthesia. *J Urol* 118:607, 1977.
36. Enberg A, Spandberg A, Urnes T: Transurethral resection of bladder tumors under local anesthesia. *Urology* 22:385, 1983.
37. Lichtwardt JR, Girgis S: Transurethral resection of prostate with intravenous sedation. *Urology* 25:112, 1985.
38. Mclaughlin MG, Kinahan TJ: Transurethral resection of the prostate in the outpatient setting. *J Neurol* 143:951, 1990.
39. Moffit NA: Transurethral resection of prostate bladder tumors: Outpatient urologic surgery. *Urol Clin North Am* 14(1):115–119, 1987.

40. Birch BRP, Anson KM, Gelister JS, Miller RA: Sedoanalgesia in urology: Technique, applications and impact. *World J Urol* 7:162, 1989.
41. Birch BRP, Gelister JS: Transurethral resection of prostate under sedation and local anesthesia (sedoanalgesia): Experience in 100 patients. *Urology* 38:P113, 1991.
42. Smith DC, Crul JF: Oxygen desaturation following sedation for regional analgesia. *Br J Anaesth* 62:106, 1989.
43. Biswas TK, Leery C: Post-operative hospital admission from a day surgery unit: A seven year retrospective survey. *Anaesth Intensive Care* 20:147, 1992.
44. Melchior J, Volk WL, Foret JD, et al: Transurethral prostatectomy computerized analysis of 2,223 consecutive cases. *J Urol* 112:634, 1974.
45. Rollema HJ, van Mastrigt R, Janknegt RA: Urodynamic assessment and quantification of prostatic obstruction before and after transurethral resection of prostate: Standardization with the aid of the computer program CLIM. *Urol Int* 47 (Suppl 1):52, 1991.
46. Meyhosf NH, Nordling J, Hald T: Economy and transurethral prostatectomy. *Scand J Urol Nephrol* 19:17, 1985.
47. Holtgrew HL, Volk W: Factors influencing the mortality and morbidity of transurethral prostatectomy: The study of 2,015 cases. *J Urol* 87:450, 1962.
48. Desmond J: Complications of transurethral prostatic surgery. *Can Anaesth Soc J* 17:25, 1970.
49. Harrison RH, Bonen JS, Robinson JR: Dilutional hyponatremic shock: Another concept of the transurethral prostatic resection reaction. *J Urol* 75:95, 1956.
50. Rhymer JC, Bell TJ, Perry KC, Ward JP: Hyponatremia following transurethral resection of the prostate. *Br J Urol* 57:450, 1985.
51. Hatch PD: Surgical anesthetic considerations in transurethral resection of the prostate. *Anaesth Intensive Care* 15:203, 1987.
52. Azar I: Transurethral prostatectomy syndrome, in *ASA Refresher Courses.* Park Ridge, IL: American Society of Anesthesiologists, 1989, vol 17, pp 1–17.
53. McGowan SW, Smith GFN: Anesthesia for transurethral prostatectomy. *Anaesthesia* 35:847, 1980.
54. McKenzie AR, Levine N, Scheinman HA: Operative blood loss in transurethral prostatectomy. *J Urol* 122:47, 1979.
55. Madson RE, Madson, PO: Influence of anesthesia forum on blood loss and transurethral prostatectomy. *Anesth Analg* 46:330, 1967.
56. Abrams PH, Shah PJR, Bryning K, et al: Blood loss during transurethral resection of prostate. *Anaesthesia* 37:71, 1982.
57. Desmond J, Gordon RA: Bleeding during transurethral prostatic surgery. *Can Anaesth Soc J* 16:217–224, 1969.
58. Hawn RG: Hemoglobin dilution method (HDM) for estimation of blood volume variations during transurethral prostatic surgery. *Acta Anaesthesiol Scand* 31:572, 1987.
59. Baker JA, Louis CJ, Rosenthal M, et al: Apparatus for measurement of blood loss during transurethral surgery. *Br J Anaesth* 60:339, 1988.
60. Smart RF: Endoscopic injection of vasoconstrictor ornithine-8-vasopressin in transurethral resection. *Br J Urol* 56:191, 1985.
61. Lombardo LN: Fibrinolysis following prostatic surgery. *J Urol* 77:289, 1957.
62. Smith RB, Riach P, Kauffman JJ: Episolon aminocaproic acid and the control of post prostatectomy bleeding: A prospective double blind study. *J Urol* 131:1093, 1984.
63. Friedman NJ, Hoag MS, Robinson AJ, Aggeler PM: Hemorrhagic syndrome fol-

lowing transurethral prostatic resection for benign atinoma. *Arch Intern Med* 123:341, 1969.

64. Harioka T, Muraka M, Noda J, et al: Effect of continuously warmed irrigating solution during transurethral resection. *Anaesth Intensive Care* 16:324, 1988.
65. Heathcoate PS, Dwer PM: The effect of warm irrigation on blood loss during transurethral prostatectomy under spinal anesthesia. *Br J Urol* 58:669, 1985.
66. Hansen RI, Iverson P: Bladder explosion during uninterrupted transurethral resection of the prostate: A case report, an experimental model. *Scand J Nephrol* 13:211, 1979.
67. Nesbutt TE, Carter DW, Tutor J, et al: Complications of transurethral prostatectomy under management. *South Med Assoc J* 59:361, 1966.
68. Oester A, Madsen PO: Determination of absorption of irrigating fluid during transurethral resection of the prostate by means of radioisotopes. *J Urol* 102:714, 1969.
69. Printess RJ, Harvery GW, Bethard WF, et al: Massive abductor muscle contraction in transurethral surgery: Cause and prevention: Development of new electrical circuitry. *J Urol* 93:263, 1965.
70. Gasparich JP, Tate MJ, Berger RE: Use of nerve stimulator for simple and accurate obturator nerve block before transurethral resection. *J Urol* 132:291, 1984.
71. Fujita Y, Kimura K, Furukawa Y, Takaior M: Plasma concentrations of lidocaine after obturator nerve block combined with spinal anesthesia in patients undergoing transurethral resection procedures. *Br J Anaesth* 68:596, 1992.
72. Kidd EE, Kennedy B: Bacteremia, septicemia and intravascular hemolysis during transurethral resection of the prostate gland. *Br J Urol* 37:551, 1965.
73. Hagstrom RS: Studies on fluid absorption during transurethral prostatic surgery. *J Urol* 73:852, 1955.
74. Haugh R, Berlin T, Lewenhaupt A: Irrigating fluid absorption and blood loss during transurethral resection of the prostate: Studies with a regular interval monitoring (RIM) method. *Scand J Urol Nephrol* 22:23, 1988.
75. Henderson DJ, Middle RG: Coma from hyponatremia following transurethral resection of prostate. *Urology* 15:267, 1980.
76. Beal JL, Freysz M, Berthelon G, et al: Consequences of fluid absorption during transurethral resection of the prostate using distilled water or glycine 1.5%. *Can J Anaesth* 36:278, 1989.
77. Wang JM, Wong KC, Creel DJ, et al: Effects of glycine on hemodynamic responses and visual evoked potentials in the dog. *Anesth Analg* 64:1071, 1985.
78. Ovassapian A, Joshi CW, Brumer EA: Visual disturbances: An unusual symptom of transuretheral prostatic resection reaction. *Anesthesiology* 57:332, 1982.
79. Roesch RP, Stoelting RK, Lingeman JE, et al: Ammonia toxicity resulting from glycine absorption during a transurethral resection of the prostate. *Anesthesiology* 58:577, 1983.
80. Fahey JL: Toxicity of blood ammonia rise resulting from intravenous amino acid administration in man: The protective effect of l-arginine. *J Clin Invest* 36:1647, 1957.
81. Mebus WK, Brady TW, Volk WL: Observations on cardiac output blood volume central venous pressure, fluid and electrolyte changes in patients undergoing transurethral prostatectomy. *J Urol* 103:632, 1970.
82. Harrison RH, Broen JS, Robinson JR: Dilutional hyponatremia: Another concept of the transurethral prostatic resection reaction. *J Urol* 75:95, 1956.
83. Deutsch S: Anesthesia for urologic surgery, in *ASA Refresher Course Lectures.* Park Ridge, IL: American Society of Anesthesiologists, 1991, vol 151, pp 1-4.

84. Haughn RG: Relations between irrigation absorption rate and hyponatremia during transurethral resection of the prostate. *Acta Anaesthesiol Scand* 32:53, 1988.
85. Maluf NSR, Born JS, Brandes GE: Absorption of irrigating solution and associated changes upon transurethral electro resection of prostate. *J Urol* 75:824, 1956.
86. Ayus JC, Krothapalli RK, Arieff AI: Changing concepts and treatment of severe symptomatic hyponatremia: Rapid correction and possible relation to central pontine myelinolysis. *Am J Med* 78:897, 1985.
87. Desmond, DJ: Serum osmolality and plasma electrolytes in patients who develop dillutional hyponatremia during transurethral resection. *Can J Surg* 13:116, 1970.
88. Hosking MP, Lobdell CM, Warner MA, et al: Anesthesia for patients over 90 years of age: Outcomes after regional and general anesthetic techniques for two common surgical procedures. *Anaesthesia* 44:142, 1989.
89. Case PH, Styles JA: The effect of various surgical positions on vital capacity. *Anesthesiology* 7:29, 1946.
90. Weber W, Chaussy C, Madler C, et al: Cardiocirculatory changes during anesthesia for extracorpeal shock wave lithotripsy. *J Urol* 131:571, 1984.
91. Abbott MA, Samuel JR, Webb DR: Anaesthesia for extracorporeal shock wave lithotripsy. *Anaesthesia* 40:1065, 1985.
92. Mays N, Challah S, Pates S, et al: Clinical comparison of extracorporeal shock wave lithotripsy and percutaneous nephrolithotomy in treating renal calculi. *Urology* 297:253, 1988.

CHAPTER 19

Anesthesia for Ear, Nose, and Throat Procedures in Geriatric Patients

Susan H. Noorily
Allen D. Noorily

INTRODUCTION

This chapter describes the anesthetic management of ear, nose, and throat (ENT) procedures commonly performed on geriatric patients and the problems and complications that may be encountered.

HEAD AND NECK CANCER

Epidemiology

As the geriatric population grows in number, more people are at risk for diseases previously seen in only a small segment of the population. Cancer of the head and neck, which is classically seen in the sixth decade and beyond, is one such disease.

In general, repeated or prolonged exposure to specific carcinogens is required for the development of a cancer. Additionally, impairment of the immune system makes an individual more susceptible to this disease. Thus, it is not surprising that cancer is a common disease in the elderly population.

Irradiation from the sun is the most common carcinogen. Therefore, it affects more people than does any other carcinogen.[1] It is because of this exposure that skin cancers often plague the elderly. These skin cancers include basal cell carcinomas, squamous cell carcinomas, and melanomas.

The largest single causative factor in the development of cancer today is tobacco use, primarily in the form of cigarette smoking.[1] Tobacco use is associated with the development of cancers in the aerodigestive tract. Tobacco is a known carcinogen that directly contacts the oral cavity when chewed and mixes with inspired air when smoked. The combination of tobacco use and heavy alcohol consumption poses an even higher risk. The carcinogenic effects of these two substances appear to be synergistic.[1] Several theories have been suggested to explain the carcinogenic effects of alcohol, including malnutrition, intracellular changes, hepatic damage, and impairment of the immune system. Patients presenting with tumors of the aerodigestive tract frequently have systemic illnesses related to both heavy smoking and drinking.

In the past, elderly patients presenting with tumors of the head and neck were treated nonsurgically. It was thought that geriatric patients had an unacceptably high perioperative risk when they underwent radical surgical procedures because of their increased incidence of cardiopulmonary and systemic illnesses. Unfortunately, many patients who were refused surgical treatment developed incurable metastatic disease.

More recently, it was discovered that geriatric patients can tolerate radical head and neck operations without an increased risk of postoperative complications if they are carefully selected and prepared preoperatively.[2–4] In a retrospective study of major head and neck operations, the risk of surgical complications did not differ between patients over 70 years of age and those under 70 years of age, although the older group had an 8 percent increase in medical complications. In addition, there was increased mortality in patients over 80 years of age, primarily as a result of pulmonary and cardiovascular complications.[2] More important, the hospital mortality for head and neck cancer patients who experience surgery has been reported to be lower than the mortality in patients who are admitted for nonsurgical treatment.[5]

Preoperative Evaluation

All patients presenting for head and neck surgery should have a thorough history and physical examination. Geriatric patients have a higher incidence of organ dysfunction and preexisting disease, and as was previously discussed, patients with head and neck cancers are more likely to have problems associated with long-term tobacco and alcohol use, such as cardiopulmonary disease and hepatic abnormalities.

Patients scheduled to have outpatient procedures should be evaluated as early as possible, ideally before the day of surgery. The perioperative complication rate during outpatient surgery appears to increase with lengthy surgical procedures and in patients with coexisiting medical disease.[6] In general, outpatient ENT procedures in the elderly should be limited to less than 3 h and reserved for patients without serious preexisting medical conditions.[7]

When performing the history and physical examination, one must remember that head and neck cancers are often accompanied by inflammation and/or airway obstruction. If patients have undergone any radiation therapy, they are more likely to have inflammation and fibrosis of the airway structures. Therefore, signs of airway compromise must be elicited. In most cases, the surgeon in the preoperative clinic has visualized the airway using indirect laryngoscopy and can describe the existing anatomy and pathology. These findings should be discussed before the induction of anesthesia.

Geriatric head and neck cancer patients have a high incidence of chronic obstructive pulmonary disease, chronic aspiration, hypertension, and coronary artery disease. In addition to routine lab tests, chest x-rays, and electrocardiograms (ECGs), symptomatic and high-risk patients should have pulmonary function and cardiovascular tests as indicated to address specific concerns. Echocardiography can noninvasively evaluate myocardial function and valvular disease. An exercise tolerance test or dipyridamole (Persantine) thallium study can be performed to evaluate ischemic heart disease. Other laboratory tests should be individualized.

Many head and neck cancer patients have a history of alcohol abuse. If this is the case, the physician should be prepared for the possibility of withdrawal symptoms. These patients are often malnourished and dehydrated not only because of alcohol abuse but also because of dysphagia caused by tumor obstruction. Because dehydration occurs frequently, the preoperative hematocrit may be normal or elevated when the patient is actually anemic.

Head and neck cancer operations are considered "urgent" elective procedures unless acute airway obstruction is imminent. As was previously mentioned, elderly head and neck cancer patients are at risk for perioperative cardiopulmonary complications. The results of one series suggest that patients requiring laryngopharyngeal resections are more likely to develop pulmonary complications and that those requiring oral cavity resections appear to have more cardiovascular complications, but no explanations for this difference were discussed.[2] Perhaps patients in the first category have a higher incidence of pulmonary aspiration as a result of the surgical resection. Because of the risk involved, procedures must be delayed until a patient's cardiopulmonary status is defined and the medical condition is optimized. Cardiac disease is the major preoperative determinant of postoperative morbidity and mortality in elderly patients.[8]

Basics of Intraoperative Care

Premedication

Geriatric patients are more sensitive to sedatives and can become confused or agitated after their administration.[9] In addition, a small degree of sedation in a patient with airway compromise may result in acute airway obstruction. Therefore, in most cases, gentle communication is the most effective and safest "premedicant." There are exceptions to this, of course. Patients prone to alcohol withdrawal may benefit from treatment with a benzodiazepine preoperatively if sedation will not compromise the airway. Drugs other than sedatives, such as antibiotics and aspiration prophylaxis medications, may be required preoperatively. Anticholinergic drugs can be administered to patients preoperatively to dry oral secretions before airway procedures. Elderly patients tend to have fewer secretions, and this treatment may not be necessary. If an antisialagogue is required, glycopyrrolate is the best choice because it does not affect the CNS.

Monitoring

The monitors selected should be chosen with regard to the patient's medical condition and the specific surgical procedure. For short procedures, routine monitors are usually sufficient. For more lengthy procedures, a Foley catheter should be inserted to monitor urine output. An arterial line is useful to follow arterial blood gases in patients with chronic obstructive pulmonary disease (COPD) and to monitor beat-to-beat blood pressure in patients with cardiac disease and during extensive surgical procedures.

A central venous or pulmonary artery catheter should be considered in all patients with cardiac disease and patients undergoing procedures in which large fluid shifts and blood loss are expected. A right-sided heart catheter can be used to detect and treat venous air embolism. If central monitoring is required, potential sites include the subclavian and antecubital veins. Internal jugular lines are not practical because they will be located in the surgical field. Also, the tumor can involve the major vessels in the neck, and it may be necessary to sacrifice the internal jugular vein as part of the dissection. It is always safest to demonstrate appropriate placement of central catheters and the absence of pneumothorax by chest x-ray before the induction of anesthesia.

Electroencephalographic (EEG) monitoring should be considered for procedures in which the carotid artery is clamped or its blood flow is severely compromised. Because open neck veins can entrain air into the venous system, venous air embolism is a potential complication of head and neck cancer surgery, especially when it is performed in the head-up position. Monitoring for venous air emboli can be performed by using a precordial Doppler and measuring the expired nitrogen concentration. When venous air embolism is suspected, the surgeon should flood the surgical field with saline and compress the jugular veins. The patient should be placed in the Trendelenburg position and given 100% oxygen. Some surgeons prefer to place the patient in the left lateral decubitus position. If a central venous catheter is in place, it should be aspirated. Hemodynamic support should be provided as necessary.

Geriatric patients are prone to hypothermia. The elderly have a decreased metabolic rate and an impaired thermoregulatory system.[9] This can be a problem postoperatively, because shivering increases oxygen consumption and necessitates a higher cardiac output. In addition, drug elimination is slowed, and this can prolong awakening. Therefore, a core temperature should be monitored in all patients, and every attempt should be made to maintain normothermia. ENT patients are usually extensively covered in drapes, and this helps maintain body temperature. However, some patients require active warming with warm intravenous fluids, humidified gases, heated blankets, and increased room temperature. Particular care must be taken to protect dependent pressure points during long procedures, because geriatric patients have atrophic skin.

Anesthetic Technique

Some head and neck cancer operations can be performed easily under local anesthesia. There is some evidence that the complication rate in elderly patients is lower when local anesthesia, without sedation, is the chosen technique.[10] The recovery time is more rapid, and there are fewer side effects. Examples of procedures that are amenable to local anesthesia include biopsies and excision of small tumors and skin cancers. If nasal anesthesia is required, cocaine should be avoided. The potential harmful side effects of this drug may be exaggerated in the geriatric population. Unfortunately, cocaine is frequently administered by otolaryngologists for nasal anesthesia and hemostasis. A recent study in healthy volunteers demonstrated that the anesthetic and vasoconstrictive properties of a lidocaine/oxymetazoline combination are as good as, and perhaps superior to, those of cocaine.[11]

The majority of head and neck cancer operations require a general anesthetic. The choice of the specific drugs used should take into account any coexisting medical problems. No specific anesthetic technique has proved to be superior. Geriatric patients have a decreased requirement for most anesthetics, and the onset of anesthetic effect is often delayed because of a prolonged circulation time.[9] Therefore, smaller doses should be administered and adequate time should be allowed for drug effect before redosing. This is very important during the induction of anesthesia. In addition, most drugs have a prolonged duration of action in elderly patients. Therefore, short-acting agents are preferred, especially for outpatient procedures and procedures of short duration.

Before the induction of anesthesia, a decision must be made regarding the ease of intubation. Consultation with the surgeon will be important in the decision-making process. If the tumor is small and nonfriable, the anatomy is not distorted, and there is no airway compromise, tracheal intubation should not pose a problem in a patient with a normal-appearing external airway. If any uncertainty exists regarding the ease of intubation, an *awake intubation* should be performed. This can be accomplished by direct or fiberoptic laryngoscopy. If there is a friable, large, or exophytic tumor, anatomic distortion, or severe airway compromise, an *awake tracheotomy* under local anesthesia is preferred (Fig. 19-1). This prevents bleeding and the seeding of cancerous particles into the airway and avoids acute airway obstruction from sedation, stimulation, and secretions.

Any of the induction agents can be administered safely in age-appropriate doses. Ketamine, however, can increase oral secretions and adversely affect some patients with cardiac disease. It therefore may be less suitable. Some anesthesiologists prefer inhalation induction in patients with airway pathology because spontaneous ventilation is maintained. Induction must wait until after the airway is secured when an awake intubation is performed. After induction, the general anesthetic can be maintained in a variety of ways but should be

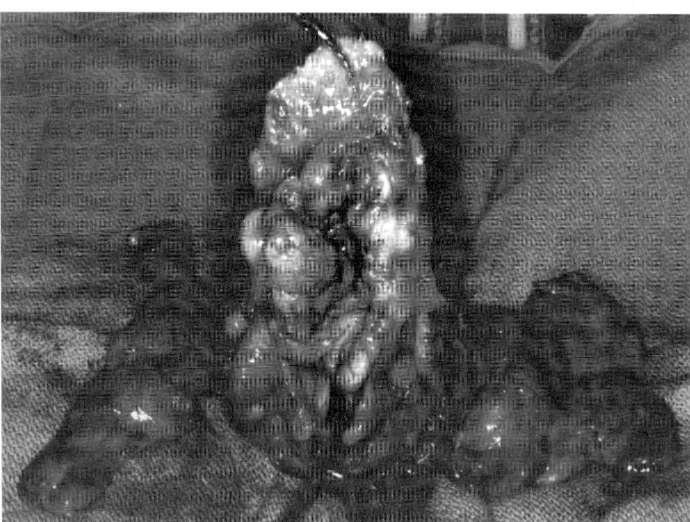

Figure 19-1 Gross specimen of a large squamous cell carcinoma of the epiglottis in a patient requiring a tracheotomy under local anesthesia before the induction of anesthesia.

based on the patient's medical condition, the length of the procedure, the intensity of postoperative monitoring, and the surgical requirements.

Specific Procedures

Tracheotomy

A *tracheotomy* is a temporary airway established directly into the trachea. This is to be distinguished from a *tracheostomy*, which is a permanent airway such as that established in a patient who has had a total laryngectomy. A tracheotomy may be required as an emergency airway in a patient who cannot be intubated in the usual orotracheal or nasotracheal fashion, will require long-term ventilatory support, or is undergoing extensive surgery of the head and neck region. Whatever the indication may be, some important anesthetic concepts must be emphasized.

In the case of a patient requiring an emergency surgical airway for the treatment of respiratory distress, local anesthesia is the safest method. The patient must be given 100% oxygen by face mask during the procedure. Sedation should be avoided. The surgeon can anesthetize the region by injecting the local anesthetic two finger breadths above the sternal notch in the midline. A horizontal skin incision is made at this site followed by a vertical soft tissue incision that is continued downward between the strap muscles in the avascular midline plane of the neck. The only vascular structure encountered is the isthmus of the thyroid gland, which directly overlies the trachea. The isthmus is divided carefully, exposing the trachea. The tracheotomy is performed, and an endotracheal tube or tracheostomy tube can be placed directly into the trachea for ventilation. If additional surgery is required, a general anesthetic can be induced after the airway is secured, breath sounds are auscultated bilaterally, and end-tidal CO_2 is documented.

If a patient has an endotracheal tube in place before surgery, a general anesthetic can be administered for the duration of the procedure, provided that the patient is hemodynamically stable. The endotracheal tube should not be removed completely until ventilation has been established via the tracheotomy. Some anesthesiologists recommend that the endotracheal tube be advanced into the right mainstem bronchus when the trachea is exposed to prevent accidental puncture of the endotracheal tube cuff and allow sealing of the airway if bleeding occurs.[12] After the trachea is incised, the endotracheal tube is partially withdrawn until the surgeon can see the tip just above the level of the tracheotomy incision. The surgical airway is placed at this time. The administration of 100% oxygen is recommended up until the time when the surgical airway is secured and breath sounds are auscultated bilaterally. This precaution will allow some oxygen reserve if the airway is lost when the endotracheal tube is withdrawn. After the tracheotomy is complete, the tracheal portion superior to the tracheotomy site should be gently suctioned because blood can pool in that region.

Complications of tracheotomy include tracheoesophageal fistula, creation of a false passage, damage to the recurrent laryngeal nerve, subcutaneous emphysema, pneumothorax, bleeding, and aspiration.

Triple Endoscopy

Triple endoscopy is a term used to describe three separate procedures performed during the staging of head and neck cancer patients: direct laryngoscopy, esophagoscopy, and bronchoscopy. Anesthetizing patients for triple endoscopy can be challenging not only because of potential abnormalities in airway anatomy but also because the procedure is usually brief and intensely stimulating. Short-acting anesthetics, narcotics, and muscle relaxants usually produce the best results.

It is prudent to discuss any plans for airway management with the otolaryngologist before the patient is brought to the operating room. As was previously discussed, some patients with head and neck cancer require awake intubations or tracheotomy under local anesthesia. If this is the case, general anesthesia cannot be induced until the airway has been secured.

Patients who can be safely induced before intubation can be given one of several intravenous induction agents. The choice depends on the patient's coexisting medical problems. Thiopental sodium, etomidate, and propofol are commonly used induction agents. Elderly patients may require a smaller dose and may take longer to respond to these medications. Some anesthesiologists prefer inhalation induction in patients with airway pathology.

In most patients, it is appropriate to administer additional medication to blunt the hemodynamic response to intubation and surgical stimulation. (Because a sterile surgical field is not possible, the procedure usually begins as soon as the endotracheal tube is secured, intubation is confirmed, and the table is turned.) Narcotics (fentanyl and alfentanil), short-acting beta blockers (esmolol), and lidocaine can be effective for this purpose. One group of investigators found alfentanil 10 μg/kg to be an excellent agent for blunting the hemodynamic response to endotracheal intubation in elderly patients. It was also found that this dose does not result in excessive myocardial depression.[13]

Muscle relaxation is required during endoscopy to decrease the risk of trauma to the teeth and the aerodigestive tract tissues.[14] Many endoscopy patients are given ultra-short-acting muscle relaxants such as succinylcholine and mivacurium during induction because there is always the potential for a difficult intubation. The pharyngeal muscles recover rapidly from a muscle relaxant. When a patient swallows, it makes endoscopy more difficult. If additional muscle relaxant is required for maintenance, a succinylcholine infusion can be started (in patients who received succinylcholine at induction) or a short-acting nondepolarizing muscle relaxant can be administered (atracurium, mivacurium).

The anesthetic can be maintained with a volatile agent, an intravenous agent (propofol infusion plus short-acting narcotic), or a combination of the two. The drug choice is based on the patient's underlying medical condition. For example, patients with bronchospastic disease often benefit from the administration of a volatile agent and patients with cardiac disease often benefit from a narcotic-based technique.

As with many ENT procedures, the head of the operating table may be turned 90 degrees away from the anesthesiologist to give the surgeons access to the patient's head. Good communication is essential whenever there is a "shared airway."

During *direct laryngoscopy*, a rigid endoscope is used to examine the structures of the upper aerodigestive tract, including the palate, tonsils, tongue, pharynx, and larynx. The examining surgeon will request that a small endotracheal tube be placed so that the larynx can be easily examined. A 6.0 to 7.0-mm-internal-diameter endotracheal tube is adequate. Once it is in place, the endotracheal tube should be taped onto the left side of the patient's face to improve surgical access. It is crucial that the endotracheal tube position be continuously monitored during endoscopy, because migration or dislodgement of the tube can occur during the procedure. Dysrhythmias can also result from stimulation of the larynx. If this occurs, the surgeon should be asked to stop momentarily until the abnormal rhythm clears. If the dysrhythmia recurs upon reinsertion of the laryngoscope, intravenous lidocaine can be administered or the superior laryngeal nerve can be blocked. One review suggests that it may be safer to reschedule the procedure when recurrent dysrhythmias present and recommends superior laryngeal nerve block before anesthetic induction on the next occasion.[14]

For *esophagoscopy*, a rigid scope is passed orally into the esophagus to the level of the gastroesophageal junction. The endotracheal tube cuff may have to be deflated temporarily to facilitate passage of the esophagoscope. Again, the position of the endotracheal tube must be monitored carefully. When the esophagoscope passes the aortic arch, some patients develop reflex bradycardia, requiring intervention.[12] Perforation of the esophagus, with subsequent mediastinitis, is a potentially life-threatening complication of esophagoscopy. Unfortunately, the perforation is not easily recognized intraoperatively. More commonly, a patient with an esophageal perforation goes into the recovery room and develops chest pain, fever, tachycardia, and possibly pneumomediastinum or pneumothorax. The diagnosis of perforation is confirmed by chest x-ray and contrast studies. These patients then require immediate evaluation by a thoracic surgeon.

During *bronchoscopy*, a rigid scope is used to examine the subglottic airway, trachea, and bronchi. The bronchoscope is positioned past the larynx in one of two ways. If the endotracheal tube is small enough, the cuff can be deflated and the bronchoscope can be slipped alongside the endotracheal tube. The other method requires removal of the endotracheal tube. In this case, a ventilating bronchoscope is positioned above the true vocal cords, the endotracheal tube is removed, and the bronchoscope is placed in the trachea. Ventilation can resume through the bronchoscope. The endotracheal tube is replaced upon completion of the procedure.

Although standard anesthetic induction, intubation, and ventilation through an endotracheal tube are used for most endoscopic procedures in geriatric patients, some anesthesiologists and otolaryngologists prefer that a *jet entila-*

tion technique be implemented for microlaryngeal surgery.[15] The advantage is an unobstructed surgical field. Jet ventilation is accomplished by attaching a needle to the proximal end of a bronchoscope to make a jet injector.[16] This needle delivers intermittent bursts of oxygen at high pressure. With this system, a Venturi effect is created, using room air. Good chest expansion can occur and results in satisfactory ventilation at normal inflation pressures in patients with normal lungs. The danger of excessive pressure is minimal in adults because air can leak back around the bronchoscope through the glottis.[17] Anesthesia must be maintained with intravenous agents. Several drugs can be used for total intravenous anesthesia. The combination of propofol, alfentanil, and a muscle relaxant has been shown to be ideal for microlaryngeal procedures when jet ventilation is used.[15] The risks of jet ventilation include barotrauma (e.g., subcutaneous emphysema, mediastinal emphysema), inflation of the stomach, aspiration, and mucosal dehydration.

Laser surgery of the airway is rarely performed in geriatric patients for laryngeal tumor excision. This type of surgery has inherent safety hazards because the laser beam can ignite flammable materials such as the endotracheal tube, the breathing circuit, drapes, and lubricants. In addition, human tissue can be burned. Safety precautions can prevent most serious injuries.[18] Eye protection is required for the patient and the operating room personnel when a carbon dioxide laser is in use. Exposed areas of the patient's skin must be covered with moist towels. The endotracheal tube must be "protected" with metallic tape and moist cottonoids, or a metal tube can be used. The endotracheal tube cuff should be filled with saline and protected with a saline-soaked gauze that can be positioned by the surgeon before laser use. Ideally, the oxygen concentration administered should be kept as low as possible. Helium or air can be used to lower the oxygen concentration. Alternative techniques that avoid the risk of endotracheal tube fire include jet ventilation through a metal needle (see above) and apneic laser ablation.[18–20] With any technique, the use of muscle relaxants is recommended because it is very important that the patient not move.

In the event of an endotracheal tube fire, the following steps should be taken:

1. Stop the gas flow.
2. Disconnect the patient from the breathing system and extubate the patient.
3. Ventilate through a mask until reintubation is possible.
4. Reintubate.
5. Perform bronchoscopy immediately to assess the extent of the injury.
6. If the injury is severe, perform a tracheotomy.
7. Administer steroids (and antibiotics if indicated).
8. Admit the patient to the intensive care unit.

Injury to the tracheobronchial tree occurs as a result of both the burn and toxicity from the products of combustion and smoke inhalation.

Biopsy of a tumor during endoscopy often produces tissue edema. Intravenous steroids help minimize the amount of airway swelling. Sometimes there is bleeding from the biopsy site, and this can irritate the larynx and lead to laryngospasm. Therefore, extubation must be performed with caution. It is best to make postoperative airway management decisions jointly with the surgeon.

Total Laryngectomy and Composite Resection

Cancer of the head and neck is best treated with surgical ablation. Most major surgical procedures for such cancers fall into two broad categories: total laryngectomy and composite resection.

Total laryngectomy requires removal of the larynx. A permanent tracheal stoma is created through which the patient can breathe or be ventilated. In the operating room, this is best accomplished by placing a flexible endotracheal tube (anode tube) into the stoma. A tracheostomy tube is not required when the patient is awake and breathing well. A patient who has had a total laryngectomy cannot be intubated orally, because the stoma is the only airway.

Composite resection is a general term used to describe the removal of a portion of a patient's tongue, floor of mouth, or tonsil in combination with some mandibular bone (Fig. 19-2). All patients receiving a composite resection require a tracheotomy postoperatively.

Metastatic tumors of the head and neck tend to spread to the lymphatics in the neck. Therefore, most head and neck cancer operations incorporate a unilateral or bilateral neck dissection as part of the definitive therapy. The removal of lymphatic tissue requires surgical manipulation near the carotid bulb. This can cause dysrhythmias and blood pressure fluctuations that may be poorly tolerated in elderly patients. When this occurs, the surgeon can infiltrate the tissues near the carotid sinus with a local anesthetic to prevent this response.[21]

Blood loss can be difficult to estimate during head and neck oncological surgery, because much of the blood lost will not be in the suction cannisters.

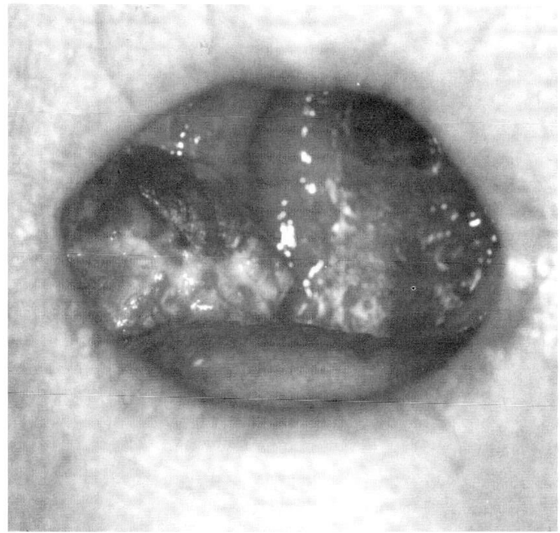

Figure 19-2 Large right tonsillar cancer in an 86-year-old woman.

Typically, blood is lost as a "slow ooze" throughout the duration of the procedure. On occasion, however, blood loss can be rapid because of the close proximity of the carotid artery and the internal jugular vein. The use of controlled hypotension to minimize blood loss during head and neck surgery is controversial and cannot be recommended for the majority of geriatric patients undergoing these procedures. The average blood loss in major head and neck oncological procedures is in the range of 750 to 1500 ml. The average procedure takes 6 to 10 hours to complete.

Most patients undergoing extensive head and neck operations will have a tracheotomy or tracheostomy postoperatively. Patients who do not require a surgical airway usually can be extubated postoperatively. All these patients require close observation postoperatively and are often admitted to an intensive care unit.

Parotid Surgery

Both benign and malignant tumors of the parotid gland occur in elderly patients; therefore, superficial parotidectomy is an operation commonly performed on geriatric patients. Anesthetic management is similar to that described for other head and neck operations, but there are a few special considerations. After induction, the endotracheal tube should be secured on the contralateral side of the face. The surgeon will electrically stimulate the facial nerve during the surgical dissection and will have to observe the ipsilateral eyelid. Therefore, tape should not be placed over the ipsilateral eye.

Muscle relaxants can be administered during the induction of anesthesia but are best avoided during the surgical procedure. This can be difficult in elderly patients, who may not tolerate a deep inhalation anesthetic, especially when a head-up position is required. Narcotics can be useful in this situation because they suppress ventilatory drive and inhibit coughing without causing profound decreases in blood pressure. If the surgeon is agreeable, a short-acting muscle relaxant at less than the full dose may provide an acceptable compromise.

FACIAL PLASTIC AND RECONSTRUCTIVE SURGERY

A growing number of geriatric patients are seeking facial plastic surgery to improve their normal function and appearance.[22] Examples of frequently performed procedures include blepharoplasty, facial lifting, chemical face peeling, and reconstructive surgery after the excision of facial skin cancers (Fig. 19-3).

Many of these procedures are routinely performed under local anesthesia. As was previously discussed, geriatric patients have fewer perioperative complications when procedures are performed using only local anesthesia. Therefore, intravenous sedation should be used sparingly. Some reconstructive

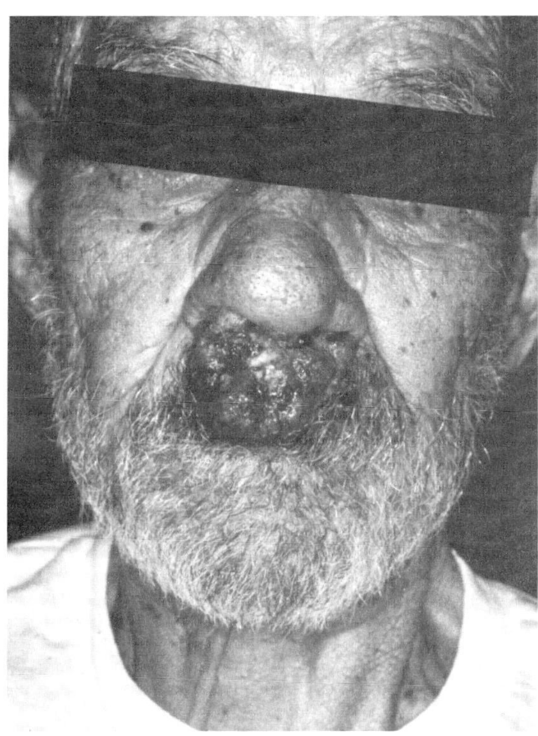

Figure 19-3 Squamous cell carcinoma of the upper lip in a 105-year-old man.

procedures require general anesthesia, and the same principles discussed for head and neck cancer operations apply.

Chemical Face Peeling

Chemical peeling is performed on geriatric patients to remove wrinkles and other skin imperfections. During the process, a combination of substances (including phenol) is applied to the facial skin. The procedure is performed under local anesthesia, but in most cases, intravenous sedation is necessary because the skin appears to retain sensation to the insult of exfoliation despite the use of a local anesthetic.[23]

These patients require close monitoring perioperatively. High blood levels of phenol may cause cardiotoxicity, hepatotoxicity, and nephrotoxicity. Cardiac dysrhythmias can occur during the chemical treatment as a result of phenol absorption.[23] Patients with a history of cardiac dysrhythmias and those with renal or hepatic insufficiency are the most susceptible. When any abnormal cardiac rhythm appears, the current recommendation is to stop the chemical treatment until normal sinus rhythm has returned for 15 min.[23] Cardiac dysrhythmias are usually transient. Hydration is important for clearance of phenol from the bloodstream via the kidney.

OTOLOGIC PROCEDURES

Although hearing loss is a common problem in geriatric patients, it is usually not amenable to surgical treatment. Most otologic procedures in the geriatric population are performed to treat chronic ear disease.[24]

Many ear operations, such as those on the tympanic membrane, can be done under local anesthesia. An advantage of this method is that an awake patient may be able to perceive a change in hearing during the procedure so that the success of the operation may be predicted.[25] More commonly, ear operations are done under general anesthesia. The following sections discuss general anesthetic considerations for otologic surgery.

Nitrous Oxide

Nitrous oxide (N_2O) is 34 times more soluble than nitrogen. This can cause problems in a closed space because N_2O enters the space faster than nitrogen can escape. If the closed space is compliant, the volume of the space will expand. If the closed space is noncompliant, the pressure will increase.

The middle ear is an air-filled noncompliant space. Several studies have demonstrated increases in middle ear pressure during use of N_2O (Fig. 19-4).[26,27] Conversely, cessation of N_2O use may result in negative pressure. The eustachian tube helps decompress the middle ear under normal circumstances. If there is underlying ear disease or edema from surgical trauma, normal equalization of pressure does not occur. This helps explain how tympanic membrane

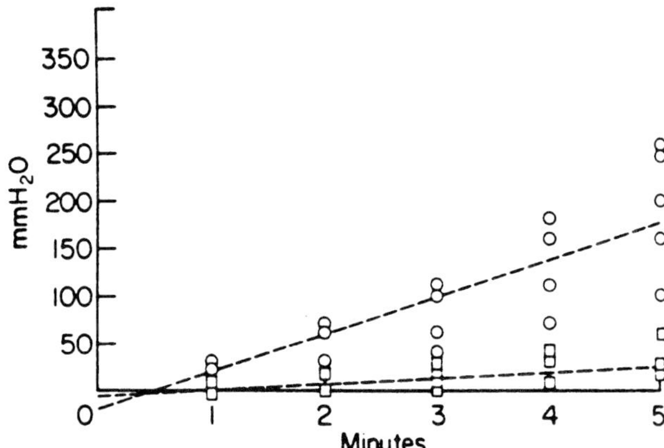

Figure 19-4 **Rate of increase of middle ear pressure. □—□ Group A: spontaneous ventilation with oxygen and halothane. ○—○ Group B: spontaneous ventilation with oxygen, halothane, and nitrous oxide.** ***(Reproduced with permission from Casey WF, Drake-Lee AB: Nitrous oxide and middle ear pressure: A study of induction methods in children. Anaesthesia 37:896, 1982.)***

rupture and displacement of surgical grafts have occurred during N_2O use. Reports of such cases exist in the literature but are rare.[28]

During middle ear operations, a closed space does not exist until the surgeon begins to close the middle ear. Each otolaryngologist will have a preference regarding the use of N_2O during middle ear surgery. It is prudent to discuss these concerns with the surgeon before N_2O is used. If N_2O is an important part of the anesthetic, it can be used as long as it is discontinued 30 min before closing begins or any time the surgeon has difficulty with graft placement.[21] N_2O is a relatively insoluble gas, and its uptake and washout from the blood are rapid.

N_2O may have other adverse effects on patients with ear disease. Several cases of sensorineural hearing loss have been attributed to pressure changes in the middle ear induced by N_2O. However, the patients involved had undergone previous stapedectomy operations.[25]

Neuromuscular Blocking Agents

Facial nerve preservation is an important part of otologic surgery. However, facial nerve stimulation is not necessary for most otologic procedures. Therefore, the use of muscle relaxants usually is not contraindicated. Immobility of the patient is essential during microsurgery because small movements are magnified under the microscope. Although volatile anesthetics are ideal in healthy patients undergoing middle ear surgery because N_2O and narcotics (which may increase nausea) can be avoided, many geriatric patients cannot tolerate a deep inhalational anesthetic.

Induced Hypotension

A bloodless operative field is desirable during microsurgery of the ear because a very small amount of blood can diminish visualization. Induced hypotension has been advocated to achieve this goal, although some investigators were unable to find any correlation between the degree of hypotension and the perceived operating conditions.[29] Geriatric patients may experience compromised perfusion of vital organs when this technique is used.

Other measures that can be used to improve operating conditions include elevation of the head of the operating table and infiltration of the tissues with epinephrine. These measures also have limitations. Head elevation increases the risk of venous air embolism, and epinephrine absorption can result in hemodynamic changes and dysrhythmias. Good anesthetic management can help improve operating conditions by preventing acute elevations in central venous pressure. For example, positive end-expiratory pressure (PEEP) can raise venous pressure and increase the amount of bleeding. PEEP should therefore be avoided.[12]

SUMMARY

Many ENT surgical procedures are performed on geriatric patients. Some ENT procedures are performed to diagnose and treat head and neck cancers. Others are performed to treat chronic ear disease or improve patient appearance and function. Elderly patients have altered drug requirements and may have coexisting diseases that affect the anesthetic management. In all cases, good communication and cooperation between the anesthesiologist and the surgeon are essential.

REFERENCES

1. Cantrell RW: Etiologic factors in the development of cancer, in Goldstein JC, Kashima HK, Koopmann CF (eds): *Geriatric Otolaryngology*. Burlington, Ontario: B.C. Decker, 1989, pp 148–157.
2. McGuirt WF, Loevy S, McCabe BF, Krause CJ: The risks of major head and neck surgery in the aged population. *Laryngoscope* 87:1378, 1977.
3. Tucker HM: Conservation laryngeal surgery in the elderly patient. *Laryngoscope* 87:1995, 1977.
4. Koopmann CF: Otolaryngologic (head and neck) problems in the elderly. *Med Clin North Am* 75(6):1373, 1991.
5. Leopold DA, Lagoe RJ: Hospital mortality for otolaryngologic disorders in New York state. *Arch Otolaryngol Head Neck Surg* 114:416, 1988.
6. Natof HE: *FASA Special Study I*. Alexandria, VA: Federated Ambulatory Surgery Association, 1985.
7. Pasternak LR: Anesthetic considerations in otolaryngological and ophthalmological outpatient surgery. *Int Anesthesiol Clin* 28(2):89, 1990.
8. Dauchot PJ, Lina AA: Geriatric anesthesia, in Brown DL (ed): *Risk and Outcome in Anesthesia*, 2d ed. Philadelphia: Lippincott, 1992, pp, 527–540.
9. McLeskey CH: Anesthesia for the geriatric patient, in Barash PG, Cullen BF, Stoelting RK (eds): *Clinical Anesthesia*, 2d ed. Philadelphia: Lippincott, 1992, pp 1353–1387.
10. McLeskey CH, Nibel DM: Anesthesia for the geriatric outpatient, in White PF (ed): *Outpatient Anesthesia*. New York: Churchill Livingstone, 1990, pp 343–367.
11. Tarver CP, Noorily AD, Sakai CS: A comparison of cocaine vs. lidocaine with oxymetazoline for use in nasal procedures. *Arch Otolaryngol Head Neck Surg* 109:653, 1993.
12. Brown ACD: Anesthesia, in Cummings CW, Fredrickson JM, Harker LA, et al (eds): *Otolaryngology—Head and Neck Surgery*. St. Louis: Mosby, 1986, pp 185–214.
13. Kirby IJ, Northwood D, Dodson ME: Modification by alfentanil of the haemodynamic response to tracheal intubation in elderly patients: A dose-response study. *Br J Anaesth* 60:384, 1988.
14. Norton ML, Strong MS: Anesthesia for endoscopic diagnosis and surgery. *Otolaryngol Clin North Am* 14(3):687, 1981.
15. De Grood PMRM, Mitsukuri S, VanEgmond J, et al: Comparison of etomidate and propofol for anaesthesia in microlaryngeal surgery. *Anaesthesia* 42:366, 1987.

16. Sanders RO: Two ventilating attachments for bronchoscopes. *Del Med J* 39:170, 1967.
17. Spoerel WE, Grant PA: Ventilation during bronchoscopy. *Can Anaesth Soc J* 18(2):178, 1971.
18. Hermens JM, Bennett MJ, Hirschman CA: Anesthesia for laser surgery. *Anesth Analg* 62:218, 1983.
19. Weisberger EC, Miner JD: Apneic anesthesia for improved endoscopic removal of laryngeal papillomata. *Laryngoscope* 98:693, 1988.
20. Hawkins DB, Joseph MM: Avoiding a wrapped endotracheal tube in laser laryngeal surgery: Experiences with apneic anesthesia and metal laser-flex endotracheal tubes. *Laryngoscope* 100:1283, 1990.
21. Feinstein R, Owens WD: Anesthesia for ear, nose, and throat surgery, in Barash PG, Cullen BF, Stoelting RK (eds): *Clinical Anesthesia*, 2d ed. Philadelphia: Lippincott, 1992, pp 1113–1124.
22. Tardy ME, Toriumi D, Broadway D: Facial plastic and reconstructive surgery in an aging population: A critical overview, in Goldstein JC, Kashima HK, Koopmann CF (eds): *Geriatric Otolaryngology*. Burlington, Ontario: B.C. Decker, 1989, pp 168–183.
23. McCollough EG, Langsdon PR: The maskless chemical face peel. *Dermatol Clin* 5(2):381, 1987.
24. Korper SP: Epidemiologic and demographic characteristics of the aging population, in Goldstein JC, Kashima HK, Koopmann CF (eds): *Geriatric Otolaryngology*. Burlington, Ontario: B.C. Decker, 1989, pp 19–28.
25. Jahrsdoerfer RA: Anesthesia in otologic surgery. *Otolaryngol Clin North Am* 14(3):699, 1981.
26. Casey WF, Drake-Lee AB: Nitrous oxide and middle ear pressure: A study of induction methods in children. *Anaesthesia* 37:896, 1982.
27. Davis I, Moore JRM, Lahari SK: Nitrous oxide and the middle ear. *Anaesthesia* 34:147, 1979.
28. Owens QD, Gustave F, Sclaroff A: Tympanic membrane rupture with nitrous oxide anesthesia. *Anesth Analg* 57:283, 1978.
29. Eltringham RJ, Young PN, Fairbairn MD, et al: Hypotensive anaesthesia for microsurgery of the middle ear: A comparison between enflurane and halothane. *Anaesthesia* 37:1028, 1982.

CHAPTER 20

Outpatient Anesthesia in the Geriatric Population

Mary Ann Gurkowski

INTRODUCTION

Ambulatory surgery in the elderly is a fairly new practice for the medical profession. To lower health care costs, particularly Medicare expenditures, the government has begun reviewing the required length of stay for all surgical procedures. It has mandated that several procedures that previously were performed only on an inpatient basis be performed in an outpatient setting. Before the mandate, there were no clinical studies showing the safety of this approach. Therefore, this idea can be viewed as experimental, and only in time will the feasibility and safety become apparent. Even now there is very little scientific literature regarding the cost-effectiveness, feasibility, and safety of ambulatory surgery in the elderly.

There is information regarding patient satisfaction. According to a 1989 report by the Office of the Inspector General, regardless of sex, surgical setting, procedure, or relative age, elderly patients prefer an ambulatory setting to an inpatient setting (Fig. 20-1).[1]

Historically, all patients about to undergo a surgical procedure were admitted to the hospital 1 or 2 days before surgery. This allowed a fairly thorough preoperative evaluation to be performed, and if necessary, the opinions of other consultants could be obtained. After the operation, patients would remain in the hospital for at least 24 h and usually longer.

In the past, a patient having a breast biopsy would stay postoperatively over 3 days and hernia operations had postoperative stays in excess of 5 days.

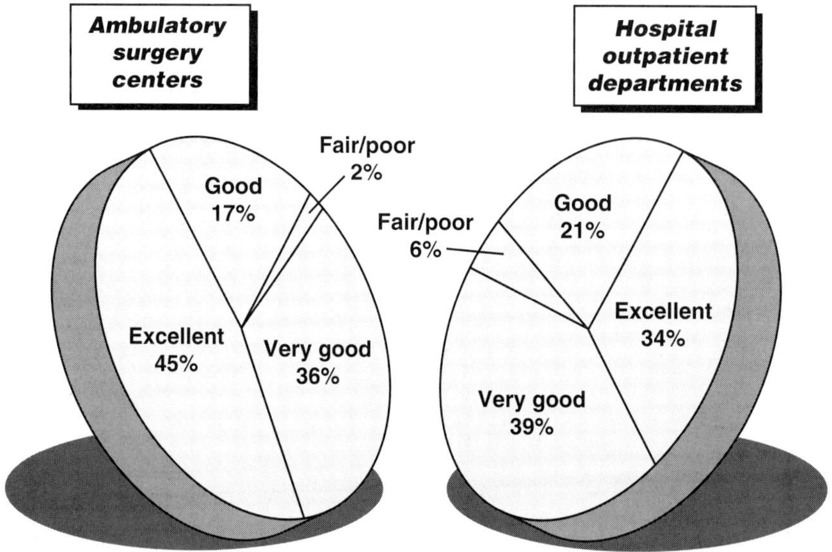

Figure 20-1 How do the elderly rate ambulatory surgical care? *(From Koska MT: Ambulatory surgery gets high marks from the elderly. Hospitals 64:55, 1990. Reprinted from Hospitals, Vol. 64, No. 7, by permission, April 5, 1990, Copyright 1990, American Hospital Publishing, Inc.)*

Patients undergoing colonoscopy were admitted the day before surgery to receive a bowel prep, which now is performed by the patient at home.

In the 1990s, almost every surgical subspecialty has a procedure that can be performed on an outpatient basis. These subspecialties include but are not limited to gynecology, ophthalmology, orthopedics, podiatry, otorhinolaryngology, urology, gastroenterology, plastic surgery, and general surgery.

PATIENT SELECTION

It is important to remember that aging is a multifactorial process that every patient experiences daily. This aging process eventually leads to an impaired ability to adapt to sudden changes because of the gradual decline in functional reserve of the body's organ systems. When one is considering whether a patient is an acceptable candidate for outpatient surgery, several factors must be analyzed. The first is the patient's physical status. In general terms, the patient should be in reasonably good health. Using the American Society of Anesthesiologists' Physical Status Classification (Table 20-1) can provide a common ground that allows both the anesthesiologist and the surgeon to communicate. This classification views a patient not as an age but as a state of health. Age no

Table 20-1 The American Society of Anesthesiologists' physical status classification

Classification	Description
Class I	A healthy patient Example: Inguinal hernia in an otherwise healthy patient
Class II	A patient with mild systemic disease Examples: chronic bronchitis, moderate obesity, diet-controlled diabetes mellitus, old myocardial infarction, mild hypertension
Class III	A patient with severe systemic disease that is not incapacitating Examples: coronary artery disease with angina, insulin-dependent diabetes mellitus, morbid obesity, moderate to severe pulmonary insufficiency
Class IV	A patient with incapacitating systemic disease that is a constant threat to life Examples: organic heart disease with marked cardiac insufficiency, unstable angina, intractable arrhythmias, advanced pulmonary, renal, hepatic, or endocrine insufficiency
Class V	A moribund patient not expected to survive 24 h with or without operation Example: ruptured abdominal aneurysm with profound shock
Emergency (E)	The suffix "E" is used to denote the presumed poorer physical status of any patient in one of these categories who is operated on as an emergency (e.g., 2E).

SOURCE: Wetchler BV: *Anesthesia for Ambulatory Surgery*, 2d ed. Philadelphia: Lippincott, 1991, p 99. With permission.

longer appears to be a limiting factor to outpatient surgery, as it was years ago. Meridy[2] stated that his data confirmed previous studies that found that the extremes of age are not a deterrent in the selection of ambulatory surgical patients. In the 1920s, some physicians suggested that "an elective operation for inguinal hernia repair in a patient older than 50 years was not justified." Just 10 years ago, only physical status class I and class II patients were considered candidates for outpatient surgery; now it is not uncommon to have class III patients present for outpatient surgery. The classic example is a centenarian who has insulin-dependent diabetes, moderate hypertension, and mild chronic obstructive pulmonary disease and is scheduled for cataract surgery.

The essential consideration in evaluating a patient for outpatient surgery is how stable is the patient's illness. The down side to relaxing the selection criteria is an increased percentage of unplanned hospital admissions, ranging from 0.02 to 0.6 percent for physical status class I and class II patients to 0.5 to 1.5 percent for physical status class III patients.[3]

The second factor is that the patient must be agreeable to having surgery as an outpatient. The patient must also be able to understand the process fully. An otherwise healthy patient with organic brain syndrome will not be able to follow the preoperative and postoperative instructions. Many elderly patients feel uneasy about returning home after an operation because they will have to provide their own postoperative care.

The third factor is the need for a responsible person to care for the patient postoperatively. Both sedative drugs and general anesthetics can create an impaired mental ability for many hours postoperatively. For this reason, it is preferable that the designated responsible person not only transport the patient home but also supervise the first 24 h of home care. Therefore, this person needs to be intellectually and physically capable of providing the required care and following the postoperative instructions given upon discharge from the facility.

The fourth factor is postoperative hospitalization. Some surgeries require a postoperative stay even if the patient comes in as an outpatient, for example, a patient undergoing laparoscopic cholecystectomy. Integrated hospital outpatient facilities can usually accept somewhat sicker patients much more easily than can a freestanding facility.

To summarize, an elderly patient who is a candidate for outpatient surgery should want to have the surgery performed in this manner, be in physically stable condition, and be able to provide a responsible person for postoperative care.

SPECIAL CONCERNS

Special concerns need to be considered in dealing with the geriatric patient population. These patients usually take longer than a younger patient to accomplish required tasks. Such tasks include getting from the parking lot to the outpatient waiting area, filling out the register and hospital questionnaires, and changing clothes. Because of these delays, it is important to ask an elderly patient to arrive earlier on the morning of surgery. Patience on the part of the caretaker is vital. An elderly patient should not be hurried or made to feel as if he or she were slowing down the process. These patients are often less able to adapt to a new environment and may become agitated or confused if left alone. Therefore, it is important to provide them with constant interaction with the staff or a family member.

In addition to these psychological concerns, the elderly are more likely to have physical handicaps. In general, they are less agile and require assistance with tasks such as changing clothes and climbing onto a stretcher. They may not want to ask for this assistance, and so one should plan on helping without waiting to be asked. Providing the right kind of equipment aids can also be helpful. Elderly patients may have problems getting in and out of chairs that are low and do not have armrests. They will also need a footstool with a handle in order to climb onto and off of the stretcher.

PREOPERATIVE EVALUATION

The preoperative evaluation ideally should be performed first by the surgeon to determine whether the patient is a candidate for outpatient surgery. If there is any doubt, an anesthesia preoperative consult should be obtained. Most elderly patients can benefit from seeing the anesthesiologist before the morning of surgery, but this is not always practical or feasible. Therefore, it is important that the patient's medical problems be addressed in a systematic fashion so that nothing is overlooked. This evaluation should include a careful review of the medical record, an in-depth conversation with the patient, and a review of the patient's recent laboratory values and preoperative tests. In obtaining the history, it is important to be aware that the patient may not hear or see well. Therefore, the physician should position himself or herself in good light and speak slowly and directly to the patient. It is often helpful to ask if the patient has a hearing impairment and, if so, which ear hears better. When providing the patient with preoperative instructions, it is then very important to stop and ask if the patient understood what the physician just told him or her. If the physician is unsure of the patient's understanding, the patient should be asked to repeat the instructions. If the patient is medically stable and there is no need for further workup, additional treatment, or medication adjustment, it is appropriate to proceed with surgery on an outpatient basis.

PREOPERATIVE LABORATORY TESTS

In the past, laboratory tests were requested primarily for screening purposes: A battery of tests would be performed to search for unsuspected disease. The rationale was that finding an abnormality would be beneficial to the patient as early diagnosis. This approach is now considered inappropriate, expensive, and unjustified. Studies that have looked at this method of laboratory screening often compare the usefulness with the cost-effectiveness of bulk testing.[4,5] Many of these studies have reached a similar conclusion. Abnormal test results occur occasionally but generally much less often than would be expected. The great majority of the abnormalities identified do not lead to a new diagnosis, being either lab errors or false-positive tests, and even in the few patients in whom a new diagnosis is established, there is generally no reason to alter the agreed on surgical plan.[6] Therefore, it is currently recommended that all preoperative laboratory tests be ordered after completion of the history and physical examination. No routine laboratory or diagnostic screening should be performed. Instead, the tests ordered should be guided by the abnormalities noted during the preoperative evaluation or the nature of the surgery to be performed. Other physicians have stated that tests should be obtained only when their results will actually be part of the decision-making process.[6] According to Cochrane,[7] "When considering whether to order a test, ask yourself what you would do if the test results were positive and what you would do if they were negative. If the answers are the same, don't order the test." Whether a list of mandatory preoperative tests is created should be based on the patient population using the outpatient surgery facility. The more homogeneous the population is, the more effective the cost-benefit ratio will be. For example, at the author's county hospital, because there is such a high incidence of diabetes and obesity in this population, almost every patient over 40 years of age has a baseline electrocardiogram performed. The more heterogeneous the patient population is, the more efficient the cost-benefit ratio becomes when laboratory tests are not mandatory but, as was stated earlier, are based on the history and physical examination. Table 20-2 provides a schema for minimal preoperative testing.

PREOPERATIVE MEDICATION

The rationale for using preoperative medication, especially in an age of rapidly expanding new anesthetics, should not be based on tradition. The fact that an anesthesiologist was trained to always give a premedicant such as glycopyrrolate does not mean that it needs to be given. It is important in the 1990s to tailor pharmacologic preoperative medications to fit the outpatient's needs both intraoperatively and postoperatively. It is important to remember that these patients will be going home the same day, possibly only a few hours after their arrival. Medications, dosages, and routes of administration must be practical and short-acting so that they do not prolong the length of stay in the postanesthesia care unit (PACU). The goals for a preoperative pharmacologic preparation need to be tailored to the patient's physical and psychological condition at the time of surgery. The most commonly given preoperative medications include benzodiazepines, opioids, anticholinergics, antacids, and H_2-receptor antagonists. It

Table 20-2 A recommended schema for minimal preoperative testing

Test to be obtained	HGB M	F	WBC	PT / PTT	PLT BT	Elect	Creat/ BUN	Blood Gluc	SGOT/Alk PTASE	X-ray	ECG	Preg.	T/S
Preoperative conditions													
Suspected													
Surgical procedure													
With blood loss	X	X											X
Without blood loss													
Neonates	X	X											
Age <40		X											
Age 40–59		X									±		
Age >60	X	X								X	X		
Cardiovascular disease							X			X	X		
Pulmonary disease										X	X		
Malignancy	X	X	*	*									
Radiation therapy			X							X	X		
Hepatic disease				X					X				
Exposure to hepatitis									X				
Renal disease	X	X				X	X						
Bleeding disorder				X	X								
Diabetes						X	X	X			X		
Smoking ≥20 pack-years	X	X								X			
Possible pregnancy												X	
Diuretic use						X	X						
Digoxin use						X	X				X		
Steroid use						X		X					
Anticoagulant use	X	X		X									

M = male; F = female; HGB = hemoglobin; WBC = white blood count; PT = prothrombin time; PTT = partial thromboplastin time; PLT = platelet count; BT = bleeding time; Elect = electrolytes; Creat/BUN = creatinine or blood urea nitrogen; SCOT/ALK PTASE = serum glutamic oxaloacetic transaminase phosphatase; Preg = pregnancy test; T/S = blood typing and screening for unexpected antibodies; ± = possibly; * = leukemias only; X = obtain.

SOURCE: Reprinted with permission from Orkin FK, Gold B: Selection, in Wetchler BV (ed): *Anesthesia for Ambulatory Surgery*, 2d ed. Philadelphia: Lippincott, 1991, p 112.

is extremely important to verify that the patient has taken (antihypertensive) or not taken (insulin) his or her chronically administered medications on the morning of surgery. It is important to allow at least 1 h for absorption, which may require a delay before suctioning the oral gastric tube. The decision to administer any of these premedicants should be based on the patient's medical problems and the anesthetic plan. It is vital that the benzodiazepine and opioids be titrated to the desired effect. Since many elderly patients have a slower circulation time than their younger counterparts, it is advisable to wait a couple of minutes before dosing the patient again intravenously.

MONITORING

All patients undergoing a general anesthetic, regional anesthetic, or monitored anesthesia care on an outpatient basis require the same monitoring standards used with an inpatient. The American Society of Anesthesiologists has a list of required standard monitors (Table 20-3). The need for monitoring beyond these standards should be based on the patient's physical status and the nature of the surgery. For example, patients with stable coronary disease in whom significant blood loss is possible may benefit from the placement of an arterial line. A patient with stable angina may also benefit from monitoring two leads on the electrocardiogram (ECG), such as leads II and V5. Just as the ordering of preoperative lab tests should not be based solely on the fact that a patient is elderly, neither should the decision to perform intraoperative monitoring.

ANESTHETIC TECHNIQUES

Before considering the advantages and disadvantages of the various anesthetic techniques, it is important to remember that the older the patient, the greater the physical frailty. Older patients' skin, as well as their veins, can be very thin and delicate. The adhesive tape and bandages used for younger patients can tear the skin in the elderly. An older patient is also much less agile and flexible than a younger patient. Therefore, care should be taken when positioning the patient on the operating room table. Extra padding around the bony protuberances is recommended to prevent compression sores and nerve injury.

Monitored Anesthesia Care

Local Anesthesia

Surgeries that can be performed under local anesthesia without sedation generally provide a greater margin of safety because the physiological trespass with local anesthesia is less. Evidence suggests that geriatric patients have an improved prognosis if the surgical procedure is performed under local anesthe-

Table 20-3 Standards for basic anesthetic monitoring

STANDARDS FOR BASIC ANESTHETIC MONITORING
(Approved by House of Delegates on October 21, 1986, and last amended on October 13, 1993)

These standards apply to all anesthesia care, although in emergency circumstances, appropriate life support measures take precedence. These standards may be exceeded at any time based on the judgment of the responsible anesthesiologist. They are intended to encourage quality patient care, but observing them cannot guarantee any specific patient outcome. They are subject to revision from time to time, as warranted by the evolution of technology and practice. They apply to all general anesthetics, regional anesthetics, and monitored anesthesia care. This set of standards addresses only the issue of basic anesthetic monitoring, which is one component of anesthesia care. In certain rare or unusual circumstances, (1) some of these methods of monitoring may be clinically impractical, and (2) appropriate use of the described monitoring methods may fail to detect untoward clinical developments. Brief interruptions of continual[@] monitoring may be unavoidable. *Under extenuating circumstances, the responsible anesthesiologist may waive the requirements marked with an asterisk* (*); it is recommended that when this is done, it should be so stated (including the reasons) in a note in the patient's medical record. These standards are not intended for application to the care of an obstetric patient in labor or in the conduct of pain management.

[@] Note that "continual" is defined as "repeated regularly and frequently in steady and rapid succession," whereas "continuous" means "prolonged without any interruption at any time."

STANDARD I
Qualified anesthesia personnel shall be present in the room throughout the conduct of all general anesthetics, regional anesthetics, and monitored anesthesia care.

Objective
Because of the rapid changes in patient status during anesthesia, qualified anesthesia personnel shall be continuously present to monitor the patient and provide anesthesia care. In the event there is a direct known hazard, e.g., radiation, to the anesthesia personnel that might require intermittent remote observation of the patient, some provision for monitoring the patient must be made. If an emergency requires the temporary absence of the person primarily responsible for the anesthetic, the best judgment of the anesthesiologist will be exercised in comparing the emergency with the anesthetized patient's condition and in the selection of the person left responsible for the anesthetic during the temporary absence.

STANDARD II
During all anesthetics, the patient's oxygenation, ventilation, circulation, and temperature shall be continually evaluated.

(*continues*)

Table 20-3 (*continued*)

OXYGENATION

Objective
To ensure adequate oxygen concentration in the inspired gas and the blood during all anesthetics.

Methods
1. Inspired gas: During every administration of general anesthesia using an anesthesia machine, the concentration of oxygen in the patient breathing system shall be measured by an oxygen analyzer with a low oxygen concentration limit alarm in use.*
2. Blood oxygenation: During all anesthetics, a quantitative method of assessing oxygenation such as pulse oximetry shall be employed.* Adequate illumination and exposure of the patient are necessary to assess color.*

VENTILATION

Objective
To ensure adequate ventilation of the patient during all anesthetics.

Methods
1. Every patient receiving general anesthesia shall have the adequacy of ventilation continually evaluated. While qualitative clinical signs such as chest excursion, observation of the reservoir breathing bag, and auscultation of breath sounds may be adequate, quantitative monitoring of the CO_2 content and/or volume of expired gas is encouraged.
2. When an endotracheal tube is inserted, its correct positioning in the trachea must be verified by clinical assessment and by identification of carbon dioxide in the expired gas.* End-tidal CO_2 analysis, in use from the time of endotracheal tube placement, is strongly encouraged.
3. When ventilation is controlled by a mechanical ventilator, there shall be in continuous use a device that is capable of detecting disconnection of components of the breathing system. The device must give an audible signal when its alarm threshold is exceeded.
4. During regional anesthesia and monitored anesthesia care, the adequacy of ventilation shall be evaluated, at least, by continual observation of qualitative clinical signs.

CIRCULATION

Objective
To ensure the adequacy of the patient's circulatory function during all anesthetics.

Methods
1. Every patient receiving anesthesia shall have the electrocardiogram continuously displayed from the beginning of anesthesia until preparing to leave the anesthetizing location.*

(*continues*)

Table 20-3 (*continued*)

2. Every patient receiving anesthesia shall have arterial blood pressure and heart rate determined and evaluated at least every 5 mins.*
3. Every patient receiving general anesthesia shall have, in addition to the above, circulatory function continually evaluated by at least one of the following: palpation of pulse, auscultation of heart sounds, monitoring of a tracing of intraarterial pressure, ultrasound peripheral pulse monitoring, or pulse plethysmography or oximetry.

BODY TEMPERATURE

Objective
To aid in the maintenance of appropriate body temperature during all anesthetics.

Methods
There shall be readily available a means to continuously measure the patient's temperature. When changes in body temperature are intended, anticipated, or suspected, the temperature shall be measured.

SOURCE: "Standards for Basic Anesthetic Monitoring" is reprinted with permission of the American Society of Anesthesiologists, 520 N. Northwest Highway, Park Ridge, IL 60068-2573.

sia rather than general or major regional anesthesia.[8] It has also been shown that patients who receive local anesthesia spend a significantly shorter period in the PACU than does the rest of the population, and significantly fewer of these patients have to be admitted to the hospital.[2] It is vital to remember that the patient is awake and that a kind, reassuring word is often all that is needed if the patient becomes anxious. It is important to tell the patient before the surgery starts that he or she will feel traction and pressure but nothing sharp. If the patient feels pain, he or she should tell the care giver and more local anesthetic can be injected. It is important to remember that infiltration by local anesthetics does not work instantaneously; once an injection is made, several minutes must elapse before the surgery can continue. It is also important to calculate the maximum allowable milligrams of the local anesthetic and compare this with the amount being given. The surgeon should be kept informed so that a toxic amount is not administered. Local anesthetics are not benign and can have profound effects on the CNS and the cardiovascular system. Tucker[9] looked at the pharmacokinetics of local anesthetics and concluded that old age uncomplicated by disease has a relatively minor effect on the kinetics of the drug. However, concomitant illnesses that affect the liver, kidneys, or cardiovascular system and may impair an elderly person's ability to metabolize or excrete the drug are important and can lead to toxicity.

As was mentioned in the introduction to this chapter, positioning of the patient is very important. Unlike a general anesthetic, where positioning is vital in the prevention of nerve damage, positioning in an awake patient is done for comfort. An older patient finds it difficult to lie still on an operating room table for lengthy periods without padding. The use of a jelly pad or foam pad can lessen the hardness of the table. A pillow under the knees helps minimize the lumbar lordosis and lends slight flexion to the hips to reduce discomfort. Extra padding such as soft foam to the arm pads provides comfort to the joints of the upper extremities. In addition, if the arms can be folded over the upper chest, this may be more comfortable than having them abducted. Most important, before prepping and draping, the patient should be asked how he or she feels and what can be done to help him or her feel more comfortable.

Conscious Sedation

Local anesthesia is often combined with conscious sedation. This helps the patient tolerate the injection of the local and provides the immobility the surgeon often requests. Elderly patients often have an increased sensitivity to sedative drugs. For instance, midazolam has been shown by Harper and colleagues[10] to have an increased elimination half-life in patients over age 50. In older patients, it is safest if the drug chosen for sedation is titrated to the desired effect, using small increments. It is important to wait a couple of minutes between dosings to be sure that the peak effect has been reached. Elderly patients often have a very slow circulation time, thus delaying the onset of sedation. A very commonly used combination of drugs for sedation is midazolam and fentanyl. The judicious use of an opioid can help with the pain in an area that has been difficult to anesthetize (e.g., scar tissue). Propofol, because of its short $t_{1/2}$, may have advantages compared with other sedative drugs in the elderly. It has been demonstrated that propofol used for a general anesthetic in patients older than age 80 can result in reduced postanesthetic mental impairment compared with a control group.[11] Although this study looked at general anesthesia, there is no reason to think the results would differ for conscious sedation. Oxygenation is usually unaffected by local anesthetic alone, but when sedative drugs are added, desaturation may occur.[12] Therefore, the use of supplemental oxygen is recommended during conscious sedation in the elderly. An exception to this recommendation is a patient who is known to have chronic obstructive pulmonary disease and a hypoxic ventilatory drive.

Regional Anesthesia

Many types of regional anesthetic techniques have been used in elderly outpatients. The more commonly performed blocks include retrobulbar blocks, wrist blocks, ankle blocks, axillary nerve blocks, subarachnoid blocks, and epidurals. The selection of an anesthetic technique should be influenced not only by the patient's medical condition and surgical needs but also by the anesthesiologist's experience and skill. One of the primary advantages of regional anesthesia in the elderly is that minimal to no sedation is needed if the block is effective. This reduces the postoperative incidence of mental confusion. It has been demonstrated that relatively modest doses of sedative agents can produce mental impairment postoperatively, similar to that resulting from general anesthesia.[13]

Once again, it is important to remember that oversedation can lead to hypoventilation and hypoxemia, and so the addition of supplemental oxygen is highly recommended. The incidence of diabetes increases with age. Regional anesthesia techniques allow diabetic patients to drink and eat earlier in the postoperative period, interfering less with their normal routine.

Other advantages of performing certain surgical procedures in the elderly under regional anesthesia rather than general anesthesia include (1) reduced postoperative negative nitrogen balance, (2) amelioration of endocrine stress responses to surgery, (3) reduction in blood loss, and (4) reduced incidence of postoperative thromboembolic complications.[14]

It is important to discuss subarachnoid block in more detail here. Spinal anesthesia has been widely used in the elderly, but the decision whether to use it in outpatients is controversial. One of the advantages often mentioned regarding spinal or epidural is the opportunity to converse with the patient during the surgery. This provides an assessment of intellectual function that may serve as a gauge of the adequacy of cerebral perfusion. Similarly, allowing a patient to remain conscious during a subarachnoid block or epidural allows patient recognition of an angina attack. Another advantage is that the patient can clear his or her own secretions and benefits from the protection of functional ciliary epithelium.[15] McKenzie and Wishart showed that the Pa_{O_2} was greater immediately postoperatively in patients undergoing lower extremity surgery under spinal versus general anesthesia.[16] One often cited disadvantage of spinal anesthesia in an outpatient is the potential occurrence of postspinal headache. Although postspinal headaches are much less common in the elderly than they are in younger patients, they can still be troublesome, especially in an elderly patient with a history of congestive heart failure. A narrow window may exist between the ability to force fluid intake or provide intravenous hydration to treat the headache and the development of the symptoms of fluid overload. Some anesthesiologists advocate an immediate epidural blood patch rather than conservative therapy with fluid and hydration in an elderly patient who develops a postspinal headache. Another disadvantage is that spinal anesthesia in the geriatric population usually lasts longer; therefore, there is a delay in ambulation because of prolonged sympathetic blockade, postural hypotension, and urinary retention. Because of this postoperative delay, it is wise to schedule these surgeries early in the morning to allow for a longer recovery time.

General Anesthesia

Even though the above information on regional anesthesia mentioned some of the disadvantages of general anesthesia in elderly patients, outcome studies have found that there is no difference in long-term survival of patients given general versus spinal anesthesia.[17] The superiority of spinal over general anesthesia in the elderly has not been proved. The opinions are usually based on impressions and tradition, not on prospective studies.[18]

When one is administering a general anesthetic, it is important to remember that with aging, significant changes occur that affect drug uptake, distribution, and elimination. For example, there is a reduction in lean body mass and an increase in the percentage of adipose tissue as one ages. The latter change is more significant in females. Therefore, lipid-soluble drugs such as diazepam have a larger volume of distribution and slower elimination. In addition, renal and hepatic blood flow may be reduced, which again slows the elimination of most drugs. The distribution of drugs may be slowed because of a depressed cardiac output. This results in early high serum levels and a potential for excessive CNS and cardiovascular depression. There is also a reduction in the minimum alveolar concentration of inhalational anesthetics with advancing age and a greater variability of response.[19]

These are only a few of the physiological changes that can affect the administration of a general anesthetic in a geriatric patient. All these factors need to be considered when one is choosing the drugs to administer, especially in elderly outpatients. It is best to choose drugs with a short elimination half-life and with few metabolites, minimal cardiovascular effects, and minimal CNS side effects. In the last 5 years, there has been an explosion of drugs that fulfill one or more of these criteria. These drugs include desflurane, sevoflurane, propofol, alfentanyl, vecuronium, mivacurium, and atracurium. To reemphasize earlier statements, the key to the administration of any drug in the elderly is titration. One must avoid boluses calculated on the basis of milligrams per kilogram. Standard dosages per kilogram frequently produce unwanted depression. For example, Peacock and colleagues showed that slower administration of propofol to elderly patients allowed the investigators to observe that half the calculated dose injected rapidly was sufficient to induce anesthesia in this population.[20] Similarly, mivacurium produces a fall in blood pressure when administered rapidly in the elderly that can largely be avoided by administering it slowly over 30 s to a minute.

It is also important to realize that elderly patients are more prone to aspiration. Their airway reflexes are depressed, and they have a higher incidence of gastric reflux and esophagitis.[21] Therefore, it is wise to consider intubation rather than a mask technique and to provide aspiration prophylaxis to geriatric outpatients undergoing a general anesthetic.

RECOVERY

Even though the logistics of where to have an outpatient recover may vary depending on the anesthetic administered and the type of outpatient facility, the goals are the same. An elderly outpatient must not be discharged until he or she is "home-ready."

A patient who has received a general anesthetic in the author's institution is given humidified oxygen on arrival to the PACU. Vital signs are taken at least every 15 min. As soon as the patient is fully awake, he or she is gradually elevated to a semisitting position. If this is tolerated the patient is transferred to a wheelchair and given ice chips. The patient must fulfill the criteria on the

Table 20-4 Aldrete scoring system

Postanesthesia recovery score	In	15	30	45	Hours	Out
Activity						
Able to move voluntarily or on command						
4 extremities	2	2	2	2	2	2
2 extremities	1	1	1	1	1	1
0 extremities	0	0	0	0	0	0
Respiration						
Able to deep breathe and cough freely	2	2	2	2	2	2
Dyspnea, shallow or limited breathing	1	1	1	1	1	1
Apneic	0	0	0	0	0	0
Circulation						
Preoperative blood pressure ____ mm						
BP ± 20 mm of preanesthesia level	2	2	2	2	2	2
BP ± 20 to 50 mm of preanesthesia level	1	1	1	1	1	1
BP ± 50 mm of preanesthesia level	0	0	0	0	0	0
Consciousness						
Fully awake	2	2	2	2	2	2
Arousable on calling	1	1	1	1	1	1
Not responding	0	0	0	0	0	0
Color						
Normal	2	2	2	2	2	2
Pale, dusky, blotchy, jaundiced, other	1	1	1	1	1	1
Cyanotic	0	0	0	0	0	0
Dismissal criteria: total score of 10, plus stable vital signs						
A physician's order is required for discharge with lower score						
				Total		____

SOURCE: Wetchler BV: *Anesthesia for Ambulatory Surgery*, 2d ed. Philadelphia: Lippincott, 1991, p 378. With permission.

Aldrete Scale (Table 20-4) and achieve a score of 10 before being released from the PACU. The patient is then transported back to the outpatient suite and placed in a comfortable reclining chair. The patient's sponsor or family member is now able to assist in the postoperative care. Oral intake is started. When the patient can tolerate oral intake and ambulate to the toilet and void, the patient is ready for discharge. All the patient's prescriptions are filled and brought to the outpatient area to facilitate discharge.

Some outpatient facilities do not require oral intake or voiding as a prerequisite for discharge. As long as the patient's vital signs are stable, ambulation is documented, and the patient is free of vomiting and has only minimal pain, the patient is considered ready for discharge. The patient is then taken by wheelchair to a waiting car and helped inside. It is important to provide the patient not only with verbal but also with written postoperative orders. These orders should also be given to the patient's sponsor or family member. Elderly patients require a longer time to synthesize the instructions, and this problem can be minimized by repetition.

SUMMARY

Outpatient surgery is a valid option for the elderly population. It can be performed safely, providing an elderly patient with a convenient cost-saving alternative. Ambulatory surgery can be a potentially positive experience because separation from familiar surroundings, family members, and friends is kept to a minimum. Outpatient surgery is no longer limited to American Society of Anesthesiologists (ASA) I and ASA II patients: Stable ASA III patients can also be candidates. All these patients require special care and handling. Patience on the part of the operating room, recovery room, and outpatient facility personnel is essential. Anesthetic techniques need to take into account the changes in metabolism and drug uptake and elimination that occur in geriatric patients. It is important not only to adjust the drug doses but also to titrate the drugs to the desired effect.

REFERENCES

1. Koska MT: Ambulatory surgery gets high marks from the elderly. *Hospitals* 64:55, 1990.
2. Meridy HW: Criteria for selection of ambulatory surgical patients and guidelines for anesthetic management: A retrospective study of 1553 cases. *Anesth Analg* 61:921, 1982.
3. Wetchler BV: Anesthesia for outpatients, in Mauldin BC (ed): *Ambulatory Surgery: A Guide to Perioperative Nursing Care.* New York: Grune & Stratton, 1983, pp 111–158.
4. Kaplan EB, Sheiner LB, Boeckman AJ, et al: The usefulness of preoperative laboratory screening. *JAMA* 253:3576, 1985.
5. Johnson H, Knee-Loli S, Butler TA: Are routine preoperative laboratory screening tests necessary to evaluate ambulatory surgical patients? *Surgery* 104:639, 1988.
6. Orkin FK, Gold B: Selection, in Wetchler BV (ed): *Anesthesia for Ambulatory Surgery.* Philadelphia: Lippincott, 1991, chap 3, pp 81–125.
7. Cochrane AL: *Effectiveness and Efficiency: Random Reflections on Health Services.* London: Nuffield Provincial Hospital Trust, 1972, chap 5, pp 26–44.
8. Backer CCL, Tinker JH, Robertson DM, Vleistra RE: Myocardial reinfarction following local anesthesia for ophthalmic surgery. *Anesth Analg* 59:257, 1980.
9. Tucker GT: Pharmacokinetics of local anaesthetics. *Br J Anaesth* 58:717, 1986.
10. Harper KW, Collier PS, Dundee JW, et al: Age and operation influence: The pharmacokinetics of midazolam. *Br J Anaesth* 57:866, 1985.
11. Servin F, Pommereau R, Rowan C, et al: Comparison of intraoperative course and

recovery with etomidate or propofol in patients over 80 years. *Anesthesiology* 73:A318, 1990.
12. Muravchick S, Johnson R: Oxygenation of peripheral tissues in young and elderly patients during spinal anesthesia. *Reg Anaesth* 7:7, 1986.
13. Chung FF, Chung A, Meier RH, et al: Comparison of perioperative mental function after general anaesthesia and spinal anaesthesia with intravenous sedation. *Can J Anaesth* 36:382, 1989.
14. McLeskey CH: Anesthesia for the geriatric patient, in Barash PG, Cullen BF, Stoelting RK (eds): *Clinical Anesthesia*, 2d ed. Philadelphia: Lippincott, 1992, pp 1301–1337.
15. Sullivan DR, Siker ES: The pros and cons of regional anesthesia, in Stephen GR, Assaf RA (eds): *Geriatric Anesthesia Principles and Practice.* London: Butterworth, 1986, chap 12, pp 277–290.
16. McKenzie PJ, Wishart HG: Comparison of the effects of spinal anaesthesia and general anaesthesia on postoperative oxygenation and perioperative mortality. *Br J Anaesth* 51:49, 1980.
17. Valentin N, Lomhalt B, Jensen JS, et al: Spinal or general anaesthesia for surgery of the fractured hip? A prospective study of 578 patients. *Br J Anaesth* 58:284, 1986.
18. Apfelbaum JL, Surinder KK, Wetchler BV: Adult and geriatric patients, in Wetchler BV (ed): *Anesthesia for Ambulatory Surgery.* Philadelphia: Lippincott, 1991, chap 5, pp 197–307.
19. Roizen ME, Horrigan R, Frazer B: Anesthetic doses blocking adrenergic (stress) and cardiovascular responses to incision—MAC BAR. *Anesthesiology* 54:390, 1981.
20. Peacock JE, Lewis RP, Reilly CS, et al: Effect of different rates of infusion of propofol for inducing anaesthesia in elderly patients. *Br J Anaesth* 60:346, 1990.
21. Pontoppidan H, Beecher HK: Progressive loss of protective reflexes in the airway with advanced age. *JAMA* 118:77, 1961.

CHAPTER 21

Postoperative Analgesia in Geriatric Patients

Kelly Gordon Knape

INTRODUCTION

There is now increased awareness of the importance of adequate postoperative pain control in elderly surgical patients. The scope of this awareness includes not only the humane aspects but also the costs in terms of clinical outcome and monetary expense. With regard to postoperative pain, the significance of providing good analgesia is becoming more apparent, especially in complicated patients. No patients have a greater potential for being complicated than those from the geriatric population. The historical practice of minimizing postoperative pain medication in the elderly for fear of complications is giving way to a more rational multimodal approach to providing analgesia.

Many concerns must be addressed before one determines the form of pain relief to provide to an elderly patient postoperatively. These include psychological factors and the nature of the surgical procedure. It is also important to review the specific anatomic, physiologic, and pharmacologic considerations of age as they relate to analgesic techniques. An outline of recommendations for the management of postoperative pain in geriatric patients is provided in Table 21-1.[1]

Table 21-1 Guidelines for the rational use of analgesics

1. Choose a specific drug based on type of pain, its intensity, patient's age, and prior opioid exposure
2. Know the clinical pharmacology of the drug prescribed
   - Duration of analgesic effect
   - Pharmacokinetic properties of drug
   - Equianalgesic doses for route of administration
3. Administer analgesic on a regular basis after initial titration
4. Use drug combinations that provide additive analgesia or reduce side effects (opioid + nonopioid, opioid + hydroxyzine, opioid + amitriptyline)
5. Avoid drug combinations that increase sedation without enhancing analgesia
6. Adjust the route of administration to type of pain, patient status, and available routes
7. Watch and treat side effects appropriately
   - Respiratory depression
   - Sedation
   - Nausea and vomiting
   - Constipation
   - Multifocal myoclonus and seizures
8. Know the differences between tolerance, physical dependence, and psychological dependence

SOURCE: Adapted from Foley KM: Pain management in the elderly, in Hazzard WR, Andres R, Bierman EL, Blass JP (eds): *Principles of Geriatric Medicine and Gerontology*, 2d ed. New York: McGraw-Hill, 1990, p 287.

PSYCHOLOGICAL OVERLAY

All patients, including the elderly, have preexisting emotional factors that have an impact on the effectiveness of analgesia and the overall outcome. By the time patients have reached an advanced age, pain-related behaviors and patterns of dependency are usually well established. Dealing with loss or the presence of depression also commonly affects the success of all the therapies involved. Determining dosing and the adequacy of pain control is difficult when these factors exist.[2]

Patients usually have preconceived ideas about how much pain they should be able to tolerate without medication. Some are stoic or afraid of taking potent pain medications. Fear of addiction is not uncommon and must be considered. These patients need to be reassured that addiction is rare and that pain relief can minimize other problems, including nausea. Other patients tolerate little if any pain and become demanding. Time-contingent dosing (medications given on a fixed schedule) and patient-controlled devices are usually helpful in these cases.

The treatment of patients who have chronic problems related to pain or depression is potentially more difficult. If these patients are already on medications, the medications should be continued whenever possible. In managing the pain of these individuals, it may be necessary to consult the patient's psychiatrist or a chronic pain specialist. Patients with chronic pain and depression present a challenge when those problems are compounded by perioperative stresses, including acute pain.

"Loss" is a common complicating factor in managing patients postoperatively. The need to deal with the loss of an extremity or organ occurs more frequently in older patients because of their increased incidence of vascular disease, diabetes, and cancer. These patients are also more likely to be concerned with death and may feel that surgery is the prodrome. Common to almost all patients is the loss of control felt when one has to be hospitalized and is seemingly forced to depend on the decisions and care of others.

As often as possible, patients should feel included in decision making and in their own care. It is especially important to ask the patient to provide input about which medications and modalities for pain have been effective in the past and which have caused bothersome side effects. Techniques are available that allow patients to determine dosing frequency independently of the nurse or physician in the form of bedside preprogrammed dispensing devices such as patient-controlled analgesia (PCA) pumps.

PAIN INTENSITY BY SURGICAL SITE

Knowing the location of the surgical site can help one predict the severity of postoperative pain. Superficial procedures are usually the least painful, while truncal surgery is the most painful. With respect to thoracic incisions, a thoracotomy is more painful than is a sternotomy. Upper abdominal incisions, especially subcostal (open cholecystectomy) and flank, are much more uncomfortable than are lower abdominal incisions. Laparoscopy has helped minimize the need for large painful incisions. Orthopedic procedures, particularly those performed on large joints, can also cause significant discomfort. Total knee arthroplasty appears to be more painful than are total hip procedures.[3] If one understands the potential degree of postoperative pain, it is possible to plan an optimal analgesic regimen and initiate it early.

THE ARMAMENTARIUM

Anesthesiologists often have the greatest knowledge about analgesic drugs and techniques, making them the most qualified to manage pain. They are well suited to manage elderly patients and their specific needs and problems. The multiplicity of modalities available postoperatively will not be covered in depth in this chapter but is summarized in Table 21-2.

Table 21-2 Medical, anesthetic, surgical, and behavioral approaches to pain

Type of approach	Indications
Drug therapy	
Nonopioid analgesics	Mild to moderate somatic and visceral pain
Opioid analgesics	Moderate to severe somatic and visceral pain
Anesthetic approaches with local anesthetics	
Trigger point injections	Local myofascial pain
Joint capsule injections	Local inflammatory joint pain
Epidural	Perioperative and postoperative pain control or peripheral vascular disease
Intrathecal	Perioperative pain control
Physical therapy approaches	
Bracing, splinting, and mechanical devices	Arm, leg, or joint support to minimize pain and facilitate activity
Transcutaneous nerve stimulation	Manage mild peripheral nerve point pain
Full ROM* and ADL+ programs	Reduce limitations at joints secondary to extremity pain
Behavioral approaches (cognitive-behavioral)	
Relaxation Biofeedback Hypnosis	Comprehensive approach to manage the psychological consequences of pain, the meaning and the impact of pain on mood

*ROM = range of motion; +ADL = activities of daily living.

SOURCE: Adapted from Foley KM: Pain management in the elderly, in Hazzard WR, Andres R, Bierman EL, Blass JP (eds): *Principles of Geriatric Medicine and Gerontology*, 2d ed. New York: McGraw-Hill, 1990, pp 285–286.

SYSTEMIC ANALGESICS: ORAL AGENTS

Whenever possible, oral analgesics should be used because of their relative safety compared with parenteral medications and more invasive modalities. The limitations of oral administration include inadequacy of analgesia for severe pain, existing postoperative ileus, and gastrointestinal irritation. Oral agents should be considered as first-line therapy after superficial and peripheral surgical procedures when pain is expected to be mild to moderate in intensity (Table 21-3).

Opioids

Because of their efficacy in alleviating moderate to severe pain, opioids are commonly used to control postoperative pain (Table 21-4). Of course, postoperative intubation and the presence of an ileus preclude the use of the oral route. For most major surgery, oral opiates are initiated after a few days, when the analgesic regimen is being changed from parenteral or continuous regional techniques.

Anti-inflammatory Drugs

Nonsteroidal anti-inflammatory drugs (NSAIDs) are effective nonnarcotic analgesics that can be used postoperatively for moderate pain or in combination with narcotics to help minimize their side effects. NSAIDs should be included in the analgesic regimen if the pain is related to inflammation, as is commonly seen in elderly patients with inflammatory joint disease. In addition to the analgesic effect, the anti-inflammatory effect has been shown to decrease the complication of heterotopic bone formation after total hip replacement and thus the incidence of reoperation.[4] Diclofenac sodium has been shown to be effective in significantly reducing and shortening the postoperative inflammatory response observed after cataract extraction. The side effects were negligible.[5]

The side effects of NSAIDs are noteworthy. Potential problems include gastrointestinal (GI) irritation, bleeding, and renal insufficiency. GI reactions may be as minimal as an upset stomach or as serious as bleeding or perforation. Risk factors for developing serious GI events include not only previous use (especially during the first 3 months of therapy), a previous history of GI problems, and corticosteroid use but also age above 60 years. In fact, there appears to be a 10-fold greater risk for GI surgery in the elderly patient using NSAIDs. With respect to the agent used, piroxicam (Feldene) tends to have the highest risk; indomethacin (Indocin) and aspirin have a very low risk; and naproxen (Anaprox, Noprosyn) and ibuprofen (Motrin) have the lowest risk.[6] Even though the decrease in platelet function is reversible, excessive bleeding is still more likely to occur. NSAIDs are generally safe when a moderate risk of bleeding is not critical. They are also safe in patients with normal kidney

Table 21-3 Analgesics commonly used orally for mild to moderate pain

Drug	Equianalgesic dose, mg*	Starting oral dose range, mg†	Comments
Nonnarcotics			
Aspirin	650	650	Often used in combination with opioid-type analgesics
Acetaminophen	650	650	Minimal anti-inflammatory properties
Ibuprofen (Motrin)	ND‡	200–400	Higher analgesic potential than aspirin
Fenoprofen (Nalfon)	ND	200–400	Like ibuprofen
Diflunisal (Dolobid)	ND	500–1000	Longer duration of action than ibuprofen; higher analgesic potential than aspirin
Naproxen (Naprosyn)	ND	250–500	Like diflunisal
Ketorolac (Toradol)	ND	5–10	Like ibuprofen; do not exceed 40 mg daily; do not exceed 120 mg (PO + IM) on day of transition from IM; bioavailability 80–100 percent
Morphinelike agonists			
Codeine	32–65	32–65	"Weak" morphine; often used in combination with nonopioid analgesics; biotransformed, in part to morphine
Oxycodone	5	5–10	Shorter acting; also in combination with aspirin (Percodan) or acetominophen (Percocet), which limits dose escalation
Meperidine (Demerol)	50	50–100	Shorter-acting; biotransformed to normeperidine, a toxic metabolite
Propoxyphene (Darvon)	65–130	65–130	"Weak" narcotic; often used in combination with nonopioid analgesics; long half-life biotransformed to potentially toxic metabolite (norpropoxyphene)

(*continues*)

Table 21-3 (*continued*)

Drug	Equianalgesic dose, mg*	Starting oral dose range, mg†	Comments
Mixed agonist-antagonist			
Pentazocine (Talwin)	50	50–100	In combination with nonopioid; in combination with naloxone to discourage parenteral abuse; causes psychotomimetic effects

*For these equianalgesic doses, the time of peak analgesia ranges from 1.5 to 2 h and the duration from 4 to 6 h. Oxycodone and meperidine are shorter-acting (3–5 h), and diflunisal and naproxen are longer-acting (8 to 12 h).

† These are the recommended starting doses from which the optimal dose for each patient is determined by titration and the maximal dose is limited by adverse effects.

‡ ND = not determined.

SOURCE: Adapted from Foley KM: Pain management in the elderly, in Hazzard WR, Andres R, Bierman EL, Blass JP (eds): *Principles of Geriatric Medicine and Gerontology*, 2d ed. New York: McGraw-Hill, 1990, p 228.

function. However, prostaglandin inhibition may reduce prostaglandin-regulated renal blood flow. This is clinically significant in patients with heart failure, liver disease, or preexisting renal compromise. NSAIDs should be employed perioperatively only if used in the short term and if there are no other risk factors present that may contribute to renal impairment.[7]

Acetaminophen

Acetaminophen is one of the most commonly used oral agents, especially for mild pain. It is used in combination with an opioid in treating moderate postoperative pain. It has minimal anti-inflammatory effects, though it does have antipyretic effects. Acetaminophen should be used with caution postoperatively, as it can mask a developing infection-related fever. The elderly are less able to mount a significant febrile response, and so the use of a drug with an antipyretic effect can delay the diagnosis of a serious infection.

SYSTEMIC ANALGESICS: PARENTERAL AGENTS

Parenteral administration usually refers to an intramuscular (IM) injection, an intravenous (IV) injection or infusion, and occasionally cutaneous or subcutaneous (SQ) injection or transdermal delivery. IM "shots" have traditionally been the easiest to administer, usually not requiring a registered nurse (RN),

Table 21-4 Oral and parenteral opioid analgesics for moderate to severe pain

Drug	Equianalgesic dose, mg	Duration, h*	Plasma half-life, h	Comments
Ketorolac	15–30 IM†	6	4.7–8.6	Loading dose 3–60 mg; use half loading dose for maintenance; if less than 50 kg, use lowest IM doses; do not exceed 120 mg (PO + IM) on day of transition from IM; do not exceed 40 mg PO daily
	5–10 PO	4–6	4.7–8.6	
Narcotic agonists				
Morphine	10 IM	4–6	2–3.5	Standard for comparison; also available in slow-release tablets; reduce dose in elderly and in renal failure
	30–60 PO	4–7		
Codeine	130 IM	4–6	3	Biotransformed to morphine; useful as initial opioid analgesic
	200 PO	4–6		
Oxycodone (Percodan, Percocet)	15 IM	?	?	Short-acting; available alone or as 5-mg dose in combination with aspirin and acetaminophen
	30 PO	3–5	?	
Levorphanol (Levo-Dromoran)	2 IM	4–6	12–16	Good oral potency; requires careful titration in initial dosing because of drug accumulation; use cautiously in elderly
	2–4 PO	4–7	12–16	
Hydromorphone (Dilaudid)	1.5 IM	4–5	2–3	Available in high-potency injectable form (10 mg/ml) for cachectic patients and as rectal suppositories; more soluble than morphine
	4–7.5 PO	4–6	2–3	
Oxymorphone (Numorphan)	1 IM	4–6	2–3	Available in parenteral and rectal-suppository forms only
	10 PR	4–6	2–3	
Meperidine	75 IM	3–4	3–4	Contraindicated in patients with renal disease; accumulation of active toxic metabolite normeperidine produces CNS excitation
	300 PO	4–6	12–16	

Methadone hydrochloride (Dolophine)	10 IM 5–20 PO	? ?	15–30 ?	Good oral potency; requires careful titration of the initial dose; drug accumulation occurs
Mixed agonist-antagonist drugs				
Pentazocine (Talwin)	60 IM 180 PO	4–6 4–7	2–3 2–3	Limited use for chronic pain; psychotomimetic effects with dose escalation; available only in combination with naloxone, aspirin, or acetaminophen; may precipitate withdrawal in physically dependent patients
Nalbuphine (Nubain)	10 IM ? PO	4–6 ?	5 ?	Not available orally; less severe psychotomimetic effects than pentazocine; may precipitate withdrawal in physically dependent patients
Butorphanol (Stadol)	2 IM	4–6	2.5–3.5	Not available orally; produces psychotomimetic effects; may precipitate withdrawal in physically dependent patients
Partial agonists				
Buprenorphine (Buprenex)	0.4 IM	4–6	?	No psychotomimetic effects; may precipitate withdrawal in tolerant patients

*Based on single-dose studies in which an intramuscular dose of each drug listed was compared with morphine to establish the relative potency. Oral doses are those recommended when changing from a parenteral to an oral route. For patients without prior narcotic exposure, start with the lowest dose.

†IM = intramuscular; PO = oral; PR = rectal.

SOURCE: Adapted from Foley KM: Pain management in the elderly, in Hazzard WR, Andres R, Bierman BL, Blass JP (eds): *Principles of Geriatric Medicine and Gerontology*, 2d ed. New York: McGraw-Hill, 1990, p 290.

as with IV injection. IM absorption can be unpredictable, especially in an obese or muscle-wasted patient or if a patient is cold, which is a common problem in the elderly in the immediate postoperative period.[8] Time to effect is also limited by the fact that the patient has to wait for the nurse to respond and then retrieve the medication. Also, the IM route is painful and becomes more so when multiple injections are required (Table 21-4 discusses IM dosing). IV routes are preferred because of their predictability and relative ease, though nursing policy may limit their use if they are ordered "IV push." Continuous infusions are seemingly ideal in that a constant plasma level may be maintained, though side effects, particularly opioid-related respiratory depression, may be more common. For example, when fentanyl infusions were used at a dose of 125 μg/h, a third of the patients developed respiratory depression.[9] The rate must be titrated carefully, especially as pain levels start to diminish after the first 24 to 48 h postoperatively.

Nonnarcotics: Ketorolac

Ketorolac (Toradol) is a parenteral NSAID that is very effective for moderate pain. It can be used to supplement IV or neuraxial narcotic regimens, with the potential to help minimize their side effects. Although approved only for IM administration, it has been used successfully in otherwise healthy patients via the IV route. Reports have emerged, however, of patients developing acute renal compromise after IV use. Therefore, the same caveats apply to ketorolac administration as apply to other NSAIDs (see above). The important consideration is that this drug provides a means of utilizing the advantages of NSAIDs in patients who cannot take oral medications in the immediate postoperative period.

Opioids

Opioids are commonly used via the IM (Table 21-4) or IV route to treat moderate to severe postoperative pain. Analgesia can also be provided via a transdermal system with fentanyl to provide constant blood levels, with results not unlike those obtained by a continuous infusion. These patches slowly release drug into the skin, and the drug is absorbed into the circulation. Even after the patch is removed, the skin acts as a depot, with continued absorption and effective analgesia for 12 to 24 h. The patches should be placed (usually on the upper chest) at least 12 h before the completion of surgery to allow for their latency. This will ensure an adequate postoperative analgesic blood concentration. Supplementation with additional narcotic may still be needed, especially in the first 12 to 24 h postoperatively. For abdominal procedures, the recommended rate is 50 to 75 μg/h patch release. Depending on the adequacy of analgesia or the side effects, the dose is increased or decreased on the second day. The patch is usually removed on the third postoperative day. Nausea is common, though it may be related to pain caused by not placing the patch early enough. As with a continuous infusion, the potential for respiratory depression still exists.[10] The manufacturer of the fentanyl patch warns of its risks when used for acute postoperative pain. It is FDA-approved only for chronic pain. The FDA recommends starting at the lowest dose (25 μg/h) for patients who have not been previously exposed to opioids, and not using the patch for outpatients.

Intravenous PCA is the preferred parenteral route because of its ease of administration and effectiveness. PCA generally uses less opioid and thus reduces the incidence of nausea. Patient satisfaction is also the highest compared with other techniques because of the patient's ability to have some control over his or her care and the elimination of anxiety related to delay in pain relief. It also saves on nursing demands, resulting in improved care. Most pumps have three options that have to be set: bolus or demand dose, lockout period in minutes, and maximum dose per unit of time. A background infusion may also be programmed on some devices. The benefits of an infusion in addition to the demand PCA dose is debatable. It has the potential to reduce demands, especially in the first few hours postoperatively, and therefore can provide better analgesia during that period. Analgesia also may be better in patients who would otherwise underdose themselves as a result of poor understanding or fear of overdose or addiction. Side effects, including excessive sedation, nausea, and respiratory depression, can develop if the background infusion is not titrated carefully.[11]

Morphine and meperidine are the most commonly used PCA narcotics, but fentanyl can also be used (Table 21-5). When fentanyl is used with PCA plus a background infusion, age does not appear to be a factor in the dose requirement. In regard to the operative site, abdominal procedures require higher doses than do peripheral vascular procedures.[12]

Problems that occur with PCA devices most commonly are due to programming errors or misunderstandings about their use. Respiratory depression also can occur. Especially in the elderly, it is usually related to a very large bolus or loading dose, which can also be programmed into most pumps.[13] The patient should be instructed initially and repeatedly to ensure understanding and proper use. Often patients underdose themselves for fear of side effects or the development of dependence. The family members and friends of patients should be instructed that only the patient is allowed to push the demand button. Being too caring has led to overdoses when someone else activated the PCA while the patient was sleeping comfortably.

With regard to the pharmacokinetics of opioids in the elderly, there appears to be a greater sensitivity compared with younger patients. This is related to

Table 21-5 Recommended programming for intravenous PCA devices

	PCA dose	Lockout, min	Infusion	Hourly maximum
Morphine	1 mg	6–10	1 mg/h	6 mg
Meperidine	10 mg	6–10	—	—
Fentanyl	20 μg	5	20 μg/h	180 μg

higher plasma levels caused by a reduced cardiac output (particularly morphine),[14] and a reduced clearance resulting in longer elimination (fentanyl). A decreased dose with age is required with fentanyl and alfentanil to produce a shift in the electroencephalogram (EEG). These facts are incongruous with studies of the same two drugs that show that there is no consistent change with age with regard to the doses required for pain relief. Therefore, it is important to treat the individual (rather than the "average") geriatric patient and to titrate analgesics, especially opioids, carefully.[15]

Adjuncts: Promethazine, Hydroxyzine, Sleeping Aids

Commonly used adjuncts to IM narcotics include promethazine (Phenergan) and hydroxyzine (Vistaril). These agents are added to allow reduction of the narcotic dose required and to control nausea, but they can also make injections more painful (Vistaril). Both drugs have the potential, particularly in an elderly patient, to increase sedation and the risk of respiratory depression.

Sleeping aids can be beneficial in optimizing patient comfort, although they should be used with caution. Some agents, such as the benzodiazepines, carry the risk of causing excessive sedation in older patients when used along with opioids. Respiratory depression also may be potentiated, though this is unlikely with antihistamine-based sleeping pills such as diphenhydramine (Benadryl). Amitriptyline (Elavil) may be useful when given at bedtime and has analgesic as well as antidepressant effects.

REGIONAL ANALGESIA: PERIPHERAL TECHNIQUES

Peripheral techniques utilize analgesics, usually local anesthetics, which are administered into the skin and layers of the operative site, or at the nerve or nerves supplying the painful area. Usually the longest-acting agent available is preferred; bupivacaine can provide up to 10 to 12 h of analgesia when injected peripherally. This helps minimize analgesic demand during the early postoperative period. When bupivacaine is administered before the incision, analgesic use may be reduced for even longer periods—a "preemptive" effect. Despite the potential benefit, it is important in an elderly patient to avoid toxicity, especially with bupivacaine (3 mg/kg). Therefore, calculation of the maximum dose per ideal body weight and limitation of the amount injected to this dose are among the anesthesiologist's chief responsibilities.

Nerve Blocks

Nerve blocks can be used to provide both anesthesia and postoperative analgesia, either alone or as a supplement, to reduce the need for other agents. This technique is especially useful in outpatients having superficial or distal procedures (e.g., retrobulbar block for cataract extraction and axillary block for hand surgery). The sedation and narcotics required are minimal, and therefore the patient can usually be sent home earlier. The patient will need to be instructed to take oral analgesics when discomfort first begins.

Supplemental nerve block can have additional benefits in the elderly. When intercostal blocks of T_6–T_{10} were performed for postcholecystectomy pain, the degree of desaturation was significantly reduced compared with IV morphine infusions (Fig. 21-1).[16] However, the risk of toxicity from multiple-site injections must be weighed against the relatively short (12 h) period of effective pain relief. In an extremely compromised and/or obese elderly patient with severe chronic obstructive pulmonary disease (COPD), the ability to cough in the immediate postoperative period may make such a technique very valuable.

Intraarticular Analgesia

There is evidence that peripheral opiate receptors exist and that peripheral administration of narcotics such as morphine can produce quality analgesia that is not due to systemic absorption. This has been mostly studied in patients undergoing knee arthroscopy. Doses of 0.5 to 1.0 mg of morphine in 40 ml of saline injected intraarticularly produce analgesia with a duration of 3 to 6 h

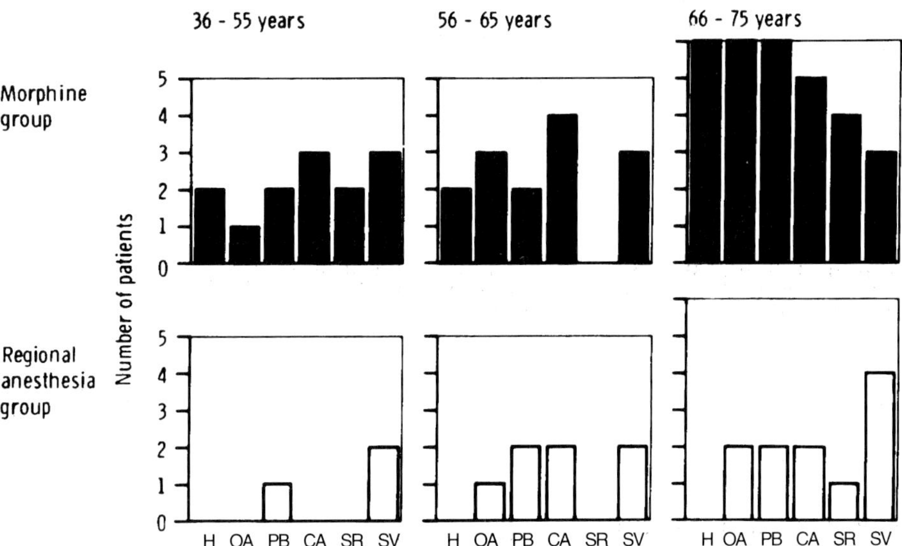

Figure 21-1 **The effect of age on the incidence of respiratory disturbances in patients receiving morphine infusions and patients receiving regional anesthesia. H = hypoxemia (Sa_{O_2} < 80 percent); OA = obstructive apnea; PB = paradoxical breathing; CA = central apnea; SR = slow respiratory rate; SV = small tidal volumes.** ***(Reprinted with permission from Catley DM, Thornton C, Jordan C, et al: Pronounced, episodic oxygen desaturation in the postoperative period: Its association with ventilatory pattern and analgesic regimen. Anesthesiology 63:20, 1985.)***

without side effects. These patients required significantly less supplemental analgesics. This analgesic effect was negated when 0.1 mg of naloxone was included in the solution.[17] Bupivacaine (30 ml, 0.25%) can be substituted for the saline to ensure complete and longer-lasting analgesia.

REGIONAL ANALGESIA: NEURAXIAL TECHNIQUES

Neuraxial techniques, both epidural and subarachnoid, have become increasingly popular because of their ability to provide postoperative analgesia, particularly when extended from intraoperative anesthesia. These modalities may reduce postoperative problems, though these findings have been inconsistent. Studies have shown reduced morbidity and lower hospital costs after combining general and epidural anesthesia with postoperative epidural analgesia in the high-risk (mostly elderly) patient population.[18,19] Postoperatively, the benefits, especially with regard to epidural analgesia, include reduced thromboembolic sequelae, less sedation, and improved mobilization while providing very good analgesia compared with parenteral narcotic techniques.

Side Effects, Management, and Monitoring

Side effects of these techniques can create problems. The most frequent is pruritus, though urinary retention and nausea and vomiting also can occur. Respiratory depression is rare but a matter for concern. Carefully titrated naloxone in doses of 40 μg IV is effective in managing these problems and will avoid complete reversal of analgesia. As a result of naloxone's short duration, side effects may reappear. Mixed agonist-antagonists such as nalbuphine (Nubain) and butorphanol (Stadol) can cause problems when they are used for the reversal of side effects because of additional sedation and dysphoria, respectively. Diphenhydramine can be used initially to treat pruritus. Although also sedating, it is much less likely to potentiate respiratory depression.

Patients, especially the elderly, who receive neuraxial narcotics require special nursing attention in the form of hourly observation. Apnea monitors are not very helpful because of frequent false alarms and because a decreased respiratory rate is a late sign of respiratory depression. Frequent assessment of the level of consciousness will more reliably detect hypercapnia-related sedation. Pulse oximetry may be added for reassurance. Oxygen supplementation is also beneficial. As a result of their age and greater potential for other medical problems, the elderly are more sensitive to the respiratory depressant effects of neuraxial narcotics.

Supplemental analgesics may still be necessary with these techniques. Generally, parenteral narcotic supplementation is discouraged because of the increased probability of potentiating respiratory depression. With proper monitoring and precautions, supplemental parenteral narcotics are not absolutely contraindicated. Mixed agonist-antagonists may be used for additional analgesia by effectively binding to kappa or sigma opiate receptors while antagonizing mu receptor side effects. NSAIDs can also be given for breakthrough pain without fear of additional respiratory depression. In fact, when ketorolac was given every 6 h combined with patient-controlled epidural analgesia (PCEA) using fentanyl, it resulted in lower pain scores, less fentanyl use, earlier return of bowel function, and less painful ambulation than was the case when PCEA fentanyl was used alone.[20]

Intrathecal Analgesia: Opioids

The administration of subarachnoid or intrathecal morphine not only accomplishes improved intraoperative anesthesia but also provides long-lasting analgesia with a very small dose. Always obtained as a preservative-free preparation, it is injected at the same time as the local anesthetic during the placement of a subarachnoid block. Older patients seem to have good analgesia even at doses lower than the standard adult dose of 0.005 mg/kg (Table 21-6). The duration of analgesia is often as long as 24 h. If a continuous spinal catheter is in place, it can be redosed as often as every 12 h, though most patients should have up to 24 h of analgesia with a single dose.

Side effects may become troublesome with intrathecal morphine even in geriatric patients. The common side effects of pruritus, nausea, and urinary retention may be minimized by using the lowest doses. Patients after transurethral resection of the prostate had virtually no nausea with a dose of 0.1 mg[21] and no difference in the incidence of pruritus with 0.05 mg compared with saline.[22] Respiratory depression is a concern, especially at higher doses. Sustained elevation of Pa_{CO_2} to as high as 58 mmHg for 12 to 16 h (but not requiring treatment) has been documented with doses as low as 0.15 mg.[23] Clinically significant depression usually becomes a problem at doses greater than 0.5 mg. The incidence of respiratory depression has been reported to be 0.36 percent, and risk factors include not only larger doses but age over 65 years and American Society of Anesthesiologists (ASA) class III to IV.[24] Therefore, use in high-risk geriatric patients must be carefully considered and monitored.

Though underutilized for thoracic procedures, intrathecal morphine can be beneficial and without serious side effects in older patients. Postlobectomy patients had lower pain scores, were more alert, and required significantly less supplemental IV meperidine with 0.012 mg/kg of subarachnoid morphine com-

Table 21-6 Intrathecal morphine dose in relation to surgical site*

Surgical incision	Total dose, mg
Thoracic	0.5 (0.012 mg/kg max*)
Upper abdominal	0.06–0.12
Lower abdominal/extremity	0.05–0.10

*Intensively monitored for at least 24 h.

pared with those receiving only IV meperidine.[25] Patients who received 0.5 mg of intrathecal morphine during coronary artery bypass surgery required significantly less supplemental morphine and significantly less nitroprusside for blood pressure control than did patients who did not receive intrathecal morphine.[26] After thoracic surgery, because of the comparatively large doses needed for adequate pain control, these patients generally require intensive care monitoring.

Fentanyl also may be administered via the subarachnoid route. As a result of its short duration (4–6 h), its usefulness for postoperative analgesia is limited when it is administered as part of a single-shot spinal. It does improve the quality of intraoperative anesthesia. It can be used with repeated doses or by infusion if a continuous spinal catheter is in place. Bolus doses of 12.5 to 25 μg have been used safely in older patients (average age, 68–70 years).[27]

Side effects can also be a problem with intrathecal fentanyl. Mild pruritus, sedation, and nausea and vomiting are the most common in order of frequency. Significant respiratory depression can occur because of passive migration by cephalad cerebrospinal fluid (CSF) flow,[28] despite the rapid binding of this lipid-soluble opioid to local nervous tissue.

Subarachnoid narcotic infusions also can be used with relative safety in the geriatric population. Both fentanyl and morphine have been used after hip arthroplasty (average age, 67–72 years).[29] The doses used were 120 μg over 24 h (5 μg/h) and 0.2 mg over 24 h (8.33 μg/h), respectively. Morphine was more efficacious than fentanyl, though both required supplementation with IM opioids. The incidences of side effects (nausea, vomiting, urinary retention, and most frequently pruritus) were similar. Respiratory depression was not found to be a problem. If a subarachnoid catheter is left in place for intermittent dosing or infusion, label it "Continuous Spinal" to avoid confusion with epidural.

Epidural Analgesia

Epidural anesthesia/analgesia is the most popular continuous neuraxial technique. This technique was first used for labor analgesia, and the flexibility provided by having an epidural catheter in place may explain why it is so commonly used. It may be used as the sole anesthetic or used in concert with general anesthesia. It can be extended after intraoperative use or initiated postoperatively for analgesia, using only preservative-free agents, usually by a continuous infusion or connected to a PCA device to provide PCEA. Ultimately, the use of perioperative epidural anesthesia and analgesia can result in an improved outcome, especially in elderly and complicated patients, as was described previously. To optimize its safety, it is extremely important that the epidural catheter and pump tubing be labeled "Epidural" at the injection ports to avoid accidental injection of other drugs.

Among all the epidural opioids, morphine has been used the longest, particularly because of its reliable efficacy. As a result of its low lipid solubility, it also has the longest duration and provides the greatest spread to higher dermatomes after lumbar administration. It is this rostral spread that has made it notorious for respiratory depression, even though the incidence is very low (0.09 percent) in the general population.[24] It is the aged and infirmed who most often develop respiratory depression. One should start with the lowest recommended adult dose of preservative-free morphine when treating geriatric patients. For example, for lower abdominal[30] and lower extremity procedures, 2 mg should be used. This can last as long as 48 h without side effects. The lack of sedation and confusion is noteworthy. Urinary retention is still a problem, especially in elderly men. For abdominal procedures and thoracic procedures, the initial dose range is 3 to 4 mg and 4 to 5 mg, respectively. The higher the dermatome requiring coverage, the shorter the duration of adequate analgesia generally reported with a given dose.

Continuous infusion of epidural opioids is also popular, as it allows not only for convenience but also for the maintenance of analgesia for longer periods. Shorter-acting agents can then be used to minimize the risk of cumulative side effects. Fentanyl is the preservative-free narcotic most commonly used for PCEA, though sufentanil, hydromorphone, and meperidine also have been used safely in older patients. If a programmable patient-controlled infusion device is connected to the epidural catheter (PCEA), both safety and patient satisfaction should be improved by allowing self-titration. The same instructions and precautions should be taken as with IV PCA. The recommended doses of infusions or PCEA are listed in Table 21-7.

Fentanyl and sufentanil, by virtue of their short duration and rapid onset, are easily titratable. When one is delivering fentanyl specifically, the best results are achieved when the epidural catheter is in the vicinity of the nerve roots from which the pain originates (i.e., low thoracic for abdominal procedures and middle to high thoracic for thoracic surgery).[31] With such placement, it is possible to achieve a decreased length of hospital stay, shortened time to first

Table 21-7 Epidural opioids by infusion and PCEA*

	Initial bolus	Infusion concentration	Infusion rate
Morphine	2 mg	0.15 mg/ml	3–6 ml/h
	2 mg	0.05 mg/ml	4 ml/h
Hydromorphone	0.8–1.5 mg	0.05 mg/ml	3–6 ml/h
Meperidine	20–25 mg	2.0 mg/ml	7–10 ml/h
Fentanyl	1.0 μg/kg	4–6 μg/ml	0.5–1 μg/kg/h
	PCEA dose = 12.5–20 μg	20–25 μg/ml Lockout = 5–10 min	20–30 μg/h
Sufentanil	10–15 μg		
	PCEA dose = 3–5 μg	1.5–6.2 μg/ml Lockout = 5–10 min	5 μg/h

*Use higher doses after thoracic operations; maintain for 2–3 days postoperatively.

bowel movement, and improved pulmonary function.[32] It is important to note that as a result of its high lipid solubility, significant plasma levels can be achieved with epidural administration. Therefore, the potential for respiratory depression still exists. Sufentanil behaves similarly to fentanyl, though, in part because of its greater potency, sedation is more likely.[33,34]

Hydromorphone (Dilaudid) and meperidine (Demerol) also may be used. Dilaudid has the advantage over morphine of less pruritus and respiratory depression,[35] in part as a result of less cephalad spread. Epidural Demerol infusion has been shown to improve mood and participation compared with IM injections while decreasing the need for supplemental opioids, regardless of age.[36]

When one is using a local anesthetic with an opioid, pain is controlled by two different mechanisms, potentially requiring lower doses than when either is used alone. Adding low concentrations of bupivacaine to epidural opioid infusions not only provides excellent analgesia but has also been shown repeatedly to allow reductions in the opioid utilized, reducing the potential for the associated side effects. A 0.25% solution with 0.05 mg/ml morphine (after a 2 mg bolus intraoperatively) infused at 4 ml/h (0.2 mg/h) both intraoperatively and postoperatively after major abdominal surgery resulted in better analgesia with movement to the sitting position and coughing and less supplemental narcotic requirement than did epidural morphine alone.[37] When this same dose regimen was used, there were no cardiovascular or respiratory complications observed in a related study that looked at two groups of patients whose mean age was 68 and 70 years, respectively.[38] Lower concentrations (i.e., 0.03125%, 0.0625%, and 0.125%) may be used to avoid the persistent sensory block seen with 0.25% solutions. Fentanyl (2–5 μg/ml; 0.5–1.0 μg/kg per hour) and sufentanil (0.5 μg/ml; up to 0.1 μg/kg per hour) also may be used with these low concentrations of bupivacaine to provide more complete analgesia. Although the total narcotic requirement is reduced, the risk of respiratory depression is still present, especially in the geriatric population, and so appropriate monitoring is needed.

Preservative-free injectable clonidine also may be added to epidural infusions. As an $alpha_2$ agonist, it has analgesic effects through these receptors. It is more effective as an adjunct to epidural fentanyl and allows for reduction of the fentanyl dose. When clonidine was administered at a rate of 0.3 μg/kg per hour with fentanyl 0.5 μg/kg per hour epidurally (in a volume of 5 ml/h), analgesia was equal to 1 μg/kg per hour of fentanyl alone and the duration of desaturation was shorter. Hypotension is potentially a problem, though only single, easily managed episodes occurred in 23 percent of patients.[39]

SUMMARY

Geriatric patients require special attention with regard to postoperative analgesia. As a result of age-related changes in physiology and coexisting diseases, analgesia must be administered carefully to ensure a good outcome and decrease the likelihood of side effects (especially respiratory depression and sedation). The goal of safe, quality analgesia is to provide the "3 L's": lowest effective dose, longest duration, and least side effects. This applies especially to the elderly. It has become apparent that the best way to achieve these goals is to provide combination therapy. When one controls the various components of pain with a specific modality for each, lower doses are needed, minimizing the side effects. Continuous and PCA/PCEA techniques provide an extended duration of analgesia while optimizing comfort and satisfaction.

REFERENCES

1. Foley KM: Pain management in the elderly, in Hazzard WR, Andres R, Bierman EL, Blass JP (eds): *Principles of Geriatric Medicine and Gerontology*, 2d ed. New York: McGraw-Hill, 1990, pp 281–295.
2. Peck CL: Psychological factors in acute pain management, in Cousins MJ, Phillips GD (eds): *Acute Pain Management*. New York: Churchill Livingstone, 1986, pp 251–274.
3. Albert TJ, Cohn JC, Rothman JS, et al: Patient-controlled analgesia in a postoperative total joint arthroplasty population. *J Arthroplasty* 6:S23, 1991.
4. Gebuhr P, Soelberg M, Orsnes T, Wilbek H: Naproxen prevention of heterotopic ossification after hip arthroplasty. *Acta Orthop Scand* 62:226, 1991.
5. Ronen S, Rozenman Y, Zylbermann R, Berson D: Treatment of ocular inflammation with diclofenac sodium: Double-blind trial following cataract surgery. *Ann Ophthalmol* 17:577, 1985.
6. Gabriel SE, Jaakkimainen L, Bombardier C: Risk for serious gastrointestinal complications related to use of nonsteroidal anti-inflammatory drugs: A meta-analysis. *Ann Intern Med* 115:787, 1991.
7. Katz JA: Ketorolac: side effects and complications. *ASRA News*, Dec. 5, 1993, pp 5–6.
8. Mangat PS, Jones JG: Postoperative pain control in the elderly, in Dodds C (ed): *Bailliere's Clinical Anaesthesiology International Practice and Research: Anaesthesia and the Geriatric Patient*. London: Bailliere Tindall, 1993, pp 169–193.
9. Holley FO, Van Steennis C: Postoperative analgesia with fentanyl: Pharmacokinetics and pharmacodynamics of constant rate i.v. and transdermal delivery. *Br J Anaesth* 60:608, 1988.
10. Gourlay, GK, Kowalski SR, Plummer JL, et al: The transdermal administration of fentanyl in the treatment of postoperative pain: Pharmacokinetics and pharmacodynamic effects. *Pain* 37:193, 1989.
11. McCoy EP, Furness G, Wright PMC: Patient-controlled analgesia with and without background infusion: Analgesia assessed using the demand:delivery ratio. *Anaesthesia* 48:256, 1993.
12. Gourlay GK, Kowalski SR, Plummer JL, et al: Fentanyl blood concentration—analgesic response relationship in the treatment of postoperative pain. *Anesth Analg* 67:329, 1988.
13. White PF: Mishaps with patient-controlled analgesia. *Anesthesiology* 66:81, 1987.
14. Stoelting RK: *Pharmacology and Physiology in Anesthetic Practice*. Philadelphia: Lippincott, 1987.
15. Hug CC: Opioids and hypnotics in the geriatric patient. *ASA Ann Refresh Course Lect* 273:1, 1993.

16. Catley DM, Thornton C, Jordan C, et al: Pronounced, episodic oxygen desaturation in the postoperative period: Its association with ventilatory pattern and analgesic regimen. *Anesthesiology* 63:20, 1985.
17. Stein C, Comisel K, Haimerl E, et al: Analgesic effect of intraarticular morphine after arthroscopic knee surgery. *N Engl J Med* 325:1123, 1991.
18. Yeager MP, Glass DD, Neff RK, Brinck-Johnsen T: Epidural anesthesia and analgesia in high-risk surgical patients. *Anesthesiology* 66:729, 1987.
19. Tuman KJ, McCarthy RJ, March RJ, et al: Effects of epidural anesthesia and analgesia on coagulation and outcome after major vascular surgery. *Anesth Analg* 73:696, 1991.
20. Grass JA, Sakima NT, Valley M, et al: Assessment of ketorolac as an adjuvant to fentanyl patient-controlled epidural analgesia after radical retropubic prostatectomy. *Anesthesiology* 78:642, 1993.
21. Kirson LE, Goldman JM, Slover RB: Low-dose intrathecal morphine for postoperative pain control in patients undergoing transurethral resection of the prostate. *Anesthesiology* 71:192, 1989.
22. Brown RA, Ong B, Greengrass R, Morgan T: Very small dose intrathecal morphine for postoperative pain after prostate resection. *Anesthesiology* 79:A886, 1993.
23. Yamaguchi H, Watanabe S, Motokawa K, Ishizawa Y: Intrathecal morphine dose-response data for pain relief after cholecystectomy. *Anesth Analg* 70:168, 1990.
24. Rawal N, Arner S, Gustafsson LL, Allvin R: Present state of extradural and intrathecal opioid analgesia in Sweden: A nationwide follow-up survey. *Br J Anaesth* 59:791, 1987.
25. Neustein SM, Cohen E: Intrathecal morphine during thoracotomy: II. Effect on postoperative meperidine requirements and pulmonary function tests. *J Cardiothorac Vasc Anesth* 7:157, 1993.
26. Vanstrum GS, Bjornson KM, Ilko R: Postoperative effects of intrathecal morphine in coronary artery bypass surgery. *Anesth Analg* 67:261, 1988.
27. Varrassi G, Celleno D, Capogna G, et al: Ventilatory effects of subarachnoid fentanyl in the elderly. *Anaesthesia* 47:558, 1992.
28. Gourlay GK, Murphy TM, Plummer JL, et al: Pharmacokinetics of fentanyl in lumbar and cervical CSF following lumbar epidural and intravenous administration. *Pain* 38:253-259, 1989.
29. Niemi L, Pitkanen MT, Tuominen MK, Rosenberg PH: Comparison of intrathecal fentanyl infusion with intrathecal morphine infusion or bolus for postoperative pain relief after hip arthroplasty. *Anesth Analg* 77:126, 1993.
30. Moskovitz B, Bolkier M, Ginesin Y, et al: Epidural morphine: A new approach to combined anesthesia and analgesia in urological patients. *Eur Urol* 12:171, 1986.
31. Chien BB, Burke RG, Hunter DJ: An extensive experience with postoperative pain relief using postoperative fentanyl infusion. *Arch Surg* 126:692, 1991.
32. Guinard JP, Mavrocordatos P, Chiolero R, Carpenter RL: A randomized comparison of intravenous versus lumbar and thoracic epidural fentanyl for analgesia after thoracotomy. *Anesthesiology* 77:1108, 1992.
33. Geller E, Chrubasik J, Graf R, et al: A randomized double-blind comparison of epidural sufentanil versus intravenous sufentanil or epidural fentanyl analgesia after major abdominal surgery. *Anesth Analg* 76:1243, 1993.
34. Swenson JD, Hullander RM, Bready RJ, Leivers D: A comparison of patient controlled epidural analgesia with sufentanil by the lumbar versus thoracic route after thoracotomy. *Anesth Analg* 78:215, 1994.
35. Chaplan SR, Duncan SR, Brodsky JB, Brose WG: Morphine and hydromorphone

epidural analgesia: A prospective, randomized comparison. *Anesthesiology* 77:1090, 1992.
36. Blythe JG, Hodel KA, Wahl TM, et al: Continuous postoperative epidural analgesia for gynecologic oncology patients. *Gynecol Oncol* 37:307, 1990.
37. Dahl JB, Rosenberg J, Hansen BL, et al: Differential analgesic effects of low-dose epidural morphine and morphine-bupivacaine at rest and during mobilization after major abdominal surgery. *Anesth Analg* 74:362, 1992.
38. Dahl JB, Hansen BL, Hjortso NC, et al: Influence of timing on the effect of continuous extradural analgesia with bupivacaine and morphine after major abdominal surgery. *Br J Anaesth* 69:4, 1992.
39. Delauney L, Leppert C, Dechaubry V, et al: Epidural clonidine decreases postoperative requirements for epidural fentanyl. *Reg Anesth* 18:176, 1993.

CHAPTER 22

Myofascial Pain in the Elderly

R. Brian Smith

INTRODUCTION

A large number of syndromes have been described for the symptoms and signs of pain associated with muscles and connecting structures. These syndromes include fibrositis, myalgia, myositis, fibromyositis, muscular rheumatism, idiopathic myalgia, and fibropathic syndrome. The syndrome of myofascial pain is now considered to cover this large group of mainly muscle disorders.

PATHOPHYSIOLOGY

Myofascial pain is characterized by "trigger points" (TP), which are areas of hypersensitivity within the muscles or the adjacent connective tissue. This syndrome is associated with muscle spasm, pain, and tenderness. With advancing age and reduced physical activity, the incidence of myofascial pain increases. It has been estimated that myofascial pain accounts for the symptoms of up to 85 percent of patients attending pain clinics.

Two pathways for the pathophysiological development of TP were proposed by Raj[1] (Table 22-1). First, muscle fibrils are damaged by overstretching during acute muscle strain. This creates a breakdown in the sarcoplasmic reticulum, with the resultant release of calcium ions. The surrounding fibers are then exposed to the excess calcium, together with adenosine triphosphate, and develop a sustained contracture. Metabolism is increased in the muscle, and the body responds by local vasoconstriction followed by decreased circulation and shortening of muscle fibers. The result is a taut band in the muscle that acts as a stimulus to the sympathetic nervous system. In the second mechanism, substances such as histamine, serotonin, kinins, and prostaglandins may be released into the muscle. This increases ischemia and the accumulation of metabolic products, which in turn create a TP.

Trigger point development also can be initiated by any type of chronic muscle spasm, including herniated disks and arthritis. Trigger points are common in patients with advanced cancer, which causes an unusual degree of stress on muscles secondary to nerve or tissue injury. Stresses and body conditions that may lead to the onset of myofascial pain are shown in Fig. 22-1.

CLINICAL FEATURES

In acute myofascial pain, the patient's history often includes an incident that caused muscle injury. Typically, an event such as slipping in the shower, prolonged standing, or lifting a heavy object will be volunteered. The patient may present with muscle spasm and pain over the affected muscle. In more chronic myofascial pain, trigger areas may have been initiated by nerve injury, muscle fatigue, or another neuromusculoskeletal disorder. Other chronic debilitating diseases, such as infection and arthritis, also can initiate the development of

Table 22-1 Pathophysiology of a trigger point

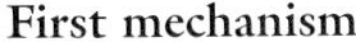

First mechanism

Acute muscle strain
Damages sarcoplasmic reticulum
↓
Ca^{++} ion release and accumulation
Presence of ATP and excess Ca^{++}
↓
Initiates and maintains sustained contracture
Produces a region of uncontrolled metabolism
↓
Body responds with local vasoconstriction
There is now a region of increased metabolism, decreased circulation, and shortened muscle fiber
↓
Taut and palpable band in the muscle
↓
Trigger point

Second mechanism

Tissue injury
↓
Releases histamine
Serotonin
Kinins
Prostaglandins
↓
Further ischemia
Increased metabolism with reduced circulation
↓
Accumulation of metabolic products
↓
Increases further sensitizing products
↓
Active trigger point

SOURCE: Reprinted with permission from Raj PP: Myofascial trigger point injection, in Raj PP (ed): *Practical Management of Pain*. Chicago, London: Yearbook, 1986, chap 33, p 570.

trigger areas. Commonly located trigger areas and the pain patterns associated with them have been identified by a number of workers. Such commonly located trigger areas are shown in Figs. 22-2 through 22-9. There is usually a deep tenderness over the trigger area. Frequently, a tight band of muscle may be felt by palpation, with the pain referred, as shown in Figs. 22-2 through 22-9.

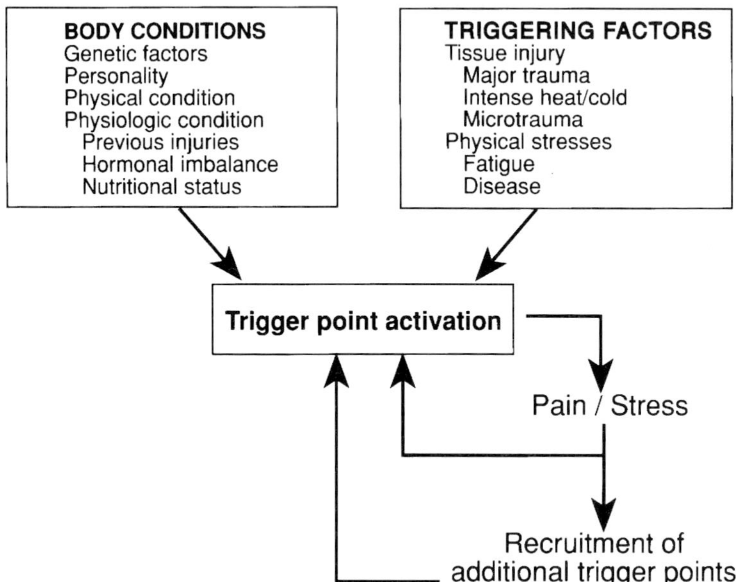

Figure 22-1 Stresses and body conditions that may lead to the onset of myofascial pain. *[Reprinted with permission from Sola AE, Bonica JJ: Myofascial pain syndrome, in Bonica J (ed): The Management of Pain, 2d ed. Philadelphia: Lea & Febiger, 1990, vol 1, chap 21, p 352.]*

Palpation also frequently elicits the "jump sign," a sudden movement by the patient caused by the painful stimulation. Stimulation of the trigger area produces pain, tenderness, and muscle spasm in the areas of reference. The referred pattern is fairly consistent and does not follow the dermatomal structure or peripheral nerve distribution. Because the referred pattern has no anatomically explainable distribution, this has led to skepticism among physicians. There is, however, overwhelming evidence that these distributions of pain patterns have been found consistently by different clinicians. Not infrequently, large segments of muscle can be felt in spasm in addition to the trigger area. Often, more than one trigger area may be found. Physical examination should include the normal range of motion of muscle groups and the patient's posture and gait. Individuals who have contributed significantly to this field include Travell,[2] Gutstein,[3] Correll,[4] and Bonica.[5]

Before one establishes the diagnosis of myofascial pain, a thorough workup must be made to rule out other treatable pathological causes. Most important is a complete neurological examination to rule out CNS pathology as a cause of the pain. This may be followed by computerized tomography, magnetic resonance imaging, and electromyography.

It is important to assess the mental health of the patient, as chronic pain is frequently associated with some degree of depression. This is particularly important in elderly patients, in whom depression seems to occur more frequently with pain. Most multidisciplinary pain clinics include psychiatrists and/or psy-

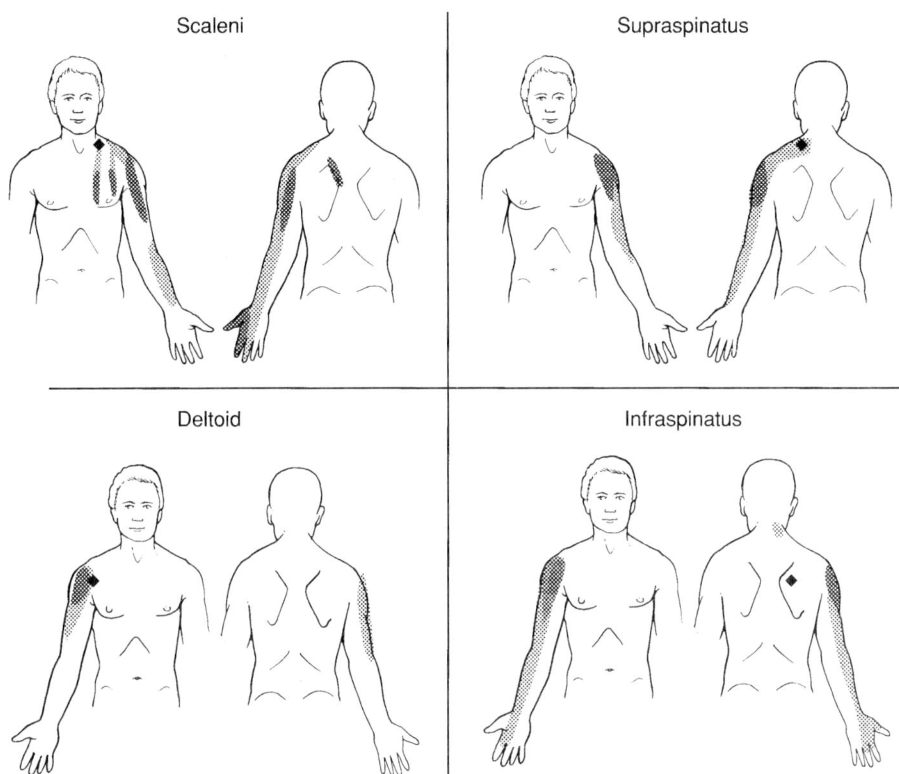

Figure 22-2 **Scaleni, supraspinatus, deltoid, and infraspinatus trigger points and referred pain patterns.** *(Reprinted with permission from Travell J, Rinzler SH: The myofascial genesis of pain. Postgrad Med 11:425, 1952.)*

chologists on the staff. Magni and colleagues[6] studied pain as a symptom in elderly depressed patients. Pain was a significant complaint in 70 percent of these patients. It was highest in patients with dysthymic disorders and atypical depression. Patients with major depression and an adjustment disorder had the fewest complaints of pain. Patients with both chronic pain and depression have greater pain intensity and exhibit more significant pain behavior. They become less active and more impaired in their daily activities than do other chronic pain patients. These patients also tend to be older than nondepressed pain patients.

The recent advent of positron emission tomography (PET) has provided a new tool for examining how pain is represented in the human cerebral cortex. Talbot and coworkers[7] examined eight subjects under PET scanning with pain stimulation and pain placebo. Peaks of activity in the contralateral anterior cingulate, primary somatosensory cortex, and secondary somatosensory cortex were observed. Previously the cingulate was thought to be involved in the emotional process but had not been linked to pain.

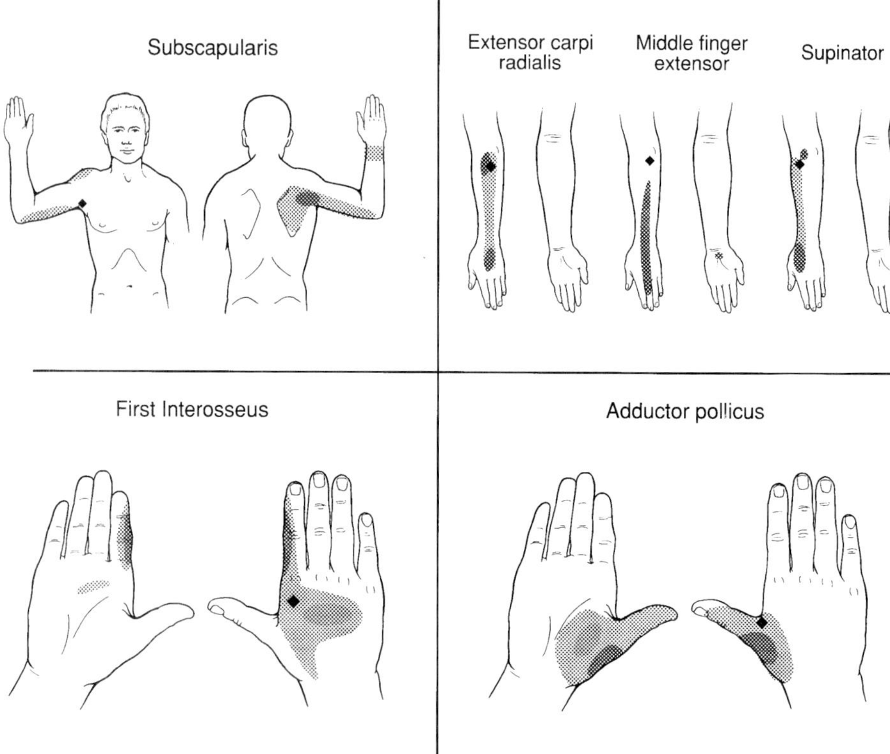

Figure 22-3 **Subscapularis, extensor carpi radialis, middle finger extensor, supinator, first interosseus, and adductor pollicus trigger points and referred pain patterns.** *(Reprinted with permission from Travell J, Rinzler SH: The myofascial genesis of pain. Postgrad Med 11:425, 1952.)*

A frequently used thorough objective psychometric test is the Minnesota Multiphasic Personality Inventory (MMPI), which consists of 566 written statements that the person being tested assesses as true or false as applied to him or her. Because this is a very time-consuming test, simpler screening tests have been developed. One is the Beck Depression Inventory,[8] a 21-item self-report measure that yields a numerical estimate of depression severity. Patients select for each item, one of four or five statements ranked in order of severity. Scores range from 0 to 63, with high scores indicating greater depression. For example, a score of 13 indicates mild depression, while 21 indicates moderate depression.

TREATMENT

The goal of treatment is to interrupt the pain cycle. The gate control theory of pain describes the modulation of sensory nerve impulses by an inhibitory

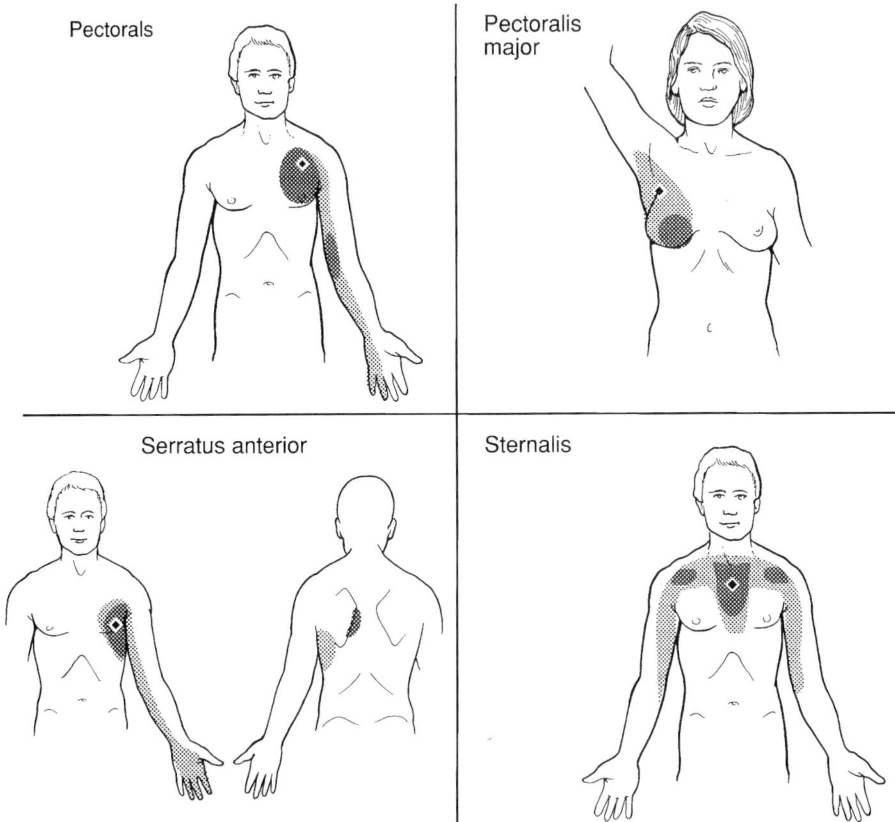

Figure 22-4 Pectorals, pectoralis major, serratus anterior, and sternalis trigger points and referred pain patterns. ***(Reprinted with permission from Travell J, Rinzler SH: The myofascial genesis of pain. Postgrad Med 11:425, 1952.)***

mechanism in the CNS. The termination of pain by hyperstimulation or local injection of an anesthetic normalizes function, which helps prevent recurrences of abnormal neural activity. Modulation of sensory input by trigger point injection may be more effective in reducing pain than is surgical interruption of the sensory input. This can be done by eliminating the TP. Two techniques are widely used to achieve TP elimination: trigger point injection (TPI) and the "stretch and spray" technique. Frequently, the stretch and spray technique immediately follows TPI.

Trigger Point Injections

For TPI, the patient is recumbent to lessen the risk of a vasovagal response. The TPs are localized and held firm with the index finger and thumb. A 22-gauge needle is inserted into the TP. There have been a number of reports on the success of "dry needling." This consists of penetrating the TP by using a

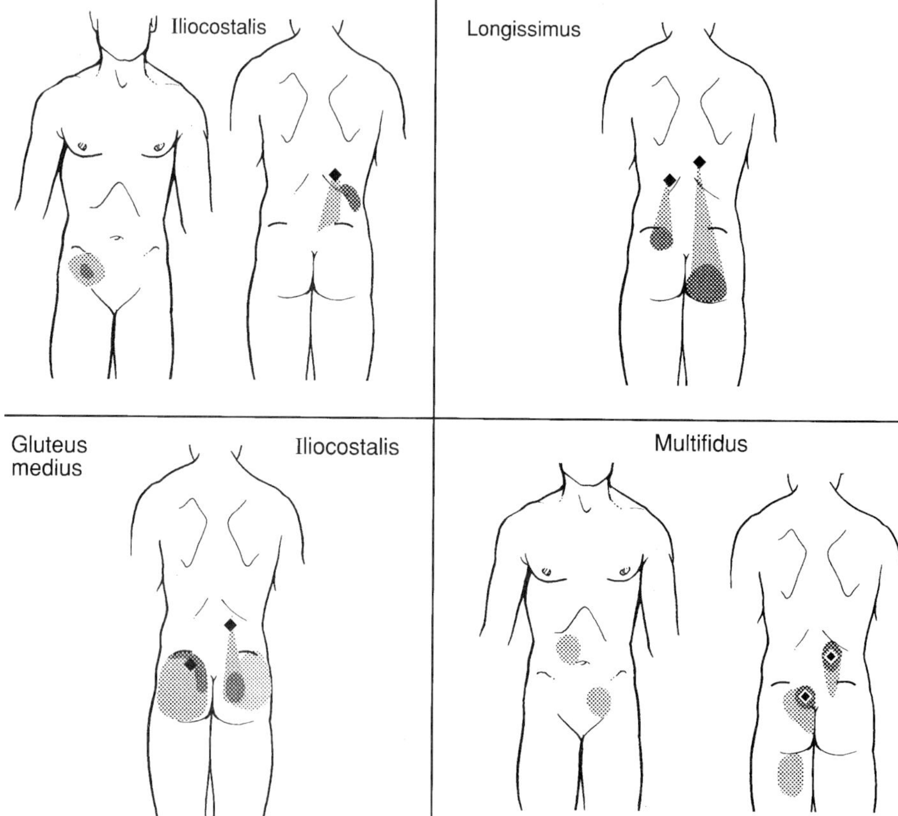

Figure 22-5 **Iliocostalis, longissimus, gluteus medius, and multifidus trigger points and referred pain patterns.** *(Reprinted with permission from Travell J, Rinzler SH: The myofascial genesis of pain. Postgrad Med 11:425, 1952.)*

"fanning" technique and not injecting solution. Most commonly, 2 to 5 ml of local anesthetic solution is injected with the fanning technique. The concentrations of lidocaine used are usually 0.25% to 0.5%; bupivacaine concentrations are 0.125% or 0.25%. Some workers have claimed good results after injecting saline alone. Also, steroids have been used alone or in combination with local anesthetics. When using multiple injections, one must be careful not to exceed a safe maximum dose of local anesthetic.

Stretch and Spray

The rationale underlying the use of the stretch and spray techniques is to eliminate TPs by maximally stretching the affected muscle. This probably should be the first technique tried. It may precede or follow TPI. Stretching is particularly useful when a single muscle is affected. When the muscle is not in spasm, stretching will occasionally initiate spasm. To prevent spasm, the af-

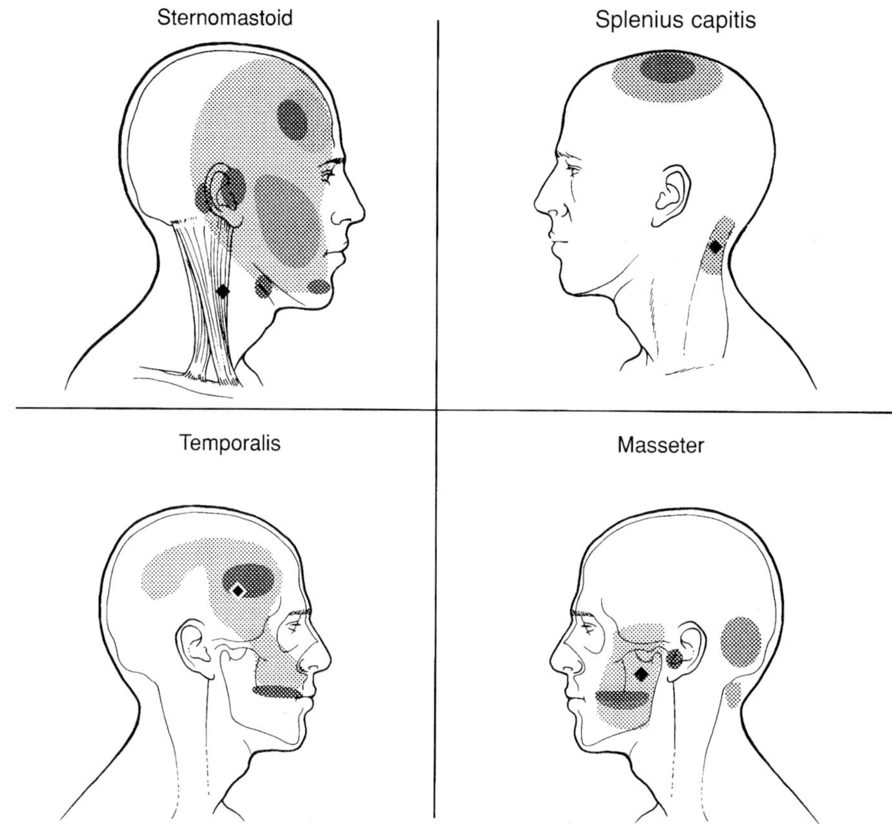

Figure 22-6 Sternomastoid, splenius capitis, temporalis, and masseter trigger points and referred pain patterns. *(Reprinted with permission from Travell J, Rinzler SH: The myofascial genesis of pain. Postgrad Med 11:425, 1952.)*

fected muscle can be sprayed with a vapor coolant spray before and during the stretching period. This will also reduce the pain of stretching. Either fluoromethane or ethyl chloride can be used as a vapor coolant. Ethyl chloride is flammable, is a potent inhalation anesthetic agent, and has a tendency to freeze the skin, which is highly undesirable. Fluoromethane is commercially available (Gebauer Chemical Co., Cleveland, OH 44104) and consists of 15% dichlorodifluoromethane and 85% trichloromonofluoromethane. The technique of spraying is shown in Figs. 22-10 and 22-11. Spraying is done along the lines of muscle fibers toward the areas of referred pain.

Physical Therapy

A number of physical therapy modalities can play a role in the treatment of myofascial pain. Massage treatments applied by qualified physiotherapists can be helpful. The use of massage during the acute phase of myofascial pain, such as muscle spasm, is somewhat controversial. Some workers believe that it may ex-

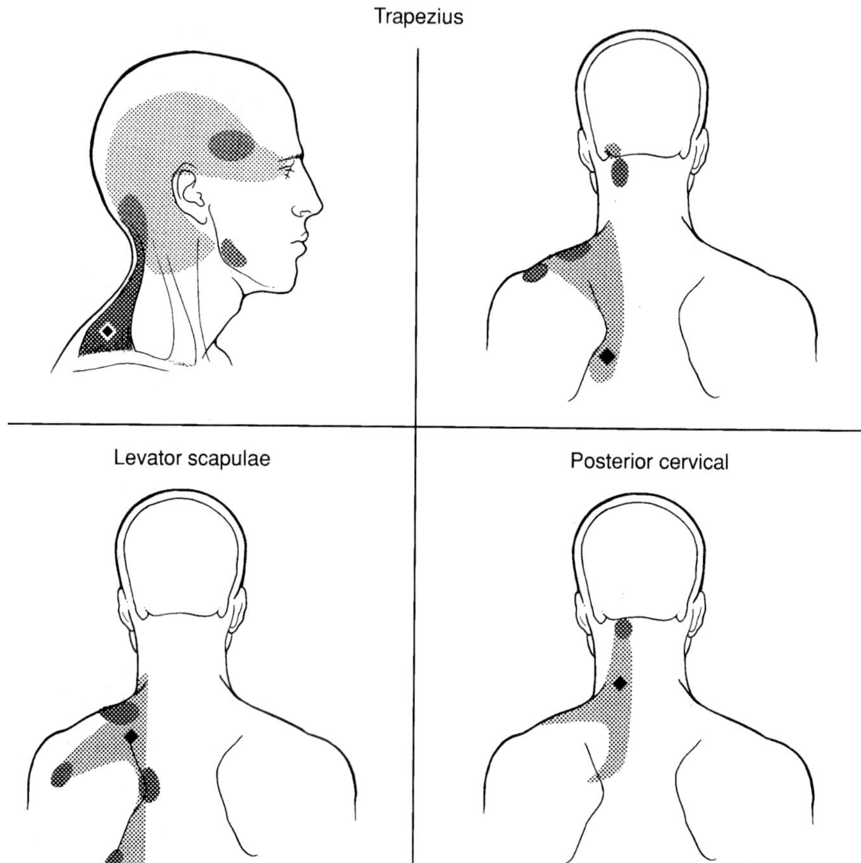

Figure 22-7 **Trapezius, levator scapulae, and posterior cervical trigger points and referred pain patterns.** *(Reprinted with permission from Travell J, Rinzler SH: The myofascial genesis of pain. Postgrad Med 11:425, 1952.)*

acerbate trigger point reflexes. Massage probably plays a more useful prophylactic role, particularly in the elderly. Heat treatments in the form of ultrasound are frequently used by physiotherapists. Ultrasound is produced by electrical stimulation of a quartz or artificial crystal, which vibrates in response. The ultrasound devices on the market produce outputs between 800,000 and 3 million cycles per second. The rapid vibration of the tissues by these sound waves produces heat, with the maximum effect occurring at the junction of the bone and muscles. The tissue penetration is thought to increase blood flow. It has been found to be useful in the treatment of conditions such as "frozen shoulder."

Transcutaneous Electrical Nerve Stimulation

Electrical stimulation in the form of transcutaneous electrical nerve stimulation (TENS) can be used to treat myofascial pain. It is used mostly in chronic

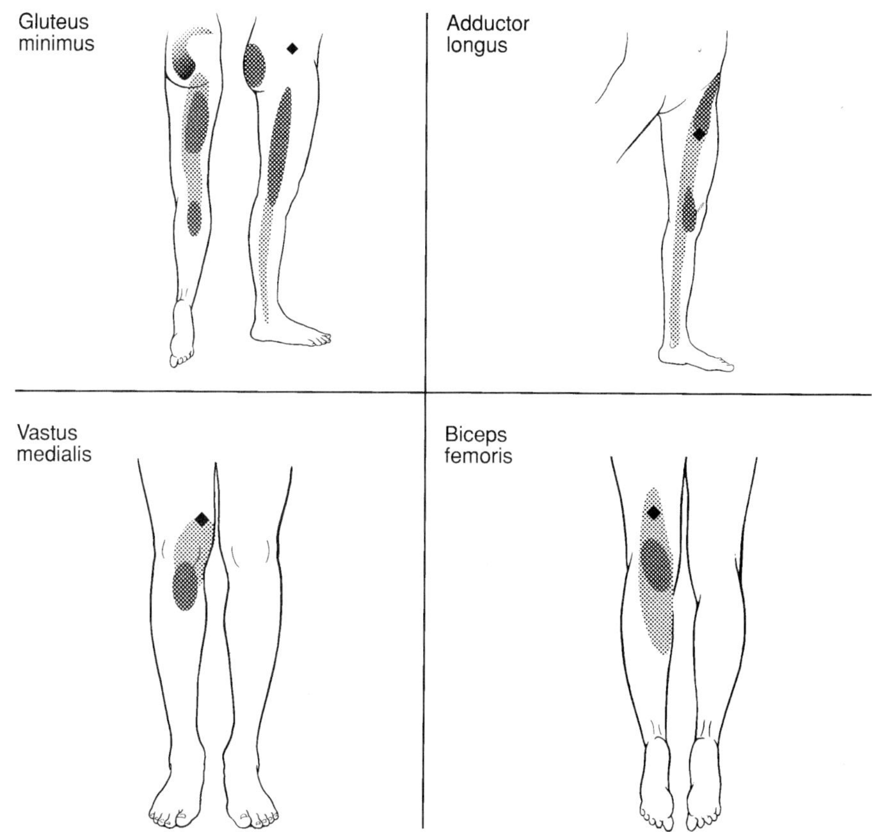

Figure 22-8 **Gluteus minimus, adductor longus, vastus medialis, and biceps femoris trigger points and referred pain patterns.** *(Reprinted with permission from Travell J, Rinzler SH: The myofascial genesis of pain. Postgrad Med 11:425, 1952.)*

cases when other modalities have failed. Electrical stimulation is provided with either direct current (DC) or alternating current (AC). DC devices were the first to be widely used but now are generally employed only for stimulation of denervated muscle and to drive subcutaneous medication (iontophoresis). Most of the devices on the market today use some form of AC current with the wave form electronically modified to the desired parameters. AC devices produce very low total current (milliamps) and do not produce the thermal or chemical effects of DC current. Most AC devices produce high-voltage output (arbitrarily designated as over 150 V) with a monophasic wave form and allow the adjustment of various parameters, such as intensity, pulse rate, and pulse width. The manner by which TENS works is not clear. According to the "gate theory" proposed by Wall and Melzak,[9] stimulation of the large nerve fibers may overwhelm the input of the smaller c pain fibers at the spinal level. Other studies with TENS have shown it to have effects that are reversible with opiate antagonists, leading to speculation that it somehow stimulates the production of endogenous endorphins. Depletion of this system is one explanation for the

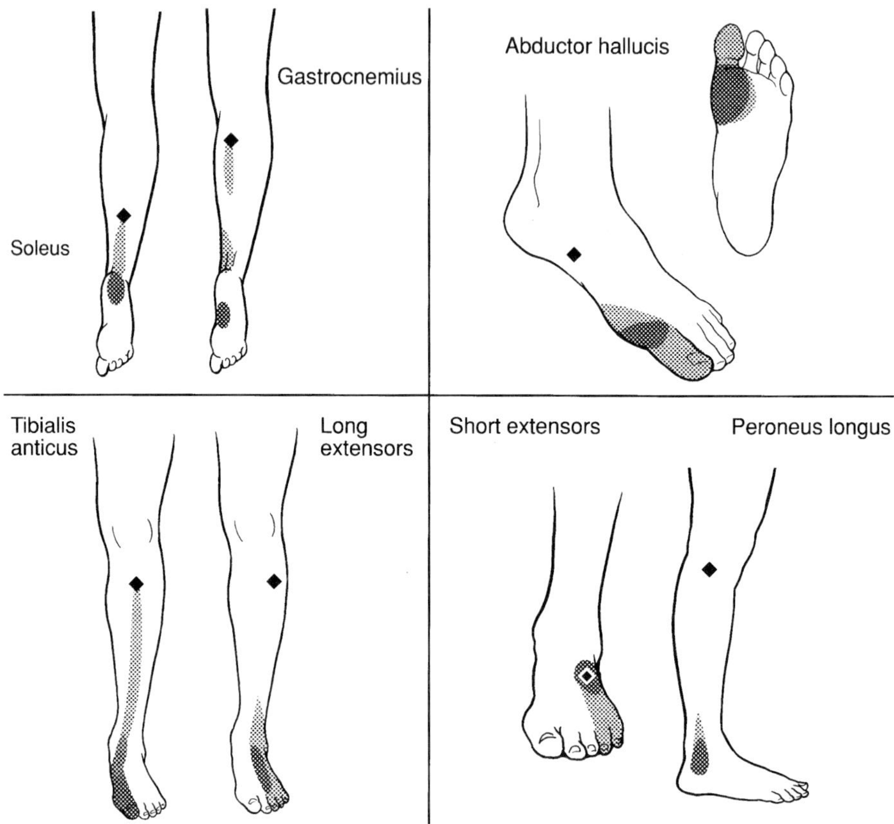

Figure 22-9 Soleus, gastrocnemius, abductor hallucis, tibialis anticus, long extensors, short extensors, and peroneus longus trigger points and referred pain patterns. ***(Reprinted with permission from Travell J, Rinzler SH: The myofascial genesis of pain. Postgrad Med 11:425, 1952.)***

observed fact that TENS loses its effectiveness in many patients after prolonged use. A controlled trial of TENS and exercise in the treatment of chronic low back pain did not show any benefit over exercise alone.[10]

Clinically, a number of other factors can determine the success of using TENS apart from the larger question of how it works in the first place. Assuming the efficacy of TENS, the proper points for stimulation must be found. Charts with specific sites for various problems are common, but it is usually necessary to try several combinations of points to get good results. Most units have adjustable pulse rate and width as well as automatic modulation modes that vary one or both of these factors. The theory states that if the stimulus is constantly changing, the body will not be able to accept the pain impulse as it would with an unchanging stimulus. Different combinations of the above may be more or less effective with individual patients. The electrodes themselves may cause skin irritation and may or may not adhere with activity. The unit and wires may not be cosmetically pleasing to some patients. Finally, the

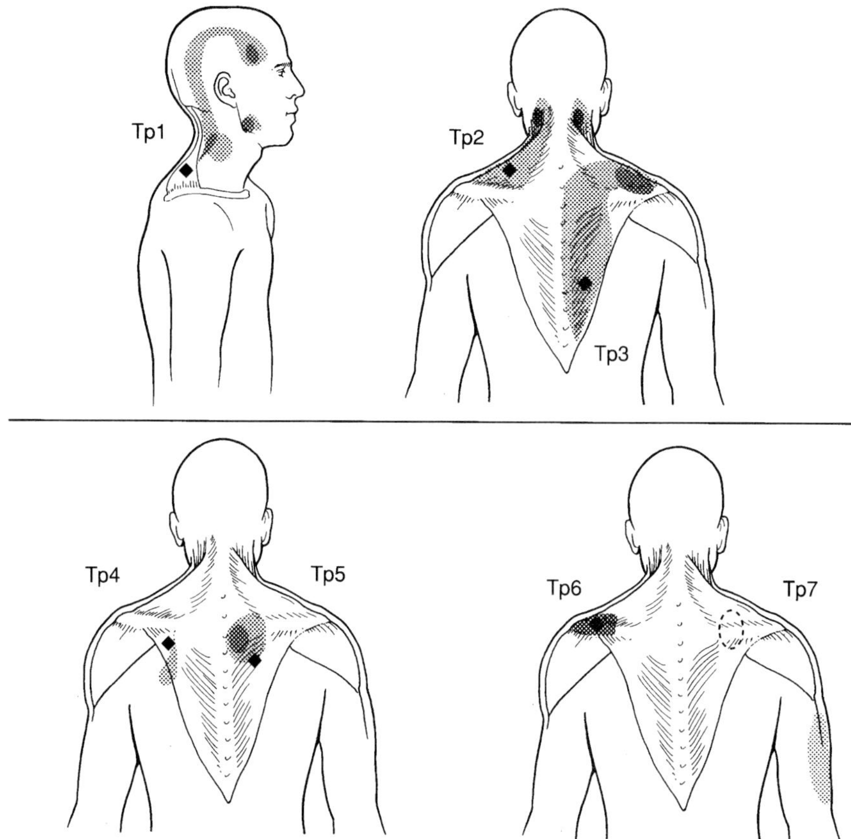

Figure 22-10 Determination of trigger points (1–7) for the stretch and spray technique. *[Reprinted with permission from Sola AE, Bonica JJ: Myofascial pain syndrome, in Bonica J (ed): The Management of Pain, 2d ed. Philadelphia: Lea & Febiger, 1990, vol 1, chap 21, p 352.]*

amount of relief given to the patient may not be worth the bother of batteries, wires, and patches.

Nonsteroidal Anti-inflammatory Drugs

The drugs discussed below have a mechanism of action different from that of opioid narcotics and anti-inflammatory steroids. These drugs are a heterogeneous group of compounds that may not be chemically related. They do, however, have common therapeutic effects. The best known of these drugs is aspirin. A term commonly used for the group is nonsteroidal anti-inflammatory drugs (NSAIDs).

The mechanism underlying the anti-inflammatory process has been the focus of much research in recent years, and considerable progress has been made on its elucidation. This in turn has led to a search for drugs that interrupt or modify

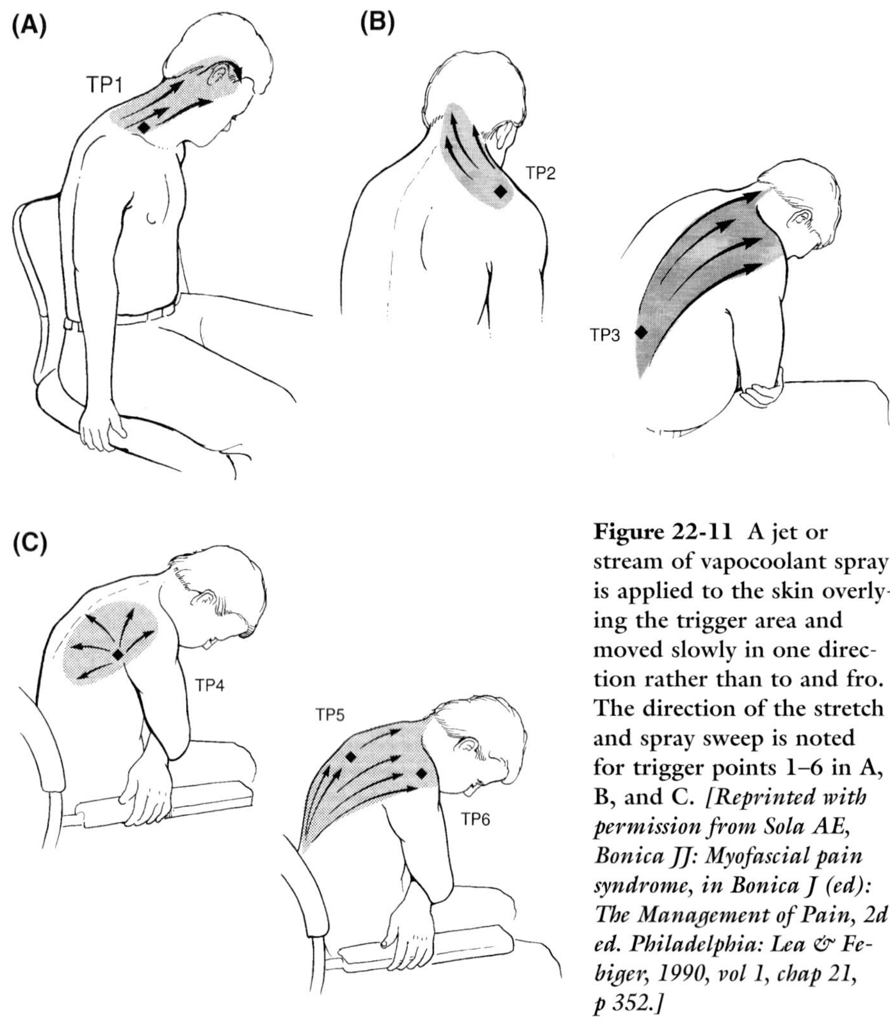

Figure 22-11 A jet or stream of vapocoolant spray is applied to the skin overlying the trigger area and moved slowly in one direction rather than to and fro. The direction of the stretch and spray sweep is noted for trigger points 1–6 in A, B, and C. *[Reprinted with permission from Sola AE, Bonica JJ: Myofascial pain syndrome, in Bonica J (ed): The Management of Pain, 2d ed. Philadelphia: Lea & Febiger, 1990, vol 1, chap 21, p 352.]*

the process in an effort to reduce pain. Important inflammatory mediators include prostaglandin E_2 (PGE_2) and prostacyclin (PGI_2). Both have the ability to counteract the vasoconstrictor effects of norepinephrine and angiotensin. Other inflammatory mediators include bradykinin, histamine, and leukotriene C_4. A potent chemotactic substance is leukotriene B_4, which is a product of the lipoxygenase pathway of arachidonate metabolism.

Aspirin-like drugs inhibit prostaglandin biosynthesis by inhibiting the enzyme cyclooxygenase, which prevents the conversion of arachidonic acid to the unstable endoperoxide intermediate PGG_2. This does not imply that all anti-inflammatory drugs have exactly the same mode of action. There are, for example, numerous forms of cyclooxygenase. Some drugs may work directly on the enzyme, and some may work through competitive inhibition.

Gastrointestinal Damage Associated with NSAIDs

NSAIDs can damage the gastrointestinal tract and cause peptic ulceration and life-threatening bleeding. The inhibitory effects of NSAIDs on the endogenous biosynthesis of prostaglandin are considered to be the major mechanism for their therapeutic effect. Prostaglandins play a significant role in the defense of the gastrointestinal mucosa. Prostaglandins of the E series have gastric antisecretory and mucosal protective properties. NSAID inhibition of gastric mucosal prostaglandin synthesis is thought to be largely responsible for much of the gastrointestinal tract toxicity.

Allison and colleagues[11] examined the stomach, duodenum, and small intestine of 713 patients postmortem. Among these patients, 249 had had NSAIDs prescribed during the 6 months before death. The remainder had no history of taking NSAIDs. Ulcers of the stomach or duodenum were found in 21.7 percent of users compared with 12.3 percent of nonusers ($p < 0.001$). Nonspecific small intestinal ulceration was found in 8.4 percent of the NSAID users compared with 0.6 percent of nonusers ($p < 0.001$). Three patients died from perforated nonspecific small intestinal ulcers.

Misoprostol, a synthetic prostaglandin E_1 analogue, is effective in preventing NSAID-induced gastric ulcers and duodenal lesions. Another effective antiulcer drug, sucralfate, increases the release of endogenous prostaglandin from the gastric mucosa. A study comparing the effectiveness of these two drugs in preventing gastric ulcers was performed by Agarwal and associates.[12] In patients receiving chronic NSAID therapy for osteoarthritis, treatment with misoprostol for 3 months was associated with a significantly lower frequency of gastric ulcer formation compared with treatment with sucralfate.

A number of NSAIDs were compared in regard to the risk of developing peptic ulcer disease (Table 22-2). Ibuprofen appeared to have the lowest risk, and meclofenamate the highest.

NSAIDs are usually used either alone or in combination with antidepressant drugs. They also may be used also in conjunction with trigger point injections and/or the stretch and spray technique.

A list of NSAID drugs appears in Table 22-3, which shows a classification together with dosage and time to peak effect, plasma half-life, analgesic effect, anti-inflammatory effect, antipyretic effect, and antiplatelet effect. A logical way to choose an NSAID is to look for one that is best suited to the patient's condition, low in undesirable side effects, and low in cost. In addition to gastrointestinal damage, the side effects of NSAID are many, and some can be life-threatening. Many of these side effects are listed in Table 22-3. Interactions of NSAIDs with other drugs are shown in Table 22-5. The high cost of some of the newer NSAIDs must be considered. Salicylates [aspirin (acetylsalicylic acid), magnesium trisilicate, salicylsalicylic acid or salicylate, and diflunisal] still head the list as the least expensive drugs that are effective and have minimal side effects. Of the nonsalicylate drugs, ibuprofen is probably the most widely used drug, because it costs less and has fewer side effects than do many other NSAIDs.

Table 22-2 Relative risk for development of peptic ulcer disease

Drug	Standard dose mg/24 h	Total	
		Case Patients n	Relative Risk (95% CI)
Ibuprofen	1200	83	2.3 (1.8 to 3.0)
Indomethacin	50	30	3.8 (2.4 to 6.0)
Sulindac	300	37	4.2 (2.8 to 6.3)
Naproxen	500	121*	4.3 (3.4 to 5.4)
Fenoprofen	900	34	4.3 (2.8 to 6.6)
Piroxicam	20	109*	6.4 (4.8 to 8.4)
Tolmetin	600	21*	8.5 (4.5 to 16.1)
Meclofenamate	200	21*	8.7 (4.6 to 16.4)

SOURCE: Reproduced with permission from Griffin MR et al: Non-steroidal anti-inflammatory drug use and increased risk for peptic ulcer disease in elderly persons. *Ann Intern Med* 114:257, 1991.
*Different from ibuprofen ($P<0.05$), adjusted for multiple comparisons.

Opioid Analgesics

There is probably little use for opioids in the management of myofascial pain. They offer no long-term solution, they are addictive, and their side effects are highly undesirable in the elderly (i.e., constipation and nausea). On occasion, though, the use of opioids can be justified, for example, in treating severe myofascial pain in a terminal cancer patient. When opioids are used in the elderly, the dose must be modified. Bellville and coworkers[13] studied acute postoperative pain relief in 712 patients. Age proved to be highly correlated with pain relief reports in that the older age group reported more pain relief. From their study, the authors concluded that it is important to adjust the dose of an opioid analgesic in relation to a patient's age rather than in relation to height, weight, or other characteristics. There was no correlation between sedation score and age. This virtually rules out the idea that the results can be based on altered absorption and distribution. It is also difficult to explain the results on the basis of the effects of the aging process on the CNS, particularly when sedation is not increased with age. Many hypotheses have been advanced to explain the phenomenon of decreased pain sensitivity with aging. It may be a manifestation of a more general phenomenon associated with changes in pain perception with aging. As shown in Fig. 22-12, there is a marked reduction in the dose of the narcotics pentazocine and morphine used to relieve pain in the seventh decade of life.

Antidepressant Drugs

It is well known that depression is frequently seen in patients with chronic pain. Studies have shown the incidence as low as 10 percent and as high as 100

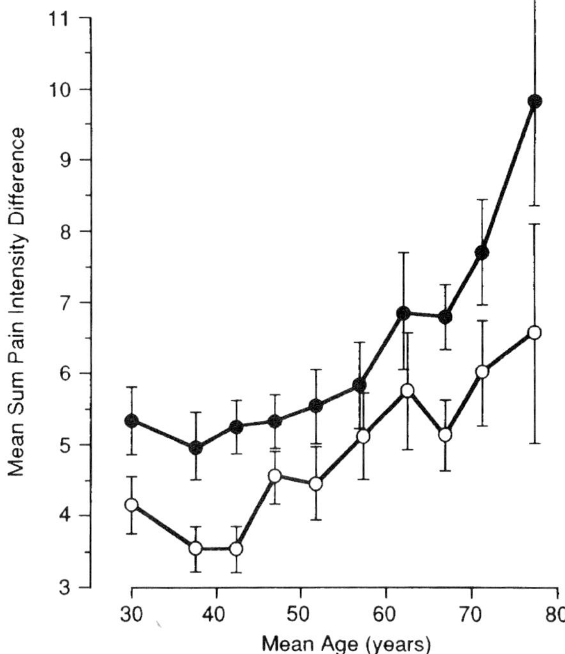

Figure 22-12 Mean sum pain intensity difference vs mean age (year) for the 10 age groups of the population. Patients received 20 mg of pentazocine (○) or 10 mg of morphine sulphate (●). (Reprinted with permission *from Bellville JW, Forrest WH, Miller E, Brown BW: Influence of age on pain relief from analgesics. JAMA 217:1835, 1971. Copyright 1971, American Medical Association.)*

percent. According to Hendler,[14] all chronic pain patients pass through a period of depression. He describes four stages in Table 22-4.

In addition to their antidepression properties, drugs of the tricyclic antidepressant group act as unconventional analgesics in pain management. The drug most widely studied is amitriptyline. A number of controlled studies support the analgesic properties of the tricyclic antidepressant drugs, particularly in diabetic neuropathy, facial pain, and postherpetic neuralgia.

The mode of action of the analgesic properties is not clear. These drugs block $alpha_1$ adrenergic, muscarinic, and H_1 histamine receptors. Serotonin and norepinephrine reuptake is also blocked. One theory is that the analgesic effects may be due to interference with 5-hydroxytryptamine (5HT) systems in the synapse, which may cause an increase in the pain threshold. An increase in 5HT occurs in the synaptic cleft by blocking reuptake by the presynaptic neurons. This in turn produces antinociception by activity in the descending pain inhibitory pathways. It appears that the analgesic effects occur with a lower dose of drugs than is required to produce antidepression. The onset of analgesia also occurs more rapidly than does the onset of antidepression.

McQuay and associates[15] studied the use of low doses of amitriptyline in the treatment of chronic pain. They compared the analgesic efficacy of amitriptyline (25 mg) to a placebo in 41 patients with chronic nonmalignant pain of more than 3 months' duration. This was a double-blind, randomized, multidose, crossover design with a 3-week treatment period. Their results

Table 22-3 Nonsteroidal anti-inflammatory drugs

Class/Drug	Usual dose (mg PO)	Peak effect (h)	Plasma T½ (h)	Analgesic effect	Anti-inflammatory effect	Anti-pyretic effect	Anti-platelet effect	Comments
Nonacidic NSAIDs								
Para-aminophenol								
Acetaminophen	325–1000 mg q4–8h	0.5–1h	1–4h	Yes +++	None 0	Yes +++	None 0	Minimal GI, renal side effects. Extensive hepatic metabolism. OD can cause hepatic damage with increased liver function tests.
Acidic NSAIDs								
Salicylates								
Acetylsalicyclic acid (aspirin)	325–1000 mg q4–6h; "ceiling dose" 1300 mg/dose	2h	0.25h	Yes +++	Yes +++	Yes +++	Yes +++	Prodrug hydrolyzed by plasma esterase to salicylate, active for m. Irreversible platelet inhibition, must discontinue 7–14 days prior to surgery. Tinnitus, decreased hearing, dyspepsia, nausea/vomiting are signs of toxicity.
Choline magnesium trisalicylate (Trilisate)	870–1740 mg q3–4h	0.5–1h	9–17h	Yes +++	Yes +++	Yes +++	Min +/−	Advantage = minimal antiplatelet effect. Fewer side effects.
Salicylsalicylic acid (Salsalate) (Disalcid)	500–750 mg q12h			Yes +++	Yes +++	Yes +++	Yes +	Minimal Gl and antiplatelet activity.

Diflunisal (Dolobid)	200–500 mg q12h	1–2h	8–20h	Yes +++	Yes ++	Yes +	Yes +	
Indoleacetic acids								
Indomethacin (Indocin)	25–75 mg q6h	2h	2–3h	Yes +++	Yes +++	Yes +++	Yes +++	Contraindicated in patients with psychiatric disorders, epilepsy, parkinsonism, and renal disease. Headache, confusion, dizziness, seizures, nausea/vomiting, syncope, signs of toxicity.
Sulindac (Clinoril)	150–200 mg q12h	1–2h	7–18h	Yes +++	Yes +++	Yes +++	Yes +++	Prodrug metabolized to active form by liver. Minimal renal side effects. Use for patient with renal disease.
Phenylacetic acid								
Diclofenac (Voltaren)	50–75 mg q12h	1.5–3h	2h	Yes +++	Yes +++	Yes ++	Yes ++	Risk of hepatotoxicity. Should check baseline and q8 weeks transaminases.
Pyrroleacetic acid								
Tolmetin	200–400 mg q6–8h	0.5–1h	1–3h	Yes ++	Yes +++	Yes ++	Yes ++	Frequent GI side effects. Increased risk of hepatotoxicity. Watch transaminase levels.
Pyrazole								
Phenylbutazone	100–200 mg q6h	2h	60–100h	Yes ++	Yes ++++	Yes ++	Yes +++	Very limited use in U.S. owing to toxicity, especially blood dyscrasias.
Fenamates								
Mefenamic acid (Ponstel)	500 mg q6–8h	2h	3–4h	Yes ++	Yes ++	Yes +	Yes ++	Not recommended for use beyond 1 week because of toxicity. Hemolytic anemia.

Table 22-3 (*continued*)

Class/Drug	Usual dose (mg PO)	Peak effect (h)	Plasma T½ (h)	Analgesic effect	Anti-inflammatory effect	Anti-pyretic effect	Anti-platelet effect	Comments
Propionic acid								
Ibuprofen (Motrin)	**200–800 mg q6–8h**	**1–2h**	**2h**	Yes +++	Yes +++	Yes ++	Yes +++	**Monitor for hepatic toxicity with prolonged high dose. Over-the-counter so easy to obtain.**
Naproxen (Naprosyn) (Anaprox)	**250–500 mg q12h**	**2h**	**12–15h**	Yes +++	Yes +++	Yes ++	Yes +++	**GI side effects are common. Caution in patient with renal disease.**
Fenoprofen (Nalfon)	**300–600 mg q6–8h**	**2h**	**2–3h**	Yes ++	Yes +++	Yes +	Yes +++	**Monitor for renal toxicity (BUN, creatinine q month)**
Ketoprofen (Orudis)	**50–100 mg q6–8h**	**1–2h**	**1–35h**	Yes ++	Yes +++	Yes +	Yes +++	**High incidence of GI side effects.**
Benzothazine (Oxicam)								
Piroxicam (Feldene)	**20 mg q12–24h**	**2–4h**	**30–45h**	Yes +++	Yes +++	Yes +	Yes +++	**Longest T½. Good for noncompliant patient.**

0 = no effect, +/− = minimal to none, + = minimal, ++ = moderate, +++ = severe, ++++ = maximal effects.

SOURCE: From Kenworthy K: Non-steroidal anti-inflammatory drugs, in Ramamurthy S, Rogers JN (eds): *Decision Making in Pain Management*. St. Louis: Mosby, 1993. With permission.

Table 22-4 Four stages of depression

Stage 1: Acute	The patient is hopeful that the pain will get better. No depression is observed (0–2 months).
Stage 2: Subacute	The patient worries more about the pain and seeks more help. Again, there is no obvious observable depression (2–6 months).
Stage 3: Chronic	The patient begins to believe that the pain is permanent and feels depressed and despondent (6 months–8 years).
Stage 4: Subchronic	The patient moves toward accepting the reality of the pain as being chronic and starts to make changes to cope with the physical, social, and psychological aspects of the condition. Patients may improve in terms of their depression if they try to begin coping sooner (3–12 years). It should be noted that these observations are based primarily on clinical experience and that valid studies are lacking.

SOURCE: Hendler NH: The four stages of pain, in Hendler NH, Long DM, Wise TN (eds): *Diagnosis and Treatment of Chronic Pain*. Littleton, MA: John Wright PSG, 1982, pp 1–8.

showed a significant analgesic effect with amitriptyline compared with the placebo within 1 week. Interestingly, no difference was found in mood scores between the two groups. The same authors[16] later studied the dose-response curve for the analgesic effect of amitriptyline in patients with chronic pain. The doses studied were 25, 50, and 75 mg. In 29 patients with chronic pain, 75 mg provided significantly greater pain relief than did 25 or 50 mg. There was no difference between mood scores using the different doses, but sleep was significantly better with a dose of 75 mg compared with 25 mg. The incidence of the side effects dry mouth and drowsiness was also higher with the 75-mg dose.

There are a large number of antidepressant drugs to choose from. A number of these drugs and their recommended doses are shown in Table 22-6. The choice of drug is frequently influenced by the side effects, as well as the drug's efficiency. The side effects of tricyclic antidepressants are shown in Table 22-7. The most common side effect is drowsiness. For this reason, when one selects a drug such as amitriptyline, it is wise to start the patient on a low dose, particularly in elderly patients.

One of the goals in treating the elderly, in addition to achieving pain relief, is to keep the patient active and mobile. Overtreatment with medication can easily cause more harm than good and can create "the cascade to dependency," as demonstrated in Fig. 22-13, which shows the hazards of bed rest in the elderly. Increased bed rest will occur with untreated myofascial pain or overtreatment with tricyclic antidepressants. Either cause can in turn lead to other medical complications and to dependency. Another problem with the overuse of sedatives, antidepressants, and analgesics in the elderly is increased sensory

Table 22-5 Interactions of NSAIDs with other drugs

Drug affected	NSAID implicated	Effect	Approach to management
		Pharmacokinetic interactions	
NSAID affecting other drug			
Oral anticoagulants	Phenylbutazone Oxyphenbutazone Apazone	Inhibition of metabolism of S-warfarin, increasing anticoagulant effect	Avoid NSAID if possible, or use careful monitoring.
Lithium	Probably all (except possibly sulindac and aspirin)	Inhibition of renal excretion of lithium, plasma lithium concentrations and risk of toxicity	Use sulindac or aspirin of NSAID must be used. Monitor lithium concentration carefully and make appropriate dose reduction.
Oral hypoglycemic agents	Phenylbutazone Oxyphenbutazone Apazone	Inhibition of metabolism of sulfonylurea prolonging their half-life and increasing rhe risk of hypoglycemia	Avoid these NSAIDs if possible; if not, monitor blood glucose level closely.
Phenytoin	Phenylbutazone Oxyphenbutazone	Inhibition of metabolism of phenytoin, increasing plasma phenytoin concentration and risk of toxicity	Avoid these NSAIDs if possible; if not, intensify therapeutic-drug monitoring.
	Others	Displacement of phenytoin from plasma protein, reducing total concentration for the same unbound (active) concentration	Interpret total plasma concentration of phenytoin carefully; measuring the unbound concentration may be helpful.
Methotrexate (high, nonrheumatologic dose)	Probably all	Reduced clearance of methotrexate (by unknown mechanism), increasing plasma methotrexate concentration and risk of toxicity	Simultaneous dosing is contraindicated. Use of NSAIDs between cycles of chemotherapy is probably safe. Interaction not seen with rheumatologic doses of methotrexate.
Sodium valproate	Aspirin	Inhibition of valproate metabolism, increasing plasma valproate concentration	Avoid aspirin; monitor plasma valproate concentration closely if another NSAID is used.

Digoxin	All	Potential reduction in renal function (particularly in very young and very old patients), reducing digoxin clearance and increasing plasma digoxin concentration and risk of toxicity (no interaction if renal function normal)	Avoid NSAIDs if possible; if not, measure plasma digoxin and creatinine concentrations frequently.
Aminoglycosides	All	Reduction in renal function in susceptible persons, lowering aminoglycoside clearance and increasing plasma aminoglycoside concentration	Monitor plasma aminoglycoside concentration closely and adjust the dose accordingly.
Other drug affecting NSAID			
Antacids	Indomethacin Others	Variable effects of different preparations: rate and extent of absorption of indomethacin reduced by aluminum-containing antacids, but increased by sodium bicarbonate	No action required unless markedly reduced absorption results in a poor response to the NSAID: dose may need to be increased. Rate of absorption of other NSAIDs can be slowed by antacids.
Probenecid	Probably all	Reduction in metabolism and renal clearance of NSAIDs and acyl glucuronide metabolites, which are hydrolyzed back to parent drug	
Barbiturates	Phenylbutazone, possibly others	Increased metabolic clearance of NSAID	May require higher dose of phenylbutazone.
Caffeine	Aspirin	Increased rate of absorption of aspirin	No action required.
Cholestyramine	Naproxen and probably others	Anion-exchange resin binding of NSAIDs in gut, reducing rate (and possibly of extent) absorption	Separate dosing times by 4 h; may need larger-than-expected doses of NSAID.
Metoclopramide	Aspirin and others	Increased rate and extent of absorption of aspirin in patients with migraine	

Table 22-5 (*continued*)

Drug affected	NSAID implicated	Effect	Approach to management
		Pharmacodynamic interactions	
NSAID affecting other drug			
Antihypertensive agents			
Beta-blockers Diuretics Angiotensin-converting-enzyme inhibitors	Indomethacin Others (possibly except sulindac)	Reduction in hypotensive effect, probably related to inhibition of prostaglandin synthesis in kidneys (producing retention of salt and water) and blood vessels (producing increased vasoconstriction)	Avoid all NSAID use in patients receiving treatment for hypertension if possible; if not, use sulindac preferentially. Check blood pressure measurements repeatedly after starting NSAID. Additional antihypertensive therapy may be needed.
Diuretics	Indomethacin Others (possibly except sulindac)	Reduction in natriuretic and diuretic effects; may exacerbate congestive cardiac failure	Avoid NSAID use in patients with cardiac failure if possible; use sulindac and monitor clinical signs of fluid retention.
Anticoagulants	All	Damage to mucosa of gastrointestinal tract and inhibition of platelet aggregation, both increasing risk of gastrointestinal bleeding in patients taking anticoagulants	Avoid all NSAIDs, if possible.
Hypoglycemic agents	Salicylate (high dose)	Potentiation of hypoglycemic effects (by unknown mechanism)	Monitor blood glucose level.
Combination with increased risk of toxicity			
Diuretics			
General	All	Combination associated with increased risk of hemodynamic renal failure	Avoid combination if possible.
Triamterene	Indomethacin	Potentiation of nephrotoxicity, even in subjects with normal renal function	Combination contraindicated.
Potassium-sparing	All	Potassium retention and hyperkalemia	Avoid combination; monitor plasma potassium level.

SOURCE: From Brooks PM, Day RO: Non-steroidal anti-inflammatory drugs—differences and similarities. *N Engl J Med* 324:1716, 1981. Reprinted by permission of the *New England Journal of Medicine*.

Table 22-6 Antidepressant drugs: Dosage forms and doses

Monproprietary name	Trade names	Dosage forms*	Usual daily dose *(mg)*†	Extreme daily dose *(mg)*†‡
Tricyclics				
Amitriptyline HCl	Elavil, others	O,I	50–150	40–300
Amoxapine	Asendin	O	200–300	50–600
Desipramine HCl	Norpramin, Pertofrane	O	75–200	25–300
Doxepin HCl	Adapin, Sinequan	O,L	75–150	25–300
Imipramine HCl	Janimine, Tofranil, others	O,I	50–200	30–300
Maprotiline HCl	Ludiomil	O	75–150	25–200
Nortriptyline HCl	Pamelor	O,L	75–100	20–150
Protriptyline HCl	Vivactil	O	15–40	15–60
Trimipramine maleate	Surmontil	O	50–150	50–300
Atypical				
Fluoxetine HCl	Prozac	O	40–60	20–80
Trazodone HCl	Desyrel	O	150–200	50–600
Monoamine oxidase inhibitors				
Isocarboxazid	Marplan	O	10–30	10–30
Phenelzine sulfate	Nardil	O	15–30	15–90
Tranylcypromine sulfate	Parnate	O	20–30	10–40

* Dosage forms: O = oral solid; I = injection; L = oral liquid.

† Oral dose.

‡ Extreme doses are for very young and very elderly patients at the low end and for hospital use in severe or treatment-resistant depression at the high end. In addition, owing to the long biological half-life of MAO inhibition, small doses of MAO inhibitors are used after several days to weeks of treatment.

SOURCE: From Baldessarini RJ: Drugs and the treatment of psychiatric disorders, in Gillman AG, Rall TW, Nies AS, Taylor P (eds): *The Pharmacological Basis of Therapeutics*, 8th ed. New York: Pergamon Press, 1990, chap. 18, p 411. With permission.

deprivation. This is particularly bad for an elderly patient who may already have visual and hearing problems.

Table 22-7 Side effects of tricyclic antidepressants

Type	Minor (early)	Major
Sedative	Lassitude Fatigue	Sleepiness Impaired consciousness with alcohol and other drugs
Sympathomimetic	Tachycardia Tremor Sweating	Agitation Insomnia Aggravation of psychosis
Anticholinergic	Blurred vision Constipation Urinary hesitancy Fuzzy thinking	Aggravation of glaucoma Paralytic ileus Urinary retention Delirium
Cardiovascular	Orthostatic hypotension ECG abnormality	Delayed cardiac conduction Prolongation of P-R interval Widening of the QRS complex Flattening or inversion of the T wave Dysrhythmias Sudden death
Neuropsychiatric	Confusion Delirium	Central anticholinergic syndrome Withdrawal
Allergic/toxic		Cholestatic jaundice Agranulocytosis
Metabolic/endocrine	Weight gain Sexual disturbance	Gynecomastia Amenorrhea
Neurogenic	Tremor Paresthesia EEG alteration	Seizures Neuropathy

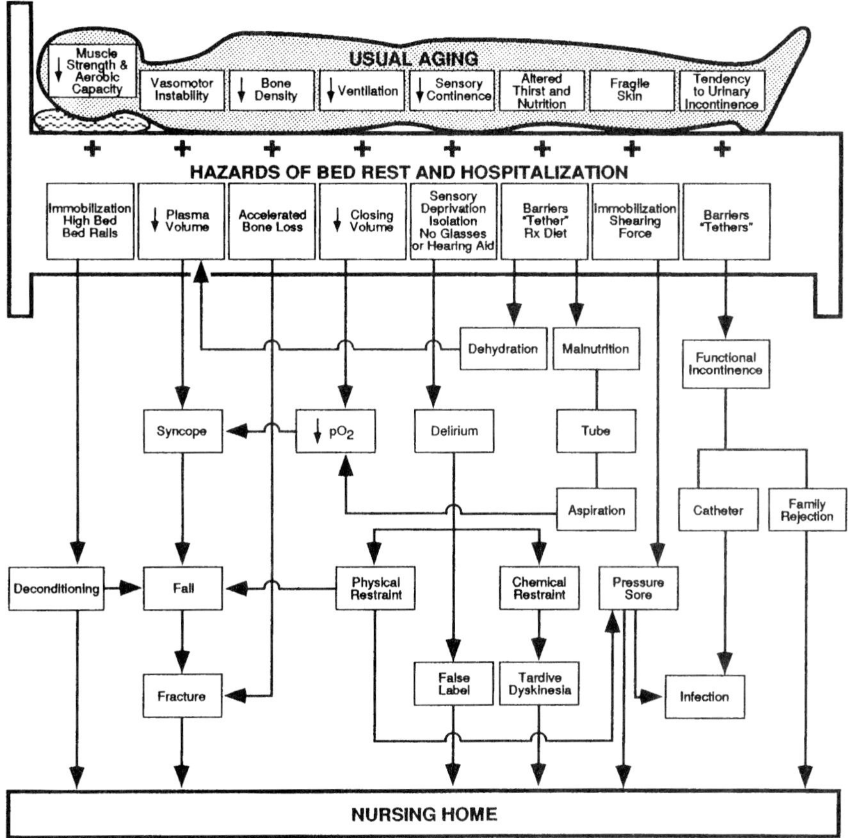

Figure 22-13 **Hazards of hospitalization of the elderly. The cascade to dependency.** *(Reproduced with permission from Creditor MC: Hazards of hospitalization in the elderly. Ann Intern Med 118:219, 1993.)*

SUMMARY

Myofascial pain accounts for the symptoms of the majority of patients who attend pain clinics. Evaluations in addition to the physical examination must include psychological evaluations. Treatment modalities include trigger point injection, stretch and coolant spray techniques, TENS, anti-inflammatory drugs, and analgesics. It is most important to keep geriatric patients active and mobile. Overtreatment with medication can easily cause more harm than good.

REFERENCES

1. Raj PP: Myofascial trigger point injection, in Raj PP (ed): *Practical Management of Pain*. Chicago, London: Yearbook, 1986, chap 33, pp 569–577.

2. Travell J: Management of pain due to muscle spasm. *NY State J Med* 45:2095, 1945.
3. Gutstein M: Diagnosis and treatment of muscular rheumatism. *Br J Phys Med* 1:302, 1938.
4. Correll RL: Treatment of skeletal pain with procaine injections: Analysis of 295 cases in general practice. *Am J Surg* 63:102, 1944.
5. Bonica JJ: Management of myofascial pain syndrome in general practice. *JAMA* 164:732, 1957.
6. Magni G, Schifaro F, Deleo D: Pain as a symptom in elderly depressed patients. *Eur Arch Psychiatry Neurol Sci* 235:143, 1985.
7. Talbot JD, Marreit S, Evans AC, Meyer E: Multiple representations of pain in human cerebral cortex. *Science* 251:1355, 1991.
8. Beck AT, Ward CH, Mendelson M, et al: An inventory for measuring depression. *Arch Gen Psychiatry* 4:53, 1961.
9. Wall PD: Introduction, in Wall PD, Melzack R (eds): *Textbook of Pain*, 2d ed. Edinburgh: Churchill Livingstone, 1989, pp 1–16.
10. Deyo RA, Walsh NE, Martin DC, et al: A controlled trial of transcutaneous electrical nerve stimulation (TENS) and exercise for chronic low back pain. *N Engl J Med* 322:1627, 1990.
11. Allison MC, Howatson AG, Torrance CJ, et al: Gastrointestinal damage associated with the use of nonsteroidal anti-inflammatory drugs. *N Engl J Med* 327:749, 1992.
12. Agarwal NM, Roth S, Graham DY, et al: Misoprostol compared with sucralfate in the prevention of nonsteroidal anti-inflammatory drug-induced gastric ulcer: A randomized, controlled trial. *Ann Intern Med* 115:195, 1991.
13. Bellville JW, Forrest WH, Miller E, Brown BW: Influence of age on pain relief from analgesics. *JAMA* 217:1835, 1971.
14. Hendler NH: The four stages of pain, in Hendler NH, Long DM, Wise TN (eds): *Diagnosis and Treatment of Chronic Pain*. Littleton, MA: John Wright PSG, 1982, pp 1–8.
15. McQuay HJ, Carroll D, Glynn CJ: Low dose amitriptylene in the treatment of chronic pain. *Anaesthesia* 47:646, 1992.
16. McQuay HJ, Carroll D, Glynn CJ: Dose-response for analgesic effect of amitriptyline in chronic pain. *Anaesthesia* 48:281, 1993.

CHAPTER 23

Low Back Pain and Medical Rehabilitation in the Elderly

Nicolas E. Walsh
Diane M.L. Gilbert
Gregory D. Powell

INTRODUCTION

The lifetime incidence of a degree of low back pain ranges from 60 to 90 percent, with only 14 to 20 percent of cases being reported as significant back pain.[1,2] Previous episodes of low back pain may predispose the elderly to exacerbation and chronic low back pain problems.[3] National statistics from the U.S. population indicate a yearly prevalence of low back pain of 15 to 20 percent. Prevalence studies of low back pain in the elderly suggest an overall prevalence of 20 to 40 percent in patients over 65 years of age.[4–7] Fifteen to 40 percent of these individuals reported specific functional limitations caused by low back pain.

Back pain is a pervasive problem for which the young and the old often seek the care of a physician. It is the third most frequently mentioned symptom by patients age 75 or older and the most commonly mentioned musculoskeletal symptom.[6] Among chronic conditions that cause limitations among individuals in the United States, impairments of the back and spine are the most frequent in persons under age 45 years and third after heart disease and rheumatologic disorders in persons 45 to 64 years of age.[2]

The major goal in the rehabilitation of a geriatric patient with low back pain is to restore maximal physical function and return the patient to maximum capacity for the activities of daily living.

FUNCTIONAL ANATOMY OF THE LUMBAR SPINE

The alterations of structure and function of the lumbar spine constitute a continuous process of aging. A significant degree of the spinal disk shock absorbancy is lost with age. Decreased water content and altered biochemical structure decrease the resilience to compression.[8] With aging, decreased nutritional diffusion results in accelerated intervertebral disk degeneration.[9] In addition to the biochemical deterioration, long-term mechanical wear and tear on the apophyseal joints, spinus ligaments, and joint capsules results in impaired biomechanical function of the lumbar spine.

Three-Joint Complex

The human spinal column consists of 26 separate bones: 7 cervical vertebrae, 12 thoracic vertebrae, 5 lumbar vertebrae, the sacrum, and the coccyx. The vertebrae form a bony ring—the vertebral canal—that protects the spinal cord and nerve roots. Each vertebra in the lumbar spine is composed of the vertebral body anteriorly, pedicles, transverse processes, laminae, and the posterior spinous process, which completes the ring of the vertebral canal. From the posterior aspect of the pedicles arise the paired superior and inferior articular processes. Three joints make up the interface between each set of vertebrae in the lumbar spine and define the motion possible at each level. This so-called three-joint complex[10] is defined as the intervertebral joint anteriorly and a pair of zygapophyseal or facet joints posteriorly.

Basic Biomechanics

There are six primary motions in the lumbar spine: forward flexion, extension, bilateral side bending, and bilateral rotation. The actual motion of each three-joint spinal segment is generally quite limited; however, in combination, considerable functional motion is possible.[11]

As the vertebral bodies of the lumbar spine progress from cephalad to caudad, the vertebral bodies are found to be larger in all dimensions. This is necessary for them to fulfill their role as the primary weight-bearing structure of the lumbar spine. As the normal human spine begins to assume an axial load, the trabecular arrangement of the bone spicules within the vertebral bodies deforms and safely transmits the load.[12] The intervertebral disks play a role in this process as well.

As an axial load develops in the intervertebral disk, the vertebral endplates compress the gelatinous nucleus pulposus. The nucleus in turn diverts a portion of the axial load into horizontal stress as it lies within an enclosed space. This horizontal load is then borne by the lamellar fibers of the annulus fibrosis and are dispersed safely.[8]

The three-joint complex acts in concert to provide a component of each primary motion at each vertebral segment. While much of the allowable motion comes from the anterior vertebral segment and is the responsibility of the intervertebral disk, it is the facet joints in the posterior elements that define the allowable motion at each segment by restricting allowable motion. The facets are multiplanar and generally lie in an oblique fashion,[13] narrower anteriorly and wider posteriorly.[14] Their geometric relation, lying between the sagittal and coronal planes, allows considerable motion in flexion but significantly restricts extension, side bending, and rotation. Indeed, up to 20 degrees of forward flexion is possible at an individual vertebral segment, but extension is limited to about 5 degrees and rotation is limited to only 2 to 3 degrees on either side.[8,14,15] Additionally, because of the multiplanar nature of the joints, a coupling of motions occurs, resulting in forced rotation during side bending.[8]

AGE CHANGES IN THE LUMBAR SPINE

Anatomic Changes: Normal versus Pathological

Much controversy ensues when the age-related changes of the lumbar spine are discussed. Certainly, many changes of the intervertebral disks and vertebrae are known to take place in a majority of individuals as they age. It has not been determined if these individual changes result from normal processes or occult preventable injury and the anatomic response to such insults. The progression of aging of the lumbar spine in normal individuals over time needs to be differentiated from known pathological entities that can cause lumbar pain and disability.

Disk

Many of the age-related changes of the normal adult lumbar spine originate at the level of the intervertebral disk. Over time, the intervertebral disks lose their resiliency and become more fibrous.[16] As a result, the intervertebral joints lose range of motion and the spinal column as a whole becomes less flexible.[11,17,18]

The derangements of the intervertebral disk combined with the changes in the vertebral bodies subsequently are responsible for compensatory anatomic changes in the posterior elements.

Nucleus Pulposus

As the human spine begins to age, a cascade of changes begins with alteration of the biochemical composition of the nucleus pulposus,[8] which begins to exhibit a relative increase in collagen fibers[19] and a decrease in proteoglycans.[20] The remaining proteoglycans are known to be shorter and subsequently less deformable. In contrast to early life, when the nucleus is highly elastic and rubbery, as time progresses, it becomes more fibrous and less resilient.

Water content was previously thought to be the primary change with age in the intervertebral disk. It was known that at birth, the water content of intervertebral disks averages 88 percent. This drops to 65 to 72 percent by age 65.[8] More recent information, however, has shown that much of the water lost by the intervertebral disk is lost in late childhood and adolescence, much too early to account for the entirety of the biomechanical changes that occur with aging. In fact, the actual hydration of the nucleus decreases by only about 6 percent throughout adulthood.[21]

Annulus Fibrosis

Considerable changes in the annular fibers of the intervertebral disk occur with aging. The fibers lose their elasticity as a result of a relative loss of elastin, which in turn makes them more prone to microtrauma with normal repetitive motion. Fissures and tears (both radial and circumferential) begin to appear and ultimately coalesce as aging takes place.[22]

The annulus seems to widen as concurrent changes take place in the nucleus pulposus, and the distinct boundary between the two becomes more blurred.[8] The unit as a whole becomes more homogeneous and loses a degree of the structural advantage that is present in earlier life. These changes further accelerate the progression of aging.

Disk Height

The intervertebral disk increases in size as the body ages. The anteroposterior diameter increases from 2 percent to 10 percent.[21] Disk height increases by an average of 10 percent in most individuals.[21] Therefore, loss of axial height is largely a result of decreased vertebral body size and is a bony rather than a soft tissue change. Most important, however, this implies that loss of disk height on radiographic examination is not a normal consequence of aging.

Vertebral Body and Endplate

The human spine is commonly known to decrease in height with aging. This decrease in axial height accounts for the bulk of the decrease in height seen with normal aging. The primary site of the loss of axial height of the skeleton is the vertebral bodies. As the body ages, the vertebrae begin to show a decrease in both bone density[23] and strength.[24] This is a result of a primary loss of trabecular bone throughout the vertebral bodies.[8] The loss of trabecular bone translates to an increased reliance on less resilient cortical bone for the primary purpose of weight bearing. The vertebrae become more injury-prone with this change.

The vertebral endplates also go through numerous changes as the body ages. They begin to lose osteocytes and decrease in both density and thickness.[22] Vascular channels through this region, those primarily responsible for the nutritional support of the intervertebral disks, progressively become obliterated.[9] While this is not thought to be the initiating factor in the biochemical changes taking place in the disk, it clearly begins to alter the disk's ability to recover from injury and accelerates its age-related changes.

Facet Joints

The morphological changes of the facet joints are secondary to the normal aging of the anterior elements. With time, pathological changes include a reactive thickening of the cortical bone underlying the articular cartilage and the calcification of the insertion of the synovial membrane into the bone surrounding the joint cavity.[8] The formation of osteophytes from this calcification is currently thought to be a consequence of normal spinal aging, as it is present in the vast majority of elderly individuals and demonstrates no correlation with the presence or absence of lumbar pain.[3,8]

Biomechanical Changes

As the lumbar spine begins to age, distinct biomechanical changes begin to occur in a predictable fashion. As the intervertebral disks are largely responsible for the ability of the lumbar spine to move through space, when they lose their elasticity, this motion becomes more limited. The changes present in any one vertebral level may be as small as a degree or two of motion, but when they are combined together as a unit, considerable loss of motion may occur.

Along with the decrease in the axial height of the vertebral bodies there is a progressive decrease in the height of the anterior elements relative to the posterior elements. This results in a progressive decrease in the amount of lumbar lordosis and an increase in the amount of thoracic kyphosis.[8] These changes subsequently alter the anatomic orientation of the facet joints and further restrict motion in the aging spine.

CLINICAL EVALUATION

The vast majority of low back pain is of mechanical etiology in the elderly. It is essential to distinguish patients with a mechanical etiology for low back pain from patients with a serious nonmechanical etiology (Table 23-1).

Table 23-1 Classification of low back pain in the elderly

Mechanical
Neurological
Disk herniation
Lumbar spinal stenosis
Fracture
Spondylolisthesis
Vertebral
Musculoskeletal
Degenerative disk disease (spondylosis)
Osteophytosis (facet joint)
Degenerative joint disease
Myofascial
Systemic
Cardiovascular
Aortic aneurysm
Claudication
Gastrointestinal
Pancreatitis
Cholecystitis
Penetrating ulcer
Urologic
Prostatitis
Pyelonephritis
Infectious
Osteomyelitis
Tuberculous spondylitis
Herpes zoster
Subacute bacterial endocarditis
Epidural abscess
Metabolic
Osteoporosis
Osteomalacia
Paget disease
Neoplastic
Metastatic lesions to the spine
Multiple myeloma
Spinal cord and retroperitoneal tumors
Lymphoma
Rheumatologic
Spondyloarthropathies
Rheumatoid arthritis
Polymyalgia rheumatica
Psoriatic spondylitis

The history and physical exam must be relied upon when one is developing a systematic clinical approach to an older patient complaining of low back pain. The purpose of this section is to familiarize the clinician with the most sensitive and specific items in the history and physical examination of the low back and to provide a framework useful for devising a differential diagnosis. A thorough review of the low back examination is beyond the scope of this chapter, and so the reader is referred to several other sources.[25,84]

History

Acute low back pain is typically defined as lasting less than 1 month, while chronic low back pain has a duration of more than 3 months. Low back pain in the elderly, as in other age groups, is most commonly a result of musculoskeletal dysfunction. In dealing with an elderly patient who presents with back pain, one must have a heightened awareness of the more serious causes of back pain. Unfortunately, low back pain may be a manifestation of a systemic illness in over 60 diseases.[26,27] In a geriatric patient, it is not unusual for a concomitant illness to be present that may be a component of the patient's low back pain.

The most valuable aspect of the exam is the history. To categorize back pain, the outline listed in Table 23-2 should be employed to answer the following questions: (1) Is a systemic disease causing the pain? (2) Is there neurological compromise? (3) Is the pain musculoskeletal in origin? (4) Is there evidence of psychological factors exacerbating the pain?

Timing of Pain

Onset immediately after trauma suggests an acute fracture, muscular tear, or strain. Vertebral body collapse can be acute, occurring after lifting or other types of exertion and precipitating acute, severe pain. This presumably reflects sudden collapse of the vertebra. Some patients may have a more gradual onset, with a period of dull, aching back pain that subsequently may increase markedly.[28] However, the pain usually improves with time, and supine positioning usually provides relief.

Metastatic vertebral collapse can be insidious. The pain may gradually escalate, culminating in unbearable pain. Nighttime pain or pain that increases with recumbency raises the suspicion of malignancy. Stiffness in the morning with improvement with activity may indicate rheumatalogic disease.

Location of Pain

The patient may describe the pain as localized to a single level or side or diffuse. Pain diagrams that the patient fills out himself or herself can provide more information. Pain that radiates down the leg below the knees to the foot suggests a radiculopathy.

Table 23-2 Medical history in the diagnosis of spine disease causing low back pain

Diseases	Source	Medical history	Sensitivity	Specificity
Cancer	Deyo and Diehl (1988)	Age ≥ 50 years	0.77	0.71
		Previous history of cancer	0.31	0.98
		Unexplained weight loss	0.15	0.94
		Failure to improve after a month of therapy	0.31	0.90
		No relief with bed rest	>0.90	0.46
		Duration of pain > 1 month	0.50	0.81
		Age ≥50 *or* history of cancer *or* unexplained weight loss *or* failure of conservative therapy	1.00	0.60
Spinal osteomyelitis	Waldvogel and Vasey (1980)	Intravenous drug abuse, urinary tract infection, or skin infection	0.40	Not available
Compression fracture	Deyo (1992)	Age ≥50 years	0.84	0.61
		Age ≥70 years	0.22	0.96
		Trauma	0.30	0.85
		Corticosteroid use	0.06	0.995
Herniated disk	Deyo and Tsui-Wu (1987), Sprangfort (1972)	Sciatica	0.95	0.88
Spinal stenosis	Turner et al (1992)	Pseudoclaudication	0.60	NA
		Age ≥50 years	0.90	0.70
Ankylosing spondylitis	Gran (1985)	Four of five positive responses*	0.23	0.82
		Age at onset ≤40 years	1.00	0.07
		Pain not relieved when supine	0.80	0.9
		Morning back stiffness	0.64	0.59
		Pain duration ≥3 months	0.71	0.54

*The five screening questions were (1) Onset of back discomfort before age 40 years? (2) Did the problem begin slowly? (3) Persistence for at least 3 months? (4) Morning stiffness? (5) Improved by exercise?

SOURCE: Modified from Deyo et al.[29] Copyright 1992, American Medical Association.

Quality, Quantity, or Severity of Pain

Pain can be described as constant, intermittent, radiating, lancinating (herpes zoster), or throbbing. Aching of the buttocks, thighs, or calves is suggestive of vascular claudication. Constant increasing pain may raise suspicions of cancer, while intermittent sharp pain associated with motion suggests muscular-ligamentous injury. Visual analogue scales provide an accurate reference for changes in pain intensity. A patient with an unstable spine secondary to degenerative spondylolisthesis may describe a slight movement of the spine that causes imbalance in standing or walking.

Onset of Pain

The initiation of pain is often related to a minor incident by the patient, but careful questioning may reveal an earlier onset. It is important to understand the exact mechanism of the suspected trauma. Was excessive hyperextension, flexion, torquing, or rotational loading present? Although workmen's compensation may not be as large an issue in the elderly, there may be pending litigation that may affect the prognosis.

Factors That Aggravate or Relieve Pain

Muscular strain is aggravated by stretching the involved muscle. Radiculopathies are often exacerbated by coughing, sneezing, or other actions, resulting in a Valsalva maneuver. Disk disease may be worse with weight bearing. The physician should inquire about the most comfortable position for the patient at rest or the position used to relieve the pain. This can be extremely useful in the differentiation of neurogenic from vascular claudication. With pseudoclaudication, patients usually relate standing, sitting, or crouching in a flexed forward position, while in those with vascular claudication, simple standing still or sitting upright often relieves discomfort. Patients with osteoporotic body collapse are often more comfortable supine. Pain related to degenerative processes that affect posterior elements is affected most significantly by positions that extend the spine, with back pain and leg pain made worse with standing or going downstairs while there is usually improvement when the patient is seated. Facet dysfunction can be exacerbated by end capsular movement. Lhermitte's sign is typically described as intermittent lightninglike pain traveling down the back, sometimes into one or both arms or legs with flexion of the neck. It usually occurs with lesions in the cervical spine but can occur at lower sites, presumably from irritation of the spinal cord by a compressive lesion.[28]

Associated Manifestations

The importance of eliciting a history of any bowel, bladder, or sexual dysfunction cannot be overemphasized. Any of these conditions indicates a potential medical emergency. These alterations imply spinal cord compression or cauda equina involvement. In patients with epidural metastasis, functional status at the start of effective treatment has a direct relation to outcome: Among those initially ambulatory, 75 percent retain the ability to walk; among those initially too weak to walk but not plegic, 30 to 50 percent retain the ability to walk; and only 10 percent of those with paraplegia initially retain the ability to walk.[28] The first sign of an epidural metastasis may be saddle anesthesia or impotence.

Personal hesitancy when questioning the sexual function of the elderly should not be a deterrent. Bladder involvement may be benign prostatic hypertrophy (BPH). Constipation may result from narcotic pain medication instead of sphincter dysfunction; therefore, a rectal exam is necessary.

Prior History of Low Back Pain

Lowback pain may be an exacerbation of a previously known dysfunction. The physician should establish the progression of pain or disability over the years.

Past Medical History

It is important to search for any history of cancer, no matter how remote. Breast cancer, prostate cancer, and melanoma can present many years after being presumed to be eradicated. Multiple myeloma is very common in the elderly. In patients with cancer, radicular pain results from epidural extension of a spinal neoplasm in about 70 percent of cases.[28] Other items to be investigated include unexplained weight loss, history of intravenous drug use, and history of urinary tract infection or skin infection resulting from the association with osteomyelitis.

Prior Treatments

A thorough history of the medications that have been prescribed and the current regimen of usage, especially the use of corticosteroids, must be obtained. Physical modalities such as superficial or deep heat, manipulation, and mobilization and any exercise programs that have been tried by the patient should be described. The physician should ascertain at what level the home program is being done. It is important to ask about chiropractic treatment and other holistic treatment modalities, as this information may not be volunteered.

Functional History

What may be perceived in a younger population as a minor inconvenience may be a functional limitation in the elderly. The physician should establish at what level the low back pain interferes with activities of daily living or social activities.

Physical Examination

It is good medical practice to undertake a general physical examination of all patients over age 50 with new-onset back pain. This should be a thorough exam of both the musculoskeletal system and the neurological system, including the basic elements of inspection, palpation, and observation. What follows is a recommended screening exam for an elderly patient complaining of low back pain.

Observation of Gait Pattern and Posture

The physician should observe the posture for evidence of lordosis, kyphosis, or scoliosis. Dowager's hump (thoracic kyphosis) may be a sign of underlying osteoporosis or osteomalacia. Compensatory curves occur in the cervical and lumbar spine to balance the spine in the saggital plane. The gait pattern may indicate a specific pattern of weakness: hip hiking—abductors; genu recurvatum—quadriceps; foot slap—dorsiflexors; lack of toe off—gastrocnemius/soleus complex. Asymmetry of the buttocks suggests an inferior gluteal nerve lesion or L5, S1–S2 root involvement.

Range of Motion

Spinal range of motion (ROM) is of limited diagnostic value but may be useful in planning or monitoring physical therapy in patients with low back pain of any etiology.[29] The physician should measure ROM of flexion, extension, and lateral bending both grossly and with an inclinometer and note which position aggravates the pain. Flexion pain suggests a paraspinous muscle injury or a herniated nucleus pulposus (HNP). Lateral bending pain suggests abnormalities in the paraspinal muscles, intervertebral disk, or apophyseal joints. Pain located to the opposite side from lateral motion is frequently muscular in origin. Ipsilateral radiating leg pain is related to HNP with nerve impingement or apophyseal joint irritation. Facet pain may be increased with direct pressure. Abnormalities of the ROM of the hips and knees may result in an altered gait that may cause or exacerbate low back pain.

Palpation

Spinal tenderness is suggestive of cancer. The physician should palpate the spinal column to locate any area of tenderness, tightness, or spasms over paraspinal muscles. Tenderness over muscles that are firm to palpation suggests spasm secondary to local injury or referred pain. Isolated tenderness over bone has systemic implications (compression fracture, tumor, infection).

Straight Leg Raise

A straight leg raise (SLR) test attempts to replicate the patient's pain by stretching the nerve. The fifth lumbar and sacral nerve roots are maximally tightened at 30 to 70 degrees. The extended leg is raised slowly, with the typical positive test reproducing the patient's pain. Patients with spinal stenosis may need to exercise before SLR is performed to exacerbate their symptoms.

The crossed straight leg raising sign is performed when the patient's well leg is raised and the patient's pain is elicited in the involved leg. This test is less sensitive but is highly specific to HNP.

To document tension in the upper lumbar roots (L2–L4) secondary to less common upper lumbar disk herniations, a femoral stretch test (reverse SLR) is performed. The patient is placed in either a prone or a supine position with the affected limb placed below the level of the table. Pain in the anterior thigh suggests impingement on L2–L3, while pain in the medial thigh suggests impingement on L4. Facet disease may be exacerbated by this maneuver.

Neurological Exam

A careful examination of the data in Table 23-3 suggests that a directed neurological examination is both sensitive and specific for HNP. Examination includes manual motor testing of ankle dorsiflexors, great toe extensors, SLR, crossed SLR, and sensory testing of the medial, lateral, and dorsal foot, which would include the L4, L5, and S1 dermatomes. Changes in deep tendon reflexes help localize lesions: knee, L4; hamstring, L5; ankle, S1. Signs of myelopathy

Table 23-3 Physical examination in the diagnosis of spine disease causing low back pain

Test	Source	Sensitivity	Specificity	Comments
Ipsilateral straight leg raising	Kosteljanetz et al (1984), Hakelius and Hindmarsh (1972)	0.80	0.40	Positive test result: leg pain at <60°
Crossed straight leg raising	Spangfort (1972), Hakelius and Hindmarsh(1972)	0.25	0.90	Positive test result: reproduction of contralateral pain
Ankle dorsiflexion weakness	Spangfort (1972), Hakelius and Hindmarsh (1972)	0.35	0.70	HNP* usually at L4–5 (80%)
Great toe extensor weakness	Kortelainen et al (1985), Hakelius and Hindmarsh (1972)	0.50	0.70	HNP usually at L5–S1 (60%) or L4–5 (30%)
Impaired ankle reflex	Spangfort (1972), Hakelius and Hindmarsh (1972)	0.50	0.60	HNP usually at L5–S1; absent reflex increases specificity
Sensory loss	Kortelainen et al (1985), Kosteljanetz et al (1984)	0.50	0.50	Area of loss poor predictor of HNP level
Patellar reflex	Aronson and Dunsmore (1963)	0.50	...	For upper lumbar HNP only
Ankle plantar flexion weakness	Hakelius and Hindmarsh (1972)	0.06	0.95	
Quadriceps weakness	Hakelius and Hindmarsh (1972)	<0.01	0.99	

*HNP herniated nucleus pulposus.

SOURCE: Modified from Deyo et al.[29] Copyright 1992, American Medical Association.

(hyperreflexia, Babinski's sign, and clonus) require evaluation of upper motor neuron disease in the CNS above the cauda equina.

Pinprick tests the spinothalamic tracts, proprioception examines the posterior dorsal columns, and light touch tests both. It is necessary to differentiate dermatomal sensory changes from stocking-glove changes associated with a peripheral neuropathy.

Manual muscle testing can be simplified by asking the patient to rise up on the toes and then the heels and then to squat. Unfortunately, this may be beyond the capabilities of some elderly patients. The typical myotomal patterns of weakness are knee extensors, L3–L4; hip abductors, dorsiflexors, extensor hallucis longus, L4–L5; knee flexors, ankle evertors, hip extensors, L5–S1; plantarflexors, S1–S2.

SPINAL IMAGING

The radiological examination of a geriatric patient has significant limitations because of the often asymptomatic evidence of long-term wear and tear.[8] Radiographic findings in a geriatric patient must have a high degree of clinical correlation as conventional x-rays, computed tomography scan, and magnetic resonance imaging routinely demonstrate structural abnormalities in asymptomatic as well as symptomatic patients.[30–32]

Plain Films

The plain radiograph is an excellent tool for identifying and evaluating the bony integrity of the entire lumbar spine. Radiographs provide valuable information related to bone density and are useful in identifying osteoporosis, fractures, decreased disk height, and primary and metastatic bone tumors (Table 23-4).

Table 23-4 Indications for imaging procedures in geriatric patients with acute low back pain

Rule out fractures
Osteoporosis
Over age 70
Prolonged steroid use
Recent trauma
Rule out tumor or infection
Elevated erythrocyte sedementation rate
History of cancer
Prolonged steroid usage
Pain not relieved by bed rest
Recent fever of unknown origin
Severe symptoms

The usual studies requested include both anteroposterior and lateral views of the lumbar spine with a coned lateral view of the sacrum and coccyx to improve resolution through the increased soft tissue in this region. Oblique lateral views, although not ordered routinely, can be useful in evaluating spondylolysis without spondylolisthesis and visualizing the facet joint space directly.

Bone Scan

A bone scan or radionuclide scintigraphy is a particularly sensitive test for the evaluation of disorders that result in an increase in the osteoclast activity of bone. Large areas of the bony skeleton in general and of the spine in particular can be visualized at once and screened for the presence of a tumor, infection, or fracture. A bone scan is appropriate in a geriatric patient with low back pain when a tumor, infection, or fracture is suspected. This examination, while more expensive than plain radiographs, is an important tool in the evaluation of more refractory pain in the elderly population.

Computed Tomography

Computed tomography (CT) examination offers a unique perspective on the spine through computer reconstruction of radiographs to produce transverse planar images. This allows the physician to assess the intervertebral canal and the neural foramen much more completely. As this technique uses x-rays, it is much better at delineating bony pathology than at demonstrating pathology of the disk or the neural elements. CT is appropriate in a geriatric patient with low back pain when a fracture or bony tumor is suspected. Visualization of neural elements can be enhanced by the addition of a myelographic radiopaque contrast solution before the study. Because of the degree of radiation exposure necessary to examine each segment and the cost of the procedure, it is generally not a useful screening tool.

Magnetic Resonance Imaging

Magnetic resonance imaging (MRI) can image the spinal column in any plane. Most commonly, longitudinal and transverse images are used to evaluate the patency of the intervertebral canal and the neural foramina. This technique is particularly useful in the imaging of the soft tissues and neural elements and as such is an excellent technique for imaging nerve root or cauda equina compression and identifying nonosseous tumors of the spinal axis. Findings suggesting cauda equina syndrome or progressive major motor weakness are indications for prompt evaluation utilizing MRI or CT myelography. Emergent surgical consultation is recommended to plan the imaging and possible surgical management of these serious problems.

Regardless of whether the plain x-rays are positive or negative, the use of a bone scan, CT, or MRI is appropriate in a geriatric patient with low back pain when a tumor, infection, or fracture is suspected. MRI with gadolinium is often the most appropriate imaging technique for patients with low back pain who have had prior surgery to distinguish disk herniation from scar tissue caused by prior surgery.

ELECTRODIAGNOSIS

Electromyography with Nerve Conduction Studies

Electrodiagnostic evaluation, including electromyography and nerve conduction studies, is useful in the evaluation of lumbar pain that is thought to be secondary to nerve root compression. This is a direct examination of the functional integrity of the nerves from the lumbar spine to the lower extremities. It is quite sensitive in delineating lumbar radiculopathy (trained hands) but has a degree of false negativity if sensory fibers are selectively involved in the root compression.

Somatosensory Evoked Potentials

Somatosensory evoked potentials (SSEPs) are becoming increasingly popular for the diagnosis of lumbar spine nerve root pathology. SSEPs are extremely sensitive but must be interpreted with caution as they are rather nonspecific. SSEPs evaluate the functional integrity of the peripheral nerve, nerve root, cauda equina, root entry zone, posterior columns, thalamus, and sensory cortex. An isolated lesion in these pathways will probably produce a positive test, but localization, particularly proximal to the peripheral nerve, is technically difficult; thus, the usefulness of this examination is limited, especially in untrained hands.

FORMULATING A DIFFERENTIAL DIAGNOSIS

A geriatric patient with low back pain must be carefully evaluated for serious life-threatening disease. The clinical evaluation of a geriatric patient is often difficult as a result of concomitant chronic diseases and disabilities.

Even with the most thorough history and physical exam, symptoms, pathological changes, and imaging results do not lead to a definitive diagnosis in up to 85 percent of patients.[33,34] It is assumed that many of these cases are related to musculoligamentous injury or degenerative changes.[29,35] Deyo and associates noted that in the primary care setting 4 percent of patients with back pain will prove to have a compression fracture, 3 percent will have spondylolisthesis, 2 percent will undergo surgery for a disk herniation, 0.7 percent will have spinal malignant neoplasms (primary or metastatic), 0.3 percent will have ankylosing spondylitis, and 0.01 percent will have spinal infection. The prevalence of spinal stenosis is not known.[29]

While the vast majority of cases of low back pain in the geriatric population are of mechanical etiology, it is imperative that the 10 percent resulting from other etiologies be rapidly identified and appropriately treated. The nonmechanical or systemic causes of low back pain are potentially devastating disease processes. A geriatric patient with a systemic etiology of low back pain often manifests signs and symptoms not related to mechanical low back pain (Table 23-5).

Systemic Causes of Low Back Pain

In evaluating a geriatric patient with low back pain for underlying systemic disease, the most useful items are age, history of cancer, unexplained weight loss, duration of pain, and responsiveness to previous therapy.[29]

Malignant Neoplasm

Malignant neoplasm is the most common serious systemic disease affecting the spine, and a previous history of cancer has such high specificity (0.98) that cancer should be suspected as the cause of low back pain until proved otherwise. Symptoms of fever, weight loss, pain with recumbency, extended morning

Table 23-5 Nonorganic physical signs in low back pain

Category	Test	Comments
Tenderness	Superficial palpation	Skin tender to light pinch over a generalized area of lumbar region
	Nonanatomic	Deep tenderness over a generalized area is not localized to one structure and often extends to the thoracic spine, sacrum, or pelvis
Stimulation	Axial loading	Low back pain is reported with vertical loading on the head
	Rotation	Low back pain is reported when shoulders and pelvis are passively rotated together in the same plane with the patient standing
Distraction	Straight leg raising	Physician asks seated patient to straighten knee; patient shows marked improvement in sitting straight leg raise (SLR) compared with supine SLR
Regional disturbances	Motor	Diffuse motor weakness noted that cannot be explained on a localized neurological basis
	Sensory	Diminished nonanatomic sensory findings that cannot be explained on a localized neurological basis
Overreaction		Disproportionate verbalization, facial expression, muscle tension and tremor, collapsing, or sweating during examination

stiffness, acute bone pain, or pain associated with gastrointestinal (GI) or genitourinary (GU) dysfunction should raise the index of suspicion for cancer. By far the most common tumor of the lumbar spine is a metastasis from a distant cancerous site. The most common metastatic tumors of the spine are from lung, breast, prostate, kidney, and GI tract cancer. Therefore, the exam should be directed at the lungs, abdomen, rectum, and pelvic areas as well as the kidney if a suspicion of cancer exists. Multiple myeloma is the most common primary spinal tumor. Serum immunoelectrophoresis and analysis of the urine for Bence Jones protein assist in screening for myeloma. The combined sensitivity of age >50 years with an associated history of cancer, unexplained weight loss, and failure of conservative therapy was 100 percent; that is, no cancer was found if those items were all negative.

Osteomyelitis

Osteomyelitis does not always present with fever, but fever has a specificity of 0.98. Vertebral tenderness and very limited spinal ROM are also common in spinal infections but have decreased specificity as they are also common in back pain without infection. In spinal osteomyelitis, 40 percent of the cases can be traced to intravenous drug abuse, urinary tract infection, or skin infection. An elevated erythrocyte sedimentation rate (ESR) and white blood count (WBC) would be supportive data.

Vascular

Vascular abnormalities may be an important cause of back pain in the older population. The signs and symptoms include diminished pulses and bruits over arteries, cutaneous signs of ischemia, skin ulcers, hair loss pattern, and sudden changes in the pain pattern.

Among all the causes of acute onset of intense lumbar pain in the middle-aged and elderly population, the most life-threatening is the referred pain of the impending rupture of an abdominal aortic aneurysm. An aortic abdominal aneurysm may cause pain as a result of ischemia in the back, buttock, or lower aorta during exercise. An episode of hypotension may herald an impending extension or rupture of the aneurysm. This pain is generally described as tearing in nature, and a pulsatile mass is usually appreciated on palpation of the abdomen. Prompt surgical referral is generally necessary.

Viscerogenic

Viscerogenic pain may refer to the lower back. Pancreatic lesions and posterior penetrating duodenal ulcers refer pain to the upper lumbar and lower thoracic area. Bowel or urinary tract lesions may refer to the midlumbar area, while pelvic disorders refer to the lower lumbar area or the sacral area.

Osteoporosis

Compression fractures most often occur in patients with generalized osteoporosis. A history of long-term corticosteroid use has a specificity of 0.99 for compression fracture. A history of acute onset of pain exacerbated by any motion, with the maximum pain localized over a vertebra, is suggestive of a compression fracture.

The diagnosis of vertebral compression fractures is common in the geriatric population, particularly in postmenopausal women. Estrogen and progesterone combined with weight-bearing exercise are critical in the maintenance of adequate bone density in this population. These fractures, commonly of the upper lumbar or lower thoracic vertebral bodies, are generally apparent on plain roentgenograms of the spine as a significant loss of vertebral body height, frequently with wedging anteriorly. Because of the mechanism of this injury and the forces generated by falls, the compression fracture is generally constrained by the anterior and posterior longitudinal ligaments and rarely results in compromise of the neural elements.

Ankylosing Spondylitis

Ankylosing spondylitis has its onset at age $\leq$ 40 years, but the diagnosis may be made at a later date. The five screening questions listed in Table 23-2 have been reported to have variable sensitivity and specificity in the literature, reflecting the low predictive value of a positive test for a rare disease.

Nephrolithiasis

Another cause of acute lumbar pain that increases in incidence in the geriatric population is nephrolithiasis. The pain in this disorder is primarily a unilateral flank pain associated with the acute onset of disabling pain. Special radiological studies and urologic referral are required when this diagnosis is suspected.

Mechanical Causes of Low Back Pain

The bulk of low back pain cases in geriatric patients are mechanical in origin. Within this classification, two small subsets of pain with neurological compromise and pain secondary to fracture may be identified. The remainder constitutes the vast but ill-defined category of low back pain caused by a musculoskeletal etiology.

Neurological Compromise

A small percentage of geriatric patients with low back pain consists of those with neurological compromise. These patients may require immediate imaging or surgical consultation.

Lumbar disk herniations with sciatica can be evaluated by using a thorough history and the physical exam techniques listed in Tables 23-2 and 23-3, along with their sensitivities and specificities. The typical presentation of discogenic low back pain is pain exacerbated by flexion activities, activities that increase shear stress across the annulus (e.g., twisting), and activities that cause a Valsalva maneuver (e.g., coughing, sneezing).

Lumbosacral radiculopathy from herniation of the nucleus pulposus usually occurs in a posterolateral direction, where the annular fibers are not well protected by the posterior longitudinal ligament and where shear forces are greatest with forward and lateral bending.[36]

Neurogenic claudication resulting from spinal stenosis caused by mechanical factors presents with increased frequency in the elderly. Frequently, osteophyte formation around the vertebral bodies and the lumbar facet joints encroaches on the vertebral canal, allowing less room for the passage of the nerve roots of the cauda equina and eventually resulting in ischemic injury to those neural elements. The resultant problems can include neurogenic claudication, decreased exercise tolerance, kyphotic postures, and ultimately bowel and bladder incontinence and lower extremity weakness.

Cauda equina syndrome, when present, requires urgent surgical care. Bladder dysfunction (usually urinary retention or overflow incontinence), saddle anesthesia, major limb motor weakness, and unilateral or bilateral leg pain and weakness are all significant signs and symptoms.

Fracture

Mild trauma cannot be dismissed as a possible provoking event in elderly patients. Spinal fractures occur with an increased incidence in the elderly as a result of a progressive loss of bone density and strength with age. While motor vehicle accidents and falls still result in traumatic fractures and often paraplegia or quadriplegia in this population, this diagnosis tends to be obvious from the history, physical examination, and imaging studies. More commonly, however, the practitioner is faced with an elderly individual who has fallen at home and has developed acute pain localized to the lumbar region without neurological compromise.

Musculoskeletal

Excluding the approximately 10 percent of patients with systemic disorders, most patients with nonradicular complaints have musculoskeletal back pain. These pain problems are often exacerbated by movement. Even though nearly all patients over 50 years of age demonstrate degenerative changes of the lumbar spine, little evidence exists to link any low back structure or specific changes from the aging process to musculoskeletal pain.[35,37]

Any mechanical dysfunction that can occur in the normal adult population can also occur in the elderly. Ligamentous strains, muscle injury, and repetitive trauma to the annulus fibrosis and facet joints occur in great numbers in the elderly. Indeed, disuse atrophy of the lumbar musculature secondary to the inactivity of the geriatric population can contribute significantly to the risk of such injuries. Facet dysfunction and myofascial disorders are also entities common to the younger populations of patients with lumbar pain and are amenable to common interventions appropriate for the diagnosis.

Psychosocial Factors

Pain has never been shown to be a simple function of the amount of physical injury; it is extensively influenced by multiple psychosocial factors. The motivational, affective, and cognitive components can never be underestimated in terms of their impact on the appropriate management of a patient with acute or chronic pain.

A psychosocial history includes necessary information such as substance abuse and depression, a history of failed treatment, and socioeconomic information such as work status, typical job tasks, educational level, pending litigation, worker's compensation, and disability. This information is helpful in planning therapy and prognosticating.

In patients with *chronic pain*, Waddell's inappropriate signs may be helpful in identifying psychological distress as a result of or as an amplifier of low back pain (Table 23-5).[38]

REHABILITATION

Rehabilitation treatments should not be initiated for geriatric patients with low back pain without a comprehensive history and physical examination, as outlined above. The treatment plan is often based on the patient's signs and symptoms, since the underlying etiology is unclear in over 85 percent of these patients because of weak correlations between symptoms, pathological findings, and imaging data.[29,39] The rehabilitation of a geriatric patient with low back pain is limited by the individual's ability to participate in physical activity and the restrictions imposed by any concomitant illness. The purpose of the rehabilitation process is to decrease pain and increase function.

The vast majority of low back pain in geriatric patients may be classified as regional musculoskeletal low back disorders. In 80 to 90 percent of adults with limiting low back problems, spontaneous recovery occurs within a month of onset.[26,40–42] It has been estimated that 80 percent of patients with acute low back pain are free of discomfort within 2 weeks.[43] Thus, it is not surprising that the bulk of low back pain problems resolve with conservative management and minimal intervention. Although patients often recover spontaneously from acute episodes of low back pain, 70 percent suffer recurrence and subsequent injuries are often more severe and longer lasting.[44]

Most studies that have looked at treatment efficacy have primarily involved a nongeriatric population and therefore may not always apply to geriatric patients with low back pain. Careful evaluation of the physical, psychological, and medical tolerance of the patient to these interventions is recommended.

Anesthetic Procedures

Trigger point injections, sympathetic blocks, and regional blocks are discussed elsewhere in this book (see Chaps. 22, 24, and 25). These anesthetic procedures are used in concert with the rehabilitation procedures described in this chapter.

Bed Rest

The use of bed rest in the elderly must be evaluated in regard to its negative impact on the patient's well-being. For patients with low back pain without accompanying neurological deficits, multiple studies suggest that brief (1–2 days), if any, bed rest is sufficient.[45,46] Previous studies have shown that there are only slight differences in disk pressures between upright posture and side-lying posture.[47]

The potential side effects from immobilization through bed rest include (1) muscle atrophy (1–1.5 percent of muscle mass lost per day), (2) cardiopulmonary deconditioning (15 percent loss in aerobic capacity in 10 days), (3) bone demineralization with hypercalciuria and hypercalcemia, (4) increased anxiety, (5) depression, and (6) increased risk of thromboembolism.[48] There are also social side effects, such as the perception of severe illness.[49] Thus, prolonged bed rest should be avoided because of the possibility of permanent loss of function.

Education and Changes in Lifestyle

After significantly reducing the probability of serious nonmechanical etiologies of low back pain, it is important to provide assurance to the patient in regard to the diagnosis.[50] Geriatric patients with low back pain should be provided information regarding the probability of rapid recovery and recurrence of symptoms, appropriate methods of symptom control, activity modifications, methods of preventing recurrent low back pain, and indications of serious nonmechanical problems (Table 23-6). Educational programs have been utilized in the form of verbal, video, and handout material. These programs have been shown to be successful in helping patients understand low back pain and have led to more appropriate utilization of medical resources.[51] Providing patients with appropriate information regarding their medical problems increases compliance with treatment and decreases patient apprehension.[52]

Education of the patient to utilize proper body mechanics and maintain appropriate posture is essential in avoiding back strain resulting in exacerbation of low back pain. Patients need to reduce the risk factors for low back pain, which include cigarette smoking, inactivity, and obesity. The use of assistive devices and activities of daily living aids, such as a cane, may be appropriate in a geriatric patient.[3,53]

Formalized back schools teach the principles of appropriate posture and use of the back in daily activity, activities that result in increased functional capac-

Table 23-6 Indicators of serious nonmechanical etiology of low back pain in the elderly

Spinal fracture
History of trauma or fall
Age over 70
Prolonged use of corticosteroids
Osteoporosis
Cancer
History of cancer
Unexplained weight loss
Pain not improved with bed rest
Duration of pain greater than 1 month
Age over 50
Infection
Recent infection
Fever
Unexplained weight loss
Pain not improved with bed rest
Elevated erythrocyte sedimentation rate (20)
Intravenous drug use
Prolonged use of corticosteroids
Neurological compromise
Acute urinary retention
Acute incontinence (urine or fecal)
Loss of rectal tone
Saddle anesthesia
Major motor weakness
Dermatologic sensory loss

ity. Participants have the potential to decrease the level of pain and increase functional performance.[54]

Exercise

Exercise is one of the commonly prescribed forms of treatment for low back pain; however, there is little scientific evidence to support its efficacy. However, overall fitness has been shown to have a protective effect and to significantly decrease the incidence of low back injuries.[55] Overall fitness was significantly correlated with less physical dysfunction and fewer depressive symptoms in patients with chronic low back pain. It also correlated with pain of shorter duration and less intensity in patients with acute low back pain.[56] Good isometric endurance of back muscles may prevent first-time occurrences of low back problems.[57] Poor physical condition has been reported to be an important factor in the development and persistence of low back pain. There appears to be a significant association between physical fitness and important elements of low back pain, especially physical limitations and depression. One study revealed that the stronger an individual with persistent low back pain is physically and the higher his or her aerobic work capacity is, the less that individual is functionally limited.[58]

Strengthening the lumbar muscles has been reported to reduce low back pain significantly. The treated subjects noted less physical and psychosocial dysfunction, whereas the control group had increases in pain and physical and psychosocial dysfunction.[59] It is important to consider that there may be a significant placebo effect from spending time with the physical therapist.[60] Unfortunately, studies often do not control for concomitant or equivalent therapy.

Few controlled double-blind trials with equivalent intervention have been performed for exercise therapy. Limited data have been presented to date regarding flexion exercises commonly prescribed as Williams flexion postural exercises,[56,61,62] and while extension exercises continue to have advocates, there is a lack of appropriate controlled research to support their efficacy.[17,56,63–65]

Exercise regimes for geriatric patients with low back pain should begin with aerobic exercise programs involving minimal stress to the back during the first 2 weeks after the onset of low back problems. Aerobic exercise sessions should be scheduled three to five times per week, ranging from 20 to 40 min, and should include warm-up and cool-down periods. These activities may include walking, biking, or swimming. General stretching exercises should be initiated during this time to maintain flexibility, increase function, and provide comfort.[17,27] After the first 2 weeks, strengthening exercises for back muscles and a more rigorous stretching program should be initiated. It is essential to maintain activity to prevent disuse and inflexibility. The exercise program should be gradual with a consistent effort by the patient to increase functional capabilities. If symptoms increase, the physician should reevaluate the patient for a possible serious systemic disease. Exercise programs are best initiated in a physical therapy setting for a brief period until the patient demonstrates the ability to complete the exercise program at home. Previous findings have demonstrated that active treatment programs involving the patient in stretching protocols in the home setting are more effective than is passive participation by the patient.[78] The primary goals of exercise in the elderly are to prevent debilitation caused by inactivity, improve function, and decrease pain.

Lumbar Orthoses

Lumbosacral orthoses may provide relief in both acute and chronic low back pain patients. Orthoses decrease strain of the lumbosacral region by providing trunk support, controlling motion, maintaining proper alignment, and compensating for muscle weakness. Studies have demonstrated significant improvement in pain and decreased injury with the use of lumbosacral orthoses.[66,67] Effective usage depends on proper fit, patient compliance, and appropriate choice of orthoses. There is no evidence to suggest that abdominal muscle strength decreases with prophylactic use of a lumbosacral corset.[67]

Medications

Nonsteroidal anti-inflammatory drugs (NSAIDs) and simple analgesics are usually sufficient to control most instances of low back pain. Oral administration of medication is preferred in the treatment of all pain. A time-contingent round-the-clock schedule for pain medication is superior to an "as needed" schedule. This form of administration minimizes alterations in plasma levels and provides optimal pain control. The schedule should be based on variables such as potency, duration of analgesic effect, and efficacy of medication. It is essential to provide adequate pain control, as suboptimal dosing results in operant conditioning, craving, a sense of dependence, and anxiety about the drug wearing off.

NSAIDs include aspirin and acetaminophen. These drugs are chosen over narcotics because they minimize side effects of constipation, sedation, and dependence. There is also no development of tolerance. Acetaminophen is preferred in the geriatric population since it is comparable in efficacy to other NSAIDs in treating back problems and has fewer side effects.[68] Aspirin and other NSAIDs have the potential complication of GI upset, especially in patients with a history of peptic ulcer disease or upper GI bleeding. When the etiology of the low back pain is metastatic cancer or spondyloarthropathy, NSAIDs are recommended. When NSAIDs are used in patients with a history of gastric ulcer disease, the simultaneous administration of misoprostol often decreases the risk of gastric ulcer complications. In patients with a history of duodenal ulcer, H_2 blockers have been demonstrated to provide adequate prophylaxis.[27]

In most instances, narcotic analgesics are no more effective than NSAIDs in the relief of low back pain.[69,70] If narcotic analgesics are required for severe symptoms, the use of oral low-dose narcotics, including codeine and oxycodone, in combination with acetaminophen for no longer than 2 to 4 weeks may be indicated. Increased difficulty with balance and constipation are common side effects of narcotic medication in the elderly. Prophylactic bowel programs should be initiated in patients who are prone to constipation. A high percentage of patients using narcotics for pain control manifest decreased reaction time, clouded judgment, and drowsiness. These individuals should be warned about using narcotics while operating dangerous equipment or driving.

Muscle relaxants are not recommended for the treatment of low back pain to reduce muscle spasm in the elderly. Studies have shown that most prescribed muscle relaxants have little peripheral effect of any type on muscle spasm. There is little evidence to suggest that muscle relaxants are more effective than NSAIDs in the relief of low back pain, and they have a high potential for the side effects of drowsiness and dizziness.[71,72]

Mobilization Techniques

Lumbosacral spine mobilization and manipulation have short-term effects on reducing pain and improving daily function in patients with acute low back pain without radiculopathy.[73,74] Contraindications for joint mobilization include a neurological deficit, osteoporosis, a tumor, pregnancy, segmental instability, and an active inflammatory process in the joint.[75]

Physical Modalities

Physical modalities are valuable adjuncts to the management of acute low back pain. Therapeutic heat and cryotherapy are time-honored interventions for treating musculoskeletal pain, resulting in temporary symptomatic relief.

Heat application is a common form of pain treatment. It is generally accepted that therapeutic heat is best tolerated in the subacute and chronic phases of a disease process. The physiological responses produced by heat include increased blood flow and metabolic rate, increased collagen extensibility, and inflammation resolution. Decreases in joint stiffness, muscle spasm, and pain are also beneficial effects of heat. Contraindications to the use of heat include sensory impairment, circulatory insufficiency, malignancy, infection, and cognitive impairment.

Cold applied to an injured area in acute musculoskeletal pain reduces vasodilation, blunts the local inflammatory response, decreases edema, and reduces pain perception. Patients with low back pain have responded well in controlled trials employing cryotherapy.[76] Ice bags, ice massage, and reusable cold packs are available for cold application. Contraindications to the use of cold are sensory impairment, marked cold pressor response, Raynaud's phenomenon and disease, and peripheral vascular disease. The major precaution is to avoid tissue damage from too vigorous or prolonged cooling. The risks and benefits of treating an insensate area must be evaluated before one begins treatment.

Electrical stimulation is utilized in multiple forms of therapy for the relief of pain involving the low back. Electrical stimulation is provided with alternating current, usually producing a high-voltage monophasic waveform. These devices allow adjustment of intensity, pulse rate, and pulse width. Electrical stimulation is often used in conjunction with other modalities, including ultrasound, to provide stimulation and deep heating.

Transcutaneous electrical nerve stimulation (TENS) is a form of electrical stimulation that has been utilized frequently in the treatment of low back pain. Conceptually, TENS achieves pain relief by stimulating a large sensory afferent fiber with resultant modification of pain perception by the patient. Controlled trials that evaluate the effectiveness of TENS on patients with low back pain are limited. One study suggested that TENS relieved acute low back pain significantly more than did acetaminophen.[77] Rigorously controlled trials suggest that TENS is no better than placebo in the management of chronic low back pain.[78, 78a]

Cold laser therapy has been used empirically for a variety of painful conditions. The effectiveness of this technique has not been scientifically demonstrated, and its mode of action, if any, remains speculative. The effectiveness of laser therapy for pain control has been compared with that of a sham laser, with no statistically significant objective or subjective therapeutic effects being demonstrated.[79]

Traction

Traction for low back pain involves the use of intermittent or continuous force along the axial skeleton to increase spinal ROM and reduce interdiscal pressure. There is no evidence to suggest that traction is effective in the treatment of patients with low back pain.[80,81]

Traditional and Modern Acupuncture

Acupuncture is a dry needling technique that traditionally has used designated points (Chinese meridians) for counterstimulation. Modern techniques involve dry needling into tender areas with or without counterstimulation to relieve pain. At the present time there is no evidence to suggest that acupuncture is effective in the treatment of low back pain.[82]

SUMMARY

Low back pain is generally a self-limiting condition with a good prognosis, yet limited information is available about the effectiveness of the specific treatments applied.[83, 84]

Abnormal radiographic findings in an elderly patient with low back pain may or may not be related to the patient's symptoms. Anatomic abnormalities of the lumbar spine become more prevalent in the elderly, regardless of symptoms. Radiographic findings may require exacting clinical correlations with the medical history, physical examination, and appropriate laboratory tests. Osteoarthritic changes are more often asymptomatic than symptomatic.[3]

When treating patients with acute low back pain, one must screen appropriately for serious conditions (Table 23-6) and then manage conservatively, as the majority of patients (70–80 percent) with acute low back pain recover from the symptoms and activity limitations within a month.[84]

The major goals of rehabilitation of a geriatric patient with low back pain are a return of that individual to a maximum level of function, elimination or minimization of pain, and control of disease processes. Deconditioning results in muscle weakness, joint stiffness, decreased ROM, and impaired function. The purpose of rehabilitation is to optimize function and mobility as well as control pain. As with all pain complaints, if a significant decrease in pain is not noted after 2 to 3 weeks of conservative therapy or if different complaints develop, a thorough review of the diagnosis and treatment plan should be done. In a geriatric patient, it is important to maintain a reasonable vigilance for low back pain of systemic etiology.

REFERENCES

1. Frymoyer J, Kats-Basil WL: An overview of the incidence and costs of low back pain. *Orthop Clin North Am* 22:263, 1991.
2. Kelsey JL, Golden AL: Occupational and workplace factors associated with low back pain. *Spine: State of the Art Reviews* 2:7, 1987.
3. Swezey RL: Low back pain in the elderly: Practical management concerns. *Geriatrics* 43:39, 1988.
4. Bergstrom G, Bjelle A, Sundh V, et al: Joint disorders at ages 70, 75, and 79 years—A cross sectional comparison. *Br J Rheumatol* 25:333, 1986.
5. Kavsky-Shulan M, Wallace RB, Kohout FJ, et al: Prevalence and functional correlates of low back pain in the elderly: The Iowa 65-plus rural health study. *J Am Geriatr Soc* 33:23, 1985.
6. Svara CJ, Hadler NM: Back pain. *Clin Geriatr Med* 4:395, 1988.
7. Reischer MA, Spindler HA: Rehabilitation management of pain in the elderly, in Felsenthal G (ed): *Rehabilitation of the Aging Patient.* Baltimore: Williams & Wilkins, 1994, chap 26, pp 303–318.
8. Bogduk N, Twomey LT: *Clinical Anatomy of the Lumbar Spine*, 2d ed. New York: Churchill Livingstone, 1991.
9. Bernick S, Cailliet R: Vertebral end-plate changes with aging of human vertebrae. *Spine* 7:97, 1982.
10. Kirkaldy-Willis WH: *Managing Low Back Pain*, 2d ed. New York: Churchill Livingstone, 1988.
11. Hilton RC, Ball J, Benn RT: In-vitro mobility of the lumbar spine. *Ann Rheum Dis* 38:378, 1979.
12. Rockoff SF, Sweet E, Bleustein J: The relative contribution of trabecular and cortical bone to the strength of human lumbar vertebrae. *Calcif Tissue Res* 3:163, 1969.
13. Horowitz T, Smith RM: An anatomical, pathological and roentgenological study of the intervertebral joints of the lumbar spine and of the sacroiliac joints. *AJR* 43:173, 1940.
14. Nordin M, Frankel VH: *Basic Biomechanics of the Musculoskeletal System*, 2d ed. Philadelphia: Lea & Febiger, 1989.
15. White AA, Panjabi MM: *Clinical Biomechanics of the Spine.* Philadelphia: Lippincott, 1978.
16. Vernon-Roberts B, Pirie GJ: Degenerative changes in the intervertebral discs of the lumbar spine and their sequelae. *Rheumatol Rehab* 16:13, 1977.
17. Tollison CD, Kriegel ML: Physical therapy in the treatment of low back pain. *Orthop Rev* 17:913, 1988.
18. Twomey L, Taylor J: Sagittal movements of the human lumbar vertebral column: A quantitative study of the role of the posterior vertebral elements. *Arch Phys Med Rehab* 64:322, 1982.
19. Hirsch C, Paulson S, Sylven B, Snellman O: Biophysical and physiological investigation on cartilage and other mesenchymal tissues: Characteristics of human nuclei pulposi during aging. *Acta Orthop Scand* 22:175, 1953.
20. Gower WE, Pedrini V: Age related variation in protein polysaccharides from human nucleus pulposis, annulus fibrosis, and costal cartilage. *J Bone Joint Surg Am* 51A:1154, 1969.
21. Twomey L, Taylor J: Age changes in lumbar intervertebral discs. *Acta Orthop Scand* 56:496, 1985.
22. Andersson GBJ, McNeill TW: *Lumbar Spinal Stenosis.* St. Louis: Mosby–Year Book, 1992.

23. Twomey L, Taylor J, Furniss B: Age changes in the bone density and structure of the lumbar vertebral column. *J Anat* 136:15, 1983.
24. Taylor J, Twomey LT: Sagittal and horizontal plane movement of the human lumbar vertebral column in cadavers and in living donors. *Rheumatol Rehab* 19:223, 1980.
25. Magee T: *Orthopedic Physical Assessment.* Philadelphia: Saunders, 1993.
26. Borenstein D, Wiesel S: *Low Back Pain: Medical Diagnosis and Comprehensive Management.* Philadelphia: Saunders, 1989.
27. Borenstein DG, Burton JR: Lumbar spine disease in the elderly. *J Am Geriatr Soc* 41:167, 1983.
28. Portenoy RK: Back pain in the elderly patient. *Hosp Pract* 14:81, 1993.
29. Deyo RA, Rainville J, Kent DL: What can the history and physical examination tell us about low back pain? *JAMA* 268:760, 1992.
30. Boden S, Davis DO, Dina TS, et al: Abnormal magnetic-resonance scans of the lumbar spine in asymptomatic subjects. *J Bone Joint Surg Am* 72A:403, 1990.
31. Hitselberger WE, Witten PM: Abnormal myelogram in asymptomatic patients. *J Neurosurg* 28:204, 1986.
32. Wiesel SW, Tsourmas N, Feffer HL, et al: A study of computer assisted tomography: I. The incidence of positive CAT scans in an asymptomatic group of patients. *Spine* 9:549, 1984.
33. Frymoyer JW: Back pain and sciatica. *N Engl J Med* 318:291, 1988.
34. Miller JAA, Schmatz C, Schultz AB: Lumbar disc degeneration: Correlation with age, sex, and spine level in 600 autopsy specimens. *Spine* 13:173, 1988.
35. Kelsey JL, White AA: Epidemiology and impact of low back pain. *Spine* 5:133, 1980.
36. Weinstein SM, Herring SA: Rehabilitation of the patient with low back pain, in DeLisa JA (ed): *Rehabilitation Medicine: Principles and Practice*, 2d ed. Philadelphia: Lippincott, 1993, chap 47, pp 996–1017.
37. Kelsey JL: *Epidemiology of Musculoskeletal Pain.* New York: Oxford University Press, 1982.
38. Waddell G, McCulloch JA, Kummel E, et al: Non-organic physical signs in low back pain. *Spine* 5:117, 1980.
39. White AA, Gordon SL: Synopsis. Workshop on idiopathic low back pain. *Spine* 7:141, 1982.
40. Andersson G, Svenson H, Oden A: The intensity of work recovery in low back pain. *Spine* 8:880, 1983.
41. Andersson GBJ: Epidemiological aspects of low back pain in industry. *Spine* 6:53, 1981.
42. Nachemson A: Work for all. *Clin Orthop* 179:77, 1983.
43. Hadler NM: Regional back pain. *N Engl J Med* 315:1090, 1986.
44. Walsh NE, Dumitru D: Financial compensation in recovery from low back pain. *Spine* 2:109, 1987.
45. Deyo RA, Diehl AD, Rosenthal M: How many days of bed rest for acute low back pain? A randomized clinical trial. *N Engl J Med* 315:1064, 1986.
46. Gilbert JR, Taylor DW, Hildebrand A, et al: Clinical trial of common treatments for low back pain in family practice. *Br Med J* 291:791, 1985.
47. Nachemson AL: A lumbar spine: An orthopedic challenge. *Spine* 1:59, 1976.
48. Deyo RA: Non-operative treatment of low back disorders. Differentiating useful from useless therapy, in Frymoyer JW (ed): *The Adult Spine: Principles and Practice.* New York: Raven Press, 1991, chap 72, pp 1567–1580.

49. Bortz WM: The disuse syndrome. *West J Med* 141:691, 1984.
50. William M, Hadler NM: Musculoskeletal components of decrepitude. *Semin Arthritis Rheum* 11:284, 1981.
51. Roland MO, Dixon M: Random controlled trial of an educational booklet for patients presenting with back pain in general practice. *J R Coll Gen Pract* 39:244, 1989.
52. Bass MJ, Buck C, Turner L, et al: The physicians' actions and outcomes of illness in family practice. *J Fam Pract* 23:43, 1986.
53. Quinet RJ, Hadler NM: Diagnosis and treatment of backache. *Semin Arthritis Rheum* 8:261, 1979.
54. Klaber-Moffett JA, Chase SM, Portek BS, Ennis JR: A controlled perspective study to evaluate effectiveness of a back school in the relief of chronic low back pain. *Spine* 11:120, 1986.
55. Cady LD, Bischoff DP, O'Connell ER, et al: Strength and fitness and subsequent back injuries in fire fighters. *J Occup Med* 21:269, 1979.
56. Jackson CP, Brown MD: Is there a rule for exercise in the treatment of patients with low back pain? *Clin Orthop Rel Res* 79:39, 1983.
57. Biering-Sorenson F: One year perspective study of low back trouble in a general population. *Dan Med Bull* 31:362, 1984.
58. McQade KJ, Turner JA, Buchner DM: Physical fitness and chronic low back pain: An analysis of the relationships among fitness, functional limitations, and depression. *Clin Orthop Rel Res* 233:198, 1988.
59. Risch SV, Norvel NK, Pollock ML, et al: Lumbar strengthening in chronic low back pain patients: Physiologic and psychological benefits. *Spine* 18:232, 1993.
60. Koes BW, Bouter LM, van Mameren HE, et al: The effectiveness of manual therapy, physiotherapy, and treatment by the general practitioner for non-specific back and neck complaints: A randomized clinical trial. *Spine* 17:28, 1992.
61. Elnaggar IM, Nordin M, Sheikhzadeh A, et al: Effects of spinal flexion and extension exercise on low back pain in spinal mobility in chronic mechanical low back pain patients. *Spine* 16:967, 1991.
62. Kendall PH, Jenkins JM: Exercises for backache: A double-blind controlled trial. *Phys Ther* 54:154, 1968.
63. Davies JE, Gibson T, Tester L: The value of exercise in the treatment of low back pain. *Rheumatol Rehab* 18:243, 1979.
64. Saal JA, Saal JS: Non-operative treatment of herniated lumbar intervertebral disc with radiculopathy: An outcome study. *Spine* 14:431, 1989.
65. Stankovic R, Johnell O: Conservative treatment of acute low back pain: A perspective randomized trial: McKenzie method of treatment vs. patient education, mini-back school. *Spine* 15:120, 1990.
66. Million R, Haavik-Nilsen H, Jason MIV, et al: Evaluation of low back pain and assessment of lumbosacral corsets with and without back supports. *Rheumatol Dis* 40:449, 1981.
67. Walsh NE, Schwartz RK: The influence of prophylactic orthoses on abdominal strength in low back injury in the workplace. *Am J Phys Med Rehabil* 69:245, 1990.
68. Hickey RFJ: Chronic low back pain: A comparison of diflunisal with parcetamol. *N Z Med J* 95:312, 1982.
69. Brown FL, Bodison S, Dixon J, et al: Comparison of diflunisal and acetaminophen with codeine in the treatment of initial and recurrent acute low back strain. *Clin Ther* 9(Suppl C):52, 1986.
70. Muncie HL, King DE, DeForge B: Treatment of mild to moderate pain of acute

soft tissue injury: Diflunisal vs. acetaminophen with codeine. *J Fam Pract* 23:125, 1986.

71. Dapas F, Hartman SF, Martinez L, et al: Baclofen for the treatment of acute low back pain syndrome: A double-blind comparison with placebos. *Spine* 10:345, 1985.
72. Basmajian JV: Acute back pain and spasm: A controlled multi-center trial of combined analgesic and anti-spasm agents. *Spine* 14:438, 1989.
73. Andersson R, Meeker WC, Wirick BE, et al: A metaanalysis of clinical trials of spinal manipulation. *J Manipulative Physiol Ther* 15:181, 1992.
74. Shekelle PG, Adams AH, Chassin MR, et al: Spinal manipulation for low back pain. *Ann Intern Med* 117:590, 1992.
75. Griffin J: Physical therapy, in Ramamurthy S, Rogers JN (eds): *Decision Making in Pain Management.* St. Louis: Mosby–Year Book, 1993, pp 190–191.
76. Landen BR: Heat or cold for the relief of low back pain? *Phys Ther* 47:1126, 1967.
77. Hackett GI, Seddon D, Kaminski D: Electro acupuncture compared to paracetamol for acute low back pain. *Practitioner* 232:163, 1988.
78. Deyo RA, Walsh NE, Martin DC, et al: A controlled trial of transcutaneous electrical nerve stimulation (TENS): An exercise for chronic low back pain. *N Engl J Med* 322:1627, 1990.

78a. Langley GB, Sheppard H, Johnson M, Wigley RD: The analgesic affects of transcutaneous electrical nerve stimulation and placebo in chronic pain patients: A double-blind non-crossover comparison. *Rheumatol Int* 4:119–123, 1984.

79. Ysla R, McAvley R: Effects of low power infra-red laser stimulation on carpal tunnel syndrome: A double-blind study. *Arch Phys Med Rehabil* 66:577, 1985.
80. Matthews JA, Hickling J: Lumbar traction: A double-blind control study for sciatica. *Rheumatol Rehab* 14:222, 1975.
81. Pal B, Mangion P, Hossain MA, et al: A controlled trial of continuous lumbar traction in the treatment of backpain and sciatic. *Br J Rheumatol* 25:181, 1986.
82. ter Riet G, Kleijnen J, Knipschild: Acupuncture and chronic pain: A criteria base med-analysis. *J Clin Epidemiol* 43:1191, 1990.
83. Deyo RA: Conservative therapy for low back pain: Distinguishing useful from useless therapy. *JAMA* 250:1057, 1983.
84. *Acute Low Back Problems in Adults.* Clinical Practice Guideline Number 15. AHCPR Publication No. 94-0105. Rockville, MD: Agency for Health Care Policy and Research, U.S. Department of Health and Human Services. December 1994.

CHAPTER 24

Pain of Herpes Zoster and Postherpetic Neuralgia in the Elderly

William E. Ackerman
James H. Diede
Gabor Bela Racz

INTRODUCTION

Elderly patients are especially susceptible to chronic pain and pain-producing illnesses, including depressive disorders.[1] Chronic pain management in elderly patients can be unique because these persons may present with multiple medically related nociceptive pathological conditions in addition to postherpetic neuralgia, such as degenerative joint disease, vascular disease, rheumatoid arthritis, and cancer. The correct diagnosis must be made before any treatment is initiated. The pharmacologic management of these patients can also be difficult because elderly patients exhibit varying pharmacokinetic and pharmacodynamic responses to drugs. Diagnosing the etiology of a geriatric patient's chronic pain syndrome can be difficult because of the patient's inability to communicate his or her perception of painful symptoms to the physician. As a result, a comprehensive physical examination, in addition to a detailed history taken from the patient or a family member, may be necessary. Chronic pain associated with postherpetic neuralgia can cause severe disruption in an elderly patient's lifestyle and affect the activities of daily living. This pain may subsequently be responsible for fatigue, immobility, and insomnia. Furthermore, a severe strain may be placed on family relations.

PATHOPHYSIOLOGY OF ACUTE HERPES ZOSTER AND POSTHERPETIC NEURALGIA

Acute herpes zoster and postherpetic neuralgia are not uncommon occurrences in the elderly. Both pathological entities are sequential effects of the herpes zoster virus. Acute herpes zoster is caused by the varicella-zoster virus, a DNA virus that causes chickenpox in children. This clinical condition results from reactivation of the latent varicella-zoster virus in the dorsal root ganglia of the spinal cord. The incidence among octogenarians is 5 to 10 in 1000.[2] Acute herpes zoster is associated with a painful vesicular rash. Both the pain and the rash usually resolve within 2 to 3 weeks. When the pain persists beyond the resolution of the rash, postherpetic neuralgia exists, involving degeneration of the dorsal root ganglia of the nerve or nerves affected by the herpes zoster virus.[3]

The incidence of postherpetic neuralgia is higher in the elderly than in the younger population. Loeser[4] reported that the increased incidence in these patients may be a result of a decrease in antibody titers. Most cases of herpes zoster involve the dermatomes of the thoracic nerves (55 percent), while the cranial (25 percent), lumbosacral (17 percent), cervical (12 percent), and multiple (1 percent) nerves may also be affected.[4] The first division of the trigeminal nerve is commonly infected in geriatric patients, and this entity commonly progresses to trigeminal neuralgia and may affect a patient's vision. As a result, patients with trigeminal nerve involvement should have an ophthalmology consultation. Although both are rare, centrally the sympathetic ganglion may be involved, resulting in sympathetically maintained pain, and peripherally the nerves in the extremities may be affected, resulting in both pain and muscle weakness.

TREATMENT OF ACUTE HERPES ZOSTER

Acute herpes zoster begins with pain, paresthesia, and dysesthesia in the affected dermatomes. Subsequently, a vesicular rash may erupt with lesions that usually heal in approximately 1 month. During the acute stage, elderly patients may have more pain than do younger patients.[4] In fact, aggressive treatment of acute herpes zoster is indicated in geriatric patients. The possible treatments include the use of antiviral agents, lotions, clonidine, nonsteroidal anti-inflammatory agents, analgesics, antidepressants, muscle relaxants, corticosteroids administered systemically or by infiltration, and nerve blocks. These nerve blocks include sympathetic blocks, topical agents, subcutaneous infiltration of the lesions, somatic nerve blocks, and epidural blocks.[5]

Topical Agents

Topical agents accelerate skin healing and decrease the pain of acute herpes zoster but do not affect the incidence of postherpetic neuralgia. Topical idoxuridine has been used in the treatment of acute herpes zoster.[6] Compresses of aluminum acetate (Burrow's) solution or calamine lotion placed over the lesion also may lessen the pain associated with acute herpes zoster.

Clonidine transdermal patches placed over the area of maximum pain may decrease not only the pain associated with acute herpes zoster but especially the pain of postherpetic neuralgia.[7] These patches provide a plasma level more consistent than the peaks and troughs that can occur with oral dosing. The 0.1-mg patches may be placed on no more than two or three different locations. It is vital that the patient be warned to pay very careful attention to the signs and symptoms of hypotension. There is clinical documentation of complete resolution of pain after the use of these patches.[7]

Oral Agents

The pharmacodynamic responses of antidepressants and other psychotropic drugs commonly used in acute herpes zoster and postherpetic neuralgia are affected by changes in age. It has been reported that changes may exist in geriatric patients with respect to target organ sensitivity to various drugs.[8] The absorption of actively transported drugs, such as vitamins and carbohydrates, has been reported to decrease as age increases, while essentially no change occurred in the absorption of passively absorbed drugs such as tricyclic antidepressants and psychotropic agents.[9,10]

ACYCLOVIR Acyclovir (800 mg orally five times a day for 7 days) is an antiviral agent frequently used for the treatment of acute herpes zoster less than 72 h in duration.[11]

TRICYCLIC ANTIDEPRESSANTS Tricyclic antidepressants are used to treat a variety of chronic pain syndromes, even though the mechanism by which they exert their analgesic action is unknown. However, the analgesic effect of amitriptyline has been confirmed in an animal model in which neuropathic pain was experimentally induced around the sciatic nerve.[12] The correct initial dose of amitriptyline in elderly patients suffering from postherpetic neuralgia has not been resolved. Although higher doses definitely produce significantly greater efficacy, the incidence of adverse effects has also been reported to be significantly higher.[13] In geriatric patients, a starting dose of 10 mg is usually effective, and if no response is noted at the end of 3 weeks, the dose is increased gradually. If excessive sedation is noted with amitriptyline or doxepin, another tricyclic antidepressant should be substituted. The tricyclic antidepressants are bound to serum $alpha_1$ acid glycoproteins, whose levels change minimally with aging.[14]

BENZODIAZEPINES It may be wise to refrain from using benzodiazepines in elderly patients, especially the long-acting benzodiazepines, which can accumulate with repeated dosing. If a practitioner must prescribe benzodiazepines for severe anxiety, it is recommended that those with shorter half-lives, such as lorazepam and alprazolam, should be used. Benzodiazepines with a longer half-life require decreased doses in older patients, whereas those with a shorter half-life can approximate the doses given to younger patients.[15] Temazepam has a relatively short half-life and may have some advantages as a hypnotic in geriatric patients. The recommended dose is 15 mg orally at bedtime.

NONSTEROIDAL ANTI-INFLAMMATORY DRUGS Nonsteroidal anti-inflammatory drugs (NSAIDs) may be effective in the pain management of acute herpes zoster and postherpetic neuralgia in elderly patients. However, in older patients, pharmacokinetic variability exists among the various classes of nonsteroidal anti-inflammatory agents. Patients may receive excellent analgesia with one particular agent but have considerable side effects with another. Wide differences may exist in the pharmacokinetics and pharmacodynamics of these agents. A patient receiving NSAIDs may need the drug given on a "regular" as opposed to an "as needed" schedule. Smaller doses (e.g., ibuprofen 200–400 mg bid-qid) of NSAIDs provide analgesia, while larger doses (600 mg qid or 800 mg tid) provide an anti-inflammatory property. Ibuprofen has a short half-life and rapid absorption from the gastrointestinal tract. By contrast, piroxicam has a half-life of approximately 45 h and should be taken every other day. It is recommended that when one is prescribing higher doses of NSAIDs, stool guaiac tests be done every 2 weeks, whereas liver function tests, blood urea nitrogen (BUN), creatine, and a urinalysis should be checked every 1 to 2 months, depending on the patient's overall medical condition.[16]

NARCOTICS It is best to avoid narcotics for the treatment of acute herpes zoster and postherpetic neuralgia unless they are absolutely indicated. When one uses narcotics in elderly patients, it is best to avoid narcotics that can be associated with psychiatric side effects, such as meperidine and pentazocine. If the patient does not get adequate pain relief from a nonsteroidal anti-inflammatory agent, the use of mild narcotics such as codeine, oxycodone, and hydrocodone may be considered. Propoxyphene has also been used with success on occasion. Each of these drugs has been found to be useful in the management of chronic pain syndromes. In many instances, these drugs are combined with acetaminophen or aspirin. When the pain syndrome becomes severe, physicians have commonly used stronger agonist opioids to provide analgesia. Morphine is the most commonly prescribed opioid for severe pain. Geriatric patients with decreased renal function may be at risk for toxicity from the active metabolite of morphine, morphine-6-glucuronide.[17] Therefore, if possible, morphine should be used on a temporary basis. With reference to meperidipine, its metabolite normeperidine may also be associated with pronounced side effects. After an accumulation of normeperidine, seizures have been noted in elderly patients suffering from cancer.[18]

MUSCLE RELAXANTS Muscle relaxants such as baclofen may also be of benefit in treating pain associated with acute herpes zoster when muscle spasm is evident. Baclofen, which acts at the spinal cord, decreases the number of muscle spasms and relieves the pain associated with spasms. The dose is 5 mg PO tid for 3 days and may be increased by 5 mg daily at 3-day intervals to a maximum of 80 mg daily.

Intravenous Agents

Vidarabine (adenine arabinoside) 10 mg/kg may be given intravenously daily for 5 days to treat acute herpes zoster in immunocompromised patients.

Nutritional Concerns

Geriatric patients with persistent pain may decrease their caloric intake and consequently sustain weight loss. Other patients may gain weight after the onset of chronic pain. These patients become immobile, remain at home, and tend to overeat because of depression and/or anxiety. Poor eating habits in combination with lack of exercise may lead to decreased mobility, muscle weakness, ligament laxity, and stress on joints, which may in turn worsen a patient's chronic pain syndrome. Therefore, the inclusion of a nutritional consultation on occasion may be important in the management of chronic pain in the elderly.[19]

TREATMENT OF POSTHERPETIC NEURALGIA

When pain persists after the vesicles have healed, postherpetic neuralgia may be diagnosed. Elderly patients are more likely to suffer from this form of deafferentation pain, which involves both the CNS and the peripheral nervous system, than are younger patients.[4] The pain may be burning or lancing and may fluctuate in intensity. Unfortunately, as with the pain of acute herpes zoster, there is no definitive treatment that provides permanent relief of postherpetic neuralgia.

Drug Therapies

Intravenous lidocaine, oral anticonvulsants, and tricyclic antidepressants have all been reported to be effective in the management of postherpetic neuralgia.[20,21] Intravenous lidocaine, a cell membrane stabilizer, can provide rapid relief of postherpetic neuralgia pain. Tricyclic antidepressants can decrease the burning pain associated with postherpetic neuralgia, while anticonvulsants can attenuate the sharp shooting pain.

Topically applied agents such as capsaicin and local anesthetics may also help with the pain of postherpetic neuralgia. Capsaicin, a substance found in hot peppers, depletes and prevents the reaccumulation of substance P in peripheral neurons. Patients may complain of severe burning pain after the application of capsaicin to the skin, and such application may have to be preceded by a topical local anesthetic such as lidocaine gel 10%.

Physical Therapy

Physical therapy and the modalities associated with it are important in the management of acute and chronic pain in geriatric patients. Heat, cold, massage, biofeedback, and transcutaneous electrical nerve stimulation (TENS) may all be tried and/or used in the treatment of chronic pain in elderly patients. It is important to preserve range of motion as well as strength and function in older patients. Aquatic therapy may be beneficial for the management of chronic pain associated with postherpetic neuralgia in these patients. When indicated, occupational therapy may be used for preservation of daily living activities. Psychological counseling, relaxation techniques, and cognitive and behavioral therapies should be considered.

ASSOCIATED DISEASE PROCESSES

Trigeminal Neuralgia

Trigeminal neuralgia associated with acute herpes zoster and postherpetic neuralgia occurs primarily in older patients.[22] This disease consists of severe facial pain and may interfere with talking as well as eating. Baclofen (5 mg orally three times a day, increasing by 5 mg/day every 3 days) has been used in combination with neural blockade or neurolysis of branches of the trigeminal nerve to treat the neuralgia.[23]

Cancer Pain

Cancer pain may also affect geriatric patients and may be seen with acute herpes zoster and/or postherpetic neuralgia. Reports of patients with cancer pain have demonstrated that 50 to 70 percent of these patients suffer needlessly.[24] However, the pain from cancer must be differentiated from that of acute herpes zoster and postherpetic neuralgia to ensure that each entity receives the appropriate treatment. Cancer pain may be caused by any or all of the following: obstruction or distension of a hollow viscus, impingement of nerves and blood vessels by the progressive spread of a tumor, occlusion of blood vessels leading to edema, inflammation, tissue necrosis, and compression of peripheral nerves by a tumor or collapse of bony structures by metastatic lesions.[25] Cancer pain noted in a geriatric patient with acute herpes zoster not only may be due to the tumor but may be a result of iatrogenic interventions such as postmastectomy pain, postradiation fibrosis, and peripheral neuropathy after chemotherapy. It is also important that cancer pain be distinguished from other benign causes of pain, such as diabetic neuropathy.

NERVE BLOCKS

Pain associated with postherpetic neuralgia may fall into one of several categories: somatic, sympathetic, and central. Somatic nerve blocks with local anesthetic can be used to predict a patient's response to a neurolytic nerve block. Sympathetically mediated pain associated with postherpetic neuralgia results from a disorder of the autonomic nervous system.[26] A central pain syndrome consists of spontaneous burning dysesthesia, hyperpathia, and hyperalgia in the absence of peripheral tissue damage, and these syndromes may result from primary cortical, thalamic, or spinal cord lesions.

Acute Herpes Zoster

Nerve blocks may be used to manage the pain associated with acute herpes zoster. Subcutaneous infiltration of steroids at the site of eruption may be of value. Somatic nerve blocks of the trigeminal nerve, brachial plexus, paravertebral nerves, intercostal nerves, and the sciatic nerve are of limited value unless a neurolytic block is performed. Sympathetic nerve blocks may not only relieve the pain of acute herpes zoster but decrease the incidence of the development of postherpetic neuralgia.[27] To be most effective, they should be done within the first 2 months after onset. Stellate ganglion blocks may be used for pain in the head, neck, and arms. Thoracic epidural blocks are utilized for pain in the thoracic area, and lumbar sympathetic blocks are used for the management of pain in the lower body. TENS is another modality that may be effective on occasion in some patients who are refractory to other forms of treatment.

Postherpetic Neuralgia

Several new procedures are available to geriatric patients for the management of pain related to postherpetic neuralgia. Nerve blocks have traditionally played an important role in intractable pain management in geriatric patients and remain a primary anesthetic focus. They are utilized primarily for the interruption of nociceptive pathways and to facilitate physical therapy. Nerve blocks are used in geriatric patients when pain becomes too severe or persistent and cannot be controlled by nonnarcotic analgesics. When nerve blocks with local anesthetics are ineffective, neurolytic neural blockade should be considered as well as neurolysis with cryoanalgesia or radiofrequency thermocoagulation. If these modalities are not effective, one must consider a dorsal column stimulator or peripheral nerve stimulator. Ultimately, if significant pain relief has not been achieved with these modalities, implantation of a morphine pump must be considered.

Many types of nerve blocks and agents have been used for the management of the chronic pain associated with postherpetic neuralgia. It is beyond the scope of this chapter to list all the blocks and agents that may be used for chronic pain in geriatric patients. Injections of nerve blocks have been used therapeutically as well as diagnostically since the introduction of cocaine by Carl Koller in 1884.[28] Sihota and associates[29] and Reiestad and coworkers[30] reported on the use of an implantable interpleural catheter for the management of postherpetic neuralgia in the thoracic area. However, this technique does not provide permanent relief. A newly designed epidural catheter (Racz Cauda Cath, Medic Epimed Int.) made from spiral stainless coils coated with fluoropolymers has been introduced and is being used frequently by anesthesiologists for pain management. The advantage of this catheter is that it facilitates radiological localization during placement under fluoroscopy and can be repositioned and aspirated for repeated injections.[31]

NEUROLYTIC AGENTS

Neurolytic substances have provided pain relief for patients, including those with postherpetic neuralgia, since the 1930s. Racz and colleagues[32] reported on the utilization of the instillation of diluted solutions of phenol through special epidural catheters over a period of days. The first report of the injection of a neurolytic solution for the treatment of pain was written in 1863 by Lutton.[25] Neurolytic therapeutic blocks for chronic pain management were initially developed by neurosurgeons. In 1925 Doppler used phenol for neurolysis,[25] and Maher reported on the use of phenol subarachnoid neurolysis in 1955.[25]

Phenol produces destruction of both myelinated and nonmyelinated nerve fibers. Histological changes in nerves caused by phenol cannot be distinguished from those caused by alcohol. Phenol can cause postinjection neuritis, but the incidence is lower than that with alcohol. Phenol allegedly has a greater affinity for vascular tissue than for neural tissue. It has therefore been reported that phenol can cause damage to perineural vascular tissue.[33] However, when Racz and colleagues[31] compared morphological changes that occurred after epidural and subarachnoid injection of phenol, it was noted that no spinal cord damage had occurred when epidural phenol was administered. However, neurological tissue damage did occur after subarachnoid injection. Phenol does not pass easily through the dura, the dural sleeve, or the nerve roots. Repeated injections of 6% phenol into the epidural space were reported to be safe.[32] Therefore, phenol may be used when there is significant residual burning associated with postherpetic neuralgia. All procedures utilizing phenol should be done with two-dimensional fluoroscopy. The concentrations of phenol used at the authors' institution vary from 3% to 6%. To obtain concentrations below 6%, phenol may be mixed with saline or water. Otherwise, phenol is mixed in glycerin for neurolysis because it is soluble in glycerin. Phenol is hyperbaric if mixed with glycerol, and the painful area must be in the dependent position when one performs a nerve block. Phenol neurolysis is accomplished by means of repeated administration of the agent through an indwelling catheter. Therefore, this procedure mandates inpatient hospitalization.

NEUROLYTIC BLOCKS

Neurolytic blocks are not totally permanent blocks; essentially no neurolytic nerve block is permanent. Neurolytic blocks last from days to months, and the response varies. Pain may recur, and consequently, the block must be repeated. Because neurolytic agents result in skin sloughing if injected superficially, neurolytic procedures should be done only for deep, well-localized lesions.

Stellate Ganglion Block

In some instances, chronic pain in a geriatric patient suffering from acute herpes zoster or postherpetic neuralgia may be due to involvement of distal fibers of the sympathetic nervous system. It is not uncommon at the authors' institution to do a stellate ganglion block with a local anesthetic (bupivacaine) and/or a phenol nerve block when indicated for complex cases of postherpetic neuralgia. It is the authors' practice to mix 5 μg of sufentanil with 0.5% bupivacaine for a total volume of 5 ml. It is also standard practice to complete at least five local anesthetic stellate ganglion blocks before proceeding to a phenol stellate ganglion block. The stellate ganglion is formed by the complete or partial fusion of the inferior cervical and first thoracic sympathetic ganglia. The stellate ganglion is situated within the base of the transverse process of the seventh cervical vertebra in the back of the first rib. It lies behind the carotid sheath, anterior to the longus colli muscle, anterior and medial to the vertebral artery, and lateral to the body of the carotid artery. The ganglion is close to the subclavian artery, the inferior thyroid artery, and the first intercostal artery. Furthermore, it is near the recurrent laryngeal nerve. The pleura is in close proximity to the stellate ganglion on the right side, but on the left side it is 1 to 2 cm below. Because of the close proximity to nerves, vessels, and lung tissue, a stellate ganglion nerve block occasionally may be associated with side effects: Horner's syndrome, hoarseness, and seizures from an intravascular injection or intraspinal injection. The possibility of these side effects must be explained to the patient before the nerve block is performed.

At the authors' institution, a series of diagnostic and/or therapeutic stellate ganglion blocks initially utilizing local anesthetics are completed. Once it has been demonstrated that the local anesthetic provides an adequate but relatively short duration nerve block (providing only temporary clinical relief of symptomatology), it is acceptable to proceed to a neurolytic block with phenol under fluoroscopy. Before the performance of any neurolytic block, an informed consent is obtained that includes all potential complications. Subsequently, an intravenous line is established and monitors are placed that consist of an automated blood pressure, pulse oximeter, and electrocardiogram (ECG). Each morning, the clinic resuscitation equipment, including a defibrillator, should be checked to ascertain that it is functioning properly. Resuscitative equipment and drugs should always be available when a nerve block is being performed. When one is doing invasive nerve blocks, intravenous sedation is administered only after informed consent has been obtained. The skin in the area where the block will be performed is prepped, usually with a povidone-iodine (Betadine) solution, and then is draped in a sterile fashion. When one is doing a neurolytic procedure, two-dimensional fluoroscopy is used to maximize patient safety. When one is doing a stellate ganglion block, a 22-gauge "B" bevel needle is inserted 2 cm lateral and 2 cm caudal to the cricoid cartilage. The needle is aimed at the ventral lateral aspect of the vertebral body at C7. The needle is advanced until contact is made with the vertebral body. The needle is then stabilized with a long clamp, and a 3-ml syringe with extension tubing containing radiographic contrast medium is attached to the needle. The needle is pulled back approximately 1 mm and then aspirated, and the physician looks for cerebrospinal fluid or blood. If a negative aspirate is observed, 1 ml of nonionic contrast medium is deposited. After administration, the contrast material may spread along the surface of the longus colli muscle. Only 1 ml of contrast material is injected because larger volumes may dilute the effects of either the local anesthetic or the phenol. Once it has been ascertained by fluoroscopy and by the injection of contrast material that the needle is positioned properly, another reaspiration is performed. If it is negative, a syringe containing 1 ml of triamcinolone (40 mg), 1.5 ml of 0.5% bupivacaine, and 2.5 ml of 6% phenol-saline solution for a total volume of 5 ml is injected. This solution is injected slowly, at a rate of 1 ml per 30 s. After the injection of each milliliter, fluoroscopy is utilized to verify that the needle has not moved. After the injection of the neurolytic solution, the patient is kept in a supine position with the head slightly elevated for approximately 30 min. Over 750 stellate ganglion blocks with 3% phenol have been performed at the authors' institution for various etiologies. There have been no serious complications with this procedure. However, potential complications exist after a neurolytic phenol stellate ganglion block. These complications include permanent Horner's syndrome, hoarseness, numbness, and/or paralysis of the muscles of the upper extremity or phrenic nerve and pneumothorax. The authors have had one patient with Horner's syndrome that lasted approximately 2.5 months. Complete recovery did occur after the fourth stellate ganglion block. Another patient developed hoarseness that resolved after approximately 5 months.

Lumbar Sympathetic Block

Another nerve block that is relatively common for the management of pain associated with postherpetic neuralgia in the geriatric population is a lumbar sympathetic block. Indications for this block include sympathetic pain in the pelvic, rectal, or genital area. As was stated previously, nerve blocks may be done with local anesthetics. However, if only temporary relief is obtained with a local anesthetic lumbar sympathetic block, consideration must be given to a neurolytic block. At the authors' institution, both local anesthetic and neurolytic lumbar sympathetic blocks are done under fluoroscopy. Anatomically, the lumbar sympathetic ganglia extends from the first thoracic vertebra to the fifth lumbar vertebra. The chain lies in the anterior lateral surface of the vertebral column. The psoas fascia and psoas muscle separate the sympathetic chain from the somatic nerves. As a result, neurolytic blockade results in no loss of sensory or motor function. Performance of a lumbar sympathetic block is similar to that of a celiac plexus block. The patient is placed in the prone position on the fluoroscopy table with a pillow under the midabdominal region. The vertebral bodies of L2 and L4 are identified, and a 10- or 15-cm 22-gauge block needle is inserted 5 to 7 cm lateral from the midline of these vertebral bodies. The angulation of the needle is approximately 30 or 40 degrees. The skin and soft tissue through which the needle will traverse are anesthetized with a local anesthetic. If the transverse process of the vertebral body is encountered, the needle should be redirected either cephalad or caudad so that the needle tip may pass the transverse process. If the needle tip does encounter the vertebral body as demonstrated by fluoroscopy, the angulation of the needle is increased until the tip passes closely to the immediate anterior surface of the vertebral body. Aspiration of the needle is done to confirm that the tip is not in a major blood vessel. Subsequently, 1 to 2 ml of nonionic contrast material is administered to identify placement of the needle tip. When the dye is injected, the fluoroscopically obtained picture is observed for a characteristic linear spread over the anterior surface of the psoas muscle on the lateral fluoroscopy view and under the vertebral body silhouette on anteroposterior fluoroscopy projection. The spread of the dye linearly for three vertebral bodies should ensure adequate interruption of the sympathetic chain. If a three-vertebral body spread is not encountered, the needle tip should be repositioned. Once it has been ascertained by fluoroscopy and dye spread that the needle tip is in proper position, 6% phenol is used for neurolysis. The recommended volume is 3 to 10 ml at L2 and a similar volume at L4. Complications of this block include an intravascular injection; perforation of the aorta, vena cava, or kidney; hypotension; sexual dysfunction; and a somatic nerve root injection.

Epidural Block

An advantage of epidural phenol is its applicability for pain occupying a wide dermatomal distribution or pain that is bilateral. The injection of epidural phenol affects dorsal (sensory) nerve roots and spares the anterior (motor) roots. Phenol is the most commonly used epidural neurolytic drug. Epidural neurolytic drugs should not be administered through a needle, as the needle may migrate after the administration of a test dose, and a high risk of paralysis will occur if the neurolytic injectate is administered in the subarachnoid space. At the authors' institution, an epidural catheter is placed for epidural injection. Injections are then carried out daily until the patient's symptoms subside and do not return for at least 24 h. To perform the procedure for epidural phenol injections, the patient is taken to the fluoroscopy room and positioned with the painful side down. A Racz RK 16-gauge epidural needle (Medic Epimed Int.) is placed in the epidural space, using a paramedian approach. Then, using a loss of resistance technique with both air and saline, the needle is placed in the epidural space. At that time, using fluoroscopy, the Racz Epidural Catheter (Medic Epimed Int.) is placed one to two segments above the desired nerve root. An aspiration is performed. After a negative aspirate for blood and cerebrospinal fluid has been confirmed, 2 to 3 ml of 0.25% bupivacaine is administered as a test dose. After confirmation of no profound sensory or motor blockade, further local anesthetic is given to a total volume of 5 to 10 ml, depending on the location (cervical, thoracic, or lumbar spinal segment). It must be confirmed pharmacologically that there is no subdural or subarachnoid placement of drug, as this precludes the use of phenol. The patient should report relief of pain without evidence of extensive sensory deficit and no motor block. If motor block results, the procedure is canceled. Subsequently, on the next day, 6% phenol is injected in 0.5-ml increments until pain relief has been reported by the patient. The patient is positioned with the painful side down and repositioned head up at a 30-degree dorsal lateral tilt to facilitate the spread of phenol to the dorsal root ganglia. The patient is kept in this position for 1 h after the phenol deposition. Each daily phenol injection is preceded by aspiration of the epidural catheter. The phenol injections usually take 2 to 3 days to reach the endpoint of 24 h of pain relief. If pain returns by 10 to 12 days, a second series is carried out. Long-lasting pain relief of postherpetic neuralgia usually follows the second series of injections.

Epidural phenol administration is not without potential complications, including damage to nerve and blood vessels, headaches, paresthesias, muscular paresis, and rectal or bladder dysfunction. Patients are more prone to transient weakness in the upper lumbar nerve root area, i.e., weight-bearing muscles, but they experience very few problems in the sacral nerve roots if injections are administered unilaterally. Over 2000 epidural phenol injections have been administered at the authors' institution without any serious complications. Most of these administrations were in patients with nonmalignant painful conditions.

ALTERNATIVE TREATMENTS

Hypertonic Saline

Hypertonic saline was first used for intrathecal injection to treat intractable facial pain caused by tumors.[34] Its mechanism of action is speculative. Excellent results have been reported in the authors' institution after the administration of 10% sodium chloride in combination with local anesthetics and steroids administered epidurally for chronic painful conditions caused by postherpetic neuralgia. It is believed that this technique decreases inflammation along nerve roots and dorsal ganglia. This inflammation, which is secondary to the acute herpes zoster infection, can cause scarring around the involved nerve roots. When the pain is confined to the lower lumbar or lumbosacral area, it is recommended that a special epidural catheter [i.e., a 16-gauge Racz RK needle (Medic Epimed Int.)] be placed caudally. Once this needle has been placed into the caudal canal, an injection of 10 ml of iohexol [(Omnipaque-240) (Winthrop-Breon, New York)] is administered to produce an epiduralgram that outlines filling defects where the effective nerve roots are involved. This will identify the causation of pain. At the authors' institution, these nerve roots have been freed by threading a Racz Cauda Cath into the painful nerve roots (Fig. 24-1 and 24-2). Subsequently, 10 ml of 0.25% bupivacaine containing 4 mg/ml of triamcinolone is injected into the scarred area. Hyaluronidase 1500 units with preservative-free normal saline also may be injected into the painful nerve root area. After a latency period of 30 min, 10 ml of hypertonic sodium chloride (10%) is administered through the epidural catheter. The catheter is taped into place, and reinjection is carried out on postprocedure days 1 and 2. Repeated injections of hypertonic saline give prolonged benefits to patients compared with administering only one dose of hypertonic saline epidurally. It is particularly efficacious if the specific nerve root involved in the painful postherpetic neuralgia syndrome is determined before injection and the local anesthetic, steroid, hyaluronidase, and hypertonic saline are deposited directly

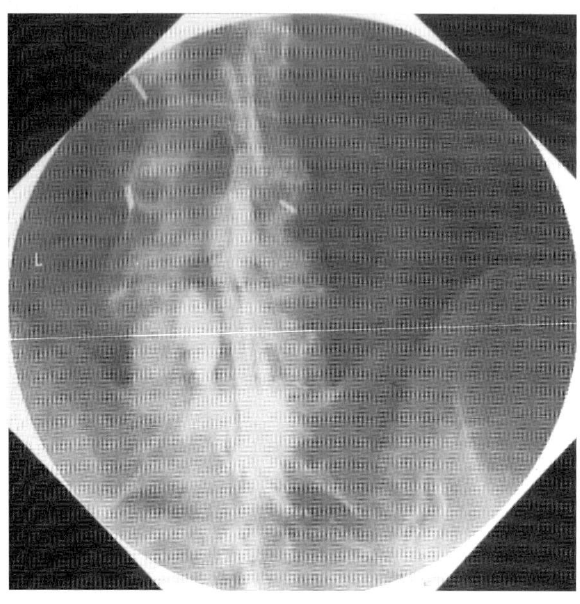

Figure 24-1 Pain from postsurgical scar formation and an inflamed nerve root may require epidurolysis to decrease pressure and inflammation at that nerve root. Dye is prevented from filling out the left L4 nerve root, which is consistent with this patient's physical exam.

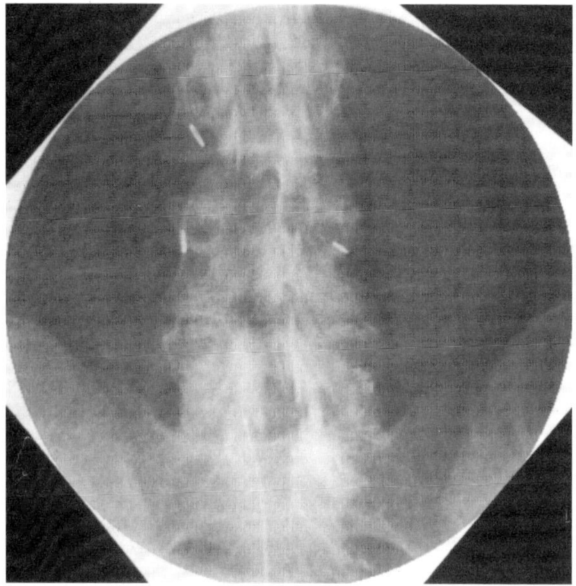

Figure 24-2 Placement of the epidural catheter to the painful nerve root for delivery of drug, which otherwise would not reach this area of pain gerneration because of either epidural scarring or inflammation.

onto it or in close proximity to it. For thoracic pain, a thoracic catheter is placed below the level of the painful area and advanced to the area of scarring demonstrated by fluoroscopy.

Radiofrequency Thermocoagulation

Radiofrequency thermocoagulation (RFTC) has been recently utilized for the management of trigeminal nerve pain caused by postherpetic neuralgia. This technique can provide a long-term interruption of the lumbar sympathetic chain as well. It is an outpatient procedure and essentially lacks the complications of chemical neurolysis. An RFTC lesion is controllable as well as discreet. To perform this procedure, the use of fluoroscopy is essential. A Teflon-coated needle (Radionics, Inc.) with a 5- or 10-mm active tip is inserted. A thermocouple electrode is placed through the SMK needle (Radionics, Inc.). Once the needle tip is in proper position, Omnipaque-240 (Winthrop-Breon, New York) is injected to verify the needle position. Once needle confirmation has been ascertained, stimulation of the sensory nerves at 50 to 70 Hz is done. Next, stimulation of motor nerves at 2 to 5 Hz is done. If no tingling or motor nerve stimulation is observed, another aspiration is performed, and 0.5% bupivacaine is administered to decrease the pain associated with RFTC. At that time, thermocoagulation is accomplished by setting the dial at 80°C for 70 s.

Nerve Stimulators

Occasionally, a dorsal column stimulator is implanted percutaneously for the treatment of persistent chronic pain associated with postherpetic neuralgia. The mechanism of action of the dorsal column stimulator is still debated. Electrical interference with multiple ascending and descending polysynaptic pathways may be the mechanism for decreasing nociception. Placement of a dorsal column stimulator for intractable pain caused by postherpetic neuralgia is effective in decreasing that pain.[35] Before the placing of a dorsal column stimulator, a trial stimulating catheter is commonly placed through a Racz RK (Medic Epimed Int.) 16-gauge epidural needle proximal to the painful area. A patient must receive at least a 50 percent decrease in pain before a permanent dorsal column stimulator is placed.

A peripheral nerve stimulator may also be used for the management of postherpetic neuralgia that affects peripheral nerves. At the authors' institution, placement of both a peripheral nerve stimulator and a dorsal column stimulator has been performed to provide adequate analgesia for postherpetic neuritis of the right proximal radial nerve in an elderly patient.

Cryoanalgesia

Cryoanalgesia may also be used to provide long-term pain relief without the use of drugs in the somatic nerves of patients with acute herpes zoster. Cryoanalgesia is indicated when a long-term reversible and peripheral nerve block is required and the nerve is accessible (e.g., an intercostal nerve). Cryoanalgesia has also been used successfully in the treatment of thoracic postherpetic neuralgia. There is no absolute contraindication except patient refusal. The procedure is applicable to any situation in which a mixed motor and sensory nerve is involved. In the authors' institution, cryoanalgesia is not performed on nerves that have a large motor component.

When one is doing cryoanalgesia, an image intensifier should be used. Accurate placement of the cryoanalgesia probe is mandatory. Using a nerve stimulator with a setting of 2 to 3 V, a muscle twitch usually is obtained when the motor nerve is in close proximity. The cryoanalgesia probe should not be removed after cryoanalgesia until it has gone through a defrost cycle. Immediate pain relief is usually obtained after the procedure and can last from 3 to 1000 days. An occasional transient area of erythema may be seen along the course of the treated nerve. A skin burn may occur if the cryoanalgesia probe is superficially placed. This skin burn will heal, but the patient may be left with a very small area of depigmentation for several months. Repeat treatments may be indicated, and there is no evidence of permanent neurological damage as a result of multiple cryoanalgesia treatments. Cryoanalgesia may be performed on an outpatient basis.

Surgical Techniques

No single standard surgical procedure is effective for the management of postherpetic neuralgia in elderly patients. Cordotomy, rhizotomy, and sympathectomy have not provided consistent pain relief. Dorsal root entry zone (DREZ) lesions may be effective for the management of postherpetic neuralgia, as is stimulation of the venteroposteromedialis.[36–38] A cordotomy is an anterolateral incision in the spinal cord. This procedure interrupts pain conduction in the lateral spinothalmic tract. A rhizotomy involves ablation of the dorsal sensory roots of the nerves involved in pain transmission. DREZ procedures involve identification of nerve rootlets involved in pain with a 2-mm incision into the dorsal horn anterior to the involved dorsal roots.[39] Venteroposteromedialis stimulation may activate the medullary nucleus raphe magnus, which may inhibit pain impulses to the cortex. This procedure involves the surgical implantation of electrodes.

It is recommended that if more conventional therapies do not provide adequate analgesia, then hypertonic epidural saline, phenol neurolysis, cryoanalgesia, or RFTC should be considered when indicated. If relief is not obtained with these modalities, one should consider using a spinal cord stimulator and, in addition, a peripheral nerve stimulator for peripheral nerve lesions related to postherpetic neuralgia if the spinal cord stimulator is not effective.

When all other modalities have failed to provide adequate pain relief for chronic intractable severe pain associated with postherpetic neuralgia, a subarachnoid catheter connected to a morphine pump implanted subcutaneously should be considered. The pump is filled periodically, and its dose is increased or decreased by telemetry as needed. Both the catheter and the pump are inserted in the operating room with sedation and local anesthesia. If a patient becomes refractory to morphine, hydromorphone may be substituted.

SUMMARY

It is felt that a geriatric patient suffering from acute herpes zoster and postherpetic neuralgia presents a challenge. Each patient's pain problem should be addressed with an understanding of the underlying pathological condition and possible relations with other medical conditions, including psychological and/or psychiatric entities. This understanding will facilitate an accurate and thorough assessment of the patient's pain and result in a more comprehensive, safe, and effective plan for the management of chronic pain in an elderly patient. Therefore, aggressive treatment of acute herpes zoster must be performed with the intention of preventing postherpetic neuralgia, which can cause physical as well as mental incapacitation. If this disease process is improperly treated, it can result in drug addiction and suicide.

REFERENCES

1. Blazer D, Hughes D, George L: The epidemiology of depression in an elderly community population. *Gerontology* 27:281, 1987.
2. Hope-Simpson RE: The nature of herpes zoster: A long term study and a new hypothesis. *Proc R Soc Med* 58:9, 1965.
3. Ghatak NR, Zimmerman HM: Spinal ganglion in herpes zoster. *Arch Pathol* 95:411, 1973.
4. Loeser JF: Herpes zoster and postherpetic neuralgia. *Pain* 25:149, 1986.
5. Katz JA, Phero JC, McDonald JS, Green DB. Herpes zoster management. *Anesth Prog* 36:35, 1989.
6. Dowber R: Idoxuridine in herpes zoster: Further evaluation of intermittent topical therapy. *Br Med J* 2:256, 1974.
7. Kraynack BJ: Topical clonidine treatment of postherpetic neuralgia. *Pain Digest* 4: 204, 1994.
8. Klotz U, Avant GR, Hoyump A, et al: The effects of age and liver disease on the disposition and elimination of diazepam in adult man. *J Clin Invest* 55:347, 1975.
9. Norris AH, Lundy T, Shock NW: Trends in selected indices of body composition in men between the ages of 30 and 80 years. *Ann NY Acad Sci* 110:623, 1963.
10. Crooks T, O'Malley K, Stevenson IH: Pharmacokinetics in the elderly. *Clin Pharmacokinet* 1:280, 1976.
11. Balfour J, Bean B, Laskin OL: Acyclovir halts progression of herpes zoster in immunocompromised patients. *N Engl J Med* 308:1448, 1983.
12. Ardid D, Guilbaud G: Antinociceptive effects of acute and chronic injections of tricyclic antidepressant drugs in a new model of mononeuropathy in rats. *Pain* 49:179, 1992.

13. McQuay HJ, Carroll D, Glynn CY: Dose-response for analgesic effect of aytroptolyline in chronic pain. *Anaesthesia* 48:281, 1993.
14. Thompson TLL, Moran MG, Nies AS: Psychotropic drug use in the elderly. *N Engl J Med* 308:134, 1987.
15. Merlis S, Koepke HH: The use of oxazepam in elderly patients. *Dis Nerv Syst* 36 (S Section 2):27, 1975.
16. Portenoy R: Drug therapy for cancer pain. *Am J Hospice Palliative Care* 67:22, 1992.
17. Osborne JR, Joel SP, Slevin, ML: Morphine intoxication in renal failure: The role of morphine-6-glucuronide. *Br Med J* 1548:292, 1986.
18. Kaiko RF, Foley KM, Grabiski PY, et al: Central nervous system excitatory effects of meperidine in cancer patients. *Ann Neurol* 13:80, 1983.
19. Jamison RN, Stetson B, Skrocco T, Parris WCK: Effects of significant weight gain on chronic pain patients. *Clin J Physiol* 6:47, 1990.
20. Hatangdi VS, Boas RA, Richards EG: Postherpetic neuralgia: Management with antiepileptic and tricyclic drugs, in Bonica JJ, Albe-Fessard D (eds): *Advances in Pain Research and Therapy.* New York: Raven Press, 1976, pp 583–587.
21. Raftery HH: The management of postherpetic pain using sodium valproate and amitriptyline. *J Irish Med Assoc* 72:399, 1979.
22. Poser CM: Facial pain: Diagnostic dilemma, therapeutic challenge. *Geriatrics* 30:110, 1975.
23. Steardo L, Leo A, Marando E: Efficacy of baclofen in trigeminal neuralgia and some other painful conditions: A clinical trial. *Eur Neurol* 23:51, 1984.
24. Daut RLL, Cleeland CS: The prevalence and severity of pain in cancer. *Cancer* 50:1913, 1992.
25. Arter OE, Racz GB: Pain management of the oncologic patient. *Semin Surg Oncol* 6:162, 1990.
26. Hogan QH: The sympathetic nervous system in postherpetic neuralgia. *Reg Anesth* 18:271, 1993.
27. Winnie AP, Hartwell PW: Relationship between time of treatment of acute herpes zoster with sympathetic blockade and prevention of postherpetic neuralgia: Clinical support for a new theory of the mechanism by which sympathetic blockade provides therapeutic benefit. *Reg Anesth* 18:277, 1993.
28. Koller C: Bor/Aufige mittheilung uber locale anasthesirung AM auge. *Klin Monatsbl Augenheilkd* 22:60, 1884.
29. Sihota MK, Ikuta PT, Holmblad BR, et al: Successful pain management of chronic pancreatitis and postherpetic neuralgia with intrapleural technique. *Reg Anesth* 13:40, 1988.
30. Reiestad F, McIlvane WB, Barnes M, et al: Interpleural analgesia in the treatment of severe thoracic postherpetic neuralgia. *Reg Anesth* 15:113, 1990.
31. Racz GB, Sabonghy M, Gintautas T: Intractable pain therapy using a new epidural catheter. *JAMA* 24B:579, 1982.
32. Racz GB, Heavner J, Haynsworth R: Repeat epidural phenol injections in chronic pain and spasticity, in Lipton S, Miles J (eds.): *Persistent Pain: Modern Methods of Treatment.* London: Grune & Stratton, 1985, pp 157–179.
33. Nour EF: Preliminary report: Uptake of phenol by vascular and brain tissue. *Microvasc Res* 2:224, 1970.
34. Hitchcock E: Osmolytic neurolysis for intractable facial pain. *Lancet* 1:434, 1969.
35. Spiegelmann R, Friedman WA: Spinal cord stimulation: A contemporary series. *Neurosurgery* 28:65, 1991.

36. Friedman AH, Nashold BS Jr: Dorsal root entry zone lesions for the treatment of postherpetic neuralgia. *Neurosurgery* 15:969, 1984.
37. Mazars GJ: Intermittent stimulation of nucleus ventralis posterolateralis for intractable pain. *Surg Neurol* 4:93, 1975.
38. Bonica JJ: Thoracic segmental and intercostal neuralgia, in Bonica JJ (ed.): *The Management of Pain*. Philadelphia: Lea & Febiger, 1953, pp 854–871.
39. Sindov M, Jeanmonod D: Microsurgical DREZ otomy for the treatment of spasticity and pain in the lower limbs. *Neurosurgery* 24:655, 1989.

CHAPTER 25

Cancer Pain in the Geriatric Patient

James N. Rogers
Chandrasekhar Doniparthi

INTRODUCTION

Cancer is a common cause of morbidity and mortality in the geriatric population, with pain being the most debilitating and incapacitating symptom of metastatic or recurrent cancer.[1] Despite the seriousness of this problem, cancer pain is often undertreated, especially in the elderly. Forty percent of all patients with cancer suffer from pain. Among patients with advanced disease, 80 percent experience moderate to severe pain.

A patient pain survey of 54 cancer treatment centers associated with the Eastern Cooperative Oncology Group evaluated cancer pain treatment. Forty-two percent of patients with pain were not given adequate analgesia. Factors reported to be predictive of inadequate analgesia included belonging to a minority, being female, and being over 70 years of age.[2] Guidelines have appeared but have not been widely adopted, and there has been considerable variability in cancer pain treatments. Despite these guidelines for cancer pain management, many patients, particularly geriatric patients, have considerable pain and receive inadequate analgesia. The U.S. Department of Health and Human Services recently released the ninth clinical practice guideline dealing with the management of cancer pain in hopes of providing better pain relief for cancer patients.[3]

One of the major goals of pain management in cancer patients is to improve their quality of life by minimizing their pain so that they can be active and as pain-free as possible. This can be accomplished when appropriate pain management techniques are used.[4] Pain medications can be self-administered easily and safely, in many instances at home, with few adverse side effects. It is important to understand the reasons for undertreatment before learning how to manage cancer pain.

There are many reasons for the undertreatment of cancer pain. Clinicians often have inadequate knowledge about effective assessment and pain management practices. Physicians do not routinely measure pain and therefore may not realize when patients have pain. Physicians are also reluctant to prescribe high doses of morphine or other narcotic analgesics because of their fear of drawing the attention, and possibly punishment, of state and federal narcotic regulatory agencies.

Patients and physicians also may be hesitant to use narcotic medications because of fear of addiction. Lack of knowledge about the clinical pharmacology of opioids and misconceptions regarding tolerance, physical dependence, and psychological dependence (addiction) have limited the effectiveness of these agents in cancer pain management. In patients who are psychologically intact, there is little risk of becoming psychologically dependent on the narcotics used to treat cancer pain.

PAIN ASSESSMENT

The assessment of pain in cancer patients is crucial to developing an effective individual program of pain management. Failure to assess pain is a major reason for undertreatment. In fact, 76 percent of physicians have reported that poor pain assessment is the single most important barrier to adequate pain control.[5] Lack of communication between those treating the cancer and those managing the pain contributes to inadequate treatment of pain. A collaborative interdisciplinary approach can improve communication not only among caregivers but also with the patient and the patient's family.

Pain assessment can cause unique problems in an elderly patient. Pain is often reported differently from the way in which younger patients report it because of physiological, psychological, and cultural differences.[6] Visual, hearing, motor, and cognitive impairments may impede the use of pain assessment instruments. Cognitive impairment, delirium, and dementia (which occurs in up to 50 percent of the institutionalized elderly)[7] can cause serious barriers to pain assessment. Behavioral observations (e.g., groaning, restlessness, agitation) may provide the clinician with clues to the presence of pain and discomfort. Because patients with cognitive impairment may have difficulty with pain recall and integration of the pain experience over time, frequent monitoring of pain is necessary.

Effective communication is often a problem for patients, particularly elderly ones. Many patients see the pain associated with cancer as inevitable, and 70 percent have reported that cancer pain is a reason to stop life-prolonging treatment or a justifiable reason for committing suicide. More than 50 percent thought that cancer patients usually die a painful death.[8] Many of these patients also have misconceptions about opioid analgesics. They feel that when opioid analgesics are prescribed, the active treatment of their disease is finished and they are near death.

Because of these factors, cancer patients are often reluctant to discuss their pain with physicians and with their families. Reporting pain may be viewed as a weakness or as drug-seeking behavior. Many patients may be afraid to report pain because of fear of the return of the cancer or of the treatments that may be necessary. Patients need to be taught that their pain can be treated effectively. They should be taught how to assess their pain and the efficacy of treatment and especially how to communicate with caregivers by using language, numerical scales, and visual scales (Fig. 25-1).

A standardized pain assessment protocol can improve communication among members of the health care team and patients. Flow sheets listing pain intensity scores and treatment side effects, similar to those used for vital signs and medications, can be of great help in assessing the effectiveness of a treatment plan. When systematic pain records are used, patients report significantly better pain control in a shorter period of time.[9] In the outpatient setting, patients can be asked to complete pain diaries. Family members may be asked to complete the diaries if the patient is incapacitated.

EVALUATION

The initial evaluation of a cancer pain patient should include a detailed history and a thorough physical examination. Particular attention should be paid to the

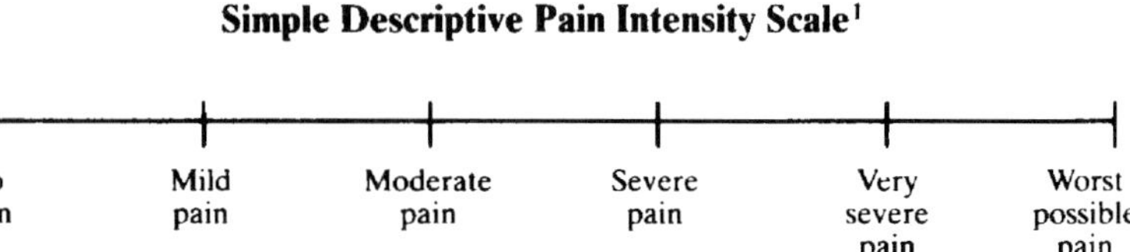

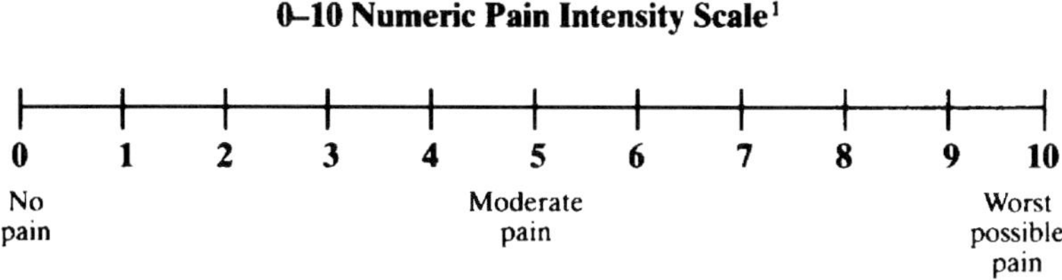

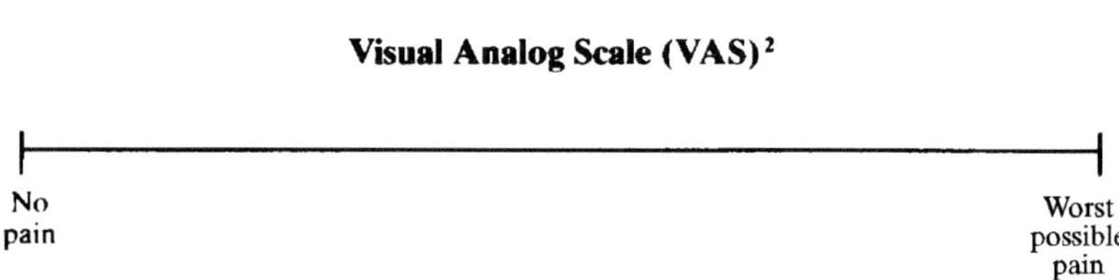

Figure 25-1 Pain intensity scales.

neurological examination and the psychosocial evaluation. Elderly patients often suffer from multiple chronic diseases and may have pain from sources separate from the cancer. Complex medication regimens may also place a geriatric patient at risk for drug-drug interactions.

Changes caused by aging also may have a significant impact on the treatment plan. Assessment of hepatic and renal function is important in older patients to evaluate routes of drug metabolism. Slower drug clearance and an increased sensitivity to undesirable side effects dictate that caution be exercised in dosing pain medications in this patient population.

Determination of the source of the pain is important in developing the most effective treatment plan. Pain in cancer patients may be caused by several different processes (Table 25-1). Pain secondary to direct tumor invasion is present in about 78 percent of cancer inpatients and about 62 percent of outpatients. Pain can result from infiltration of surrounding structures such as nerves, muscles, and visceral organs or from metastasis. Bony metastasis is responsible for pain in up to 50 percent of cancer patients.[10]

About one-quarter of cancer pain is due to the treatment of the disease. Surgical procedures, radiotherapy, and chemotherapy can all induce pain syn-

Table 25-1 Cancer pain syndromes

Pain associated with direct tumor involvement
- From bone invasion
  - Base of skull
  - Vertebral body
  - Generalized bone pain
- From invasion of nerves
  - Peripheral nerve syndromes
  - Polyneuropathy
  - Brachial, lumbar, sacral plexopathies
  - Leptomeningeal metastases
  - Epidural spinal cord compression
- From invasion of viscera
- From invasion of blood vessels
- From invasion of mucous membranes

Pain associated with cancer therapy
- Postoperative pain syndromes
  - Phantom pain syndromes
  - Postthoracotomy, postmastectomy syndromes
- Postchemotherapy pain syndromes
  - Polyneuropathy
  - Aseptic necrosis of bone
  - Steroid pseudorheumatism
  - Mucositis
- Postradiation pain syndromes
  - Radiation fibrosis of brachial or lumbosacral plexus
  - Radiation myelopathy
  - Radiation-induced peripheral nerve tumors
  - Mucositis
  - Radiation necrosis of bone

Pain indirectly related or unrelated to cancer
- Myofascial pain syndromes
- Postherpetic neuralgia
- Osteoporosis

dromes.[11] Postmastectomy syndrome, postthoracotomy syndrome, and phantom pain syndrome can occur after surgery, even curative surgery. Radiation therapy can cause fibrosis, myelopathies, bony necrosis, and radiation-induced tumors. Chemotherapeutic agents can cause diffuse neuropathies, aseptic necrosis of joints, and postherpetic neuralgia.

It is important to remember that not all the pain experienced by a patient with cancer results from the disease or its treatment. The presence of cancer does not make the patient immune to the other common causes of pain seen in the geriatric population. Localized infections can cause pain and may be difficult to identify, particularly in patients with head and neck tumors. Fever and an increased white blood cell count may not be present because of the effects of the cancer or its treatment.[12] Other causes of pain may include osteoporosis, degenerative joint disease, diabetic neuropathies, claudication, myofascial pain, and headaches. These pain syndromes should be treated aggressively as well.

PSYCHOSOCIAL EVALUATION

The various contributions of psychosocial factors, psychological characteristics, and environmental factors to pain manifestations are poorly understood. No set of psychological characteristics correlates with the development, exacerbation, and/or maintenance of cancer pain. This lack of consistency, however, does not preclude the role of psychological factors in cancer pain.[13] Anxiety and depression are often associated with an increase in pain intensity.

The patient's social situation should also be evaluated to ensure adequate support at home. Home hospice care should be considered when patients have less than 6 months of life expectancy. Hospice care can be especially helpful in providing terminally ill patients with pain relief and family support.

PHARMACOTHERAPY OF CANCER PAIN

Drug therapy is the cornerstone of the cancer pain management therapies. It is effective, inexpensive, and relatively low risk. It should be remembered that pain is an individual experience and that the treatment regimen should be individualized for each patient. Before one chooses drugs to treat the pain, it is important to identify the specific causes of the pain and then select the drugs accordingly. The three major classes of drugs used in managing cancer pain are nonsteroidal anti-inflammatory drugs (NSAIDs), opioids, and adjuvant analgesics. It is best to choose the simplest dosage schedule.

In 1990 the World Health Organization (WHO) devised a simple, well-validated, and effective therapy rationale for the treatment of cancer pain. The WHO ladder has been shown to be effective in relieving pain in 90 percent of patients with cancer.[14] The essential features of this analgesic ladder are by mouth, by the clock, by the ladder, individualization, and attention to detail.

It is important to remember that elderly patients are at increased risk for drug-drug and drug-disease interactions. Close attention to doses, concurrent medications, and side effects is required. Elderly patients are at particular risk for both under- and overtreatment. Few studies of analgesic dose requirements are performed in elderly patients, with most studies systematically excluding patients over age 65. Fewer than 1 percent of the reports on pain published annually focus on pain experience or syndromes in the elderly.[15]

Nonsteroidal Anti-Inflammatory Drugs

The first rung of the ladder is the use of NSAIDs for mild to moderate levels of pain. NSAIDs are effective and often are easily obtained. They do not produce tolerance or dependence (physical or psychological) the way narcotics can. Pain relief occurs because of inhibition of the arachidonic acid cascade, reducing the levels of inflammatory mediators. Although there may be a central action of NSAIDs, they do not activate opioid receptors. NSAIDs therefore produce analgesia by a different mechanism. The concurrent use of NSAIDs or acetaminophen with opioids often produces a greater level of analgesia than does either drug class alone. Acetaminophen is included in this group because even though it is not an anti-inflammatory drug, it has similar analgesic effects and pharmacologic characteristics (Table 25-2).

Although effective, NSAIDs are more likely to cause gastric and renal toxicity in elderly patients. Platelet inhibition may pose a significant bleeding risk in elderly patients, who are already at greater risk of sustaining falls.

Table 25-2 Acetaminophen and NSAID doses in adults

Drug	Dose	Comments
Acetaminophen and over-the-counter NSAIDs		
Acetaminophen	50 mg q 4 h or 975 mg q 6 h	No peripheral anti-inflammatory or antiplatelet effects
Aspirin	650 mg q 4 h or 975 mg q 6 h	Irreversible platelet inhibition
Ibuprofen	400–600 mg q 6 h	
Prescription NSAIDS		
Carprofen	100 mg tid	
Choline magnesium trisalicylate	100–1500 mg tid	Minimal antiplatelet activity
Choline salicylate	870 mg q 3–4 h	Minimal antiplatelet activity
Diflunisal	500 mg q 12 h	
Etodolac	200–400 mg q 6–8 h	
Fenoprofen calcium	300–600 mg q 6 h	
Ketoprofen	25–60 mg q 6–8 h	
Ketorolac tromethamine	10 mg q 4–6 h (max 40 mg/day)	Same GI effects as other NSAIDs
Magnesium salicylate	650 mg q 4 h	
Meclofenamate sodium	50–100 mg q 6 h	Coombs-positive autoimmune hemolytic anemia with prolonged use
Mefenamic acid	50 mg q 6 h	
Naproxen	250–275 mg q 6–8 h	
Naproxen sodium	275 mg q 6–8 h	
Sodium salicylate	325–650 mg q 3–4 h	
Parenteral NSAIDSs		
Ketorolac tromethamine	60 mg initially, then 30 mg q 6 h (intramuscular)	Should not exceed 5 days; same GI effects as other NSAIDs

Aspirin causes an irreversible inhibition of platelet aggregation. Acetaminophen and the nonacetylated salicylates such as salsalate, sodium salsalate, and choline magnesium trisalicylate do not affect platelet function and do not alter bleeding times. Other NSAIDs produce a reversible platelet inhibition. With the exception of acetaminophen and the nonacetylated salicylates, NSAIDs should be avoided in patients who are thrombocytopenic, have a bleeding disorder, or are at risk for falls or other injuries.

Besides bleeding, the adverse effects of NSAIDs include renal failure, hepatic dysfunction, and gastric ulceration. These effects occur more frequently in the geriatric population and require close monitoring. The addition of a gastric protective agent such as misoprostol may reduce the risk of gastric ulceration.

No single NSAID has been shown to be superior to others in providing pain relief. It is also impossible to predict which NSAID will be best tolerated by an individual patient. When a specific agent has been selected, it should be titrated until pain relief is obtained. If the maximal dose has been reached or the side effects become intolerable, another NSAID should be selected. NSAIDs exhibit a ceiling effect to their efficacy, and exceeding the recommended maximal dose usually is not helpful. The choice of an NSAID should be based on efficacy, safety, and expense. In general, the least expensive NSAID should be chosen.

Narcotics

Opioids are the mainstay of management for moderate to severe cancer pain. They are very effective, are easily titratable, and have a favorable risk-benefit ratio. Commonly used opioids include morphine, hydromorphone, codeine, oxycodone, hydrocodone, methadone, levorphanol, and fentanyl. Opioid drugs are classified by their activity at opioid receptors. Full-agonist opioids do not have a ceiling to their analgesic efficacy. Partial agonists such as buprenorphine have a lower intrinsic activity at opioid receptors and demonstrate a ceiling effect to analgesia. Mixed agonist-antagonists also exhibit a ceiling effect to analgesia. Patients who are receiving full-agonist opioids should not be given mixed agonist-antagonist drugs because this may precipitate withdrawal symptoms and increase pain (Table 25-3).

Elderly patients may be more sensitive to the analgesic effects of opioid drugs. They experience a higher peak drug concentration and a longer duration of pain relief.[16] They can also be more sensitive to sedation and respiratory depression resulting from changes in the distribution and excretion of the drug. Elderly patients generally have an increased fat-to-lean body mass ratio and a reduced glomerular filtration rate. Biologically active metabolites such as morphine-6-glucuronide and normeperidine can accumulate and produce significant cognitive and neuropsychiatric dysfunction. Normeperidine, the metabolite of meperidine, accumulates when meperidine is used for more than several days and can cause CNS stimulation that can result in seizures.

Table 25-3 Adult opioid analgesic agent doses*

Drug	Approximate equianalgesic dose		Usual starting dose for moderate to severe pain	
	Oral	Parenteral	Oral	Parenteral
Opioid agonists†				
Morphine	30 mg q 3–4 h (for around-the-clock dosing) 60 mg q 3–4 h (for single dose or intermittent dosing)	10 mg q 3–4 h	30 mg q 3–4 h	10 mg q 3–4 h
Controlled-release morphine	90–120 mg q 12 h	Not available	90–120 mg q 12 h	Not available
Hydromorphone	7.5 mg q 3–4 h	1.5 mg q 3–4 h	6 mg q 3–4 h	1.5 mg q 3–4 h
Levorphanol	4 mg q 6–8 h	2 mg q 6–8 h	4 mg q 6–8 h	2 mg q 6–8 h
Meperidine	300 mg q 2–3 h	100 mg q 3 h	Not recommended	100 mg q 3 h
Methadone	20 mg q 6–8 h	10 mg q 6–8 h	20 mg q 6–8 h	10 mg q 6–8 h
Oxymorphone	Not available	1 mg q 3–4 h	Not available	1 mg q 3–4 h
Combination opioid-NSAID preparations				
Codeine	180–200 mg q 3–4 h	75 mg q 3–4 h	60 mg q 3–4 h	60 mg q 2 h (IM or SC)
Hydrocodone	30 mg q 3–4 h	Not available	10 mg q 3–4 h	Not available
Oxycodone	30 mg q 3–4 h	Not available	10 mg q 3–4 h	Not available

*Published equivalent dose to morphine data varies. Clinical response should be used when adjustments are necessary. Incomplete cross-tolerance may be present. It is recommended to use a lower dose than the equianalgesic dose when one is changing drugs and adjusting according to the clinical response. Doses do not apply to patients with renal or hepatic insufficiency or other conditions that may affect drug metabolism and pharmacokinetics.

†For morphine, hydromorphone, and oxymorphone, rectal administration is an alternative route for patients unable to take oral medications. Equianalgesic doses may vary because of pharmacokinetic differences.

Meperidine should not be used on a continuous basis for cancer pain management.

Opioid dosage titration requires the physician to take into account not only the analgesic effects but also the side effects that may occur in this patient population. Besides cognitive impairment, opioid side effects that may be present in elderly patients include urinary retention, constipation, intestinal obstruction, respiratory depression, and exacerbation of Parkinson's disease.

Opioid tolerance and physical dependence can be expected with long-term opioid pain management and should not be confused with psychological dependence (addiction). Opioid tolerance may require an increased dose to achieve the same level of pain relief over time. Progressive disease is more likely to require dose increases. Physical dependence may manifest as anxiety, irritability, chills, hot flashes, joint pain, lacrimation, rhinorrhea, diaphoresis, nausea, vomiting, abdominal cramps, and diarrhea if opioids are withdrawn. Mild withdrawal symptoms may resemble a viral flulike syndrome.

The correct dose of an opioid should be one that controls pain with the fewest side effects. Medication should be scheduled to prevent pain rather than allowing pain to break through. Side effects should be treated aggressively. Constipation is a common problem and should be treated prophylactically. Increased fiber and mild laxatives should be administered on a regular schedule. A stimulating cathartic or hyperosmotic agent may be necessary to treat severe constipation. Antiemetics may be needed for opioid-induced nausea and vomiting but may increase sedation and other CNS side effects in the elderly.

Adjuvants

Adjuvant agents can be used to enhance the analgesic effects of opioids or to treat other symptoms of the disease or the side effects of the opioids. They can be used at any point on the WHO ladder (Table 25-4).

Tricyclic antidepressants are helpful in treating pain of neuropathic origin, potentiating opioid analgesia, and elevating mood. Orthostatic hypotension, anticholinergic side effects (dry mouth, constipation, urinary retention), and sedation can be significant problems in geriatric patients. The most extensive experience has been with amitriptyline. Treatment should be started at a low dose (10–25 mg orally) and increased slowly as tolerated. This approach minimizes the risk of falling from orthostatic hypotension. Analgesic effects are often seen at doses lower than those needed to treat depression.

Anticonvulsants are also useful in treating neuropathic pain, which is often described as lancinating, shooting, and burning pain. Anticonvulsants are thought to provide pain relief by suppressing spontaneous neuronal firing. Carbamazepine should be used with caution in patients receiving bone marrow–suppressive chemotherapeutic agents. Systemically administered local anesthetic-antiarrhythmic agents such as intravenous lidocaine, oral mexiletine,

Table 25-4 Adjuvant analgesic drugs

Class and drug	Approximate dose range	Administration	Use
Corticosteroids			
Dexamethasone	16–96 mg/day	Oral or intravenous	For pain associated with brain metastasis and epidural spinal cord compression
Prednisone	40–80 mg/day	Oral	
Anticonvulsant agents			
Carbamazepine	200–1600 mg/day	Oral	For neuropathic pain
Phenytoin	300–500 mg/day	Oral	
Antidepressant agents			
Amitriptyline	25–150 mg/day	Oral	For neuropathic pain
Doxepin	25–150 mg/day	Oral	
Imipramine	20–100 mg/day	Oral	
Trazodone	75–225 mg/day	Oral	
Neuroleptic agents			
Methotrimeprazine	40–80 mg/day	Intramuscular	For analgesia, sedation, and as an antiemetic agent
Antihistamines			
Hydroxyzine	300–450 mg/day	Intramuscular	Potentiates opioids; relieves anxiety, insomnia, and nausea
Antiarrhythmic agents			
Lidocaine	5 mg/kg/day	Intravenous or subcutaneous	For neuropathic pain
Mexiletine	450–600 mg/day	Oral	
Tocainide	20 mg/kg/day	Oral	
Psychostimulants			
Dextroamphetamine	5–10 mg/day	Oral	Improves opioid analgesia, decreases sedation
Methylphenidate	10–15 mg/day	Oral	

and tocainide have also been used to treat neuropathic pain,[17] although there is no current FDA-approved indication for these drugs for pain.

Psychostimulants such as dextroamphetamine and methylphenidate can be used to improve opioid analgesia and treat excessive sedation from opioid medications. Antihistamines may reduce anxiety, insomnia, and nausea. Corticosteroids may elevate mood and provide anti-inflammatory, antiemetic, and appetite stimulation effects in cancer patients.

ROUTES OF ADMINISTRATION

The oral route of administration should be the preferred route for delivering analgesic medications. It is the most convenient and cost-effective method of administration. If the patient cannot take analgesic medications orally, other minimally invasive routes, such as rectal or transdermal, should be tried. Fentanyl, a synthetic opioid, is available in a transdermal delivery system that provides up to 3 days of constant, steady serum blood levels. NSAIDs, opioids, and many adjuvant agents are available in both oral and suppository preparations.

If noninvasive routes are not tolerated or dose requirements make it impossible to meet the patient's analgesic needs, more invasive routes of administration may be used. These include the intravenous, subcutaneous, epidural, and intraspinal routes. These routes have been used primarily to deliver opioid medications, although adjuvant agents such as local anesthetics, clonidine, and baclofen have also been administered in this manner. Intramuscular administration should be avoided because it is painful and inconvenient and because absorption is unreliable.

A major advantage of epidural and intrathecal narcotic management is the opportunity to perform a preimplantation trial. An epidural or intrathecal drug delivery system should not be considered without verification that it will alleviate the patient's pain.

Preimplantation considerations should include a successful trial, no active infection, and no clotting disorders. Behavioral and psychological abnormalities may interfere with the assessment of pain relief. Cost is a factor that should not be overlooked. Support systems, concurrent therapies, and life expectancy should be evaluated before one considers implantation.

Standard percutaneous epidural catheters can be used to provide short-term pain relief. Subcutaneous tunneling of epidural and intrathecal catheters is useful in patients in whom several weeks to months of pain relief are necessary. Infection is a major concern, and careful attention to sterile technique is crucial. Prophylactic antibiotics should be considered during the placement of implanted systems. In patients with a life expectancy greater than 3 to 6 months, it is often cost-effective to place a totally implantable infusion pump. With careful patient selection and screening, continuous intraspinal drug infusion of morphine has been especially helpful in managing lower body pain in up to 90 percent of patients.[18]

INVASIVE THERAPIES

Noninvasive treatments should be exhausted before invasive approaches are attempted. Neurolytic peripheral neural blockade should be considered only after more conservative therapeutic modalities for treating the patient's pain have proved to be inadequate, poorly tolerated, or clinically inappropriate.

Nerve blocks with local anesthetics can be used to identify the source of the pain and provide prognostic information to predict the outcome of permanent neurolysis. Patients should be evaluated for their ability to understand the risks associated with the procedure and their ability to cooperate during the procedure. Radiographic guidance is especially helpful in ensuring precise anatomic positioning of the needle before the injection of a neurolytic agent (Table 25-5).

Peripheral neurolysis can be accomplished by means of the injection of neurolytic agents such as alcohol and phenol or by means of thermocoagulation or cryoanalgesic techniques. Pancreatic cancer is particularly responsive to neurolytic celiac plexus blockage.[19] Complications from neurolytic blockade may include hypotension, paresis, paralysis, and bowel or bladder dysfunction.

If a patient becomes pain-free after neurolysis, narcotics should not be stopped abruptly, as this may precipitate narcotic withdrawal. Opioids should be tapered slowly to avoid withdrawal.

SUMMARY

Elderly patients with cancer require comprehensive assessment and aggressive management of their pain. However, this patient population is at risk for undertreatment of pain. Issues that are important when one is treating geriatric cancer include the following.

Concurrent Medical Diseases and Noncancerous Pain

Elderly patients often suffer from a wide variety of chronic diseases and may be on complex medication regimens that increase their risk of drug-drug and drug-disease interactions.

Table 25-5 Regional anesthetic techniques used in cancer pain

Pain source	Regional technique
Head and neck	Somatic nerve blocks
Mandibular/maxillary invasion	Cervical epidural
Pancoast's tumor	Stellate ganglion block
Thoracic pain	
Pleural involvement	Thoracic epidural
Single rib metastases	Paravertebral somatic nerve block, intercostal nerve block
Multiple rib metastases	Thoracic epidural
Mediastinal involvement	Thoracic epidural
Abdominal malignancy	Celiac plexus block
Lower extremity metastases	Lumbar epidural/intrathecal
Perineal and pelvic malignancy	
With colostomy and urethrostomy	Epidural/intrathecal phenol neurolysis
With intact bladder and bowel function	Intrathecal morphine pump

Physical and Cognitive Impairment

Pain assessment may be more difficult in patients with physical and cognitive impairment. It may be necessary to use behavior-based assessment tools to evaluate pain levels and the efficacy of pain management. Family members can also be taught how to assess pain.

Side Effects

Elderly patients are more likely to develop side effects from NSAIDs because of impaired metabolism and excretion related to age. Alternative NSAIDs with fewer gastrointestinal effects, such as choline magnesium trisalicylate, or the addition of misoprostol should be considered to reduce the risk of gastric toxicity. Increasing the dosage beyond the recommended dose is unlikely to improve pain relief and increases the risk of side effects. A different NSAID should be chosen if the first compound is poorly tolerated or pain is not relieved.

Efficacy of Opioids

Opioids can provide significant pain relief in patients with cancer. Older patients may be more sensitive to opioids because the peak opioid effect is higher and the duration of pain relief is longer. The initial dosing requires caution and careful titration to achieve pain relief while providing frequent monitoring for undesirable side effects.

Adjuvant Agents

Adjuvant agents are used to enhance analgesia and lessen side effects in pain patients. When they are combined with NSAIDs and opioids, cancer pain can often be relieved satisfactorily with a minimum of complications.

Route of Administration

The oral route is the preferred route of administration. In some patients, however, this route cannot be used. Alternatives include the rectal, subcutaneous, transdermal, intravenous, and intraspinal routes. Intramuscular injections should not be used to administer medication on a chronic basis.

Invasive Procedures

Invasive procedures such as peripheral and central neurolytic blockade and neuroablative surgical procedures should be considered only when other conservative methods have failed or the side effects cannot be tolerated. When appropriate, invasive procedures can alleviate pain and reduce opioid requirements. Informed consent is critical. The effects of permanent neurological interruption may be more undesirable to the patient than is the pain itself.

Cancer pain is a significant problem in the geriatric population. It can be adequately treated in most patients with careful use of medications, following the WHO analgesic ladder: NSAIDs for mild to moderate pain and increasingly potent opioids for more severe pain. Adjuvant agents can be used at any point on the ladder to enhance analgesia, treat side effects, and elevate mood. Each patient should have an individual pain management plan developed to allow for individual variations in the pain experience.

Frequent reassessment of the pain management regimen is necessary in elderly patients to ensure continued adequate analgesia and monitoring for potentially devastating side effects. With care, most patients can receive significant relief of pain with minimal and tolerable side effects.

REFERENCES

1. Bonica JJ: Treatment of cancer pain: Current status and future needs, in Fields HL, Dubner R, Cervero F (eds): *Advances in Pain Research and Therapy.* Proceedings of the Fourth World Congress on Pain. New York: Raven Press, 1985, vol 9, pp 589–616.
2. Cleeland CS, Gonin R, Hatfield AK, et al: Pain and its treatment in outpatients with metastatic cancer. *N Engl J Med* 330:592, 1994.
3. *Management of Cancer Pain.* Clinical Practice Guideline, vol 9. U.S. Department of Health and Human Services, March 1994.
4. Payne R: *Current Strategies in Cancer Pain Assessment and Cancer Pain Syndromes.* Syllabus for Postgraduate Course, Memorial Sloan-Kettering Cancer Center, New York, 1992.
5. Von Roenn JH, Cleeland CS, Gonin R, et al: Physician attitudes and practice in cancer pain management. *Ann Intern Med* 119:121, 1993.
6. Fordyce WE: Evaluating and managing chronic pain. *Geriatrics* 33:59, 1978.
7. Kane RL, Ouslander JG, Abrass IB: *Essentials of Clinical Geriatrics,* 2d ed. New York: McGraw-Hill, 1989.
8. Cleeland CS: Research in cancer pain: What we know and what we need to know. *Cancer* 67(Suppl):823, 1991.
9. Faries JE, Mills DS, Goldsmith KW, et al: Systematic pain records and their impact on pain control. *Cancer Nurs* 14:306, 1991.
10. Twycross RG, Fairfield S: Pain in far-advanced cancer. *Pain* 14:303, 1982.
11. Koeller JM: Understanding cancer pain. *Am J Hosp Pharm* 47:S3, 1990.
12. Coyle N, Portenoy RK: Infection as a cause of rapidly increasing pain in cancer patients. *J Pain Sympt Manage* 4:266, 1991.
13. Dalton JA, Feuerstein M: Biobehavioral factors in cancer pain. *Pain* 33:133, 1988.
14. Ventafridda V, Caraceni A, Gamba A: Field testing of the WHO guidelines for cancer pain relief: Summary report of demonstration projects, in Foley KM, Bonica JJ, Ventafridda V (eds): *Proceedings of the Second International Congress on Pain.* Vol

16: *Advances in Pain Research and Therapy*. New York: Raven Press, 1990, pp 451–464.
15. Melding PS: Is there such a thing as geriatric pain? *Pain 46*:119, 1991.
16. Kaiko RF, Wallenstein SL, Rogers AG, et al: Narcotics in the elderly. *Med Clin North Am* 66:1079, 1982.
17. Brose WG, Cousins MJ: Subcutaneous lidocaine for treatment of neuropathic cancer pain. *Pain* 45:145, 1991.
18. Onofrio BM, Yaksh TL: Long-term pain relief produced by intrathecal morphine infusion in 53 patients. *J Neurosurg* 72:200, 1990.
19. Brown DL, Bulley CK, Quiel EL: Neurolytic celiac plexus block for pancreatic cancer pain. *Anesth Analg* 66:869, 1987.

INDEX

Page numbers followed by t and f refer to tables and illustrations, respectively.

ISBN 0-07-058642-X